OXFORD MEDICAL PUBLICATIONS

Oxford Handbook of
Genitourinary Medicine, HIV, and Sexual Health

Published and forthcoming Oxford Handbooks

Oxford Handbook for the Foundation Programme 4e

Oxford Handbook of Acute Medicine 3e

Oxford Handbook of Anaesthesia 4e

Oxford Handbook of Cardiology 2e

Oxford Handbook of Clinical and Healthcare Research

Oxford Handbook of Clinical and Laboratory Investigation 4e

Oxford Handbook of Clinical Dentistry 6e

Oxford Handbook of Clinical Diagnosis 3e

Oxford Handbook of Clinical Examination and Practical Skills 2e

Oxford Handbook of Clinical Haematology 4e

Oxford Handbook of Clinical Immunology and Allergy 3e

Oxford Handbook of Clinical Medicine – Mini Edition 9e

Oxford Handbook of Clinical Medicine 10e

Oxford Handbook of Clinical Pathology

Oxford Handbook of Clinical Pharmacy 3e

Oxford Handbook of Clinical Specialties 10e

Oxford Handbook of Clinical Surgery 4e

Oxford Handbook of Complementary Medicine

Oxford Handbook of Critical Care 3e

Oxford Handbook of Dental Patient Care

Oxford Handbook of Dialysis 4e

Oxford Handbook of Emergency Medicine 4e

Oxford Handbook of Endocrinology and Diabetes 3e

Oxford Handbook of ENT and Head and Neck Surgery 2e

Oxford Handbook of Epidemiology for Clinicians

Oxford Handbook of Expedition and Wilderness Medicine 2e

Oxford Handbook of Forensic Medicine

Oxford Handbook of Gastroenterology & Hepatology 2e

Oxford Handbook of General Practice 4e

Oxford Handbook of Genetics

Oxford Handbook of Genitourinary Medicine, HIV, and Sexual Health 2e

Oxford Handbook of Geriatric Medicine 3e

Oxford Handbook of Infectious Diseases and Microbiology 2e

Oxford Handbook of Integrated Dental Biosciences 2e

Oxford Handbook of Humanitarian Medicine

Oxford Handbook of Key Clinical Evidence 2e

Oxford Handbook of Medical Dermatology 2e

Oxford Handbook of Medical Imaging

Oxford Handbook of Medical Sciences 2e

Oxford Handbook for Medical School

Oxford Handbook of Medical Statistics

Oxford Handbook of Neonatology 2e

Oxford Handbook of Nephrology and Hypertension 2e

Oxford Handbook of Neurology 2e

Oxford Handbook of Nutrition and Dietetics 2e

Oxford Handbook of Obstetrics and Gynaecology 3e

Oxford Handbook of Occupational Health 2e

Oxford Handbook of Oncology 3e

Oxford Handbook of Operative Surgery 3e

Oxford Handbook of Ophthalmology 4e

Oxford Handbook of Oral and Maxillofacial Surgery 2e

Oxford Handbook of Orthopaedics and Trauma

Oxford Handbook of Paediatrics 2e

Oxford Handbook of Pain Management

Oxford Handbook of Palliative Care 3e

Oxford Handbook of Practical Drug Therapy 2e

Oxford Handbook of Pre-Hospital Care

Oxford Handbook of Psychiatry 3e

Oxford Handbook of Public Health Practice 3e

Oxford Handbook of Rehabilitation Medicine 3e

Oxford Handbook of Reproductive Medicine & Family Planning 2e

Oxford Handbook of Respiratory Medicine 3e

Oxford Handbook of Rheumatology 4e

Oxford Handbook of Sport and Exercise Medicine 2e

Handbook of Surgical Consent

Oxford Handbook of Tropical Medicine 4e

Oxford Handbook of Urology 4e

Oxford Handbook of
Genitourinary Medicine, HIV, and Sexual Health

Third edition

Edited by

Laura Mitchell

Consultant in Sexual Health
University Hospitals Plymouth NHS Trust, Plymouth, UK

Bridie Howe

Consultant in Genitourinary Medicine and HIV,
NHS Highland, Inverness, Scotland, UK

D. Ashley Price

Consultant in Infectious Diseases, Newcastle upon Tyne
Hospitals NHS Foundation Trust, Newcastle upon Tyne, UK

Babiker Elawad

Consultant Physician in Genitourinary Medicine,
Northumbria Healthcare Trust, and Honorary Consultant
in Infectious Diseases, Newcastle upon Tyne Hospitals NHS
Foundation Trust, Newcastle upon Tyne, UK

K. Nathan Sankar

Retired Consultant in Genitourinary Medicine,
formerly of Newcastle upon Tyne Hospitals
NHS Foundation Trust, Newcastle upon Tyne, UK

OXFORD
UNIVERSITY PRESS

Great Clarendon Street, Oxford, OX2 6DP,
United Kingdom

Oxford University Press is a department of the University of Oxford.
It furthers the University's objective of excellence in research, scholarship,
and education by publishing worldwide. Oxford is a registered trade mark of
Oxford University Press in the UK and in certain other countries

First Edition Published as Oxford Handbook of Genitourinary Medicine, HIV, and
AIDS 2005
Second Edition Published in 2010
Third Edition Published in 2019

Impression: 1

Published in the United States of America by Oxford University Press
198 Madison Avenue, New York, NY 10016, United States of America

British Library Cataloguing in Publication Data

Data available

Library of Congress Control Number: 2018962016

ISBN 978–0–19–878349–7

Printed and bound in China by
C&C Offset Printing Co., Ltd.

Contents

Preface _viii_

Foreword _ix_

List of colour plates _x_

Contributors _xi_

Symbols and abbreviations _xiii_

1 The genitourinary medicine service   1
2 Ethical, medico-legal, & sociocultural issues   15
3 Gender diversity   41
4 The standard clinic process and sexual health
  in primary care   47
5 Investigations and microscopy   63
6 Specific genitourinary situations   81
7 Syphilis   117
8 Gonorrhoea   137
9 Chlamydia   149
10 Non-gonococcal urethritis and mucopurulent
   cervicitis   161
11 Pelvic inflammatory disease   169
12 Prostatitis/chronic pelvic pain syndrome in men   181
13 Epididymo-orchitis   193
14 Sexually acquired reactive arthritis   201
15 Bacterial vaginosis and anaerobic balanitis   213
16 Trichomoniasis   225
17 Genital candidiasis   233
18 Tropical genital and sexually acquired infections   245
19 Endemic treponematoses   255

20 Proctocolitis and enteric sexually
    acquired infections   259

21 Urinary tract infection   267

22 Anogenital herpes   277

23 Anogenital warts   291

24 Molluscum contagiosum   305

25 Sexually acquired viral hepatitis   309

26 Other viral infections   323

27 Scabies   331

28 Pediculosis pubis   339

29 Anogenital dermatoses   345

30 Cervical neoplasia   357

31 Vulval pain   365

32 Streptococcal and staphylococcal infections   373

33 Genital anomalies   377

34 Contraception, including contraception for
    women living with HIV   381

35 Psychological aspects and sexual problems   429

36 HIV: prevention   443

37 HIV: introduction and epidemiology   449

38 Pathogenesis of HIV   457

39 Staging, classification, and natural history of
    HIV disease   465

40 HIV: diagnosis and assessment   469

41 HIV: primary infection   479

42 HIV: gastrointestinal disorders   485

43 HIV: hepatitis virus co-infection   507

44 HIV: disorders of the eye   513

45 HIV: respiratory disorders   523

46 HIV: neurological disorders   539

47 HIV: dermatological disorders 551

48 HIV: pyrexia of unknown origin 563

49 HIV: endocrine and metabolic disorders 571

50 HIV: renal disorders 581

51 HIV: cardiovascular disorders 589

52 HIV: musculoskeletal disorders 595

53 HIV: reticulo-endothelial disorders 603

54 HIV: malignancies 609

55 HIV: management 621

56 HIV: pregnancy 653

57 HIV: travel 659

Index 663

Preface

This Handbook is a comprehensive guide to all aspects of sexual health. Reflecting the mainstream move to provide integrated sexual health services, this Handbook provides a one-stop shop of information. It provides up-to-date, evidence-based guidance on diagnostics and management in genitourinary medicine, HIV, and contraception. A holistic approach to sexual health is emphasized with information on genital pain, psychological aspects, prevention, and sociocultural issues (including sections on child sexual exploitation and female genital mutilation). Although primarily aimed at those working in UK services, it is also envisaged to be of global use to all those with an interest in sexual health, whatever their level of expertise and wherever they may practice.

People with sexual health concerns or those with HIV may present first to primary care services or to healthcare professionals working in a wide variety of specialties. It is intended that the concise information in this book will address the needs of both specialists and generalists working across these different settings.

With 2017 seeing the centenary of sexual health service provision, free at the point of care, in the UK, we continue to see service provision evolve. The last 100 years have seen a plethora of changes and we continue to see more. Changes to previous editions include a chapter as an introduction to gender diversity to provide a useful background to ensure trans, including non-binary, people are able to access appropriate sexual healthcare. The HIV management chapter has been overhauled to reflect significant developments in treatment recommendations. Changes in practice in relation to developments in diagnostics for, and treatment of, *Mycoplasma genitalium* are included in all relevant chapters.

The contents start with service design, proceeding to ethical and medicolegal issues and a chapter on gender diversity. Routine patient management and flowcharts detailing common clinical situations follow, and then there is a series of chapters that adopt a systematic approach to STIs, and other infections or clinical syndromes relating to sexual health. A chapter on contraception then precedes a series of chapters on HIV. The HIV section starts with prevention and an epidemiological overview, and is followed by some key virology before taking a systemic approach to describing conditions both directly related to HIV and also opportunistic infections, prior to concluding with chapters on pregnancy and travel.

The editors would like to thank Dr Richard Pattman MBE (retired Consultant in Genitourinary Medicine) and Pauline Handy MBE (retired Lead Nurse in Genitourinary Medicine) for their work on the previous two editions of this publication.

Feedback on errors and omissions would be much appreciated. Please post your comments via the OUP website.

Foreword

The past 70 years has seen significant changes in the population's sexual behaviour, as highlighted by the three National Survey of Sexual Attitudes and Lifestyle (NATSAL) studies. The early 1980s saw the impact of the emerging 'AIDS epidemic', and national health promotion campaigns about sexual activity and a consequent disappearance of what had been common sexually transmitted infections. In 2018, we have seen the return of syphilis and gonorrhea to levels not seen since World War 2. There has been a significant decrease in HIV infections. Improved diagnostic testing has enabled 'on-line' self-taken tests to open up access to STI screening and HIV testing. Anti-retroviral drugs are now not only used to treat HIV, but also to prevent its acquisition—pre-exposure prophylaxis (PrEP). In this changing climate, the healthcare professional needs a reliable source of information to ensure they have an understanding of the fundamentals of genitourinary medicine, HIV, and sexual health, and can respond to emerging public health challenges.

This 3rd edition of the *Oxford Handbook of Genitourinary Medicine, HIV, and Sexual Health* is a comprehensive resource, which is a 'must read' for anyone interested in attaining an in-depth knowledge of genito-urinary medicine and allied conditions. Its uniqueness lies with its broad overview of the specialty, its history, and the description of differing professional roles and responsibilities involved in service delivery. The 57 chapters cover diverse topics from the individual STIs, common syndromes, HIV, the law, and sexual assault, to contraception. Each chapter is well structured giving comprehensive information in line with current guidelines and practical 'frequently asked question 'sections. New chapters cover gender diversity and *Mycoplasma genitalium*, while the chapters on HIV have been considerably updated to include PrEP and new treatment guidelines. There is excellent cross-referencing between infections/conditions throughout the book, which makes it easy for the reader to get an excellent insight into the association between diseases.

The authors are to be congratulated on bringing together this knowledge in what is a truly comprehensive new edition, which will be appreciated by its readers.

Dr Olwen E. Williams, OBE
BASHH President 2018–20

x

List of colour plates

Plate 1   Gram stain lactobacilli
Plate 2   Gram stain BV
Plate 3   Gram stain candidiasis
Plate 4   Gram stain gonorrhoea
Plate 5   Dark-ground trichomonas vaginalis
Plate 6   Ziehl–Nielsen stain Mycobacteria
Plate 7   Classic chancre
Plate 8   'Contemporary' chancre
Plate 9   Secondary syphilis
Plate 10   Condolymata lata
Plate 11   Vulval herpes
Plate 12   Chancroid
Plate 13   Granuloma inguinale
Plate 14   LGV 'groove sign'
Plate 15   Anogenital warts
Plate 16   Molluscum contagiosum
Plate 17   VIN
Plate 18   Vulval lichen sclerosis
Plate 19   Lichen planus; purple papules with Wickham striae showing
            koebnerization
Plate 20   Lichen planus; hyperkeratosis on buccal mucosa
Plate 21   Beçhet's oral ulcer
Plate 22   Pathergy reaction
Plate 23   Beçhet's genital ulcer
Plate 24   Anterior uveitis with hypopyon
Plate 25   Oral candidiasis and HIV
Plate 26   HIV: oral hairy leukoplakia
Plate 27   Oral Kaposi's sarcoma
Plate 28   Oral lymphoma and HIV
Plate 29   Chest X-ray—PCP
Plate 30   MRI—progressive multifocal leukoencephalopathy
Plate 31   CMV retinitis
Plate 32   Cutaneous Kaposi's sarcoma
Plate 33   KS on white skin
Plate 34   KS on the face
Plate 35   KS on black skin
Plate 36   Crusted 'Norwegian' scabies

Contributors

Caroline Allsop

Ch1: The genitourinary medicine service, and Ch2: Ethical, medic-legal, and sociocultural issues

Sexual Health Advisor, The Newcastle upon Tyne Hospitals NHS Foundation Trust, Newcastle upon Tyne, UK

D. Ashley Price

Editor

Consultant in Infectious Diseases, The Newcastle upon Tyne Hospitals NHS Foundation Trust, Newcastle upon Tyne, UK

Pam Barnes

Ch23: Anogenital warts

Specialty Doctor in Sexual Health, The Newcastle upon Tyne Hospitals NHS Foundation Trust, Newcastle upon Tyne, UK

Stephen Bushby

Ch4: The standard clinic process and sexual health in primary care, and Ch5: Investigations and microscopy

Consultant in Genitourinary Medicine and HIV, City Hospitals Sunderland NHS Foundation Trust, Sunderland, UK

Babiker Elawad

Editor

Consultant in Genitourinary Medicine, Northumbria Healthcare NHS Foundation Trust and Honorary Consultant in Infectious Diseases, The Newcastle upon Tyne Hospitals NHS Foundation Trust, UK

Katherine Gilmore

Ch6: Specific genitourinary situations, and Ch30: Cervical neoplasia

Specialty Trainee in Community Sexual and Reproductive Healthcare, Newcastle upon Tyne, UK

Bridie Howe

Editor

Consultant in Genitourinary Medicine and HIV, NHS Highland, Inverness, Scotland, UK

Jane Hussey

Ch12: Prostatitis/chronic pelvic pain syndrome in men, and Ch31: Vulval pain

Consultant in Genitourinary Medicine and HIV, City Hospitals Sunderland NHS Foundation Trust, Sunderland, UK

Diana Mansour

Ch34: Contraception including contraception for women living with HIV, and Ch35: Psychological aspects and sexual problems

Consultant in Community Gynaecology, The Newcastle upon Tyne Hospitals NHS Foundation Trust, Newcastle upon Tyne, UK

Laura Mitchell

Editor

Consultant in Sexual Health, University Hospitals Plymouth NHS Trust, Plymouth, UK

K. Nathan Sankar
Editor
Consultant in Genitourinary Medicine, The Newcastle upon Tyne Hospitals NHS Foundation Trust, Newcastle upon Tyne, UK (retired)

Jane Richards
Ch22: Ano-genital herpes
Associate Specialist in Genitourinary Medicine and HIV, The Newcastle upon Tyne Hospitals NHS Foundation Trust, Newcastle upon Tyne, UK

Kate Short
Ch29: Ano-genital dermatoses, and Ch47: HIV: dermatological disorders
Consultant Dermatologist, The Newcastle upon Tyne Hospitals NHS Foundation Trust, Newcastle upon Tyne, UK

Joanna Speedie
Ch34: Contraception including contraception for women living with HIV, and Ch35: Psychological aspects and sexual problems
Locum Consultant in Community Sexual and Reproductive Health, NHS Greater Glasgow and Clyde, Glasgow, UK

Daniel Weiand
Ch21: Urinary tract infection, and Ch32: Streptococcal and staphylococcal infections
Consultant Microbiologist & Educational Lead, The Newcastle upon Tyne Hospitals NHS Foundation Trust, Newcastle upon Tyne, UK

Symbols and abbreviations

➔	cross reference
ℳ	website
►	important
►►	don't dawdle
❶, ⚠	warning
☄	bomb (controversial topic)
♂	male
♀	female
∴	therefore
~	approximately
≈	approximately equal to
±	plus/minus
↑	increased
↓	decreased
→	leads to
1°	primary
2°	secondary
α	alpha
β	beta
γ	gamma
δ	delta
σ	sigma
3TC	lamivudine
ABC	abacavir
ACOG	American College of Obstetricians and Gynecologists
ACTH	adrenocorticotrophic hormone
AGH	anogenital herpes
AHU	arginine, hypoxanthine, and uracil
AIDS	acquired immunodeficiency syndrome
AIHA	autoimmune haemolytic anaemia
AIN	anal intra-epithelial neoplasia
AIS	adenocarcinoma in situ
ALO	actinomycoces-like organisms
ALP	alkaline phosphatase
ALT	alanine aminotransferase
APV	amprenavir

ARS	acute retroviral syndrome
ART	antiretroviral therapy
ARV	antiretroviral
ASCUS	atypical squamous cells of uncertain significance
AST	aspartate aminotransferase
ATL	adult T-cell leukaemia
ATT	anti-tuberculosis treatment
ATV	atazanavir
AZT	zidovudine (see also ZDV)
BAL	broncho-alveolar lavage
BASHH	British Association for Sexual Health and HIV
BCG	Bacillus Calmette-Guerin vaccine
bd	twice daily
BHIVA	British HIV Association
BMA	British Medical Association
BMD	bone mineral density
BSCC	British Society for Cervical Cytology
BV	bacterial vaginosis
BXO	balanitis xerotica obliterans
CAP	chronic abacterial prostatitis
CBP	chronic bacterial prostatitis
cccDNA	covalently closed circular DNA
CCG	Clinical Commissioning Groups
CD	cluster differentiation
CDC	Centers for Disease Control
CFT	complement fixation test
CFU	colony-forming unit
CGIN	cervical glandular intra-epithelial neoplasia
CHC	combined hormonal contraceptive
CHOP	cyclophosphamide, hydroxydaunomycin (doxorubicin), Oncovin® (vincristine), prednisolone
CIN	cervical intra-epithelial neoplasia
CMV	cytomegalovirus
C_{min}	minimum concentration
CNS	central nervous system
COBI	cobicistat
COC	combined oral contraceptive
COX-2	cyclo-oxygenase 2
CP	chronic prostatitis
CPPS	chronic pelvic pain syndrome
CPAP	continuous positive airway pressure

CRF	circulating recombinant forms
CRP	C-reactive protein
CSE	child sexual exploitation
CSF	cerebrospinal fluid
CSW	commercial sex worker
CT	computed tomography
D4T	stavudine
DAA	directly acting antivirals
DDC	zalcitabine
DDI	didanosine
DEXA	dual-energy X-ray absorptiometry
DFA	direct fluorescent antibody
DFSA	drug-facilitated sexual assault
DGI	disseminated gonococcal infection
DILS	diffuse infiltrating lymphocytosis syndrome
DLBCL	diffuse large B-cell lymphomas
DLV	delavirdine
DMARD	disease-modifying anti-rheumatic drugs
DMPA	depot medroxyprogesterone acetate
DNA	deoxyribonucleic acid
DoH	Department of Health
DSP	distal symmetric polyneuropathy
EBV	Epstein–Barr virus
EC	emergency contraception
ED	erectile dysfunction
EFV	efavirenz
EGD	endocervical gland dysplasia
eGFR	estimated glomerular filtration rate
EIA	enzyme immunoassay
EM	erythema multiforme
ENF	enfuvirtide
EO	early onset
EPP	exposure-prone procedure
EPS	expressed prostatic secretions
ERCP	endoscopic retrograde cholangiopancreatography
ESLD	end-stage liver disease
ESR	erythrocyte sedimentation rate
ESRD	end-stage renal disease
ETV	entecavir
EUA	examination under anaesthetic
FAM	fertility awareness method

FBC	full blood count
FGM	female genital mutilation
FI	fusion inhibitor
FPV	fosamprenavir
FSH	follicle-stimulating hormone
FTA	fluorescent treponemal antibody
FTC	emtricitabine
FtM	female to male
FVU	first voided urine
g	gram
G6PD	glucose-6-phosphate dehydrogenase
GALT	gut-associated lymphoid tissue
GAS	Group A β-haemolytic streptococci
GB	gamma-butyrolactone
GBL	gamma butyrolactone
GBS	group A β-haemolytic streptococci
GCSF	granulocyte colony-stimulating factor
GHB	gamma hydroxybutyric acid
GI	gastrointestinal
GMC	General Medical Council
GNDC	Gram-negative diplococci
GnRH	gonadotropin-releasing hormone
gp	glycoprotein
GRA	Gender Recognition Act 2004 (UK)
GRC	gender recognition certificate
GUD	genital ulcer disease
GUM	genitourinary medicine
HA	health adviser
HAV	hepatitis A virus
HBcAG	hepatitis B core antibody
HBeAg	hepatitis B envelope antigen
HBsAg	hepatitis B surface antigen
HBV	hepatitis B virus
HCC	hepatocellular carcinoma
HCFT	herpes complement fixation test
hCG	human chorionic gonadotrophin
HCGIN	high-grade cervical glandular intra-epithelial neoplasia
HCP	healthcare professional
HCV	hepatitis C virus
HCW	health care worker
HDL	high-density lipoprotein

HHV	human herpes virus
HIV	human immunodeficiency virus
HIVAN	HIV associated nephropathy
HLA	human leucocyte antigen
HNIG	human normal immunoglobulin
HPA	Health Protection Agency, hypothalamic–pituitary–adrenal
HPF	high power field
HPV	human papilloma virus
HR	high risk
HRT	hormone replacement therapy
HSIL	high-grade squamous intraepithelial lesions
HSV	herpes simplex virus
HT	hydroxytryptamine
HTLV	human T-cell lymphotropic virus
HZ	herpes zoster
IAP	intrapartum antibiotic prophylaxis
IC_{50}	50% inhibitory concentration
ICC	invasive cervical carcinoma
ID	identification (number)
IDU	injecting drug user
IDV	indinavir
Ig	immunoglobulin
IgM	immunoglobulin M
IHD	ischaemic heart disease
IIEF-5	International Index of Erectile Function-5
IM	intramuscular
IMB	intermenstrual bleeding
IN	intra-epithelial neoplasia
INI	integrase inhibiter
INR	international normalized ratio
IP	index patient
IRIS	immune recovery inflammatory response
ISH	Integrated sexual health
IU	international units
IUD	intra-uterine device
IUS	intra-uterine system
IV	intravenous
IVDU	intravenous drug user
JCV	John Cunningham virus
KB	keratoderma blennorrhagica
KC	Koerner code

KS	Kaposi's sarcoma
LAM	lactational amenorrhoea method
LARC	long acting reversible contraception
LBC	liquid-based cytology
LARC	long acting reversible contraception (also known as lasting and reliable contraception)
LCGIN	low-grade cervical glandular intra-epithelial neoplasia
LDH	lactic dehydrogenase
LDL	low-density lipoprotein
LFTs	liver function tests
LGE	linear gingival erythema
LGV	lymphogranuloma venereum
LH	luteinizing hormone
LIP	lymphocytic interstitial pneumonitis
LLV	low level viraemia
LNG	levonorgestrel
LPV	lopinavir
LS	lichen sclerosis
LTR	long-terminal repeat
LSIL	low-grade squamous intraepithelial lesions
LUTI	lower urinary tract infection
LUTS	lower urinary tract symptoms
MAC	*Mycobacterium avium* complex
MACE	multi-agency child sexual exploitation
MASE	multi-agency sexual exploitation
MASH	multi-agency safeguarding hubs
mcg	microgram
MCV	molluscum contagiosum virus
MDA	Mullerian duct anomalies
MDT	multi-disciplinary team
MEDFASH	Medical Foundation for HIV and Sexual Health
MHA-TP	microhaemagglutination assay for Treponema pallidum
MI	myocardial infarction
MOMP	major outer membrane protein
MOPP	mechlorethamine, Oncovin® (vincristine), procarbazine, prednisolone
MPC	mucopurulent cervicitis
MRI	magnetic resonance imaging
MRP1	multidrug resistance associated protein 1
MSM	men who have sex with men
MSSU	midstream specimen of urine

MtF	male to female
MTCT	mother to child transmission
MU	mega-unit(s)
NAAT	nucleic acid amplification test
NAM	multi-NRTI associated mutation
NASBA	nucleic acid sequence based amplification assay
NB	non-binary
NET-EN	norethisterone oenanthate
NGU	non-gonococcal urethritis
NHL	non-Hodgkin lymphoma
NHS	National Health Service
NNRTI	non-nucleoside reverse transcriptase inhibitor
NPV	negative predictive value
NRTI	nucleoside/nucleotide reverse transcriptase inhibitor
NS	necrotizing stomatitis
NSAID	non-steroidal anti-inflammatory drug
NSGI	non-specific genital infection
NSI	non-syncytium-inducing
NSU	non-specific urethritis
NUP	necrotizing ulcerative periodontitis
NVP	nevirapine
OHL	oral hairy leukoplakia
OI	opportunistic infection
OPV	oral polio vaccine
p	protein
PACE	probe assay chemiluminescence enhanced
PBS	primer binding site
PCB	post-coital bleeding
PCC	post-coital contraception
PCL	primary CNS lymphomas
PCP	*Pneumocystis jiroveci* (*carinii*) pneumonia
PCR	polymerase chain reaction
PCT	Primary Care Trust
PegIFNα	pegylated interferon alfa α
PEP	post-exposure prophylaxis
PEPSE	post-exposure prophylaxis after sexual exposure
PET	positron emission tomography
PGD	patient group directions
PHI	primary HIV infection
PI	protease inhibitor
PIC	pre-integration complex

PID	pelvic inflammatory disease
PLCS	pre-labour caesarean section
PLWH	people living with HIV
PML	progressive multifocal leukoencephalopathy
PMNL	polymorphonuclear leucocyte
PN	partner notification
POC	progesterone-only contraception
POCT	point-of-care test
POEC	progesterone-only emergency contraception
POP	progesterone-only contraception
ppt	polypurine tract
PPV	positive predictive value
PrEP	pre-exposure prophylaxis
PROM	premature rupture of membranes
PSA	prostatic specific antigen
PTH	parathyroid hormone
PUO	pyrexia of unknown origin
PVL	Panton–Valentine Leucocidin-positive
PWID	people who inject drugs
RA	rheumatoid arthritis
RAL	raltegravir
RCOG	Royal College of Obstetricians and Gynaecologists
ReA	reactive arthritis
RPV	rilpivirine
RNA	ribonucleic acid
RPR	rapid plasma reagin
RT	reverse transcriptase
rT3	reverse triiodothyronine
RTV	ritonavir
RV	right ventricular
RVVC	recurrent vulvovaginal candidiasis
SARA	sexually acquired reactive arthritis
SARC	sexual assault referral centres
SC	subcutaneous
SCC	squamous cell carcinoma
SCJ	squamo-columnar junction
SDA	strand displacement amplification
SI	syncytium-inducing
SIADH	syndrome of inappropriate secretion of antidiuretic hormone
SIL	squamous intra-epithelial lesion

SIV	simian immune deficiency virus
SJS	Stevens–Johnson syndrome
SQV	saquinavir
SRH	sexual and reproductive health
SSRI	selective serotonin re-uptake inhibitor
STD	sexually transmitted disease
STI	sexually transmitted infection
TAF	tenofovir alafenamide
TAM	thymidine analogue mutation
TasP	treatment as prevention
TB	tuberculosis
TBG	thyroid-binding globulin
TCA	trichloroacetic acid
TDF	tenofovir
TDM	therapeutic drug monitoring
TDR	transmitted drug resistance
TENS	transcutaneous electrical nerve stimulation
TFT	thyroid function test
tid	three times a day
TMA	transcription-mediated assay
TNF	tumour necrosis factor
TOC	test of cure
TOP	termination of pregnancy
TP	*Treponema pallidum*
TPHA	TP haemagglutination assay
TPPA	TP particle agglutination
TSH	thyroid-stimulating hormone
TSS	toxic shock syndrome
TV	*Trichomonas vaginalis*
TZ	transformation zone
U&E	urea & electrolytes
ULN	upper limit of normal
UPAI	unprotected anal intercourse
UPSI	unprotected sexual intercourse
UTI	urinary tract infection
UUTI	upper urinary tract infection
VBU	voided bladder urine
VD	venereal disease
VDRL	Venereal Disease Research Laboratory
VIN	vulval intra-epithelial neoplasia
VL	viral load

VLP	virus-like particle
VTE	venous thromboembolism
VVC	vulvovaginal candidiasis
VZV	varicella zoster virus
WBC	white blood count, white blood cells
WHO	World Health Organization
ZDV	zidovudine (see also AZT)
❶	*All other abbreviations are defined in the text on the page in which they appear.*

The genitourinary medicine service

Service development 2
Provision 4
Availability 6
The process 7
Sexual health promotion 12

Service development

Genitourinary medicine (GUM)

During the 1914–18 World War there was an alarming increase in legally defined venereal diseases (VDs): syphilis, gonorrhoea, and chancroid. A Royal Commission produced the Venereal Disease Regulations (1916), specifying that local authorities should provide clinics which:

- could be accessed directly (without general practitioner referral)
- enabled voluntary attendance
- assured confidentiality
- provided free treatment.

One-hundred-and-thirteen clinics were established in 1917.

During the 1939–45 World War there was a concern that troops were being incapacitated by infection, with a core group of individuals acting as a reservoir. Therefore, doctors began to question patients about their sexual partners. An individual named by more than one person could be compelled to have treatment; failure to comply could lead to imprisonment (Defence of the Realm Act 33B 1942). This regulation was subsequently repealed in 1947, but led to the introduction of voluntary partner notification (PN) in the uk, a vital tool in the control of infection.

In the uk, there are now over 260 clinics led by consultants specializing in GUM, covering a wide range of sexually transmitted infections (STIs), including human immunodeficiency virus (HIV) and other genitourinary conditions or problems. Their name has evolved from 'VD Clinic', 'Special Clinic', or 'Sexually Transmitted Diseases Clinic' to 'Genitourinary Medicine Clinic', 'Sexual Health Clinic', or an eponymous name, and many are integrated with sexual and reproductive health (SRH) services, previously known as contraception, family planning, or contraception and sexual health services.

STIs and genitourinary conditions present in a variety of guises to different specialties (e.g. dermatology, gynaecology, urology, and infectious diseases). Therefore, cross-referral is common and allows for the establishment of multidisciplinary clinics, e.g. for vulval disorders.

Integrated sexual health (ISH) services

The National Strategy for Sexual Health and HIV (2001) identified wide-ranging differences in the provision of sexual health services throughout England. Concerns that such inequalities might adversely affect the government's attempts to ↓ the number of teenage pregnancies and rates of STIs resulted in the concept of ISH services. GUM and SRH services, which in the past have traditionally operated as separate entities, are now working closely together to provide high-quality easily accessible ISH services for all.

Robust joint training initiatives for both medical and nursing staff have resulted in dual-trained clinicians able to deal with all aspects of routine sexual health care. Specialist clinicians deal with complex STIs and contraception, medical gynaecology, psychosexual problems, erectile dysfunction and HIV care and treatment. Patients now have the opportunity to self-refer for termination of pregnancy (TOP) and information about this service must be made readily available to attendees.

The continued ↑ in infections and unwanted pregnancies may be addressed by the provision of high-quality easily understandable health promotion together with the opportunity to undergo testing in alternative locations. Point-of-care testing allows immediate results and undoubtedly encourages those who may not otherwise attend conventional sexual health services to be screened.

Provision

Aims of GUM and ISH services

The ultimate goal of GUM and ISH is to ↓ STIs within the community. This is achievable by delivering accessible and non-judgmental services, which provide free and immediate diagnosis and treatment to those who think they may have, or be at risk of having, an STI. Epidemiological control of infection remains essential to the sexual welfare of the community. However, clinics must reconcile confidentiality with a need for both 1° care and hospital services to be aware of serious chronic health problems in the individual. Health advice with good community links is important for ensuring that PN issues are dealt with efficiently and sensitively, reducing the continued transmission of STIs.

Comprehensive national surveillance programmes are essential when formulating strategies for national screening and treatment policies. Surveillance data inform clinical practice, allow the planning and allocation of resources, and help identify at-risk populations. This is largely achieved by the collection of reliable data from GUM/ISH clinics, as information on infection managed elsewhere, including 1° care, is limited.

GUM: core and specialized roles

The core function of GUM is to provide screening, surveillance, diagnosis, treatment, and PN for STIs including HIV. This is combined with sexual health promotion, teaching, training, and research.

In addition some services provide specialized clinics at their main location or at outreach venues (e.g. prisons). These are established and resourced to meet local need and may include sessions for:
- chronic or recurrent conditions, e.g. HIV, warts, herpes
- problems involving different specialties, e.g. vulval conditions, sexual assault (providing both forensic examination and infection screening), one-stop sexual health service
- related problems where service need is identified, e.g. psychosexual and sexual dysfunction
- special groups, e.g. young people; lesbian, gay, bisexual, or transgender people; ethnic minorities; commercial sex workers.

Doctors

GUM/ISH is a consultant-led service with a dedicated higher medical training programme for specialty registrars from specialty training years 3–6 (ST3–ST6). There are also training posts at the more junior levels of foundation year 2, and general practice specialty training years 1 or 2. Many non-consultant career-grade doctors, who are known as associate specialists or specialty doctors, are working either exclusively in GUM, ISH, or in association with SRH, 1° care, etc.

Nurse specialists/practitioners

The role of the nurse within GUM/ISH has continued to evolve, with specialist (and consultant) nurses now the norm. Nurse-led clinics run alongside conventional medically led services, with nursing staff working independently, taking responsibility for total patient care, including the examination of new patients under protocol and providing medication through patient group directions. No uniform model of care exists; individual centres implement their own preferred methods.

Health advisers (HAs)

In the UK, HAs are employed within GUM/ISH services. Their primary public health role is PN, which is the identification and management of partners who may have been exposed to STI(s). Their role also includes work at community and population levels, identifying local sexual health needs and ensuring that services are accessible to those with the greatest need by effective targeting and the development of innovative practice approaches. They act as advocates for health gain and work collaboratively with others to tackle the wider determinants of health (Box 1.1).

Box 1.1 Role of HAs (varies between clinics)

- Providing a holistic approach to patients, with information, education, treatment, and support.
- Comprehensive needs assessment of index patients (IPs) and other vulnerable groups (e.g. young people, ethnic minorities, those sexually assaulted), including associated social, emotional, or sexual difficulties.
- Effective PN ensuring the attendance and treatment of sexual contacts, including settings outside GUM/ISH, e.g. 1° care.
- Establishing and maintaining care pathways for patients in primary/ acute care diagnosed with STIs.
- Pre- and post-test HIV discussion.
- Counselling, information, and support to patients, including those with HIV infection and their partners, friends, and relatives.
- Sexual health education provision within GUM/ISH and the community, liaising with statutory and voluntary services.
- Research, audit, and service development.
- Support of clinical outreach in non-clinical settings to targeted groups, e.g. increasing the uptake of HIV testing in those most at risk, hepatitis B vaccination for men who have sex with men, STI screening for sex workers.
- Tackling the stigma and discrimination and prejudice often associated with sexual health.
- Helping people make informed decisions about relationships, sex, and sexual health.
- Preventive interventions that build personal resilience and self-esteem and promote healthy choices.

Availability

Referrals

The majority of patients seen in GUM or ISH, either self-refer or are seen as a result of PN. 2° referrals are seen, especially from 1° care, SRH, and rape crisis organizations, with tertiary referrals from gynaecology, dermatology, infectious diseases, urology, etc. These may be formal, with a letter, or based on verbal advice. By common acceptance, there is no correspondence unless the patient has been referred by letter. However, in certain situations, it may be in the patient's best interests for there to be an exchange of medical information between professionals providing care, but this should have the patient's agreement.

Access

Easy and timely access to the clinic should be available. When the clinic is closed, a pre-recorded telephone message detailing clinic opening hours, together with the telephone number for other local GUM/ISH services, Accident and Emergency, or NHS Direct is of benefit to anyone with an urgent problem. Appointment availability should be linked to staff numbers and experience. Ideally, patients should be seen within 48 hours. However, testing too soon after an infection risk may produce false-negative results (e.g. 2 weeks for chlamydia); therefore, this period should be extended (unless prophylactic treatment is required), or clear information should be given to patients regarding this possibility and re-testing at the appropriate time offered. If this is not possible, careful use of triage may help identify those with urgent problems.

All services should review their location and opening hours to match the needs of the local population. Some clinics provide open access without prior booking, although most utilize some form of appointment system.

Triage

In clinics operating by an appointment system, a robust triage system should be available for urgent situations. Trained staff should be able to assess and prioritize the patient's condition, including advice on optimum screening time intervals following an infection risk, and then arrange the appropriate attendance. Use of digital technology for triaging and some aspects of clinical consultation with home testing or self-testing is a recent development. Some services have introduced these to address the increasing demands for the services; further developments could see wider application of such new technology.

Disability

Any assistance required by the disabled should be highlighted when making an appointment, but accessibility facilities, such as wheelchair access, disabled toilets, minicom systems, etc., should be in place.

Interpreters

Most hospitals are able to provide an accredited interpreting service, but will need time to arrange an interpreter of the appropriate language. Alternatively, a telephone system can be used (e.g. Language Line). If possible, avoid family members, friends, or relatives acting as interpreters, as information may be withheld by the patient under these circumstances.

The process

Registration

Patients should be allowed privacy during registration by ensuring that they cannot be overheard while providing information, or by the use of self-completed registration forms or digital interface. Help must be available to those with difficulties in completing such forms or digital portals. The amount of information required at registration will differ from clinic to clinic. However, collection of the data shown in Table 1.1 may assist the clinic to contact the patient if required and help with service planning, statistics, and surveillance.

Patients who refuse to give any information about themselves may attend. The right to anonymity is accepted within GUM/ISH. The patient should be issued with an individual clinic identification (ID) number, which should be used on all specimens and request forms. They should be encouraged to provide at least their date of birth, which can be used with the ID number as an additional reference when confirming identity, test results, etc.

Appointment cards showing the patient's ID number and all booked appointments should be issued at the time of registration. Details of the clinic opening times and telephone numbers should be clearly printed on the card. These administrative processes can be digitized, and some services have already introduced digital systems as the main or an additional option.

Waiting areas are inevitably areas of stress for those wishing to remain anonymous. Issuing patients with a welcome leaflet on arrival explaining how the clinic operates will hopefully ↓ anxiety. Those who are acutely distressed should be moved into a private area. The use of a television or music system in the waiting room may help to distract the anxious patient and also reduce the risk of sensitive information being overheard.

Soundex codes

Soundex codes (Table 1.2), together with dates of birth, are commonly used within GUM/ISH to provide clinical information, while protecting individual confidentiality.

Confirmation of attendance

Letters confirming attendance for a clinic or hospital appointment should be made available for the patient to present to their employer using hospital-headed notepaper without reference to GUM/ISH. This letter should state the date and time of the visit together with the date and time of any further appointments.

Table 1.1 Useful information for registration

Name	Nationality
Address	Country of birth
Date of birth	Ethnicity
Telephone number(s)	Area of residence
General practitioner	Referral source and documentation
Employment status	Name of partner (if attending)

Table 1.2 The Soundex code

The Soundex code contains four characters, with the first being the first letter of the surname.
  The remaining three are numbers derived from the name.
  When the adjacent letters are from the same category, the second is disregarded.
  The letters A, E, H, I, O, U, Y, and W only contribute if they start the name.
An empty space is represented by a zero. Once the four-character limit has been reached, all remaining letters are redundant.

Category	Letter
1	B, P, F, V
2	C, S, K, G, J, Q, X, Z
3	D, T
4	L
5	M, N
No code	A, E, H, I, O, U, Y, W

Reimbursement of travel expenses

Patients attending GUM/ISH clinics may reclaim their travel expenses upon receipt of bus/train tickets if the distance travelled is >15 miles from home. Legislation is unclear about those who travel less than this distance. Therefore, it is suggested that discretion be used in such cases. This facility is offered to patients irrespective of individual financial circumstances (Department of Health NHS Charges HC11 2002).

Transfer to other GUM clinics

Patients leaving the area can be issued with a summary of investigations and treatments carried out while attending the initial clinic. This allows subsequent clinics to assess the need for further management.

Test results

Various systems are employed throughout the country to provide test results and include:
• returning in person or telephoning for all results
• contact by the clinic (letter, phone, text message, e-mail, secure online portal).

Informing patients that if they are not contacted the results are −ve or normal ('no news is good news') is considered poor practice. Some patients, including those working in the sex industry, may request written proof of the test result. When provided, it must be made clear that this may not cover recently acquired infections (e.g. within 'window' periods). Patients must produce a photographic identification before issue of such results.

Recall

A digital system aids the process of recall. Patients are generally reviewed for the following reasons:

- to be given positive test results and treatment
- further management (e.g. ongoing treatment, PN).

Recall usually takes the form of a letter requesting that the patient contacts the clinic, but may also be by telephone, e-mail, or text-messaging.

Health advice and partner notification

PN (see Table 1.3) is the process of contacting the sexual partners of an individual with a STI, including HIV, to advise them of their exposure to infection, and encourage them to attend for counselling, testing, treatment, and other prevention measures. PN is an essential component of STI management and control, protecting patients from re-infection, partners from long-term consequences from untreated infection, and the wider community from onward transmission. First introduced as 'contact tracing' in the 1940s in the UK, to identify, diagnose, and treat contacts of VDs, PN now applies to all sexually transmitted infections as an essential part of infection control. Guidelines produced by the World Health Organization endorse PN as an essential component of prevention and control of STIs. In the UK, PN is undertaken primarily by HAs, employed within GUM/ISH services. The guidance document, *Sexual Health Advising – Developing the Workforce* (DoH/SSHA/Unite 2008) recommends a robust programme to prepare the future HA workforce and to strengthen the public health role of HAs. This was an aim of the National Strategy for Sexual Health and HIV (DH 2001).

Aims of PN

The ultimate aim is to break the chain and transmission of STIs and rates of infection by:

- Stressing the importance of PN to those diagnosed with certain STIs.
- Providing them with information on the nature, exposure, and risk of infection. The need to have sexual partners appropriately managed before sexual intercourse resumes must be emphasized.
- Identifying, contacting, and screening sexual partners of the IP, providing information and offering treatment if appropriate.

Description of terms and methods used in PN

PN should be conducted so that all information remains confidential and the process is voluntary. Consultation with the HA should take place in an appropriate soundproofed environment, free from interruption.

- *Patient referral:* IP with an STI is encouraged to notify their sexual partner(s) of any infection risk. HAs can help the IP to decide what information should be passed on to partners and how best to do this. The process is facilitated by the issue of contact slips bearing the IP ID number, name of infection (usually in a coded form), and details of the issuing clinic. Use of digital technology for PN is a recent development.

Table 1.3 Partner notification

| Infection | PN method | | Trace period |
	Patient	Provider	s = symptomatic as = asymptomatic
Cervicitis (mucopurulent), PID, epididymitis	✓	✓	Current sexual partners
Chancroid	✓	✓	10 days from disease onset
Chlamydia	✓	✓	4 weeks (s), 6 months (as), or last partner if longer
Donovanosis	✓	✓	40 days from disease onset
Gonorrhoea	✓	✓	2 week (s) males, 12 weeks (as) males, and all females or last partner if longer
Hepatitis A	✓	✓	2 weeks prior to and 1 week after onset of jaundice
Hepatitis B	✓	✓	2 weeks prior to onset of jaundice or based on risk
Hepatitis C	✓	✓	Based on risk assessment
Anogenital herpes	✗	✗	Offer advice and STI screening
HIV	✓	✓	Risk assessment informs PN for as cases (If 1° infection—3 months)
Lymphogranuloma venereum	✓	✓	30 days from disease onset
Non-gonococcal urethritis	✓	✓	4 weeks (s), 6 months (as), or last partner if longer
Pediculosis	✓	✗	12 weeks: current partner
Scabies	✓	✓	8 weeks: current partner, household members
Syphilis (early)	✓	✓	12 weeks (1°), up to 2 years (2°, early latent)
Syphilis (late)	✓	✓	10 years; vertical transmission possible for a decade post-infection; therefore, includes children born to infected mothers
Trichomoniasis	✓	✗	Current partner
Anogenital warts/molluscum	✗	✗	Offer to screen current partners

- *Provider referral:* these are offered to those IPs who do not wish to inform their sexual partner(s) themselves. The IP provides partner details to the HA after reassurance that confidentiality will not be compromised. HAs make direct contact with at-risk sexual partner(s) based on information provided by the IP. Evidence demonstrates that provider referral is more effective than partner referral.
- *Contract referral:* this allows the IP and HA to negotiate an acceptable time span in which the IP will attempt to contact sexual partner(s). If unsuccessful, provider referral may follow by agreement.
- *No referral:* where PN is impractical (involves careful risk–benefit analysis), e.g. when there is insufficient information or a threat of violence to the IP or HA.

While partner notification remains a voluntary activity within the UK, countries such as Sweden and certain states of the usa have made it a legal requirement.

Sexual health promotion

Definition

Sexual health promotion is an activity that proactively and positively supports the sexual and emotional health and well-being of individuals, groups, communities, and the wider public, and reduces the risk of HIV transmission. The key aim is to ↓ inequalities in sexual health.

Specific aims

- ↓ Transmission of HIV and STIs (advice on safe sex)
- ↓ prevalence of undiagnosed HIV and STIs by encouraging testing
- ↓ unintended pregnancy rates
- education to bring about ↓ stigma of STIs and HIV.

Objectives include raising awareness, education and provision of information, and service-provider development.

Methods of sexual health promotion

These should be carefully chosen to match the needs of the target group. They can be divided into direct and indirect methods.

Direct methods

- National and local media health campaigns to ↑ public awareness.
- Individual one-to-one work in a sexual health setting (HAs, nurse specialists).
- Condom distribution, e.g. in youth clinics, GUM/ISH/SRH clinics and primary care.
- Screening for STIs and HIV in a variety of easily accessible settings.
- Promoting self-care, e.g. over-the-counter emergency contraception, pregnancy testing, advice on testicular self-examination.
- Targeted community work, particularly with marginalized and vulnerable groups (outreach, street, and group work).
- Dissemination of information via digital media or using materials such as leaflets, posters, and magazines which also inform clients about local sexual health services.
- Peer education programmes.
- Sex and relationship education in formal and informal educational settings.

Indirect methods

- Training courses and workshops for those involved in sexual health work. Digital media can be used to support these.
- Conferences where research and best practice can be shared.
- Development of policies and strategies, including local needs assessment.
- Inter-agency working, especially within the voluntary and community sector (e.g. Terrence Higgins Trust).
- Support and advice to groups developing sexual health services.
- Engaging in research.
- Discussion with health commissioners to enable funding and provision of services.

Settings for sexual health promotion

Can be widespread in diverse settings by trained staff from different disciplines, including:

- Schools.
- Further education, training colleges, and universities.
- Pubs, clubs, and recreational settings (e.g. gyms), including poster and leaflet displays, condom machines in toilets, etc.
- *Residential care*: for people with disabilities or learning difficulties, older adults, hostels for people seeking asylum, refuge from abuse, and people lacking permanent accommodation.
- Prison and young offenders' institutions.
- *Drug and alcohol services*: needle exchanges and methadone clinics.
- Sex venues, such as saunas and cruising areas.
- Community centres, including youth clubs and faith groups.
- Workplaces, including armed services (barracks, etc.), pharmacies, NHS.
- *Clinic settings*: GUM/ISH, 1° care, SRH, TOP clinics.

Good practice in health promotion

Accurate information should be provided that is clear, easily accessible, and up to date. It should be offered in a non-judgemental way, be sensitive and respectful to the diversity of individual and community beliefs and attitudes. Misconceptions should be challenged, and stigma and prejudice should be actively discouraged. This information should empower individuals to make responsible decisions about their sexual health. Information should be evidence based. Discussion should be encouraged to explore ideas, thoughts, and feelings. Support should be available to all, but particularly those who are vulnerable and marginalized.

Ethical, medico-legal & sociocultural issues

Introduction 16
Confidentiality 17
Consent 18
Consent: children 20
Child sexual exploitation 24
Sexual offences 27
Female genital mutilation 29
Consent: other specific issues 31
Intimate examinations and chaperones 32
Electronic technology 34
Partner notification issues 35
HIV-infected healthcare workers 36
Death 36
Writing statements and court appearances 37
Legislation pertinent to GUM 38

Introduction

This section deals with some of the ethical and medico-legal aspects specific to HIV infection and GUM. Most medico-legal problems arise from:
- failure to appreciate legal responsibilities
- problems in clinical management
- medication errors
- administrative errors
- failure of communication and inadequate clinical records.

Awareness and adherence to relevant law and General Medical Council (GMC) guidance is essential. If in doubt seek advice from experienced colleagues, professional bodies, or medico-legal defence organizations.

Confidentiality

Common law and the Data Protection Act 1998 protect personal health information. Confidentiality is central to the trust between patient and healthcare professional (HCP). Without its explicit assurance, the patient may not volunteer a full history and medical care may be compromised. It is particularly important for those dealing with STIs where patients provide highly sensitive information. This is formally recognized by the NHS Trusts and Primary Care Trusts (Sexually Transmitted Diseases) Directions 2000. These apply to any healthcare setting and not just GUM clinics.

To maintain confidentiality the following practices should be adopted:

- anonymize patient data on records/forms/specimens by using identification (ID) numbers, dates of birth, or Soundex codes (Chapter 1, Table 1.2)
- offer the patient a choice on how they would like to be called from the waiting room
- do not discuss patients outside the health team or where the conversation may be overheard by others
- ensure that any consultations are in private, e.g. triage patients in a separate room, not at reception
- disclose information to general practitioner only following consent from the patient (unless it falls within the STD Directions 2000).

Public interest

There are some situations when confidentiality may need to be broken, however, it is vital to consider any decisions in accordance with up to date GMC guidance. These instances usually include disclosures where there is felt to be a risk of harm to the patient or others.

Specific regulations apply to 'serious communicable diseases' including HIV, Hepatitis B and C, the latter two (and also Hepatitis A) being notifiable. Problems may also be encountered if the patient is unable to take responsibility for his/her management (e.g. prisoners, patients who lack capacity, children). Before sharing any confidential information, this should be discussed and explained to the patient (and ideally their consent sought) and with senior colleagues. All NHS organizations will have a Caldicott Guardian (a senior person responsible for protecting the confidentiality of patient information) and their opinion should be sought if a breach of confidentiality is being considered.

Consent

It is good practice and a legal requirement to obtain consent from a patient before treatment. Failure to do so can result in complaints to the individual's employing authority or relevant professional body, criminal proceedings for assault or indecent assault, and civil proceedings (e.g. if injuries arise following treatment without informed consent). To be valid, consent must be given voluntarily by a competent, fully informed patient. A detailed discussion, clearly recorded in the notes, is required.

Consent is required for investigations, treatment, disclosure of information, research, photography/video recording, and teaching (e.g. medical students observing a consultation). In certain circumstances, the use of a signed consent form is required. It must be made clear that refusal to participate in such activities will not compromise clinical care.

The person obtaining consent must be fully aware of the situation, ideally directly involved in it, and able to answer any queries. To help understanding, and therefore the ability to give valid consent, information should be provided clearly, using written or visual aids. If the patient cannot understand English, an interpreter, accredited if possible, should be provided and additional time set aside. In certain situations, it is helpful to involve another member of the health team, such as a HA. It may be necessary to provide time, over a number of sessions, to allow the patient to reach their informed decision.

To obtain consent for a screening test, the patient should be aware of the following points.
- Description of the test:
  • Why the test is being taken?
  • What does it involve?
- The likelihood of receiving +ve or –ve results.
- Implications of a +ve result to the person and their partner(s).
- Any medical, social, or financial implications.
- Requirement for follow-up tests/treatment.

Mental Capacity Act 2005 (enacted October 2007)

- Applies to England and Wales (similar principles apply in Scotland) to people aged 16 years and over.
- Statutory framework, largely based on common law, to empower and protect vulnerable people who may be unable to make their own decisions.

It clarifies who can decide when and how to proceed. It also enables people to plan for a time when they may lose capacity through Lasting Powers of Attorney and Advanced Decisions. It only applies if the person is shown to lack capacity. When capacity to decide is lacking, the doctor should provide treatment in the patient's best interests under the common law doctrine of necessity, unless limitations apply.

Key principles

- A person must be assumed to have capacity unless it is established that they lack capacity.
- A person is not to be treated as unable to make a decision unless all practical steps to help them to do so have been taken without success.
- A person is not to be treated as unable to make a decision merely because he/she makes an unwise decision.

- An act done or decision made under the Act for, or on behalf of, a person who lacks capacity must be done, or made, in his/her best interests.
- Before the act is done or the decision is made, regard must be had to whether the purpose for which it is needed can be effectively achieved in a way that is less restrictive of the person's rights and freedom of action.

Capacity

For the purposes of the Act, a person lacks capacity in relation to a matter if, at the material time, they are unable to make a decision for themselves in relation to the matter because of an impairment of or a disturbance in the functioning of the mind or brain. Capacity is decision specific; therefore, a person may lack capacity to make some decisions, but retain capacity to make others. It does not matter whether the impairment or disturbance is permanent (e.g. a learning disability or dementia) or temporary (e.g. alcohol/drug use, sedation or anaesthesia, mental illness). Therefore, capacity can fluctuate and the assessment made is relevant to the person's state at that time.

Capacity assessment

A person is unable to make a decision for themselves if they are unable:

- to **understand** the information relevant to the decision (the information must be presented in a way appropriate to the individual)
- to **retain** that information (if only for a short time, may still be regarded as able to make the decision)
- to **use or weigh** that information as part of the process of making the decision or
- to **communicate** their decision (whether by talking, using sign language, or any other means).

It is good practice for professionals carrying out a proper capacity assessment to record the findings in the relevant professional records.

Best interests

This has no statutory definition, but:

- Consider:
  - whether (and if so, when) person will have capacity
  - if practicable, encouraging participation
  - if possible, the person's past wishes, beliefs, values, etc.
- Take into account (if practicable and appropriate) the views of anyone named by the person to be consulted, e.g. carer, anyone interested in person's welfare, in possession of the patients' Lasting Powers of Attorney, Court Deputy.
- When in relation to 'life-sustaining treatment', not to be motivated to bring about death when considering whether the treatment is in the best interests of the person concerned.

Exceptions

- Where the person has made a valid advance decision to refuse treatment.
- In specific circumstances the involvement of a person who lacks capacity in research.

Ultimately the Court of Protection can be asked to make a decision. Always ensure that a written record is made of the process followed.

Consent: children

The age of consent for medical treatment in England, Scotland, Wales, and Northern Ireland is 16.

Competence

England and Wales

Any competent person, regardless of age, can give consent for medical treatment. A patient is competent if they can understand the choices and their consequences, including the nature, purpose, and possible risk of any treatment or non-treatment. Although parental support should be encouraged, if the patient does not wish the parent's involvement, this view should not be overridden. When establishing if a patient under the age of 16 years is competent the Fraser Ruling (Gillick competence) should be followed. The Gillick case (*Gillick v West Norfolk and Wisbech Health Authority* [1985], 3 All ER 402 HL) established the current legal position in England and Wales. Although this ruling was directed towards contraceptive services, it can be extrapolated to include the management of STIs and details the following points:

• The patient should be encouraged to inform his/her parents of the consultation.
• The patient must understand the potential risks and benefits of the treatment and advice.
• The HCP must take into account whether the patient is likely to engage in sexual activity without contraception.
• The HCP must assess whether the patient's physical or mental health, or both, are likely to suffer if they do not receive contraceptive advice or supplies.
• The HCP must consider whether the patient's best interests would require the provision of contraceptive advice or methods, or both, without parental consent.

Guidance published in 2004 highlights that where a request for contraception is made by a person under the age of 16, doctors and other HCPs should establish a rapport with the young person and give them the time and support to make an informed choice. They should do this by discussing:

• the emotional and physical implications of sexual activity, including the risks of pregnancy and STIs
• whether the relationship is mutually agreed or whether there may be coercion or abuse
• the benefits of informing their GP
• encouraging discussion with a parent or carer.

Any refusal should be respected. In the case of termination of pregnancy, where the young woman is competent to consent, but cannot be persuaded to involve a parent, every effort should be made to help her find another adult to provide support.

Scotland

Gillick competency is not relevant in Scotland. The Age of Legal Capacity (Scotland) Act 1991 gives statutory power to the minor to consent to medical or dental treatment. This act goes beyond the Fraser Ruling, stating that children <16 years have the legal capacity to consent to any surgical, medical, or dental treatment or procedure as long as that child is capable of understanding the nature and consequences of the proposed treatment or procedure. In England and Wales, if a child refuses treatment, this can be overruled by a person with parental responsibility for the child or by the court. This is not the case in Scotland where the Age of legal Capacity (Scotland) Act protects the child's right to refuse examination or treatment, presuming the child has the capacity under the legislation.

Immature patients

GMC guidelines state that if a doctor does not consider the patient to be capable of giving consent because of immaturity, the relevant information may be disclosed to an appropriate person or authority, if it is thought to be in the best interests of the patient. However, the following conditions should be met:

- the patient does not have sufficient understanding to appreciate the implications of advice or treatment
- the patient cannot be persuaded to involve an appropriate person in the consultation
- the doctor believes it is in the best medical interests of the patient.

Child protection issues

There is a duty of confidentiality to all patients, irrespective of their age. The exception is when disclosure of information is in their best medical interests, or the patient or other vulnerable person is at risk of harm. The HCP must be prepared to justify their decision to their professional body. Under such circumstances, if the patient cannot be persuaded to make a voluntary disclosure, the HCP should explain to the patient that confidentiality cannot be preserved. However, confidentiality is important for young people and it is important to ensure that there is no breach when that young person is not at risk.

The age of a 'child' for child protection purposes has been raised from 16 years to 18 years in the UK.

Social services are the lead agency for child protection with statutory responsibilities and the police have powers to intervene when there are concerns about a child's welfare.

Child abuse is almost always committed by a perpetrator known (and often trusted) by the child. Abuse may be:

- physical
- emotional
- sexual
- neglect
  - this also includes the abuse of an unborn child (e.g. drug misuse during pregnancy), which may lead to inclusion on the Child Protection Register after the 20th week of pregnancy.

Sexual activity and abuse

Although the legal age of consent for sex is 16 years for both heterosexual and homosexual sex in the uk, an estimated 25% of boys and girls are sexually active below this age.

Under 13 years

Not legally capable of consenting to sexual activity; penetrative sex is classed as rape. Any offence under the Sexual Offences Act 2003 is very serious and should be taken to indicate a risk of significant harm to the child. All cases should be discussed with the child protection lead within the organization, with the presumption that the case will then be reported to social services. There may be situations where reporting is not considered to be necessary, but all must be fully documented, including the reasons where a decision is taken not to share information.

The age of criminal responsibility in the UK is 10 years (except Scotland, where it is 8 years).

13–15 years

Sexual activity with a child aged under 16 years is an offence. Where consensual it may be less serious than if the child were under 13, and the law is not intended to prosecute mutually agreed sexual activity between young people of a similar age, unless it involves abuse or exploitation. However, it may have serious welfare consequences. In every case of sexual activity involving a child aged 13–15 years consideration should be given as to whether there should be a discussion with other agencies and whether a referral should be made to social services. The professional should make this assessment using the considerations detailed in Box 2.1. Where confidentiality needs to be preserved, a discussion can still take place as long as the child is not identified. All cases should be fully documented and include detailed reasons where a decision is taken not to share information.

16 and 17 years

It is an offence for a person to have a sexual relationship with a 16- or 17-year-old if that person holds a position of trust or authority in relation to them. Otherwise, although sexual activity is unlikely to involve an offence, it may still involve harm or the risk of harm.

Box 2.1 Child assessment for risk

The following considerations should be taken into account when assessing the extent to which a child (or other children) may be suffering or be at risk of harm and, therefore, the need to hold a strategy discussion in order to share information:

- *The age of the child*: sexual activity at a young age is a very strong indicator that there are risks to the welfare of the child (whether boy or girl) and, possibly, others.
- The level of maturity and understanding of the child.
- What is known about the child's living circumstances or background.
- *Age imbalance*: in particular where there is a significant age difference.
- Overt aggression or power imbalance.
- Coercion or bribery.
- Familial child sex offences.
- Behaviour of the child, i.e. being withdrawn or anxious.
- The misuse of substances as a disinhibitor.
- Whether the child's own behaviour, because of the misuse of substances, places them at risk of harm so that they are unable to make an informed choice about any activity.
- Whether any attempts to secure secrecy have been made by the sexual partner, beyond what would be considered usual in a teenage relationship.
- Whether the child denies, minimizes, or accepts concerns.
- Whether the methods used are consistent with grooming.
- Whether the sexual partner(s) is known to one of the agencies.

Sourced from Working Together to Safeguard Children (2018) ℘ https://www.gov.uk/government/publications/working-together-to-safeguard-children--2

Child sexual exploitation

Definition

Sexual exploitation of children and young people under 18 years of age involves exploitative situations, contexts, and relationships where young people (or a third person or persons) receive 'something' (e.g. food, accommodation, drugs, alcohol, cigarettes, affection, gifts, money) as a result of them performing, and/or another or others performing on them, sexual activities. Child sexual exploitation (CSE) can occur through the use of technology without the child's immediate recognition; e.g. being persuaded to post sexual images on the Internet/mobile phones without immediate payment or gain. In all cases, those exploiting the child/young person have power over them by virtue of their age, gender, intellect, physical strength, and/or economic or other resources. Violence, coercion, and intimidation are common, involvement in exploitative relationships being characterized, in the main, by the child or young person's limited availability of choice resulting from their social/economic and/or emotional vulnerability.

Background

CSE occurs across all social and ethnic backgrounds. Often unreported and hidden, there are many reasons why young people delay or do not disclose, particularly if the young person does not recognize that they are being exploited. Any child can be at risk and, although the majority of perpetrators are male, it can be perpetrated by women and by all ages, and may involve heterosexual and/or same-sex relationships. Furthermore, the child that is being exploited may also be involved in exploiting others. There may be many perpetrators or just one. Internal trafficking and networks may be involved. Grooming of children is common. It is the power imbalance between the perpetrator and victim that is key; this may be obvious (i.e. significant age difference), but may be more subtle.

Recognition

Box 2.2 highlights vulnerabilities that may predispose some children to CSE and Box 2.3 highlights behaviours/signs to look out for that are seen more frequently in exploited children. Routinely, questioning should therefore aim to cover these issues. Confidentiality should be explained, and capacity considered.

It is important to ensure privacy for all young people seen in a sexual health setting and to ensure they are seen alone for at least part of the consultation. Understandably, victims of CSE may find it hard to establish a rapport, particularly with people they see as having power, such as healthcare professionals. Their behaviour may be challenging. Examples of questions that can be used to explore sexual activity include: 'Are you in a relationship?' 'Can you tell me about it?' 'Are you happy?' 'What's going well?' 'How were things at the beginning of the relationship?' 'Has anything changed, such as how you feel about yourself, or how your partner treats you?' 'Are you happy with the sex you're having?' 'Do you feel good about yourself?'

Management

CSE is always a safeguarding issue. If the clinician has concerns (even in the absence of clear disclosure from a child), it is imperative that they raise these concerns with the child and share information by following local safeguarding protocols. If the clinician has any concerns about a child's physical or mental health, then these should be appropriately managed. Clear documentation is important, both for the sharing of information and for use as evidence should a court case ensue.

Box 2.2 Risk factors or vulnerabilities associated with risk of child sexual exploitation

Relationships
- Friends with young people who are sexually exploited.
- Gang association, either through relatives, peers, or intimate relationships (in cases of gang-associated child sexual exploitation only).
- Being unsure about their sexual orientation or unable to disclose sexual orientation to their families.
- History of abuse (including familial child sexual abuse, risk of forced marriage, risk of honour-based violence, physical and emotional abuse, and neglect).

Home life
- Homelessness.
- Living in a chaotic or dysfunctional household (including parental substance use, domestic violence, parental mental health issues, parental criminality).
- Living in a gang neighbourhood.
- Living in residential care.
- Living in hostel, bed and breakfast accommodation, or a foyer.
- Attending school with children and young people who are already sexually exploited.
- Young carer.
- Recent bereavement or loss.

Mental health
- Learning disabilities.
- Low self-esteem or self-confidence.

Box 2.3 Signs or behaviours indicating that someone may be affected by child sexual exploitation

Relationships
- Evidence of sexual bullying and/or vulnerability through the Internet and/or social networking sites.
- Recruiting others into exploitative situations.
- Repeat sexually transmitted infections, pregnancy, or termination of pregnancy (TOP).
- Exhibiting inappropriate sexualized behaviour for stage of development.
- Anxieties around sexual health (suggesting a lack of autonomy).
- Forming new relationships with people outside of their social circle.

Consent
- Receipt of gifts from unknown sources.
- New possessions.
- Unexplained gifts.
- New clothes or jewellery.
- Mobile phones or money that cannot be accounted for.
- Change in physical appearance.
- Rapid change in weight.
- Unkempt appearance.
- Physical or unexplained injuries.

Home life
- Missing from home or care.
- Drug or alcohol misuse.
- Involvement in offending.
- Estranged from their family.
- Absence from school.
- Deterioration in academic achievement.

Mental health
- Poor mental health.
- Self-harm.
- Thoughts of or attempts at suicide.

Sexual offences

These include both ♂ and ♀, and apply irrespective of the relationship between those involved, e.g. a ♂ can be convicted of raping his wife.

Rape

- In law, rape can only be committed using the penis; it cannot be committed with an object.
- Penetration has to be proven in order to show that intercourse has taken place.
- It is not necessary for ejaculation to have taken place in order to prove the offence of rape.
- Intentional penetration of the penis by the assailant into the vagina, mouth, or anus of another person, without that person's consent or if that person is under 13 years of age (consent irrelevant if <13 years).

Sexual assault by penetration

It is an offence for someone intentionally to penetrate the vagina or anus of another person with a part of their body or anything else without their consent. The purpose also has to be sexual, defined as:
- a reasonable person would always consider it to be so
- if a reasonable person may consider it to be sexual, depending on the circumstances and intention.

Sexual assault

Any unwanted sexual behaviour or touching of another person without reasonable belief that they consented. Touching covers all physical contact of a sexual nature (as defined previously), whether with a part of the body or anything else, or through clothing. It may include forced acts of oral sex, and forcing someone to watch pornography or masturbation.

Causing a person to engage in sexual activity without consent

This offence covers non-consensual activity not within the definition of rape or sexual assault. It applies when a person intentionally causes another to engage in sexual activity without consent. Examples: person A forces person B to masturbate; A forces B to manually stimulate a third person; A compels B to penetrate her/him.

Indecent exposure

It is an offence for someone, ♂ or ♀, to expose their genitals if they intended another person to see them, and be caused alarm or distress.

Incest: sex with a family member

In England and Wales, the Sexual Offences Act 2003 replaced the offence of incest with two new, wider groups of offences—familial child sex offences (sections 25–29) and sex with an adult relative (sections 64–65).

The Act makes illegal sexual activity or consenting to sexual activity with someone who is related as a parent (including adoptive), grandparent, child (including adopted), grandchild, sibling, half-sibling, uncle, aunt, nephew, or niece (the last four related consanguineously). Legal provisions governing child protection apply when a sexual act or encouragement of a sexual act involves those aged under 18 and cover situations where the alleged assailant lives under the same roof as the child or young person, or is in a position of trust. Criminal Law (Consolidation) (Scotland) Act 1995 and Sexual Offences (Northern Ireland) Order 2008 provide a similar legal framework in Scotland and Northern Ireland, respectively.

Female genital mutilation

Female genital mutilation (FGM) comprises all procedures that involve partial or total removal of the external female genitalia, or other injury to the female genital organs for non-medical reasons.

Procedures are mostly carried out on young girls, generally between infancy and adolescence, but occasionally on adult women, for sociocultural reasons. More than 3 million girls are estimated to be at risk of FGM annually, and >200 million girls and women alive today have been 'cut'. The practice is centred on 30 countries in Africa (predominantly west, east, and north-eastern countries), the Middle East, and Asia. As FGM may also continue as a practice among migrants from these areas, it is a global concern.

Classification
See Box 2.4

Complications
- *Immediate*: severe pain, haemorrhage, swelling, infection (tetanus, blood-borne virus), urinary retention, death.
- *Delayed*: urinary problems [dysuria, urinary tract infection (UTI)], dysmenorrhoea, scarring (keloid), dyspareunia, anorgasmia, obstructed labour, post-partum haemorrhage, neonatal death, psychological problems (depression, anxiety, PTSD, low self-esteem).

Legal issues
FGM is recognized internationally as a violation of the human rights of girls and women. It reflects deep-rooted inequality between the sexes and constitutes an extreme form of discrimination against women. It is nearly always carried out on minors and is a violation of the rights of children.

Box 2.4 Classification of FGM
- *Type 1 (clitoridectomy)*: the partial or total removal of the clitoris or more rarely only the prepuce.
- *Type 2 (excision)*: the partial or total removal of the clitoris and the labia minora, with or without excision of the labia majora.
- *Type 3 (infibulation)*: narrowing of the vaginal opening through the creation of a covering seal. The seal is formed by cutting and repositioning the labia minora or labia majora, sometimes through stitching, with or without clitoridectomy.
- *Type 4*: this includes all other harmful procedures to the female genitalia for non-medical purposes, e.g. pricking, piercing, incising, scraping, and cauterizing the genital area.
- *Deinfibulation*: refers to the practice of cutting open the sealed vaginal opening in a woman who has been infibulated, which is often necessary for improving health and well-being, as well as to allow intercourse or to facilitate childbirth.

In the UK it is a criminal offence to perform FGM, to fail to protect a girl from FGM, or to assist a non-UK person to perform FGM on a girl overseas. Any child/young woman (<18 years) either identified to have had FGM or considered to be at risk, must be reported to the police. There is a mandatory reporting duty placed on the individual regulated professional first recognizing this to do so.

Local safeguarding policies for FGM should be developed and followed.

Consent: other specific issues

Epidemiological studies

Testing for epidemiological purposes [e.g. for HIV, hepatitis C virus (HCV)] is important for planning disease management, but raises ethical issues. It generally involves screening surplus material (e.g. serum) taken for other tests to allow meaningful epidemiological data to be obtained, ensuring that it cannot be linked to the anonymous individual. However, it is acknowledged that the information gained will not directly benefit that person. It is generally agreed that the benefit to public health outweighs the ethical dilemma of testing without consent to avoid biased sampling. Written information explaining the nature of this testing should be available to patients within the clinic as leaflets or posters, which must highlight the option to refuse without prejudice.

Testing in error

GMC guidance states that mistakes should be acknowledged, with an apology and appropriate support offered. The patient must be given the choice as to whether they are given the result of the test. If the patient refuses to receive a +ve result (with health implications for that individual, partners, and others), advice should be obtained from professional bodies.

Occupational exposure to infection

In the case of a needlestick injury or other occupational exposure to a HCP, it may be important to determine whether the patient has a blood-borne infection, such as HIV. If unconscious, the GMC advises that such testing should not be requested until consciousness has been regained and agreement obtained. In the event of a patient being unable to give consent for any reason, testing should not be carried out for the sole benefit of the healthcare worker (HCW). If the source's status is not known, this should be discussed with occupational health and legal advice sought.

Post-mortem testing for sexually transmitted blood-borne infections (HIV, hepatitis B and C, syphilis)

If a member of staff has been exposed to the blood or body fluids of a deceased patient, screening is permitted, although the agreement of a close relative or next of kin should be sought. Any person who is brainstem dead and being considered for organ donation requires screening for such infections, and this should be explained to the relatives.

Where a post-mortem is required, the deceased may be screened for these infections if relevant to the cause of death. Information should be disclosed regarding a +ve diagnosis to any persons known to be at risk of the infection, e.g. sexual contacts; otherwise, it must remain confidential.

Professional duty of candour

All organizations and individuals providing care to NHS patients in the UK have a duty of candour. Healthcare professionals must tell the patient (or, where appropriate, the patient's advocate, carer, or family) when something has gone wrong, apologize to the patient (or, where appropriate, the patient's advocate, carer, or family), offer an appropriate remedy or support to put matters right (if possible), and explain fully to the patient (or, where appropriate, the patient's advocate, carer, or family) the short- and long-term effects of what has happened.

Intimate examinations and chaperones

In 2001, the GMC produced guidance on the use of chaperones (Box 2.5), which was reinforced in the Ayling Report published in 2004, recommending that trained chaperones are made available for all intimate examinations. The GMC issued revised guidance in 2006 under *Maintaining Boundaries*. It stresses the importance of patient perception as to what may be construed as being intimate. This is most likely to include examination of the breasts, genitalia, or rectum, but could also include any examination where it is necessary to touch or even be close to the patient (e.g. fundoscopy).

Chaperones

The GMC advises that, wherever possible, the patient should be offered the security of having an impartial observer (a 'chaperone') present during an intimate examination. This applies whether or not the examiner is of the same gender as the patient. A chaperone does not have to be medically qualified, but ideally should:

• be sensitive and respectful of the patient's dignity and confidentiality
• be prepared to reassure the patient if he/she shows signs of distress or discomfort
• be familiar with the procedures involved in routine intimate examinations
• be prepared to raise concerns about a doctor if misconduct occurs.

In GUM the use of friends and relatives (as endorsed in the Ayling Report) is not advised, as their use could compromise either the disclosure of important information, which may only be volunteered during the examination, or the personal relationship with the chaperone. In addition, it is unlikely that such a person will be familiar with the procedures involved and the doctor could be at risk of malicious accusations through collusion.

In GUM, it is standard accepted practice to provide a chaperone when ♀ patients are examined by ♂ doctors. In all situations it is recommended that a chaperone be offered for intimate examination in GUM, although the acceptance rate may be low. A report from an Australian sexual health clinic published in 2007 records that only 7.3% and 6% of ♂ patients expressed a desire for a chaperone when being examined by ♂ and ♀ practitioners, respectively. The equivalent figures for ♀ patients were 26.8% and 5.5%.

In some scenarios a healthcare professional may wish to be accompanied by a chaperone, but this may be declined by the patient. Guidance is clear that a chaperone cannot be enforced in this scenario, but arrangements can be made for the patient to be seen by another professional (who is happy to examine them alone), as long as any resultant delay doesn't compromise the patient's health.

Box 2.5 GMC guidance on the intimate examination and conduct

Before conducting an intimate examination
- Explain to the patient why an examination is necessary and give the patient an opportunity to ask questions.
- Explain what the examination will involve, in a way the patient can understand, so that the patient has a clear idea of what to expect, including any potential pain or discomfort.
- Obtain the patient's permission before the examination and record that permission has been obtained.
- Give the patient privacy to undress and dress, and keep the patient covered as much as possible to maintain their dignity. Do not assist the patient in removing clothing unless you have clarified with them that your assistance is required.

During the examination
- Explain what you are going to do before you do it and, if this differs from what you have already outlined to the patient, explain why and seek the patient's permission.
- Be prepared to discontinue the examination if the patient asks you to.
- Keep discussion relevant and do not make unnecessary personal comments.

Chaperones
You should record any discussion about chaperones and its outcome. If a chaperone is present, you should record that fact and make a note of their identity. If the patient does not want a chaperone, you should record that the offer was made and declined.

Electronic technology

The use of computer records, e-mails, faxes, and text messages have revolutionized the way healthcare professionals communicate with each other and also with patients. This technology, however, has the potential for breaching patient confidentiality. The GMC has guidelines for the security of personal information by electronic processing. If necessary, specialist advice should be sought on the security of such information.

Increasingly, video and telephone consultations are becoming part of clinical practice. Practitioners should check their indemnity covers them for such consultations.

To maintain patient confidentiality and confidence in the service, computerized medical record systems must overtly exhibit a high level of security. Many clinics have stand-alone systems, but if linked to a network, robust systems must be in place to ensure that sensitive patient information cannot be accessed by any unauthorized personnel, including HCPs working in other services. Individual computers should be password protected, especially for patient-related information, with the level of information accessible appropriate to the staff member involved. As with written records, patients have the right of access to all electronically held material, with the exclusion of third-party information.

Computers and fax machines should be kept in a secure setting, computer passwords should be changed regularly, and any information sent by e-mail should be encrypted as it may be intercepted. The use of pre-arranged codes can help protect confidentiality.

Recording consultations

Although the GMC expects doctors to obtain patients' consent to make a visual or audio recording, patients do not need their doctor's permission to record a consultation, because they are only processing their own personal information and are, therefore, exempt from data protection principles.

If you suspect a patient is covertly recording you, you may be upset by the intrusion, but your duty of care means you would not be justified in refusing to continue to treat the patient.

Section 36 of the Data Protection Act 1998 states: 'Personal data processed by an individual only for the purposes of that individual's personal, family or household affairs are exempt from data protection principles.'

Partner notification issues

Patient with an STI and an unaware regular sexual partner

If a person infected with an STI is reluctant to inform sexual partners, you may disclose information about a patient, whether living or dead, in order to protect a person from risk of serious harm. For example, you may potentially disclose information to a known sexual contact of a patient with HIV where you have reason to think that the patient has not informed that person and cannot be persuaded to do so. This would clearly be a difficult situation and, in such circumstances, you should tell the patient before you make the disclosure and you must be prepared to justify a decision to disclose information. In such circumstances clear documentation and discussion with colleagues, defence unions, and Trust legal teams is vital.

Patient with an STI and unaware casual sexual partners

This situation is more difficult. The patient must be counselled that they have a duty to inform any sexual partners of their infection. This is especially relevant to someone who has a chronic infection, such as HIV, or hepatitis B and C viruses, and remains infectious. It is also essential to document such advice in the patient's case records.

Ethically, the same principles apply to the other STIs, although the consequences compared with HIV infection, are generally less serious.

Criminalization of HIV transmission

Numerous prosecutions have taken place in the UK, to date, for the 'reckless' transmission of HIV, but the potential for prosecution is there for the transmission of other STIs, too. These have been based on causing grievous bodily harm under Section 20 of the Offences against the Person Act. Guidance from the Crown Prosecution includes the following criteria:

- The defendant needs to have known they were infectious to others and how the infection is transmitted. Patients with a fully suppressed viral load and those using condoms are unlikely to face prosecution.
- The defendant needs to have known they were infectious at the time of transmission or have good reason to believe they were infected, without actually being tested.
- The defendant did not disclose their HIV status to their partner prior to consensual sex.
- Phylogenetic analysis of the HIV in both must be used to show that they are probably from the same source of infection.
- Transmission must actually take place for a 'reckless' charge. However, there is a charge of 'attempted intentional transmission'.

HIV-infected healthcare workers

The GMC advises that doctors or other HCPs with a serious communicable disease, such as HIV, are entitled to the same level of confidentiality and support as any other patient.

Previously, HCWs known to be living with HIV were banned from performing exposure-prone procedures (EPPs). Since 2013, this advice has been lifted, provided that HCWs are on effective combination antiretroviral drug therapy, with a very low or undetectable viral load, and are regularly monitored by both their treating and occupational health physicians.

If there is knowledge or good reason to believe that a HCW is practising, or has practised, in a way that places patients at risk, an appropriate person in the HCW's employing authority, e.g. an occupational health physician, or a relevant regulatory body must be informed. Wherever possible, the HCW concerned must be advised before such information is passed on to an employer or regulatory body. The Public Interest Disclosure Act 1998 protects any employee who discloses concerns about a colleague in the public's best interests.

Death

Living wills

These allow competent people to give instructions about what is to be done if they subsequently lose the capacity to decide or communicate.

- *Advance statements*: these are not legally binding. They are a statement written on preferences of care, such as type of diet preferred (e.g. vegetarian) and type of bathing preferred. They can be overridden in the individual's 'best interests'.
- *Advance decisions*: these are legally binding. They document decisions to refuse certain treatments should they lose capacity. However, strict formalities are required when that treatment would be required to sustain life.
- *Lasting power of attorney*: a person can appoint another to act on their behalf if they should lose capacity in the future. The attorney is able to make both health and welfare decisions.

Death certificates

GMC guidance states that if HIV or any other STI has contributed to the death it is unlawful to omit this from the death certificate.

Writing statements and court appearances

Statements may be required for a variety of reasons—from insurance companies, solicitors, or a police statement.

Before writing a statement, the following should be established:

* *What questions the enquirer wants answered.* Exclude irrelevant information.
* Whether the information is to be provided as a *professional witness* (a factual report concerning a patient to whom the doctor has provided care) or an *expert witness* (to give an opinion concerning a patient who may not have been under the care of that individual).
* *Has the patient given consent?* Always check that the patient understands what the information is for and that they have consented to it being passed onto a third party, even if the person requesting the information states that the patient has given consent. However, consent is not required for a coroner's statement or if demanded by an order of the court.
* *Is the statement required to deal with criticism regarding the medical management of the patient?* Always consult defence organizations prior to sending any completed statement.

Doctors are usually only required in court if there is dispute as to the contents of any statements provided. If called to court because of the medical management of a patient, the doctor involved should contact his/her defence organization for advice.

Legislation pertinent to GUM

Venereal Diseases Regulations 1916

Enacted as a response to the STI epidemic affecting soldiers in the First World War, these regulations promoted the establishment of sexual health clinics, which were confidential and free (30 years before the NHS was established).

Venereal Diseases Act 1917

On 24 of May 1917, the **Venereal Disease Act 1917** was enacted. This was 'An Act to prevent the treatment of Venereal Disease otherwise than by duly qualified medical Practitioners, and to control the supply of Remedies therefor; and for other matters connected therewith.'

NHS Trusts and Primary Care Trusts (Sexually Transmitted Diseases) Directions 2000

These came into force on 1 April 2000 replacing the 1974 Venereal Diseases Regulations and apply only to England.

Confidentiality of information

Every NHS Trust and Primary Care Trust shall take all necessary steps to secure that any information capable of identifying an individual obtained by any of their members or employees with respect to persons examined or treated for any sexually transmitted disease shall not be disclosed except:

- for the purposes of communicating that information to a medical practitioner, or to a person employed under the direction of a medical practitioner in connection with the treatment of persons suffering from such disease or the spread thereof; and
- for the purpose of such treatment or prevention.

National Health Service Act 1977 (Schedule 12, Section 77)

The Act states that no charge is to be made to patients in relation to any medication or investigation required in the treatment of venereal diseases. Treatment for sexually transmitted infections (referred to as venereal disease in the text) should be available free of charge.

The Sexual Offences Act 1967

This Act permitted 'male homosexual practices' by two consenting adults in private, for the first time in the UK. The age of consent for sex between men was lowered from 21 to 18. The Sexual Offences (Amendment) Act 2000 then equalized that age of consent to 16.

Sexual Offences Act 2003 (enacted May 2004)

This act more closely defines 'consent' and the abuse of trust, especially with regard to children. The age of a 'child' set in the Protection of Children Act 1978 has been raised from 16 to 18 years. Although it should not alter normal practice, clinic staff need to be aware that 'children' up to the age of 18 years fall within its protection. It redefines 'sexual' with, for example, attention to 'grooming', use of the Internet, child pornography, prostitution, administration of a substance with intent to commit a sexual offence, and other miscellaneous offences, including voyeurism and bestiality.

It protects the public, especially children, from sexual harm. Sexual offences prevention orders replace sex offenders and restraining orders. In addition, new sexual harm and foreign travel orders have been created.

In view of concerns expressed by those providing sexual healthcare and advice to young people, a statute has been introduced to ensure that a person does not commit an offence if the action taken is to:

- protect the child from STIs
- protect the physical safety of the child
- prevent the child from becoming pregnant
- promote the child's well-being with advice.

It is conditional that such action does not cause or encourage a child's participation, and is not for the purpose of obtaining sexual gratification.

Anyone who acts to protect a child (e.g. teachers, relatives, friends), and not just HCPs, are now covered.

Public Health (Control of Diseases) Act 1984 or Public Health (Infectious diseases) Regulations 1988

These Acts list notifiable diseases. Among the many infections, it should be remembered that acute infectious hepatitis and hepatitis A, B, and C infections are all notifiable. Any doctor who makes the diagnosis is required by statute to notify the proper officer of their local authority.

Gender diversity

Introduction 42
Useful terminology 43
Sexual health for trans/non-binary people 46

Introduction

Gender identity is a person's innate sense of their own gender.

The terms *cis* or *cisgender* is used to describe someone who identifies as the gender that is the same as the sex they were assigned at birth.

Conversely for a *trans* or *transgender* person, their gender identity differs from the sex that they were assigned at birth.

People may identify with a binary gender identity (male or female) or a non-binary (neither exclusively male nor female) identity.

In the UK, the 2010 Equality Act assigns gender reassignment as a protected characteristic and, therefore, provides legislation to make any form of discrimination or harassment illegal.

Useful terminology

Gender expression

The ways in which people externally communicate their gender identity to others through behaviour, mannerisms, clothing, haircut, voice, etc.

Gender non-conforming

People whose gender expression differs from society's stereotypical expectations of their birth-assigned sex.

Gender role

The roles, activities, expectations, and behaviour assigned to people by society, based on stereotypical expectations. Most Western cultures recognize two basic gender roles—masculine and feminine. Other cultures may have three or more gender roles.

Gender dysphoria

Dysphoria (coming from the Greek 'difficult to bear'); a medical diagnostic term used to define the clinically significant distress, of >6 months duration, caused by a mismatch between birth-assigned sex and a person's gender identity, which is causing impairment in social, occupational, or other important areas of functioning.

Transsexual

A medical diagnostic term (defined in the ICD-10). This has now largely been superseded by 'gender dysphoria'. Three criteria should be fulfilled:
- The desire to live and be accepted as a member of the opposite sex, usually accompanied by the wish to make his or her body as congruent as possible with the preferred sex through surgery and hormone treatment.
- The transsexual identity has been present persistently for at least 2 years.
- The disorder is not a symptom of another mental disorder or a chromosomal abnormality.

MtF (male to female) or transwoman

A person assigned male sex at birth, who identifies and lives as a woman.

FtM (female to male) or transman

A person assigned female sex at birth, who identifies and lives as a man.

Non-binary (NB)/genderqueer

All those whose gender identity lies outside, or somewhere in between, the gender binary.

An umbrella term used for a heterogeneous group of people. Including (but not exclusive to) the following identities:
- bigender
- trigender
- pangender
- agender (no gender)

- neutrois (neutral gender)
- gender fluid (gender identity changes)
- third gender (a different gender)

NB people may identify as masculine or feminine, but there is a clear distinction between this, and being a binary male or female.

Social transition/coming out

The process of changing gender expression and role so that it matches a person's gender identity.

Steps can include 'coming out' to family/friends/colleagues, legal name change, and subsequent change in identity documents (different countries have differing legislation in relation to this).

Transition should be regarded as a process, not an event.

Medical transition

The process of changing physical characteristics to bring them more in line with a person's gender identity.

Input is highly individualized with a move away from standardized pathways.

Interventions include:
- hair removal
- *hormonal therapies*: including oestrogens, testosterone, gonadotropin-releasing hormone (GnRH) analogues
- speech and language therapy
- hair transplantation
- masculinizing chest surgery
- breast augmentation
- facial surgery
- phonosurgery
- *genital reassignment surgery*: vulvoplasty, vaginoplasty, phalloplasty, metoidioplasty.

Current guidelines recommend that genital surgery should be preceded by a social role transition of at least 12 months duration and 12 months of hormone therapy.

Genital reassignment/reconstructive surgery

It should be noted that not all trans/NB people seek genital surgery. It would not be rare for someone to seek hormonal interventions and possibly other surgical interventions, such as chest surgery, but retain their birth genitals.

- *Vulvoplasty*: involves the removal of the penis and testes and sculpting of a vulva, including the creation of a sexually responsive clitoris from the glans penis.
- *Vaginoplasty*: carried out in some in addition to vulvoplasty and involves the creation of a vagina usually by inversion of penile skin. In other countries, the lower bowel is sometimes used. Evidently, the differing surgical techniques may have implications for susceptibility to, and screening for, STIs.

- *Metoidioplasty*: involves the enhancement of the clitoromegaly that people experience on testosterone ± urethroplasty (to redirect the urethra to this tip of the phallus) vaginectomy, hysterectomy, and/or scrotoplasty with testicular implants.
- *Phalloplasty*: is the surgical formation of a larger phallus than can be achieved by metoidioplasty using a flap from either the forearm, thigh, or lower abdomen. A prosthetic inflatable erectile device may be subsequently implanted to allow an erection suitable for penetrative sex.

Gender Recognition Act (GRA) 2004 (UK)

The GRA allows transgender people, provided they meet the requirements outlined in the Act, to obtain a gender recognition certificate ('GRC'), which grants them legal recognition of their affirmed gender. It also enables them to receive a birth certificate with the correct gender marker on it.

At that point, they become their confirmed gender for all legal purposes and must be treated as such. It is not lawful to ask a person if they have applied for or have a GRC. If verification of identity is required they may show their birth certificate or other identity documentation, such as a passport. It is potentially a criminal offence, with a financial penalty, for anyone to knowingly reveal the gender history of a transgender person with a GRC without their consent.

Sexual health for trans/non-binary people

Service provision

It is important for all sexual health services to consider how appropriate their set-up is for trans and NB people who may need to attend for care. Particular consideration should be given to registration forms, waiting areas (including the leaflets and posters that are available), toilets, and clinical examination facilities.

Screening/testing

Decisions around which tests to offer should be based on an individual risk assessment and guided by anatomy (rather than gender) and sexual practise. Self-taken swabs may be preferred and should always be offered where possible.

It is important to recognize that the consultation and any necessary examination may be more distressing for trans and NB people, and sensitivity and extra time may be needed.

HIV

There is international evidence that suggests trans people are at significantly increased risk of HIV. This particularly relates to transwomen, but data for transmen is lacking. There is also evidence that late diagnosis and poorer outcomes are more likely. Pre-exposure prophylaxis (PrEP) is an appropriate consideration for trans people who meet the usual criteria.

Other issues

- *Contraception*: transmen/NB people who are sexually active with a risk of pregnancy should be offered contraception. Progesterone only methods or intrauterine devices would be most appropriate. Testosterone and GnRH analogues are not licensed contraceptives.
- *Cervical screening*: any trans/NB person with a cervix should be offered cervical screening. They may no longer be part of the routine recall if the gender marker on their NHS records is male. ➔ Chapter 30 'Screening', p. 360
- *Vaginal stenosis*: post-vaginoplasty regular dilatation, together with douching, of the vagina is required for most people to maintain patency. Without this stenosis may occur.
- *Vaginal bleeding*: following vaginoplasty this can be due to granulation tissue, which has formed along internal scar lines and can be managed with silver nitrate.
- *Vaginitis*: transmen/NB people with a vagina who access testosterone may experience atrophic-type vaginal symptoms. There is no evidence base for the management of this. Lubricants, topical oestrogens, management of any bacterial overgrowth (e.g. with clindamycin vaginal cream) could be considered as options, depending on the presentation.

The standard clinic process and sexual health in primary care

The genitourinary medicine patient 48
Types of sexual practice 50
The sexual history 52
Routine examination: general principles 54
Examination 55
Principles of management and review 59
Sexual health commissioning and sexual health in
    primary care 60

The genitourinary medicine patient

An estimated one in seven adults >16 years old in the UK has attended a GUM clinic. Many are asymptomatic, but wish to exclude an STI. Young people may attend more commonly, although a wide age range from <16 to >60 are seen. Demographic characteristics vary, depending on the risk factors of the local and commuting population, and the acceptability and accessibility of GUM services to potential users. Slightly more ♂ than ♀ attend, with sexuality and ethnicity varying geographically. People more likely to attend include:

- ♂ aged 25–34
- ♀ aged 16–24
- Those who have changed sexual partners recently
- Those having multiple sexual partners
- Those single, separated, or divorced.

Special situations

The distressed or aggressive patient
While most patients attending may feel anxious and embarrassed, some are intensely distressed. The psychological responses to STIs or risk of such include anxiety, depression, stigma, shame, guilt, low self-esteem, and anger. These emotions may hamper communication and lead to apparently irrational behaviour. To provide optimum care it is necessary to be cognisant of their emotional state. If a patient is aggressive, prioritize safety, while attempting to de-escalate the situation.

Children and young people
➔ Chapter 6, 'Child sexual assault', pp. 110–15.

Adolescents <16 years attending GUM have a high incidence of STIs and report a low use of reliable contraception. Some may also have suffered sexual abuse.

Sexual assault or rape
➔ Chapter 6, 'Sexual assault: general principles', pp. 102–4.

Victims may attend for sexual health screening and STI risk assessment. Consideration should be given to any post-traumatic stress.

Risk factors

Social and demographic
The following risk factors have been noted in various epidemiological studies. They are likely to vary over time and by geographic regions, but are useful in planning local service provision and targeting specific sexual health promotion. Clinically, they are useful in risk assessment.

- *Age <25 years*: the highest rates of gonococcal and chlamydial infections occur ♀ aged 16–19 years and ♂ aged 20–24 years.
- *Being single, separated, divorced*: associated with ↑ rates of STIs.
- ≥2 partners in preceding 6 months.
- Use of non-barrier contraception.
- Residence in inner city.
- Symptomatic partner.
- History of previous STI.

- *Ethnicity or migration*: prevalence of several infections, notably syphilis, gonorrhoea, and HIV infection, is higher in certain ethnic minority groups and immigrants.
- *Sexual orientation*: e.g. syphilis, gonorrhoea, HIV, and hepatitis B virus infections are more prevalent among MSM.
- Use of Internet geosocial networking apps.
- Chemsex.

Sexual

Certain types of physical contact carry higher risks for certain infections, e.g. penetrative sex and HIV, oral sex, and anogenital herpes.

Types of sexual practice

Knowledge of the wide range of sexual practices and vocabulary in use is of value in advising those at risk of STIs.

Sexuality and relationship

- *Heterosexual*: opposite sex relationships, 'straight'.
- *Homosexual*: same sex relationships, (♂♂ 'gay', ♀♀ lesbian).
- *Bisexual*: relationships with both sexes.
- *Pansexual*: indiscriminate sexuality.
- *Polyamorous/polygamous*: relationships involving ≥2 partners.
- *Threesome, group sex*: sex (often casual) between ≥3 individuals.
- Sex in public places, while others watch (dogging), sex parties, swinging.
- *Cruising*: searching for men who have sex with men (MSM) partners in public places, e.g. common land, saunas, toilets (cottaging).
- Use of geosocial networking apps to find casual sexual partners, e.g. Grindr, Tinder.
- *Cybersex*: use of the Internet to deliver sexual pleasure.

'Safer sex' (non-penetrative sex)

Arousal from kissing, mutual masturbation, heavy petting, body rubbing (frottage and 'dry rooting'), rubbing buttocks, feet, tickling, lap dancing, genital to genital rubbing (♀♀ tribadism or 'scissoring'). Penile stimulation between breasts, in axilla, between legs.

Genital stimulation using the mouth

- *Penile oral sex*: fellatio, 'blow-job'.
- Oral testicular stimulation ('tea bagging').
- ♀ *genital oral sex*: cunnilingus, clitoral tongue stimulation.
- *Insufflation*: blowing air into a body cavity, usually the vagina.

Anorectal stimulation

- *Anal sex*: anal penetration by penis. Practiced between ♀♂ or ♂♂. Old fashioned terms, such as buggery and sodomy, are derogatory and should not be used.
- *Oral stimulation*: rimming (anal stimulation with tongue).
- *Manual*: fisting (fist/arm into anorectal canal).

Arousal with body fluids

- *Urine*: golden shower, water sports.
- *Faeces (scat)*: arousal from rubbing faeces on body, watching defaecation, freezing faeces in condom and using as dildo (Alaskan dildo).
- *Semen*: Felching or 'snowball' (ingestion of semen from vagina or anus), ejaculating over chest/neck (pearl necklace).
- *Blood slamming*: arousal from being injected with another's blood.
- *Roman shower*: vomit and vomiting over partner.

Sadomasochism

- *Sadism*: arousal by inflicting pain.
- *Masochism*: Arousal from pain; examples include:
  - caning/flagellation;
  - bondage/strangulation (physical restraint/constriction);
  - dominatrix (dominating female in sadomasochistic activities).
- *Sexual fetishism*: sexual attraction to objects, situations, body parts or secretions that are not traditionally viewed as sexual.

Sex with animals

- *Bestiality*: sex with animals, e.g. horse, sheep, or dog.
- *Felching*: inserting animal into anus/vagina; probably an urban myth.

Use of sex toys and piercings

- *Arousal enhancers*: dildos, vibrators, butt plugs, and genital piercings (rings, bars, beads, wires, etc.).
- *Erection sustainers*: cock ring, penis vacuum pump devices.
- *Lubricants/condoms*: delay (with benzocaine to delay climax), tingle/cooling with peppermint, warming, textured condoms with bumps/ribs, flavoured.

Paraphilia

Experience of recurrent intense sexual arousal to atypical objects, situations, fantasies, fetishes, behaviours, or individuals. Listed within DSM-V and ICD-10.

Use of drugs during sex

- Amyl nitrite (poppers) for euphoria and sphincter relaxation.
- Crack cocaine ↑ desire.
- Alcohol and some tranquillizing drugs (e.g. 'rape drug' rohypnol) removes inhibitions.
- *Chemsex*: use of drugs particularly crystal methamphetamine ('tina'), mephedrone and gamma hydroxybutyric acid (GHB) or gamma butyrolactone (GBL) to facilitate sexual activity in the context of sex parties within predominantly MSM groups, often using sexual networking apps. Associated with unprotected sex with multiple partners, increasing duration of sexual activity and, hence, high acquisition of STIs, particularly HIV and HCV.
  - 'Slamming': injecting chemsex drugs.

The sexual history

Taking a sexual history is vital for assessing STI risk and sexual health issues. It must be non-judgemental and empathic, thereby promoting effective patient participation. Consultations should take place in a private, soundproof environment to maintain confidentiality. If possible, record the patient's preference as to how they wish to be called from the waiting area (first name, full name, or patient number). It is important that care is taken to ensure patient identification is correct.

When taking a sexual history:
- Put the patient at ease with proper introduction and positioning.
- Reassure regarding confidentiality.
- Explain why a sexual history is needed.
- Check if patient agrees to be asked personal questions.
- Ideally, interview the patient alone, but respect the patient's wish to have a third person present, which may help to ↓ anxiety. Students and other observers should only be present with consent of the patient.
- Avoid distractions during the consultation.
- Display a non-judgemental attitude.
- Do not make assumptions about patient's gender identity, gender history, sexuality, or sexual behaviour.
- Listen actively and maintain adequate eye contact, observing non-verbal communication.
- Use language the patient understands, avoiding jargon, with appropriate intonation, pauses, and cues to gain information.
- Reflect what patient says to clarify and confirm.

Pro formas ensure a systematic approach to history-taking (Fig. 4.1). Many integrated sexual health clinics now use electronic patient records. Asking when last sexual intercourse took place is a useful way to start the sexual history (details of sexual partners, contraception, and sexual risks). Presence of a third person, especially the sexual partner, may inhibit this. Types of sexual practices reported can help in planning which specimens to obtain. Obtain any information the patient has on the nature of a sexual partner's infection(s). Where mother-to-child transmission is relevant enquire about clinical presentations in the children.

Procedures should be in place to address the needs of those with communication issues, and this should include access to sign language interpreters and language interpreters where English is not a patients' first language, telephone interpreting services, and the use of communication aids. It is preferable to use an unrelated interpreter, but sometimes this may not be possible. Where possible, a patient's request for a clinician of a preferred gender should be accommodated.

℘ https://www.bashhguidelines.org/media/1078/sexual-history-taking-guideline-2013-2.pdf

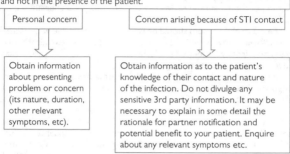

1. Introduce yourself and your position to the patient. They may be anxious or feeling guilty and, therefore, it is important to put them at ease as soon as possible.

2. Determine the presenting problem or concern. There may be information available to you (e.g. contact information), which should be accessed before and not in the presence of the patient.

Personal concern	Concern arising because of STI contact
Obtain information about presenting problem or concern (its nature, duration, other relevant symptoms, etc).	Obtain information as to the patient's knowledge of their contact and nature of the infection. Do not divulge any sensitive 3rd party information. It may be necessary to explain in some detail the rationale for partner notification and potential benefit to your patient. Enquire about any relevant symptoms etc.

Obtain relevant background information
- Past STIs, and other relevant present and past medical history
- For ♀, obtain contraceptive, gynaecological, and obstetric history
- Current/recent drug history and drug allergies
- Drug misuse

Sexual history
- *Last sexual contact*: date, relationship (regular/casual), sex (male/female), country (if relevant). More detailed information may be obtained, such as the type of contact and use of protection (condoms) although the latter merely ↓ risk and should not alter immediate clinical practice, except for HIV post-exposure prophylaxis.
- Other contacts in last 3 months (incubation/ latent period for most symptomatic STIs) and last 12 months (helpful in risk assessment).

Finally
- Thank patient for providing this information (often embarrassing to them).
- Discuss and explain further recommended investigation and management plans, based on the information available.

Fig. 4.1 Taking a sexual history.

Routine examination: general principles

Asymptomatic patients may wish to perform their own self-taken nucleic acid amplification tests (NAAT) for *Chlamydia trachomatis* and *Neisseria gonorrhoeae*, but it is recommended that genital examination should be performed for those who have genital symptoms. Prior to the examination the patient should be given an explanation on the rationale for examination and their verbal agreement obtained and documented in the clinic notes. Certain procedures require written consent (e.g. local anaesthesia, minor surgery, and clinical photography).

The examination room should be warm and comfortable with a screened area allowing privacy while the patient undresses. An examination couch with good lighting is required (with stirrups/leg rests for ♀ to allow examination in the semi-lithotomy position).

The patient should undress below the waist and be provided with drapes or gowns. Irrespective of the gender of the patient or the examiner, a chaperone must be offered (GMC Guidance, 2013), who may also be able to assist in the collection of specimens and reassure the nervous patient. The acceptance or refusal of a chaperone should be documented in the patient's notes. Chaperones should sign to confirm their attendance during the examination or evidence documented within the electronic notes. Although the GMC suggests that a patient's friend or relative could act as a sole chaperone, this is not advised in GUM as it may compromise confidentiality and the provision of relevant information to the HCP.

The examination trolley should be set up prior to the examination. Specula should be pre-warmed in water, which also acts as a vaginal lubricant. If using lubricating gel, ensure it is sterile, water-based, without bactericidal agents, which may inhibit gonorrhoea culture, and care should be taken to ensure that swabs are not contaminated. During examination the patient should be kept informed of progress, but unnecessary comments must be avoided. Convenient facilities should be available to obtain urine specimens.

Serology

A venous blood sample for syphilis and HIV should be taken with informed consent from patients at risk of an STI. Testing for hepatitis A, B, and C virus may also be required depending on risk assessment.

Examination

General

Skin rashes/lesions, generalized lymphadenopathy, hair loss, jaundice, mucosal lesions (orogenital), conjunctivitis/uveitis, and arthritis may arise from STIs, and genital problems may be features of dermatological or systemic diseases.

Symptomatic women

See Fig. 4.2.

- Inspect the entire pubic and anogenital area ensuring that the labia are parted and the clitoral hood gently retracted.
- If genial ulceration seen take appropriate STI tests (➔ Chapter 7, 'Diagnosis and investigation', pp. 125–9, and Chapter 22, 'Diagnosis', p. 282).
- Palpate the inguinal area for lymphadenopathy.
- Urethral specimens are no longer recommended unless a culture is being taken for gonorrhoea in a woman who has had a hysterectomy.
- Introduce a speculum lubricated with warm water.
- Inspect the vagina and cervix for atypical discharge, mucosal lesions, and signs of inflammation (such as muco-purulent cervicitis).

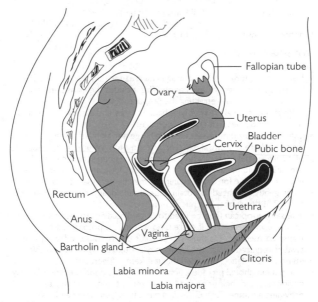

Fig. 4.2 Female genital anatomy.

- Take vaginal material from the posterior vaginal pool/vaginal walls using a loop or swab and prepare a suspension in normal saline on a slide (wet-mount) protected with a cover-slip to look for evidence of *Trichomonas vaginalis* (TV), candida, or bacterial vaginosis (BV). An additional swab should be prepared as a Gram-stained smear for candida and BV diagnosis.
- If TV is suspected either a TV NAAT or culture swab can be taken.
- Take a vulvovaginal swab (VVS) for *C. trachomatis and N. gonorrhoeae* NAAT testing by taking material from the vaginal walls and vaginal pool. Alternatively, an endocervical swab can be taken for chlamydia and gonorrhoea later in the examination by rotating a swab within the wall of the endocervical canal. VVS have been found to be more sensitive than endocervical swabs.
- If cervical cytology is required, it is best taken at this stage.
- Before microbiological sampling clean the cervix using a cotton ball held in a sponge-holder to remove vaginal material
- If gonorrhoea is suspected take an endocervical swab to prepare a Gram-stained smear and to plate onto selective medium for *N. gonorrhoeae* or send in transport medium, e.g. Amies or Stuart's charcoal.
- If there are any signs or symptoms to suggest lower abdominal or pelvic pathology, offer a bimanual pelvic and abdominal examination.
- Urine specimens should be obtained if pregnancy testing is required or a urinary tract infection (mid-stream sample) suspected. They can also be used for chlamydia and gonorrhoea testing (1st 20 mL) by NAAT, although sensitivity is lower than VVS.

Symptomatic men

See Fig. 4.3.

- Inspect the entire pubic and anogenital area for skin lesions, masses, discharges, and signs of infestation. This includes the glans penis and sub-preputial sac by retracting the prepuce.
- Palpate the inguinal area for lymphadenopathy and scrotal contents for masses, tenderness, and other anomalies.
- Examine the urethral meatus for discharge and skin lesions, especially warts. If there is urethral exudate, any symptom of urethritis, or history of penile sexual contact with gonorrhoea, a gentle scraping from the urethra should be taken using a small plastic loop and smeared onto a microscope slide for Gram-staining. It may be necessary for the urethra to be gently massaged to obtain a specimen. Ideally, samples should be taken 3–4 hours after last micturition.
- The same loop can then be used to plate directly onto selective medium for *N. gonorrhoeae* even if there is no material to prepare a slide. If a transport medium (e.g. Amies or Stuart's charcoal) is used, a separate swab is required, which the laboratory should ideally receive within 48 hours for plating, provided that it is kept refrigerated.
- The patient should provide a first-voided 20 mL urine specimen (ideally having retained their urine for 1 hour before testing). As well as providing a sample for a *C. trachomatis and N. gonorrhoeae* NAAT it can also be examined for threads, a possible indicator of urethritis.

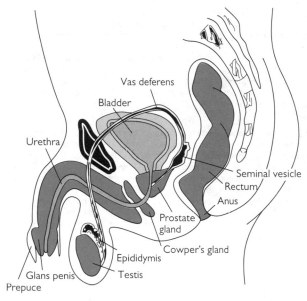

Fig. 4.3 Male genital anatomy.

- Alternatively urethral sampling for *C. trachomatis* and *N. gonorrhoeae* can be undertaken using a NAAT if the patient is unable to provide a urine sample. It is recommended that a fine urethral swab is inserted 2–4 cm into the urethra and rotated once against the urethral wall. Urethral sampling is less acceptable to the patient than urine testing.
- A second, mid-stream sample should be obtained, especially if urinary tract infection needs to be excluded. Samples can also be tested by dipstick for blood, protein, glucose, nitrites, and leucocytes as required.

Extra-genital infection

Rectum

In those at risk, such as MSM and ♀ practicing receptive anal sex, rectal screening with a *C. trachomatis* and *N. gonorrhoeae* NAAT should be offered. Self-taken samples may be more acceptable to patients, and have comparable sensitivity and specificity compared with clinician-taken specimens. If symptomatic, the anal canal and distal 5 cm of the rectum should be examined with a proctoscope to check for pus (which can be sampled and prepared as a Gram-stained smear) and other lesions (e.g. warts). This also minimizes faecal contamination when taking swabs. Water-based sterile lubricant should be used to avoid inhibiting gonorrhoea culture.

If gonorrhoea is suspected or confirmed a rectal sample should be taken for culture, either plated onto selective medium or placed into transport medium (e.g. Amies or Stuart's charcoal) to determine antibiotic sensitivities.

If chlamydia is +ve and rectal symptoms are present with evidence of proctitis, then a *Lymphogranuloma venereum* (LGV)-specific NAAT test should be performed (usually requested from the original sample). LGV testing should also be performed in all HIV+ve MSM if rectal or pharyngeal chlamydia is confirmed.

Pharynx

NAAT swabs for *C. trachomatis* and *N. gonorrhoeae* should be offered to those at risk, especially if symptomatic, in ♀ who are contacts of gonorrhoea or if gonorrhoea is found at other site(s), MSM, and those who have been sexually assaulted. The use of NAATs may require local validation as, although they are not approved for testing on pharyngeal samples they have significantly greater sensitivity than culture.

If gonorrhoea is suspected, then a swab for culture should be performed prior to treatment to determine antibiotic sensitivities. Consideration should be given to sending a *C. trachomatis* and *N. gonorrhoeae* NAAT in asymptomatic ♀ practicing fellatio.

Principles of management and review

During the consultation, the patient will require advice and information on their condition or situation, and the need for follow-up and/or additional tests. It good practice to provide written information.

Treatment

- If specific treatment is required it should:
  - be based on regularly reviewed local or national guidelines
  - recognize individual factors (e.g. co-morbidities, allergies, pregnancy, etc.)
  - meet individual patient needs to maximize adherence (especially long-term HIV treatment).
- Treatment dispensed by a nurse must be provided under local Trust ratified patient group directions (PGDs).
- Any medicine dispensed and advice given must be documented in the patient's records.

Management points

- Confirm that any test results relate to the patient and that complete information is available (e.g. antibiotic sensitivity).
- Explain the nature of the condition and its implications.
- Discuss treatment rationale, risk–benefit analysis, and specific information on recommended treatments. Obtain patient's agreement.
- Offer full STI screening, if this has not already been undertaken.
- Provide additional advice that may include:
  - avoidance of sexual intercourse even with condoms (until infection cleared and partner treated)
  - possible effects on combined hormonal contraception [e.g. post-exposure prophylaxis after sexual exposure (PEPSE)]
  - additional self-help information (providing patient information leaflets and signposting to reliable Internet resources)
  - general sexual health promotion.
- Consider sexual partner(s) and partner notification issues when indicated (with health adviser).
- Agree arrangements for obtaining results and/or further review (which may include tests of cure).

Pharmacy arrangements

Ideally, medication should be dispensed, free of charge, to the patient while he/she is in the clinic.

Free treatment

Treatment of STIs, excluding HIV/AIDS, is free without any prescription charge to all attendees at GUM clinics, irrespective of their nationality.

Sexual health commissioning and sexual health in primary care

From April 2013, following the Health and Social Care Act 2012, Local authorities became responsible for commissioning sexual health services and most sexual health interventions in England as part of a wider public health responsibility, which was previously the role of Primary Care Trusts (PCTs). PCTs were replaced by Clinical Commissioning Groups (CCGs) overseen by NHS England.

Local Authorities commission

- Contraception in specialist services and those commissioned from PCTs (Community Pharmacy and GP) under local public health contracts.
- STI testing and treatment (excluding ongoing HIV treatment and care) in specialist services and partner notification.
- Sexual health aspects of psychosexual health.
- Any sexual health specialized services, HIV prevention and sexual health promotion, outreach and services in schools, colleges and pharmacies, community chlamydia testing.
- Social care, including HIV social care and support for teenage families.

Principal responsibilities of CCGs

- Termination of pregnancy services.
- Male and female sterilization.
- Non-sexual health elements of psychosexual health services.
- Contraception for gynaecological (non-contraceptive) purposes.
- HIV testing in CCG-commissioned services.

Responsibilities of NHS England

- HIV specialized treatment and care.
- Testing and treatment for STIs in general practice, when clinically indicated as part of 'essential services' under the GP contract.
- Sexual assault referral centres.
- Cervical screening in a range of settings.
- Contraceptive services as an 'additional service' under the GP contract.
- Sexual health elements of prison health services.

Different arrangements exist within the other devolved UK nations.
- Making it Work –A guide to whole system commissioning for sexual health, reproductive health and HIV, Public Health England: https://www.gov.uk/government/publications/commissioning-sexual-health-reproductive-health-and-hiv-services

Levels of service provision

Key objectives set out in 'A Framework for Sexual Health Improvement in England' by the Department of Health in 2013:
- Continue to reduce the rate of under 16 and under 18 conceptions.
- Reduce the rate of STIs among people of all ages.
- Reduce onward transmission of HIV and avoidable deaths from it.
- Reduce unintended pregnancies among all women of fertile age.

The Medical Foundation for HIV and Sexual Health (MEDFASH) and the British Association of Sexual Health and HIV (BASHH) revised the 'Standards for the Management of Sexually Transmitted Infections' document in 2014 to take account of recent changes (Box 4.1). Sexual health services were originally divided into levels as outlined in the National Strategy for Sexual Health and HIV.

If a primary care practice is unable to provide Level 1, arrangements must be made for their patients through other community services. CCGs should identify and support primary care teams who can provide enhanced services to a high standard. GPs and nurses need to undertake specific training to develop and maintain skills. Provision of Level 2 services (Box 4.1) should be made in collaboration with GUM and SRH to meet local needs and fill gaps in existing services.

Box 4.1 Levels of service

Level 1 services

- Sexual history and risk assessment.
- Signposting to appropriate sexual health services.
- STI screening and treatment of asymptomatic infections (except gonorrhoea and syphilis) in women and men (excluding MSM).
- HIV testing (including point of care testing) and counselling.
- Contraception and sexual health information and promotion including condom distribution
- Onward referral for partner notification (or provision of partner notification).
- Testing for hepatitis B and C and hepatitis B vaccination.
- Assessment and onward referral for psychosexual problems.
- Pregnancy testing and referral.
- Contraception provision.

Level 2 services

Level 1 *plus*:
- STI testing and treatment of symptomatic, but uncomplicated infections in women and men (except MSM and pregnant women).
- Intra-uterine device insertion.
- Contraceptive implant insertion.

Level 3 services

Levels 1 and 2 *plus*:
- STI testing and treatment of MSM.
- STI testing and treatment of symptomatic men and women.
- Testing and treatment of STIs at extra-genital sites.
- STIs with complications, with or without symptoms.
- STIs in pregnant women.
- Recurrent or recalcitrant STI, or related conditions.
- Management of syphilis and blood-borne viruses.
- Tropical STIs.
- Specialist HIV treatment and care.
- Provision and follow-up of HIV post-exposure prophylaxis (PEP).

Investigations and microscopy

Laboratory testing 64
The microscope 69
Slide preparation 70
Clinic-based tests 71
Routine female microscopy 73
Routine male microscopy 74
Accuracy of microscopy 75
Rapid point of care tests (POCTs) 76
Commensals and confounders 79

Laboratory testing

Introduction

Certain infections can be detected or diagnosed within clinics or surgeries, but others require microbiological services, also essential for confirmatory and antimicrobial sensitivity testing. If on-site microscopy is unavailable, the use of air-dried swabs sent for laboratory staining and microscopy should be considered. This is applicable for vaginal discharge (e.g. bacterial vaginosis, candidiasis) and also for ♂ urethral discharge for polymorphonuclear leucocytes (PMNLs) indicating urethritis and Gram −ve intracellular diplococci, which are highly suggestive, but not diagnostic of gonorrhoea.

The optimum minimum time to take swabs for screening from asymptomatic patients following a specific incident has not been established. It will depend on the type of test used, the site screened, and the presence/absence of infected secretions. However, 14 days after a sexual risk is recommended.

The timing of serological tests should take into consideration the 'window periods' of the respective infections. Final exclusion tests must be advised at the end of this time. Baseline assays soon after the incident may be useful, especially if subsequent repeat tests are positive.

Chlamydia trachomatis

Nucleic acid amplification test (NAAT)

First-voided 20 mL of urine (especially in ♂ as variable sensitivities in ♀) or ♂ urethra, vagina/vulva (specimen of choice for ♀, 96–98% sensitivity) or endocervix. In addition, rectal samples (although unlicensed) have been shown to be useful in MSM. Important to take if MSM present with ano-rectal symptoms because of lymphogranuloma venereum. If confirmed, genotype for L1, L2, or L3. Also unlicensed for oropharyngeal sampling due to variable sensitivities, but NAAT is the most sensitive test that is widely available. In medico-legal situations, a +ve NAAT test should be confirmed using a second target.

Enzyme immunoassay (EIA)

Rarely used, but are at least 30% less sensitive than NAAT and are now generally not recommended. Not suitable for urine and vulvo-vaginal testing in ♀ and certain kits are not recommended for urine testing in ♂.

Culture

Not widely available and due to low sensitivity (60–80%) compared with NAAT testing, not now recommended in medico-legal situations. Available from Sexually Transmitted Bacterial Reference Unit for persistent infection/failed treatment.

Transport and storage

Specimens for culture should be kept refrigerated at all times. Storage of NAAT and EIA specimens for >24 hours at room temperature may result in sample degradation, although absolute data are lacking. If delays are anticipated, storage at 4°C is recommended. Manufacturer's instructions of individual commercial assays should be followed.

Neisseria gonorrhoeae

Nucleic acid amplification test

Investigation of choice to detect gonorrhoea infection. High sensitivity, >90% for all urogenital specimens (male urine, vulvovaginal, endocervical), except female urine. Single swab or urine as a dual NAAT to detect gonorrhoea and chlamydia widely available. No assay is licensed from extragenital sites, but significantly more sensitive than culture from rectum and oropharynx, and rectal and pharyngeal specimens should be considered if at risk. Positive extra-genital NAATs should ideally be confirmed with a supplementary test on a different nucleic acid target. Positive results need culture primarily for antibiotic sensitivity testing and also confirmation, but the sensitivity is lower. Transport and storage as above for chlamydia NAAT. Testing for gonorrhoea recommended in situations where it is clinically indicated (e.g. sexual history, symptomatic, contacts), whereas screening is only recommended in a population or setting where prevalence ≥1% due to a clear local public health need. NAAT test of cure recommended from positive site 2 weeks post-treatment.

Culture

Required, if possible, in all patients with a positive gonococcal NAAT test from the infected site to enable antibiotic sensitivity testing and detection of resistant strains. Culture swabs should be taken before anti-gonococcal antimicrobial therapy initiated, including situations such as treatment of contacts or treatment for microscopic identification of gonorrhoea. Sensitivities differ depending on sites sampled with a greater sensitivity from endocervix and male urethra than extragenital sites

If a carbon dioxide incubator is available, specimens can be plated directly onto selective growth medium (e.g. modified New York City culture medium), although they will need to be transported to the laboratory in a carbon dioxide-enriched environment (e.g. in candle jars).

Otherwise, specimens must be sent in a transport medium (e.g. Amies or Stuart charcoal). Their use only reduces sensitivity by ~10% (compared with direct inoculation) provided that the specimens are refrigerated and received by the laboratory within 48 hours.

Bacterial vaginosis (BV)

Swab from posterior fornix. Prepare air-dried smear from the swab or send in transport medium (Amies, Stuart), requesting a Gram stain for bacterial flora and clue cells. A result suggestive of BV does not necessarily indicate the need for treatment, which must be assessed clinically.

Herpes simplex virus (HSV)

Swabs of vesicular fluid or from ulcers

Real-time polymerase chain reaction (PCR)

NAAT is the investigation of choice to determine genital herpes. Highly sensitive (detects 11–77% more cases than culture), specific, allows typing, and is rapid. Confirmatory testing of +ve PCR samples is not recommended. Manufacturer's instructions should be consulted for transport, but less stringent storage and transport conditions required than for virus culture.

Culture

Will miss ~30% of PCR +ve samples (usually late or mild recurrent epi-sodes). Must be sent in transport medium. Standard viral transport systems should be kept refrigerated, but some commercial systems (e.g. Virocult®) can be maintained at ambient temperature as HSV will survive for up to 12 days at up to 23°C. Local laboratory or manufacturer's instructions should be consulted.

Others
- *Immunofluorescent antigen detection*: provided by some laboratories using material (sample in viral transport medium).
- *Type-specific serology*: of little diagnostic value (➔ Chapter 22, 'Diagnosis', p. 282).

Trichomonas vaginalis

Swab from posterior fornix or urethra/sub-preputial sac (if indicated) in growth medium (e.g. Feinberg–Whittington incubated at 37°C) or trans-port medium (Amies/Stuart charcoal), refrigerated, and received within 24–48 hours. Although some laboratories provide a culture service, most diagnose on slides prepared from the swabs. Newer culture systems (InPouch TV; BioMed Diagnostics, USA) offer advantages over previous media, negating the need to prepare wet preparations on a daily basis and also allowing the entire pouch to be read microscopically, rather than a pro-portion of the culture medium.

Nucleic acid amplification test

Test of choice where resources allow, vaginal or endocervical swabs in women, and urine samples from men demonstrate sensitivities of 88–97% and specificities of 98–99%. Becoming increasingly available.

Candida spp.

Swab from vaginal wall or vulva, glans penis, prepuce, anus, etc., if indi-cated, in transport medium (Amies, Stuart) without any special precautions. *Candida* spp. are common skin and genital commensals and, therefore, the need to treat must be based on clinical findings.

Mycoplasma genitalium

Routine NAAT testing is not performed in UK Sexual Health clinics, but validated commercially available assays may become more widely available in the future.

Serology

Clotted blood is required with no special arrangements needed for trans-port. Baseline assays are useful, especially if subsequent repeat tests are positive.
- *Syphilis and HIV*: seroconversion usually occurs within 2–6 weeks, but may take up to 3 months. However, 4th-generation HIV assays are now routinely used, detecting both HIV antibody and HIV p24 antigen, which can shorten the duration of detection to 4 weeks post-HIV infection. Guidelines now recommend that an HIV test at 4 weeks post-exposure is highly likely to exclude infection, but those at high risk should be retested at 3 months.

• *Hepatitis B core antibody and/or surface antigen, and hepatitis C antibody*: can usually be detected within 3 months of infection although occasionally may take longer. In high-risk situations a further test at 6 months is advisable. Additional investigations for e-Ag/eAb are performed on this sample if the initial hepatitis B surface antigen test is positive. Hepatitis C RNA test may be positive within 2 weeks and can be used to detect early infection in possible high risk exposure.

More detailed information on testing in specific situations and less common infections can be found in the relevant chapters.

Frequently asked questions
See Box 5.1.

Box 5.1 Frequently asked questions about laboratory tests

Will the tests hurt?
• ♂: Usually we only need to do a urine test, but if you have a discharge then we also use a swab to send for gonorrhoea culture and smear onto a microscope slide. You will feel some discomfort, but it should not be painful. The swabs only take a few seconds to take. You may notice slight discomfort on urinating the first time after the swab and/or loop has been taken.
• ♀: If you have no symptoms then you may wish to do your own vulvovaginal swab placed about 2 inches into the vagina and rotated for just over 10 seconds. If you have symptoms, then we use a speculum inserted into the vagina to take the swabs, similar to when having a smear taken.

We may advise that swabs be taken from your throat or rectum for gonorrhoea and chlamydia, depending on certain circumstances (e.g. sexual activity at these sites). You may be able to do some of these tests yourself.

Are you going to use the umbrella?
No. This is an old instrument used for ♂ >40 years ago. Modern swabs are taken with very fine swabs or we use a small loop to sample secretions.

Will I get the result today?
No. You will not get all your results today.

If you are ♀, microscopy at the time of your appointment may show thrush, bacterial vaginosis, or trichomoniasis. We can also sometimes detect gonorrhoea, but this needs to be confirmed by swabs taken at the same time and sent to the laboratory. One of the swabs will detect both gonorrhoea and chlamydia, another is to see if gonorrhoea can be grown in the laboratory to ensure the correct antibiotics are been given. The results for chlamydia and gonorrhoea are usually available within a week.

(Continued)

Box 5.1 *Contd.*

In ♂ we can diagnose some conditions, such as non-specific urethritis (NSU) or gonorrhoea on the day if microscopy is performed (usually in someone with a urethral discharge). A urine test also needs to be sent away, however, as a second test for gonorrhoea and to check for chlamydia, as do any swabs taken from other parts of your body (rectal or throat). All results should be available within a week.

Blood tests results take up to 7 days. However, if there is a particular concern we can obtain a preliminary result within 24 hours.

Do they need repeating?
Yes if gonorrhoea is detected we advise the patient to return in 2 weeks for a repeat urine (♂) or vaginal swab (♀), and other swabs if it was detected at other sites (throat, rectum) to check the antibiotics have worked. We rarely need to do tests of cure for chlamydia. You will be told if you may need a test of cure. Tests do not need repeating unless the first tests were taken too soon after a risk (within 2 weeks), there is a high infection risk, symptoms persist, or there is a risk of re-infection/new infection. If your test was positive and you were treated for an infection you may be invited to come back in 3–6 months for some routine repeat tests; this is good practice to ensure infections are detected and treated early.

I'm on my period. Can you still do the tests?
Yes. We can still take tests while you are menstruating. However, some prefer to wait until their period has finished.

The microscope

Two microscopes are usually required, one for direct light and phase contrast illumination, and the other for dark ground microscopy.

Objective lenses

- ×10, ×40 *(low power)*: provide overall magnification of ×100 and ×400. Suitable for screening for clue cells, trichomoniasis and candidiasis, and fungal infection, although may require high power to confirm. Also used to identify scabies mites and threadworm ova.
- ×100 *(high power)*: provides overall magnification of ×1000. Must be used with immersion oil. Used to examine specimens for PMNLs, gonococci, and other bacteria, including treponemes.
- Separate objectives are required for direct light/phase contrast and dark ground illumination.

Condensers

See Fig. 5.1.
- Direct light.
- Phase contrast (must match with the same Ph code on the objective).
- Dark ground (used with immersion oil between lens and under surface of the slide).

Microscopy: general points

- Ensure lenses are wiped clean of immersion oil and dust with a lens tissue after use.
- To avoid lens damage, ensure that high-power objective lens is not aligned when slides are moved to and from the microscope.
- When using dark ground microscopy, place a drop of oil on the condenser and raise until it just touches the slide.
- When using phase contrast, ensure that the Ph codes on the condenser and objective match.
- Start with low power to identify a good wide field, and approximate focus before moving to high power.

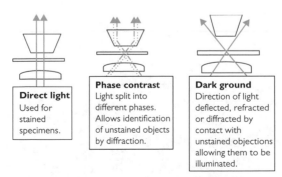

Direct light
Used for stained specimens.

Phase contrast
Light split into different phases. Allows identification of unstained objects by diffraction.

Dark ground
Direction of light deflected, refracted or diffracted by contact with unstained objections allowing them to be illuminated.

Fig. 5.1 Condensers.

Slide preparation

See Box 5.2.

> ### Box 5.2 Slide preparation techniques
>
> *Gram stain*
> - Fix the smear by heating the slide or submerging it in 95% methanol for 2 minutes.
> - Apply crystal violet, methyl violet, or gentian violet (a combination of the first two) for 15 seconds.
> - Apply an aqueous solution of iodine for 15 seconds.
> - Decolorize slide with acetone for 3 seconds.
> - Rinse slide with water.
> - Apply red counterstain (e.g. carbol fuchsin, basic fuchsin, or neutral red) for 15 seconds.
> - Rinse slide in water.
> - Carefully dry the slide.
>
> *Preparation of ulcer fluid for dark ground microscopy for T. pallidum*
> See ➔ Chapter 7, 'Diagnosis and investigation', pp. 125–9.
> - Clean the ulcer with a swab soaked in sterile saline.
> - Squeeze the lesion gently to release serum.
> - Collect serum with the edge of a cover-slip and mount in normal saline.
> - Gently press the cover-slip onto the slide.

Clinic-based tests

Examination by microscopy

Gram-stained smear

- ♂ *urethral discharge/urine threads*: PMNLs, Gram −ve intracellular diplococci.
- *Glans penis/sub-preputial sac*: yeast spores ± hyphae, mixed Gram +ve and −ve cocco-bacilli ± curved rods (generally anaerobes).
- ♀ *cervix*: PMNLs, Gram −ve intracellular diplococci.
- *Vagina*: lactobacilli (Plate 1), PMNLs, mixed Gram +ve and −ve cocco-bacilli ± curved rods (generally anaerobes), Gram +ve cocci, yeast spores ± hyphae.
- *Rectum*: PMNLs, Gram −ve intracellular diplococci.
- *Ulcers*: Gram −ve coccobacillus in shoals (*Haemophilus ducreyi*)—unusual finding.

Saline suspension

- *Phase contrast*:
  - *Vagina or sub-preputial sac/glans penis*—clue cells/motile curved rods, *T. vaginalis*, yeast spores ± hyphae;
  - *Urethra*—*T. vaginalis*.
- *Dark ground*:
  - *Ulcers*—*T. pallidum*;
  - *Vagina or sub-preputial sac/glans penis*—clue cells/motile curved rods, *T. vaginalis*, yeast spores ± hyphae'
  - *urethra*—*T. vaginalis*.

Skin samples

- Burrow material for scabies mite.
- Skin scales in 10% potassium hydroxide for mycelia (tinea/ringworm).
- Perianal transparent adhesive tape strip: threadworm ova.

Vaginal discharge

- 'Whiff test': addition of 10% potassium hydroxide releases pungent amines; rarely used now in clinical practice.
- pH >4.5.

Both are indicators of BV. Unnecessary if Hay–Ison diagnostic criteria used (➲ Chapter 15, 'Diagnosis', p. 220).

Urine

Inspection

Urine haze in ♂ (not cleared by addition of 5% acetic acid) ± threads in first pass suggests anterior urethritis. A second specimen [mid-stream specimen of urine (MSSU)] may be of value in suggesting posterior urethritis or UTI (if turbid), and is essential for culture and sensitivity. Urine may also be required for pregnancy testing (see Box 5.3).

Box 5.3 Pregnancy test (immunoassay), urine, and serum

First documented in Egypt (1350 BC) when ♀ suspecting pregnancy urinated on wheat or barley seeds for 7 days. Seed germination (probably due to ↑ levels of oestrogen) indicated pregnancy (70% accuracy demonstrated in 1963).

Pregnancy testing can be performed on urine or serum. Both tests detect β-human chorionic gonadotrophin (hCG), a hormone produced by the placental trophoblastic cells shortly after implantation. A positive result usually indicates the presence of a viable foetus.

Urine (qualitative test)

Urine sampling kits give only a +ve or −ve result. Samples can detect hCG levels >25–50 mIU/mL. Levels of urinary hCG average 100 mIU/mL following the first missed menstrual period and ↑ up to 200,000 mIU/mL at 10–12 weeks of pregnancy, after which time levels fall. Test read after 3 minutes.

Limitations of urine test

- Unable to distinguish between uterine and ectopic pregnancy.
- Occasional false-negative results in ectopic pregnancy.
- Inability to distinguish between pituitary hCG (secreted by gonadotrophs of anterior pituitary) and placental hCG.
- Positive result may be obtained in the presence of gestational trophoblastic disease.
- Certain non-trophoblastic neoplasms (e.g. testicular, liver, neuroendocrine, breast, ovarian, pancreatic, cervical, gastric) can cause higher levels of hCG, but rises are usually modest.
- 10% of pregnancies are undetectable on the first day of missed menses.
- False-positive results estimated at up to 10%.
- False-negative results may be due to dilute urine.

Serum

More accurate and should be considered if urine testing is −ve, but there is a pregnancy risk. Tests can detect hCG levels above 5–10 mIU/mL. Positive results may be obtained within 7–10 days of conception. Quantitative tests are available that allow exact measurement of serum hCG, useful in assessing the stage of pregnancy. Serum hCG doubles every 36–48 hours in the early stages. A subnormal response may indicate miscarriage or ectopic pregnancy. Extremely high levels of hCG may suggest multiple pregnancy.

Urinalysis

- *Glucose, ketones*: diabetes (recurrent candidiasis, balanitis).
- *Leucocytes, nitrites, blood*: UTI.
- *Persistent proteinuria and haematuria*: refer to nephrology.
- *Persistent haematuria*: discuss with Urology team.
- *Leucocytes ≥1 only; with symptoms of urethritis (microscopy unavailable)*: non-gonococcal urethritis (NGU).

Routine female microscopy

Vaginal Gram-stained smear

See Fig. 5.2.

1. Are there bacteria present and what are they like?

Grade 0	Grade I	Grade II
Epithelial cells only	*Lactobacilli only*	*Reduced lactobacilli and mixed bacteria*
• Post-menopause	• Normal flora	• Intermediate transitional phase
• Pre-menarche		
• Antibiotics		
• Intra-vaginal gels		

Grade III		Grade IV	
Mixed bacteria/no lactobacilli and 'clue cells'		*Gram +ve cocci only (often in chains)*	
• Indicates bacterial vaginosis		• Usually irrelevant	

Treatment for bacterial vaginosis required for Grade III (and, occasionally, Grade II) with symptoms/signs.

2. Are there any yeast spores and/or hyphae?

Usually associated with vaginal PMNLs if symptomatic.		
Hyphae +/− spores	*Usually*	*Candida albicans*
Spores alone	*Probably*	*Candida glabrata*

3. Are there vaginal PMNLs?

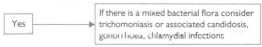

Yes → If there is a mixed bacterial flora consider trichomoniasis or associated candidosis, gonorrhoea, chlamydial infections

Fig. 5.2 Algorithm for analysing results on a vaginal Gram-stained smear.

Cervical Gram-stained smears

Are PMNLs present?

Variable depending on menstrual cycle, sexual activity, and contraception (often ↑ with hormonal methods). >30 per high-power field correlates best with gonococcal or chlamydial infections.

Are Gram −ve diplococci (GNDC) present?

Examine cervical smear for intracellular GNDC. Urethral smear of doubtful value if cervix examined and now rarely performed. Finding extracellular GNDC ↑ sensitivity by 20% but ↓ specificity by 4%.

Vaginal preparation in saline protected by a cover-slip

- Switch light source to phase contrast (or dark ground).
- Screen slide (low power) for motile protozoa, spores ± hyphae.
- If necessary, switch to high power. Place a drop of immersion oil on to cover-slip before examining. Can also be used to identify clue cells and motile vibrios (*Mobiluncus* spp.) often found in bacterial vaginosis.

Routine male microscopy

Urethral Gram-stained smear

Are PMNLs present?
Non-gonococcal urethritis diagnosed by finding:
- ≥5 PMNLs per high-power field (averaged over five fields with the greatest concentration of PMNLs)
- no GNDC.

Are GNDC present (with intracellular organisms)?
If seen, allows a working diagnosis of gonorrhoea. Generally associated with numerous PMNLs.

Gram-stained smear from urine
Useful if urine threads in first voided urine (FVU) specimen and no urethral material to sample directly. The slide can be prepared from threads or centrifuged FVU. Ideally, urine should not be passed for at least 3–4 hours before assessment.

Are PMNLs present?
Non-gonococcal urethritis diagnosed by finding:
- ≥10 PMNLs per high-power field (averaged over five fields with the greatest concentration of PMNLs)
- no GNDC.

Are GNDC present (with intracellular organisms)?
Allows a working diagnosis of gonorrhoea.

Saline suspension of sub-preputial, glans penis, or urethral material

Sub-prepuce and glans
If balanitis/balanoposthitis check for:
- yeast spores ± hyphae.
- clue cells (anaerobic balanitis).
- *T. vaginalis*.

A Gram-stained smear can also be used.

Urethra
T. vaginalis: may occasionally be seen with urethritis.

Accuracy of microscopy

See Table 5.1

Table 5.1 Accuracy of microscopy by infection and site

Infection and site	Sensitivity (%)	Specificity (%)
Gonorrhoea		
Urethral Gram stain, symptomatic ♂	90–95	95–99*
Urethral Gram stain, asymptomatic ♂	50–75	
Rectal Gram stain from MSM	35–80†	95–100*
Cervical Gram stain	23–65	88–100*
Bacterial vaginosis (Hay–Ison criteria)		
Vaginal Gram-stained specimen	97.5	96
Trichomoniasis (saline suspension)		
Suspension of vaginal discharge	40–80	If motile protozoa seen 100
Suspension of male urethral/ sub-preputial material	30	
Candidiasis		
Vaginal Gram stain if symptomatic	65	No data
Vaginal saline suspension	40–60	
Primary syphilis		
Dark ground examination of ulcer material in saline	79–86	77–100

*Excludes *Neisseria meningitidis*, which may rarely be found (indistinguishable morphologically from *N. gonorrhoeae*). †Higher level if rectal pus.

Rapid point of care tests (POCTs)

Rationale

Near patient, rapid medical diagnostic testing, usually performed by non-lab staff, and results used to inform immediate clinical decisions. Useful in resource-limited settings, where expensive laboratory facilities are not available. Some may also be used by the patient at home (see Box 5.4 for properties of an ideal POCT).

Studies have demonstrated that POCTs can lead to the treatment of a greater number of infected patients as they often do not re-attend for results assuming that results will be negative.

Significant advances have been made in rapid real-time cartridge-based NAAT testing with results available within 90 minutes for chlamydia/gonorrhoea, 40 minutes for trichomonas and <60 minutes for HIV. They enable patients to receive results and be treated on the same day. These tests have high sensitivities and specificities. Non-NAAT POCT for chlamydia and gonorrhoea are commercially available for home use, but have been largely superseded by newer NAAT tests.

Chlamydia POCTs

Immunoassays for chlamydial antigen (usually lipopolysaccharide) using anti-chlamydial monoclonal antibody. A number are commercially available for testing first-catch urine, endocervical, or vaginal swabs. Sensitivities 77–93%, specificities 97.5–100%, and result time ranges from 12 to 30 minutes. Examples include Clearview® Chlamydia *MF*, Alere™, Biostar® OIA® Quidel® Quickvue® Chlamydia, Chlamydia Rapid Test (Diagnostics for the Real World Ltd). Because of the low sensitivities of tests, it is important to obtain a confirmatory sample for NAAT testing if facilities are available.

Gonorrhoea POCTs

Rarely ever used in clinical settings with the advent of NAAT testing. Some commercially available, e.g. Biostar® Optical Immunoassay and the double-sandwich immunoassay OneStep Rapicard™ Instatest (Cortez Diagnostics). The Biostar® OIA® Gonorrhoea test identifies the L7/L12 ribosomal protein marker, which only occurs in the gonococcus and not other *Neisseria* spp. (sensitivity 87.8%, specificity 98.5%). Uses endocervical swab in ♀ and urine in ♂, results in 24 minutes. Confirmatory NAAT + culture to determine antibiotic sensitivities prior to treatment essential.

> Box 5.4 **Properties of an ideal POCT**
>
> - Easy to use.
> - Cost-effective.
> - Rapid results.
> - Easy to store, long shelf-life.
> - Sampling acceptable to the patient.
> - Suitable for ♂ and ♀.
> - Incorporate a test control.
> - High sensitivity and specificity.
> - Undergone quality assurance tests (i.e. CE marked).

Trichomonas POCTs

POCTs based on antigen detection are available, which offer quick diagnosis compared with culture, with sensitivities as high as 83–95.5% compared with culture, e.g. OSOM® Trichomonas Rapid Test, Sekisui Diagnostics.

HIV POCTs

Used widely in clinical practice. Over 60 different products are produced. Recommended in the following settings:
- Community settings/home testing.
- Source testing in exposure/needlestick incidents.
- High-risk situations in which venepuncture is refused.
- When rapid results are required.

POCTs use oral fluid, finger-prick, plasma, whole-blood, or urine.

In low-prevalence settings false-positive rates are relatively higher, with poor positive predictive value of some tests. Therefore, all positive results should be confirmed by laboratory tests. Results may not be reliable if patient is within the 'window period'.

Examples of rapid assays include particle agglutination on latex particles, immunochromatography (lateral flow) strips, and immunoconcentration (rapid vertical flow) using HIV antigens to immobilize Ab on porous membrane:
- *1st generation*: HIV antigen coated on latex particles detects HIV specific IgG. No longer used in UK.
- *2nd generation*: Synthetic peptide or recombinant antigen has ↑ sensitivity for HIV1 group O and HIV2. Used in some rapid tests.
- *3rd generation*: Synthetic peptide or recombinant protein in immunometric sandwich. Detects IgG and IgM with ↑ sensitivity during early seroconversion.
- *4th generation*: 3rd generation Ab detection + monoclonal antibodies to detect p24 Ag. Detects HIV infection before seroconversion (preferred method).

Antigens vary with individual assay, often from viral envelope (glycoprotein (gp)41, 120, 160). Some include p24 core antigen. Tests have been developed that, in addition to HIV-1, will identify HIV-2 (using gp36 antigen), appearing positive at a different location on the strip or membrane. Difficulty in some tests identifying Group O subtypes and certain HIV-2 strains. Sensitivities of 3rd and 4th generation POCTs range between 93 and 98% (oral fluid: OraQuick) 87–100% (blood: Uni-Gold Ab, INSTI HIV1/2Ab, SD Bioline Combo and Determine Combo) and specificities are similarly high, >99%, for POCTs using oral fluid and blood.

Home testing

Kits became legal to purchase in the UK in April 2014; currently, the only approved CE marked POCT in the UK is the HIV Self-Test from Biosure Ltd, which can be read in 15 minutes using a finger-prick blood sample. Sensitivity 99.7%, specificity of 99.9%, and detects HIV antibody only.

Home sampling

Some companies or agencies offer STI home sampling. The customer purchases a test kit, conducts sampling at home, then posts it back. The customer receives results, usually by text or secure online site. For some infections, e.g. chlamydia, the company may sell treatment or refers to a local sexual health clinic for treatment. Some NHS and voluntary sector initiatives now offer a free home-sampling service in parts of the UK.

Other POCT

A variety of other POCTs have been developed for syphilis (e.g. *Determine*® *TP* assay, *INSTI*™ *Multiplex Syphilis/HIV1/HIV2* assay) and for hepatitis B and C.

Commensals and confounders

Genital specimens include various micro-organisms, which may not be pathogenic. These include hydrogen peroxide producing *Lactobacillus* spp., which indicate normality, and other organisms, usually commensal, but pathogenic under certain conditions. Therefore, results of routine genital specimens should be interpreted in the clinical context and inappropriate antibiotic treatment should be avoided.

Leptothrix (leptotrichia)

Elongated chain of lactobacilli that may be mistaken for *Candida* spp. on microscopy. Usually, not clinically significant, but may be associated with vaginitis caused by candida or TV.

Group B β-haemolytic streptococci: *Streptococcus agalactiae*

Vaginal carriage rates in ♀ attending GUM clinics 12–36%; usually, not clinically significant, except in late pregnancy. Antenatal services should be informed if isolated in a pregnant woman (**➲** Chapter 32, 'Group B β-haemolytic streptococci', pp. 374–5).

Actinomyces israelii

Found in 3% of ♀ genital specimens—4% if using intrauterine device (IUD). Detectable on cervical cytology, vaginal wet mount, and Gram-stained smears. If asymptomatic, no intervention is required. However, removal (and culture) of IUD and treatment with prolonged courses of antibiotics may be indicated if otherwise unexplained symptoms, e.g. intermenstrual bleeding, dyspareunia, and pelvic pain.

Actinomycosis (suppurative upper-genital tract infection) is a rare complication, especially associated with long-term use of plastic IUDs (**➲** Chapter 11, 'Aetiology', p. 171).

Neisseria meningitidis

↑ Rates of nasopharyngeal carriage in MSM and those practising orogenital sex, reporting multiple sexual partners, or diagnosed with anogenital gonococcal infection (>20% in these groups compared with a general rate of 5–15%). High rates also found in university students (up to 34%). Anogenital carriage in up to 2% of MSM, 0.2% of heterosexual ♂, and 0.1% ♀. May rarely cause urethritis in ♂ and there are case reports of symptomatic disease in women

Other micro-organisms

- *Gardnerella vaginalis, Prevotella melaninogenica, Peptostreptococci*, and other anaerobic organisms may be detected in genital specimens because of low-level colonization without bacterial vaginosis.
- *Ureaplasma urealyticum, Bacterioides urealyticum*, and *Mycoplasma hominis* may also be found without any clinical manifestations but may cause local inflammation.
- *Corynebacterium species, Escherichia coli*, and coagulase-negative staphylococci in genital specimens are usually of no clinical significance, but rarely may be implicated in vaginitis.

- *Spirochaetes: Brachyspira aalborgi* and *Brachyspira pilosicoli* colonize colorectal epithelium in up to 30% of people in some developing countries and a similar proportion of MSM or those with HIV infection in the developed countries. In addition, *Treponema denticola, Treponema vincentii*, and other similar treponemes associated with periodontal infections and *Treponema refringens, Treponema phagedenis*, and *Treponema minutum*, found as commensals in the genitalia, need to be distinguished from *T. pallidum* in rectal, oral, or genital specimens.

Specific genitourinary situations

Men with symptoms suggesting urethritis 82
Balanitis and balanoposthitis 83
Vulval irritation/discomfort/pain 84
Altered vaginal discharge 85
Anogenital ulceration 87
Genital lumps and bumps 89
Proctitis 90
Management of sexual contacts 91
Oral sex 93
Pregnancy 98
Sexual assault: general principles 102
Sexual assault: management 105
Sexual assault: forensic assessment 109
Child sexual assault 110

Men with symptoms suggesting urethritis

Factors suggesting sexually acquired cause

- *Presentation*: ↑ likelihood if new sexual risk/suspicion about a partner with urethritis arising within 4 weeks (usually).
- *Age*: most commonly found in ♂ from late teens to 50 years.
- *Symptoms*: usually prominent dysuria and/or urethral discharge (may just be found on examination).↑ urinary frequency and systemic symptoms unusual.

Management

- *Urethral smear*: =>5 polymorphonuclear leucocytes (PMNL) per high-power field (HPF) and/or urinary thread from FVU: =>10 PMNL per HPF. Consider sending air-dried smear to lab if on-site microscopy unavailable.
- *Urethral swab* (NAAT and preferably culture) or FVU (NAAT) for *Neisseria gonorrhoeae* (urethral culture before treatment for gonorrhoea); FVU or swab using NAAT for *Chlamydia trachomatis* and *Mycoplasma genitalium*.
- Consider:
  - mid-stream sample of urine (MSSU) to exclude urinary tract infection (UTI), if relevant;
  - *exposure to other STIs*—consider screening, e.g. syphilis and HIV serology.
- Treat on microscopy findings or clinical assessment if microscopy unavailable (while awaiting lab results).
- PN/contact tracing must be arranged. Contacts of gonorrhoea, chlamydia, or mycoplasma should be treated epidemiologically. Treatment may be appropriate for contacts of NSU with negative tests for the above tests, if likely to be sexually acquired.
- Abstain from sex until treatment completed and partner(s) treated.

Factors suggesting non-sexually acquired cause: consider underlying UTI

- Sexual history: long-standing stable sexual relationship/not sexually active
- Age: >50 years (prostatism with UTI more common)
- Symptoms: ↑ frequency, loin pain, pyrexia, malaise

Management

- Consider/exclude STI:
  - urethral smear for Gram stain, specimens for *N. gonorrhoeae*, *C. trachomatis*, *M. genitalium*
  - offer syphilis and HIV serology.
- FVU and MSSU typically both opaque, failing to clear on acidification (e.g. 5% acetic acid). Dip-stick usually shows leucocytes, nitrites, protein, and blood. Send MSSU for microscopy, culture, and sensitivity.
- If suspected, manage as UTI.

Balanitis and balanoposthitis

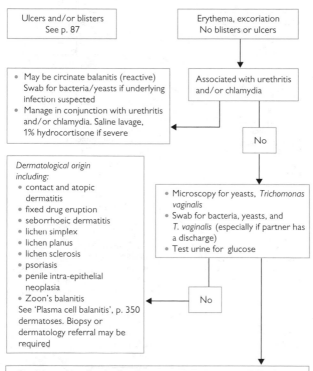

Fig. 6.1 Investigating balanitis and balanoposthitis.

Vulval irritation/discomfort/pain

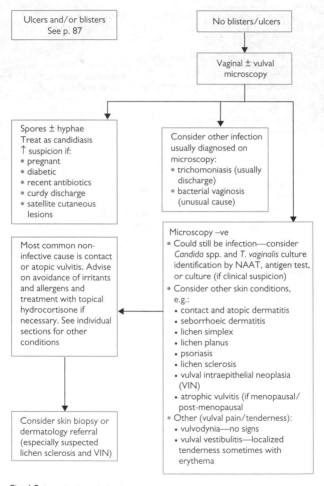

Fig. 6.2 Investigating vulval pain.

Altered vaginal discharge

The normal physiological discharge will alter with the time of the menstrual cycle, pregnancy, and sometimes hormonal contraception. Finding lactobacilli without other anomalies provides reassurance pending swab results.

Remember that it is common for infections to coexist.

Primary vaginal conditions

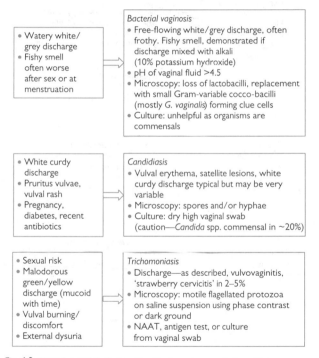

• Watery white/grey discharge • Fishy smell often worse after sex or at menstruation	**Bacterial vaginosis** • Free-flowing white/grey discharge, often frothy. Fishy smell, demonstrated if discharge mixed with alkali (10% potassium hydroxide) • pH of vaginal fluid >4.5 • Microscopy: loss of lactobacilli, replacement with small Gram-variable cocco-bacilli (mostly *G. vaginalis*) forming clue cells • Culture: unhelpful as organisms are commensals
• White curdy discharge • Pruritus vulvae, vulval rash • Pregnancy, diabetes, recent antibiotics	**Candidiasis** • Vulval erythema, satellite lesions, white curdy discharge typical but may be very variable • Microscopy: spores and/or hyphae • Culture: dry high vaginal swab (caution—*Candida* spp. commensal in ~20%)
• Sexual risk • Malodorous green/yellow discharge (mucoid with time) • Vulval burning/discomfort • External dysuria	**Trichomoniasis** • Discharge—as described, vulvovaginitis, 'strawberry cervicitis' in 2–5% • Microscopy: motile flagellated protozoa on saline suspension using phase contrast or dark ground • NAAT, antigen test, or culture from vaginal swab

Fig. 6.3 Altered vaginal discharge—Investigating primary vaginal conditions.

Other causes of altered vaginal discharge commonly seen in GUM

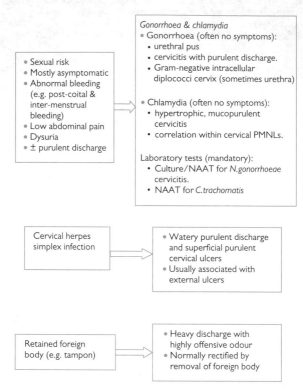

Fig. 6.4 Altered vaginal discharge—Investigating other common GUM presentations.

Anogenital ulceration

Traumatic
- Timing—immediately after incident
- Appearance (often irregular—as dermatitis artefacta)

Management
- Exclude STI cause
- Bacterial swab (if 2° infection)
- General STI screen
  Advise
- Saline lavage
- Antibiotics for secondary infection if necessary

Possible STI
- Herpes: multiple, painful, preceded by vesicles. Most common infective cause
- Syphilis: 1°chancre—typically single and painless (multiple painful ulcers now more common): 2°—'snail track', usually with skin rash
- Tropical: (suspect if travel history or exposure). Typical presentations:
  - chancroid—multiple, soft, painful ulcers
  - lymphogranuloma venereum (LGV)—usually bilateral inguinal lymphadenopathy (preceded by transient, small, painless ulcer)
  - granuloma inguinale—pruritic papule followed by granulomatous ulcer

Investigations
- Herpes—swab for herpes simplex virus
- Dark-ground examination for treponemes. Consider repeating on 3 separate days if clinically suspicious. Ensure full syphilis serology requested
- Swab for *Haemophilus ducreyi*
- Swab ulcer/bubo pus for *C. trachomatis*; blood for LGVCFT
- Biopsy for Donovan bodies

Other
- Neoplastic: progressive over weeks or months (age usually over 50 years)
- 'Dermatological', e.g. aphthous ulcers/Behçet's disease—usually chronic, relapsing associated with oral ulcers and if Behçet's other systemic symptoms

Management
Urgent urology referral if carcinoma suspected. Dermatological referral may be required for other conditions

Fig. 6.5 Investigating and managing anogenital ulceration.

The most common infective cause of anogenital ulceration in GUM is genital herpes

First episode
- *Diagnosis*:
  - *swab* – in viral transport medium
  - diagnostic confirmation important, although treatment should commence on clinical grounds
  - full STI screen advised. Internal examination in ♀ may be deferred until acute symptoms resolved.
- *Management*:
  - if clinically suspected, start oral antiviral treatment
  - analgesia may be required (e.g. 30–60 mg codeine phosphate 4–6 times a day)
  - recommend saline lavage
  - suggest micturition in warm bathwater if severe dysuria. Suprapubic catheterization may be required if urinary retention.

Recurrence
- Supportive treatment (e.g. saline bathing) unless unusually severe when oral antiviral treatment is justified
- STI screen only if new risk.

Frequent recurrence (>6 per year)
- Anticipatory episodic treatment
- Suppressive treatment.

Genital lumps and bumps

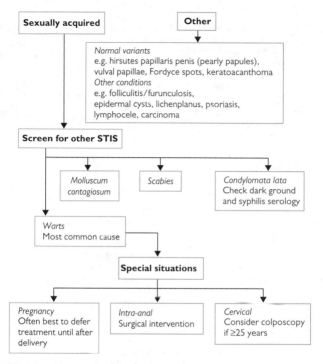

Fig. 6.6. Investigating genital lumps and bumps.

Proctitis

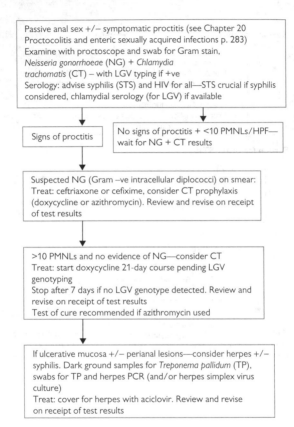

Passive anal sex +/− symptomatic proctitis (see Chapter 20
Proctocolitis and enteric sexually acquired infections p. 283)
Examine with proctoscope and swab for Gram stain,
Neisseria gonorrhoeae (NG) + *Chlamydia
trachomatis* (CT) – with LGV typing if +ve
Serology: advise syphilis (STS) and HIV for all—STS crucial if syphilis
considered, chlamydial serology (for LGV) if available

Signs of proctitis

No signs of proctitis + <10 PMNLs/HPF—
wait for NG + CT results

Suspected NG (Gram −ve intracellular diplococci) on smear:
Treat: ceftriaxone or cefixime, consider CT prophylaxis
(doxycycline or azithromycin). Review and revise on receipt
of test results

>10 PMNLs and no evidence of NG—consider CT
Treat: start doxycycline 21-day course pending LGV
genotyping
Stop after 7 days if no LGV genotype detected. Review and
revise on receipt of test results
Test of cure recommended if azithromycin used

If ulcerative mucosa +/− perianal lesions—consider herpes +/−
syphilis. Dark ground samples for *Treponema pallidum* (TP),
swabs for TP and herpes PCR (and/or herpes simplex virus
culture)
Treat: cover for herpes with aciclovir. Review and revise
on receipt of test results

Fig. 6.7 Investigation and management of proctitis.

Management of sexual contacts

See Tables 6.1 and 6.2.

Table 6.1 Epidemiological treatment for contacts of STIs

Infection of index case	Treatment need	Contact treatment
♀ candidiasis	×	
♂ candidiasis	✓	Antimycotic treatment often required
Chancroid	✓	Ciprofloxacin 500 mg bd for 3 days Ceftriaxone 250 mg single dose, IM
Chlamydia	✓	Azithromycin 1 g stat., doxycycline (100 mg bd for 7 days (recommended if likely rectal infection), erythromycin 500 mg bd for 14 days
Donovanosis	✓	Azithromycin: to current contacts and those from 30 days prior to onset of symptoms
Epididymitis (if non-gonococcal)	✓	Azithromycin, doxycycline, erythromycin (as chlamydia)
Gonorrhoea	✓	Single doses of cefixime 400 mg; ciprofloxacin 500 mg; amoxicillin 3 g + probenecid 1 g; ceftriaxone 250 mg IM
Hepatitis A	✓	Hepatitis A vaccine HNIG* – close contacts <2 weeks
Hepatitis B	✓	Specific hepatitis B immunoglobulin (<7 days). Super-accelerated active immunization
HIV	× / ✓	If <72 hours, consider post-exposure prophylaxis (PEP) with highly active antiretroviral therapy for 1 month
Lymphogranuloma venereum	✓	Doxycycline: to current contacts and those from 30 days prior to onset of symptoms
Non-gonococcal urethritis	✓	Azithromycin, doxycycline, erythromycin (as chlamydia)
Mucopurulent cervicitis and PID	✓	Azithromycin, doxycycline, erythromycin (as chlamydia). Consider anti-gonorrhoea treatment
Mycoplasma genitalium	✓	If no macrolide resistance in index patient: azithromycin 500 mg followed by 250 mg daily for 4 days,
		If macrolide resistance in index patient: Moxifloxacin 400 mg oral daily for 14 days
Pediculosis	✓	Permethrin or malathion to sex contacts
Scabies	✓	Permethrin or malathion to sex and household contacts
Syphilis—early Syphilis—late	× / ✓ ×	Consider benzathine benzylpenicillin 2.4 MU IM stat or oral doxycycline 100 mg bd for 14 days
Trichomoniasis	✓	Metronidazole 2 g single dose or 400 mg bd for 7 days

*Human normal immunoglobulin

Table 6.2 No partner treatment required

Infection	Need	Contact treatment
Bacterial vaginosis	×	Not required
Hepatitis C	×	
Anogenital herpes	×	
Anogenital warts/molluscum contagiosum	×	

NB: Tables 6.1 and 6.2 only provide information about epidemiological treatment. They do not cover the requirement to offer contacts at risk STI screening, information, and advice.

Oral sex

- *Oro-penile*: fellatio.
- *Oro-vulval*: cunnilingus.
- *Oro-anal*: anilingus (also spelt analingus).

Lifestyle reports suggest an increase in oral sex, especially among adolescents, and MSM. Factors include a younger age at sexual debut, avoidance of pregnancy, and reducing HIV risk (in MSM). Oral sex is often not regarded as sex, or as relevant to the transmission of infection, so direct questions regarding its practice must be asked when relevant (Box 6.1).

Box 6.1 Receptive oral sex or receiving oral sex

Descriptions of oral sex can be confusing because of variable interpretation:

- *Receptive oral sex* has been used in the same sense as receptive anal sex, i.e. accepting the sexual partner's penis into one's mouth.
- *Insertive oral sex* has similarly been used to describe the act of inserting one's penis into the partner's mouth.
- On the other hand *receiving oral sex* has been used to describe male or female genital stimulation by the sexual partner's mouth. *Giving or (performing) oral sex* is the opposite of 'receiving', i.e. stimulating the partner's genitals by one's mouth. In view of the greater applicability, the descriptions used in this book are:
  - *receiving oral sex*—indicates genital stimulation by the sexual partner's mouth ('insertive oral sex' in some publications).
  - *giving oral sex* to indicate stimulating the sexual partner's genitals ('receptive oral sex' in some publications).

Non-infective

Idiosyncratic reports of genital lesions arising from trauma, usually from the teeth, but also related to the use of piercings. Underlying medical conditions may aggravate, e.g. vulval haematoma in ♀ with essential thrombocytopenia. Oral injuries arising from fellatio have been reported, with the typical lesion appearing as a circular area on the soft palate consisting of erythema, petechiae, dilated blood vessels, and vesicles. A case of accidental condom inhalation has been reported in a ♀ presenting with a chronic cough, sputum, and fever with a collapse-consolidation of the right upper lobe. Videobronchoscopy revealed the presence of a condom in the right upper lobe bronchus. Case reports have associated vaginal insufflation (blowing into the vagina) with venous air embolism (through the uterine veins or subplacental sinuses) during pregnancy, and pneumoperitoneum (presenting with acute severe abdominal pain) in any ♀, including those who have undergone hysterectomy, independent of operative procedure.

Infective

Adenovirus

A probable cause of NGU associated with receiving oral sex. Adenovirus infection has also been implicated in cervicitis and genital ulceration, as well as keratoconjunctivitis. Seasonal clustering of cases is reported.

Types identified in studies are 4, 8, 9, 35, 37, and 49, and NGU typically presents with marked dysuria, mucoid urethral discharge, and meatitis. Extragenital manifestations include conjunctivitis, pharyngitis, and constitutional symptoms.

Bacterial vaginosis

There is a lack of clear reproducible evidence of an association with oral sex in general. However, a significant association has been reported with receiving oral sex in lesbians. *Mycoplasma hominis*, associated with BV, has been isolated from the throats of partners of ♀ who carried BV vaginally, and a history of having ever performed fellatio is significantly associated with *M. hominis* throat carriage.

Candidiasis

Symptomatic culture-proven recurrent vulvovaginal candidiasis (VVC) is associated with cunnilingus, although it appears that isolated episodes are not. Although *Candida* spp. are found in the mouth, saliva may have an important role in recurrent VVC, as other associated factors include recent ♀ masturbation with saliva and ♂ masturbation with saliva in the past month. It has been postulated that antimicrobial products in saliva could clear local bacteria, providing an advantage to resilient *Candida* spores, provoking recurrent VVC, have a direct irritant effect or otherwise alter the local immunological state.

Chancroid

Isolated case reports alleging orogenital transmission.

Chlamydia trachomatis

Chlamydial throat infection has been reported in 3.7% heterosexual ♂, 3.2% ♀, and 1.4% MSM, with a significant association in ♀ to ever having performed fellatio. It has also been found in patients with eye infections, which in turn could be caused by contact with infected semen or genital secretions. Symptoms arising from isolated throat infection are extremely unusual and, currently, there are no data on infections transmitted from the throat.

Cytomegalovirus

Found in saliva, semen, genital secretions. ↑ infection rates associated with a history of sexually transmitted infections. Considered to be transmitted by kissing; therefore, spread by oral sex is feasible.

Epstein–Barr virus (EBV)

Cause of infectious mononucleosis (glandular fever). Classically spread by infected saliva through kissing, EBV has also been detected in semen, cervical secretions, and vulval ulceration. Although unproven, sexual transmission, including oral sex, is a possibility.

Enteric infection

Shigella spp., *Salmonella* spp., *Campylobacter* spp., *Cryptosporidium* spp., *Entamoeba histolytica,* cytomegalovirus, *Giardia duodenalis,* and *Enterobius vermicularis* are all widely reported in MSM as being spread by oro-anal sex or fellatio after insertive anal intercourse (➲ Chapter 19, 'Endemic treponematoses', p. 254). *Isospora belli* enteritis has been reported in immunocompromised MSM following oro-anal sex.

Gonorrhoea

Oral infection usually involves the pharynx (asymptomatic in >90%), but stomatitis is also reported (following cunnilingus). In patients with gonorrhoea, pharyngeal infection is found in 10–30% MSM, 5–15% ♀, and 3–10% heterosexual ♂. Disseminated infection from a pharyngeal source has been reported. There is clear evidence supporting the transfer of *N. gonorrhoeae* from the throat to the male urethra, and case reports alleging throat infection from oro-anal sex or kissing. Gonococcal conjunctivitis can arise following contact with infected semen or genital secretions during oral sex.

Granuloma inguinale

Rare case reports of oral manifestations suggest that the mouth may be an infection reservoir, but no evidence of orogenital transmission.

Herpes simplex virus (HSV)

There has been an ongoing national and international increase in the incidence of new genital infections caused by HSV1, predominantly in ♀, compatible with the reports of greater rates of oral sex. HSV1 seroconversion in young ♀ has been shown to be directly associated with receiving oral sex and vaginal intercourse. Genital HSV1 infection is associated with receiving oral sex, with a weaker association with vaginal sex, suggesting that it is the partner's mouth that is the infection source. HSV2 infection can also be transmitted during oral sex causing oro-pharyngeal infection. However, unlike HSV1 infection, oral reactivation and viral shedding are uncommon.

As well as typical herpes infection both HSV1 and HSV2 can cause NGU without visible lesions, with HSV1 more common, and a positive association with the latter, NGU, and oral sex.

Hepatitis (viral)

Hepatitis A

RNA (ribonucleic acid) virus found in faeces and typically spread through the oro-faecal route. Studies suggest a link between oro-anal sex and hepatitis A in MSM, with some outbreaks clearly associated with this practice. In addition, hepatitis A may also be acquired by ingesting infected urine.

Hepatitis B

Hepatitis B virus antigen has been found in semen, saliva, cervical fluid, and faeces although much higher levels are found in blood. Anus-to-mouth transmission during oro-anal sex is considered to be an important factor, especially if there is any local bleeding. Although population studies have shown an association between oro-anal sex and hepatitis B infection, others have failed to confirm it.

Hepatitis C

Although sexually transmissible, its rate of transmission through this route is very small, and much less than for HIV and hepatitis B. However, it is associated with HIV infection in MSM, especially those engaging in unprotected receptive and insertive anal sex, fisting, use of sex toys, and oro-anal sex.

Human herpesvirus 8 (HHV8)—cause of Kaposi's sarcoma (KS)

Studies in MSM have shown that oro-anal sex is a risk factor for KS and HHV8; infection is associated with both giving and receiving oro-anal sex.

Human immunodeficiency virus (HIV)

Found in saliva at much lower concentrations than in semen and vaginal fluid, but probably ↑ infection risk if local oropharyngeal or anogenital inflammation, ulceration, or bleeding (even after tooth brushing or dental flossing). However, anti-HIV inhibitory factors in saliva, especially secretory leucocyte protease inhibitor from the parotid glands, have protective properties against HIV infection, contributing to >1 in 10,000 risk of transmission via oral sex. The risk is, however, increased by some factors:

- oral mucosal ulceration
- very high viral load such as during seroconversion stage in the HIV +ve partner
- ejaculation of semen into the mouth of the person giving oral sex.

These factors should be considered in assessing risk of infection from giving oral sex to a ♂ with HIV infection. Giving oral sex to a ♀ or receiving oral sex from ♂ or ♀ carry very little risk and do not warrant post-exposure prophylaxis.

Human papillomavirus (HPV)

The development of oropharyngeal warts is uncommon, but when found is usually caused by types 6, 11, 16, and 18, i.e. those most commonly causing genital infection. The development of an oral condyloma attributed to cunnilingus with an infected partner has been reported. High-risk (most commonly type 16) HPV infection is associated with HIV infection (especially cluster differentiation (CD) 4 counts <200cells/mL, oral mucosal abnormalities, and >1 oral sex partner. The natural history of oral HPV infection is similar to genital infection. In patients with oropharyngeal cancer, there is a significant association with HPV type 16 (and oral infection with any of 37 HPV types) with or without the established risk factors of tobacco and alcohol use. The data on the role of oral sex are unclear. Associations with a high lifetime number of vaginal or oral sex partners (with a 250% increased risk for those with >5 oral sex partners) and concurrent oral infection in a sexual partner have been reported. However, other studies have failed to show an association between oral sex and oral or genital HPV infection.

Lymphogranuloma venereum

There are no data associating the recent development of LGV proctitis in MSM with oral sex. However, oral lesions and cervical adenopathy due to LGV have been reported following oral sex. Ocular inoculation can give rise to a follicular conjunctivitis, often accompanied by pre-auricular lymphadenopathy.

Molluscum contagiosum

May be found on the cutaneous lip and peri-oral skin, usually in clusters, especially when immunocompromised. When extensive, often signifies advanced HIV disease.

Non-chlamydial non-gonococcal urethritis

Although the sexually transmitted nature of non-chlamydial NGU has been demonstrated, an association with oral sex has not been confirmed.

Pediculosis

Pthirus pubis may be transmitted from pubic hair to facial hair (i.e. beard, moustache, eyebrows, and eyelashes) during orogenital sex.

Respiratory tract organisms

- *Neisseria meningitidis*: case reports and series. Most common—anal infection in MSM, usually asymptomatic. Case reports of urethritis associated with fellatio and cervicitis, vulvovaginitis, and salpingitis in ♀, although asymptomatic carriage more common than with urethral infection in ♂.
- *Moraxella catarrhalis*: less common than *N. meningitidis*. Urethritis reported in ♂.
- *Streptococcal infection*: isolated case reports of acute balanitis following fellatio caused by group A streptococci. Balanitis due to group B infection appears to be related to vaginal coitus.
- *Haemophilus influenzae*: case reports of *H. influenzae*-associated septic abortion related to recent oral sex.

Syphilis

The resurgence of syphilis in the UK, W. Europe, and N. America has largely arisen in MSM and their partners. Studies have shown that over a third reported oral sex as the only risk factor, frequently not considering this to be a risk. Oral sex is much less likely to be condom protected compared with anal sex. The reporting of oral sex (often anonymous) among MSM is extremely common, and there is a significant association with higher numbers of oral sex partners, although not with particular oral practices. Kissing as a means of transmission has also been implicated.

Pregnancy

Bacterial vaginosis

Increased bacterial production of cytokines and prostaglandins and amniotic fluid/chorioamniotic infection leading to:

- chorioamnionitis
- low birth weight
- preterm birth (relative risk 1.5–2.3) from preterm labour and premature rupture of membranes
- 2nd trimester miscarriage (up to 3–6-fold risk)
- endometritis (pre/post-delivery, including Caesarean section).

History of previous premature delivery ↑ risk of further preterm birth 7-fold with BV. Risk of preterm birth higher with BV in early rather than late pregnancy.

Data from clinical trials screening for and treating BV during pregnancy have produced conflicting results. Therefore, current UK (BASHH guidelines recommend:

- Symptomatic ♀ should be treated (as if non-pregnant).
- There is insufficient evidence to recommend routinely screening and treating asymptomatic ♀ attending GUM for BV.

Candidiasis

Vaginal prevalence rate doubles in pregnancy to ~40% (↑ circulating oestrogens and vaginal glycogen). Although not usually associated with chorioamnionitis or preterm delivery, there is limited evidence that eradicating vaginal candidiasis during pregnancy may ↓ risk of preterm delivery.

Chlamydia

Associated with preterm delivery, low birth weight, premature rupture of membranes (PROM), intrapartum pyrexia, endometritis, neonatal infection (➲ Chapter 9, 'Pregnancy and the neonate', pp. 154–5) and post-abortal pelvic inflammatory disease. Screening is advised for those at risk, including those having surgical termination of pregnancy (rates of 2–30% reported). Tetracyclines, fluoroquinolones, and co-trimoxazole are contraindicated during pregnancy.

Gonorrhoea

In view of the ↑ risks of preterm delivery, low birth rate, PROM, endometritis, and neonatal infection (➲ Chapter 8, 'Sexual and non-sexual transmission', p. 140), and post-abortal pelvic inflammatory disease, screening for gonorrhoea is advisable in PROM, septic abortion, intra-/post-partum fever, or those considered to be at risk. Quinolone and tetracycline antibiotics are contraindicated during pregnancy.

Group B streptococcal infection

➲ Chapter 31, '*Streptococcus agalactiae*', p. 346.

Hepatitis B virus (HBV)

Pregnancy does not ↑ maternal morbidity or mortality from HBV infection or ↑ the risk of foetal complications, although preterm labour increases with acute HBV infection. In acute maternal infection the neonatal risk depends on gestational age with 10% transmission risk in the 1st trimester rising to 80–90% in the 3rd trimester. With chronic HBV infection, i.e. hepatitis B surface antigen (HBsAg) positive, transmission risk depends on maternal infectivity with 90% of infants born to hepatitis Be antigen (HBeAg) ♀ becoming chronic carriers compared with <5% if HBeAg –ve and HBsAg +ve. Maternal screening in pregnancy is important as neonatal passive immunization (hepatitis B immunoglobulin) given within 24 hours of birth combined with active vaccination ↓ the 90% chronic carriage rate with HBeAg +ve infection to 10–15% and with HBeAg –ve infection to <1%.

Hepatitis C virus (HCV)

~5% of infants born to HCV-infected ♀ become infected, i.e. serum HCV-RNA detected in at least two samples and/or HCV antibody reactive when the infant is at least 15 months old. Maternal HIV co-infection ↑ the risk of transmitting HCV 2–3-fold. As only 30–50% of infected infants have HCV-RNA detected at birth, it seems that the majority acquire infection at delivery. However, several studies have shown no difference in the neonatal incidence rate with regard to mode of delivery. Although there are contradictory data on breastfeeding it need not be avoided in mono-infected pregnant ♀.

Herpes simplex virus

85% of neonatal infections are acquired perinatally (exposure from infected birth canal), with 5% due to intrauterine exposure (usually ascending lower genital tract infection) and 10% postnatally (contact with family and staff). Risk of neonatal herpes is very low (probably <1%) for ♀ with recurrent herpes. Highest risk is when the mother has not seroconverted by delivery, with a 40–50% risk of neonatal herpes if primary infection is acquired in the 3rd trimester and a 20% risk for initial HSV-2 infection with previous HSV-1 infection.

Oral aciclovir should be prescribed as indicated for initial episodes and intravenous (IV) aciclovir for severe genital or disseminated infection, with case reports demonstrating significantly improved survival of the neonate. It is rarely indicated for the treatment of recurrences during pregnancy. For further information ➔ Chapter 22, 'Pregnancy and neonatal infection', pp. 286–8.

HIV

Most HIV transmission risk occurs during delivery and postpartum (breastfeeding), with antepartum (transplacental) spread uncommon. Pregnancy does not ↑ maternal morbidity or progression of infection. In ♀ with asymptomatic infection there is no ↑ in foetal malformations or antenatal mortality and only a small ↑ in spontaneous abortion, possible ↑ in low birth weight and preterm delivery. With optimized antenatal/postnatal care and antiretroviral treatment transmission rates are ↓ from 10–40% to <2%.

Sexually acquired reactive arthritis

This is uncommon in pregnancy, but if treatment is required select appropriate antibiotic (➔ Chapter 14, 'Pregnancy', p. 211), try to restrict use of non-steroidal anti-inflammatory drugs and avoid methotrexate, gold salts, and tumour necrosis factor (TNF) blockers.

Syphilis

Syphilis can be transmitted at any stage of pregnancy. In early untreated maternal syphilis preterm delivery or perinatal death will occur in 50% of all maternal 1° or 2° syphilis and 40% of those with early latent infections. With late untreated infection up to 20% prematurity/perinatal death 10% of infants develop congenital syphilis. Therefore, all pregnant ♀ should be screened for syphilis at the initial booking visit.

Early syphilis is treated with procaine benzylpenicillin G 750 mg IM daily for 10 days or benzathine benzylpenicillin, single dose in 1st and 2nd trimester with a second dose after 1 week if treated during the third trimester. Second-line treatments include oral amoxicillin 500 mg with oral probenecid 500 mg qds for 14 days, IM ceftriaxone 500 mg daily for 10 days (limited data) and oral macrolides (erythromycin 500 mg qds for 14 days or azithromycin 500 mg daily for 10 days). However, there are case reports of congenital infection with macrolides, so if used neonatal treatment is required after delivery. Late syphilis is treated as for non-pregnant patients but excluding doxycycline. See also ➜ Chapter 7, 'Management of positive syphilis serology in pregnancy', pp. 131–2).

Trichomoniasis (TV)

There is an independent association in pregnancy with premature rupture of the membranes, preterm delivery, and low birth weight. Although treatment (with metronidazole) is advocated for symptomatic ♀, there is no value in providing antenatal screening and treatment for asymptomatic ♀. There is no evidence that treatment will ↓ the risk of preterm birth and in one trial the treatment of asymptomatic ♀ with metronidazole appeared to be associated with preterm birth. The reason is unclear, and it has even been postulated that it may be due to an immune reaction elicited by the dying TV or virus released from its cytoplasm.

Urinary tract infection

More common during pregnancy with 2–10% of ♀ having asymptomatic bacteriuria. Without treatment, this persists with a third progressing to acute pyelonephritis. Complications include low birth weight/prematurity, pre-eclampsia, maternal anaemia, amnionitis, and intra-uterine death with risks reduced by treating asymptomatic bacteriuria.

Symptomatic UTI most commonly occurs towards the end of the 2nd trimester because of hormonal changes, although progression to pyelonephritis is uncommon.

All pregnant ♀ should be screened for bacteriuria, ideally by urine culture, although reagent strip testing, although less effective, is cheaper. Asymptomatic and symptomatic bacteriuria should be treated for 7-10 days (➜ Chapter 21, 'Management', pp. 275–6) avoiding aminoglycosides, quinolones, tetracyclines, and trimethoprim (1st trimester). ♀ with acute pyelonephritis should be assessed in hospital as hydration is crucial.

Warts

Commonly appear, proliferate, or enlarge rapidly during pregnancy, probably related to relative immunosuppression. There is no known association of human papilloma infection with pregnancy complications and they do not usually obstruct vaginal delivery. Occurrence of Buschke–Lowenstein tumours has been reported occurring during pregnancy.

Treatment options are limited as podophyllotoxin and podophyllin are contraindicated and imiquimod is not licensed in pregnancy, although its use has been reported. As risks are low and regression after delivery is usual, information and reassurance are appropriate for most ♀ affected.

Sexual assault: general principles

Definitions
➔ Chapter 2, 'Sexual offences', pp. 27–8.

Introduction
Sexual assault is highly prevalent and often remains undisclosed. Reasons for non-disclosure are multifactorial and may include lack of faith in the criminal justice system, feelings of guilt, fear, and the desire to protect partners and or family. Victims of sexual assault may present to GUM and sexual health services. Clinicians need to be aware of its presentation and the appropriate steps for assessment, referral, and management, including appropriate safeguarding of children and vulnerable adults.

Background
A British Crime Survey showed 19.9% of women and 3.6% of men had experienced sexual assault (including attempts). Of these, 33% of people told no one and only 17% reported the incident to the police. A perpetrator is more likely to be known to the victim than be a stranger.

Latest police recorded crime figures showed an increase of 37% in all sexual offences. The main factors thought to explain this rise are an improvement in crime recording by the police and an increase in victims coming forward to report these crimes. Sexual offences are one of the longest cases to complete in court, reflecting the complexities involved.

The impact of sexual assault on a victim is diverse. Social/interpersonal effects may manifest as strain on relationships or social isolation, but the impact may be far wider on society as a whole, e.g. fear in the community or inability of the victim to work. Associated short-term effects include physical injury (reported by 45% of victims) or other negative health effects (5% report pregnancy and 3% STIs). 61% suffer mental or emotional problems.

Perpetrators often use alcohol and or drugs—drug-facilitated sexual assault (DFSA)—to make it easier to commit sexual assault. This can compromise the victim's ability to consent to sexual activity through disinhibition and diminished capacity. Drugs used are commonly referred to as 'date rape drugs', chosen because they are quick acting, relax voluntary muscles, and have the effects of lasting anterograde amnesia for the events occurring. Alcohol is the most commonly used substance in DFSA and can potentiate the effects of drugs if taken in combination.

Presentation
Victims of sexual assault may or may not disclose the assault, and may not have any physical signs or injuries. Presentation may be acute within hours of the assault or many years after. Sexual assault referral centres (SARC) in the UK provide assessment and management of victims of sexual assault. SARC functions include:
- discussion of the options available
- taking of forensic samples/gathering evidence in a secure environment
- documentation of injuries
- signposting on for medical care and psychological support
- STI screening (in some centres) or onward referral to GUM/Integrated sexual health (ISH) services.

Multiagency work is key in the management of sexual assault with appropriate sharing of information and ongoing support/aftercare arrangements.

Coordinated approach
- Facilitates disclosure of sexual assault
- Boosts confidence in the criminal justice system
- Improves short- and long-term effects in victims
- Reduces negative health/psychological consequences
- Increases conviction rate.

Staff should have the relevant contact information for SARCs, and other local support services in order to liaise with or signpost where appropriate. These may include:
- Police stations/specialist sexual offence police units
- Child protection/safeguarding teams
- Local mental health services
- Voluntary organizations, e.g. Reach, Victim Support, Rape Crisis Centres, Respond, and others
- Multi-agency sexual exploitation (MASE) or multi-agency child sexual exploitation (MACE): these are meetings that are held to discuss safeguarding cases, and attendance by referring clinicians or those involved in the patients care may be required.
- Multi-agency safeguarding hubs (MASH) provide a link between universal services, e.g. schools, healthcare settings, and statutory services, such as police and social care. The aim is to improve multi-agency work and to prevent young people from 'slipping through the net'. Clinicians who deal with young people should have links with and an awareness of their local hub.

Acute assault: initial assessment

Some initial screening questions will aid in gathering information and inform what steps will be taken in the assessment and management of the case:
- When did the sexual assault occur?
- What type of sexual assault/act occurred?
- Did they give consent?
- Were they competent to give consent?
- Have they reported this to the police/want to report to the police?
- Are there any physical injuries that need medical attention?

In acute presentations, treatment of serious physical injury following assault must take precedence over obtaining forensic evidence. Where this is not relevant, timed samples of blood and urine are important (for alcohol and drug assays), together with oral samples (mouth washings/swabs), which should be taken as soon as possible after the attack to avoid the loss of potentially useful evidence.

The victim should have the choice of an experienced ♂ or ♀ clinician where possible. Ideally, a suitable appointment with minimum waiting time and a private waiting area should be provided. It is crucial to explore victim's needs and wishes, and ensure that arrangements are in place for anonymous reporting of incidents to the police if they do not want to make a formal charge.

Information to be provided to victim
- Reporting to the police and releasing forensic samples/information.
- Remaining anonymous but releasing forensic samples and some information to the police (3rd party reporting).
- Storing all forensic samples and information at the sexual assault referral centre (SARC), in case they want to release them at a later date (self-referral).
- Proceeding with STI screening/GUM assessment without police or forensic involvement.

Safeguarding

All clinicians working with young people should be aware of named individuals for safeguarding in their trust.

Forensic testing

Forensic examination should be only undertaken by those who are forensically trained, with the correct equipment and in a suitable environment to decrease the chance of DNA contamination. Forensic examiners have both a therapeutic and forensic role. Examination is top to toe, documenting any injuries/other findings on a detailed body chart, and taking of appropriate swabs to try and detect any DNA from the perpetrator. Colposcopic examination, where appropriate, may be performed to record any injuries in the anogenital region.

If the victim wishes to proceed with forensic examination, they should be advised about the importance of preserving evidence. Where possible, keep clothing unwashed and sanitary wear, avoid brushing teeth, drinking liquids, and bathing or washing. If DFSA is suspected, hair should not be dyed as this may interfere with hair analysis for toxicology.

'Early evidence test kits' are available from the police and in A&E, and these should be used as early as possible. The kit includes a mouthwash, mouth swab, and urine sample that can be obtained and kept for evidence where required. Advice should then be taken from the local SARC as to whether a forensic examination is appropriate.

Sexual assault: management

If reporting the sexual assault to the police, defer examination and screening for STIs until after forensic examination to protect evidence. It is possible to have a forensic examination at the local SARC without police involvement (self-referral).

The management of victims of sexual assault should include:

- Screening for STIs.
- Consideration of emergency contraception.
- Psychological support.

Medical evidence may be required in court and well-written documentation in the notes is vital. Use of a *pro forma* can ensure all necessary information is recorded and no vital areas of management are missed.

History-taking

In addition to the standard history, detailed information is needed regarding the assault and should be approached in a calm and sensitive manner. Asking a patient to give full details of an assault can be very distressing and the patient should only disclose as much information as they feel comfortable with.

Sexual assault: history checklist

- *Presenting/associated symptoms*: e.g. vaginal/anal pain, bleeding, bruising.
- *Date/time of assault*: essential for determining when STI screening should occur and the need for emergency contraception.
- *Location of assault*: to assess the background prevalence of certain STIs, especially if the attacker is a stranger.
- *Perpetrator(s) details*: Assessing the risk of the acquisition of STIs:
  • number of perpetrators
  • known or stranger
  • if known—any risk factors in perpetrator for blood-borne viruses, HIV, hepatitis B/C.
- *Associated physical violence*.
- *Was assault reported to police? Does the victim want to report?*
- *Has a forensic examination been performed?* Important as forensic examination should be performed prior to STI screening.
- *Were alcohol/drugs taken prior to attack? To establish the possibility of DFSA.*
- *Is the GP aware of the assault and/or a rape support agency been contacted?* To assess any treatment given and psychological support arranged.
- *Details regarding type of attack*: to determine the exact nature of the attack for legal purposes and the risks/sites of possible STIs or injury:
  • Physical injury (new or old)
    — Vagina, anal, oral, digital/penile penetration
    — Ejaculation
    — Condom use
    — Sexual history (before/after assault).

NB: Those assaulted may be too upset to recall this information or may have blanked out the detail as a means of coping. Therefore, it is wise to offer screening from all sites and this may provide additional assurance to the patient.

Other areas of history taking
- Past medical/surgical history.
- Gynaecological, contraceptive, obstetric history.
- Psychiatric history.
- *Medications*: prescribed, over the counter, drugs of abuse, and allergies.
- *Social history*:
  - *Family circumstances, children*—it is important to ensure that the patient is safe from further assault once they go home.
  - *If the victim has children*—their safety must also be considered and, where relevant, a discussion had with the local safeguarding team.

Examination

This should be performed sensitively and in privacy, with the victim's consent. In recent assault cases, the presence or absence of visible trauma should be clearly documented with the use of body mapping/diagrams.
- General state, including any signs of intoxication; general behaviour.
- Height, weight, body mass index.
- *Observations*: blood pressure, heart rate.
- *Both sexes*: examine the mouth in cases of recent forced oral penetration to look for signs of injury, e.g. haemorrhages on the palate.
- *Female*: examination of the genitalia looking for signs of injury or infection. This may include Cusco's speculum to inspect for internal signs of infection or injury.
- *Male*: examination of external genitalia and perianal area looking for signs of injury or infection. Offer proctoscopy if recent forced anal penetration for any signs of trauma or infection.

More detailed examination: signs to look for
- *Anogenital injury*: in post-pubertal, anogenital injury is found in up to a third of those sexually assaulted. Severity of assault is a poor predictor of anogenital injury. However, presence of anogenital injury is considered to carry more weight in obtaining a conviction. The site should be recorded using a 'clock-face'.
- *Bruising*: bruising may be difficult to interpret. Appearances may assist in the interpretation of its cause (e.g. bruising from finger-tips).
- *Leakage of blood into skin due to blunt trauma*:
  - *Petechiae*—bruises <2 mm due to increased pressure (strangulation, etc.), oblique blunt trauma, suction, blunt trauma through fabrics, medical causes (infection, coughing, medication, blood disorders)
  - *Purpura*—larger haemorrhages within the skin
  - *Haematoma*—blood collection beneath the skin.
- *Abrasions (scratches—linear, grazes—broad)*: involve only outerskin layers
- *Lacerations (tears)*: full-thickness splitting of skin, usually irregular and often associated with bruising
- *Others*: incision, stab wounds, thermal (dry heat or moist heat (scald), electrical, friction, cigarette, fracture.

Investigations

It is rare for the presence of an STI to legally reinforce a case of rape. It is advisable to do a full screen at presentation to detect any pre-existing STIs. However, it is recommended that tests are repeated 2 weeks after the assault, as early sampling may miss recently acquired infection. (i.e. the window period.) See Table 6.3 for the investigations by site after sexual assault.

Ensure that the patient fully understands what investigations/tests are recommended and their implications. Where possible the 'chain of evidence' should be implemented (i.e. every handover of the specimen must be signed, dated, and timed).

As well as a standard STI screen and microscopy, additional specimens should be considered. If the patient does not want serological testing at presentation a serum specimen can be stored. This may help to clarify the timing of any subsequent seroconversion.

Table 6.3 Investigations by site after sexual assault

Female consenting to examination	Investigation	Site
	NAAT for C. trachomatis and N. gonorrhoeae	From any site of penetration vulvovaginal, throat, rectum. NAAT for N. gonorrhoeae screening is highly sensitive, but should be confirmed by culture for medico-legal purposes
	Culture for N. gonorrhoeae	From any site of penetration: endocervical, throat, and rectum (advised even in the absence of forced anal penetration)
	Microscopy: only if symptomatic	Vaginal, endocervical, and rectal smears for N. gonorrhoeae
		Vaginal preparations for yeasts, bacterial vaginosis, and T. vaginalis
	Culture or NAAT (if available) for T. vaginalis	Vaginal (only if symptomatic)
Female not consenting to examination	Self-taken NAAT for C. trachomatis and N. gonorrhoeae	From any site of penetration vulvovaginal, throat, rectum
	Self-taken culture for N. gonorrhoeae	Vaginal, throat, rectum
	Self-taken culture	Vaginal (only if symptomatic). For yeasts, bacterial vaginosis, and T. vaginalis
Male consenting to examination	NAAT for C. trachomatis and N. gonorrhoeae	From any site of penetration: urethral swab or urine, throat, rectum
	Culture for N. gonorrhoeae	From any site of penetration: urethral, throat, and rectum
	Microscopy: only if symptomatic	Urethral and rectal smears for N. gonorrhoeae

(Continued)

Table 6.3 (Contd.)

Male not consenting to examination	*Self-taken NAAT for C. trachomatis and N. gonorrhoeae*	From any site of penetration: urine, throat, rectum
	Culture for N. gonorrhoeae	From any site of penetration: urethral, throat, and rectum
Male and female	Syphilis serology	
	HIV serology	4th-generation test HIV antibody and p24 antigen
	Hepatitis B virus	
	Hepatitis C virus	If victim has risk factor, assailant unknown, or if assailant known to have risk factor
	Storage bloods	If victim does not wish baseline testing.

Management
- Offer treatment for any infection detected.
- Assess mental state and suicide risk.
- A health adviser can reinforce information given, provide links for psychological support, and clarify the follow-up arrangements. Provide contact numbers of agencies able to provide further psychosocial/ emotional support.

Sexual assault: management checklist
- Treat any infection found.
- *Emergency contraception*: if indicated.
- *Prophylactic antibiotics*: consider for chlamydia and gonorrhoea if the patient cannot tolerate an examination or requires an intra-uterine device for emergency contraception. Disadvantages include unnecessary treatment, risk of re-infection if source was not the perpetrator and no PN performed.
- *Hepatitis B immunization*: hepatitis B infection is very rare post-sexual assault, but immunization may prevent development of infection for those at risk if given within 6 weeks following an assault.
- *HIV prophylaxis*: individual risk assessment needed, including type and location of assault and assailant risk factors. If offered, this should be within 72 hours of the sexual assault.
- *Support*: may be provided by a health adviser, specialist nurse, or other agencies.
- *Obtain consent to write to general practitioner*: important for the sharing of information.
- *Review*: for follow-up of any infection detected, repeat investigations (to cover 'window periods'), hepatitis immunization, and psychological support.

Sexual assault: forensic assessment

Purpose

To establish:
- exact documentation of injuries
- identification and retrieval of any possible evidence
- relevant illnesses/previous trauma that may affect the interpretation of injuries/evidence.

Consent

Document in notes discussion of the concept of confidentiality and the potential disclosure of any documented information to the police if the assault is reported to ensure informed consent is obtained.

Consent must be given for both non-genital and genital examination, and the recording of findings (including photography), the retention of relevant items of clothing, the collection of forensic evidence, and disclosure to police, Crown Prosecution Service, and Crown Court.

Forensic assessment

Timing

An understanding of forensic timescales can help to advise patients and facilitate referral for forensic testing when requested/appropriate.

The sooner that forensic examination occurs, the better will be the evidence obtained. If the assault is recent (i.e. <14 days,) then a discussion should take place with the SARC, regarding the collection of evidence and documentation of injuries even if the patient does not wish to report to the police.

Timeframe for DNA evidence

- *Mouth*; <48 hours.
- *Skin*: <48 hours.
- *Digital penetration*: <12 hours.
- *Anal*: <72 hours.
- *Vaginal*: <7 days.
- *Blood for toxicology*: <72 hours.
- *Seminal fluid/soil/fibres in skin*: 2 days; 7 days if unwashed
- *Urine for toxicology*: <14 days
- *Head hair*: 6 months
- *Documentation of injuries*: <21 days

Child sexual assault

Definition

'Forcing or enticing a child or young person to take part in sexual activities, not necessarily involving a high level of violence, whether or not the child is aware of what is happening. The activities may involve physical contact, including assault by penetration (for example, rape or oral sex) or non-penetrative acts such as masturbation, kissing, rubbing and touching outside of clothing. They may also include non-contact activities, such as involving children in looking at, or in the production of, sexual images, watching sexual activities, encouraging children to behave in sexually inappropriate ways, or grooming a child in preparation for abuse (including via the Internet). Sexual abuse is not solely perpetrated by adult males. Women can also commit acts of sexual abuse, as can other children.'

Reproduced from HM Government. Working together to safeguard children (2015) under the Open Government Licence v3.0.

Approach to sexual abuse

When a young person presents with a STI, sexual health-related problem or for sexual health advice, consideration should be given as to whether they are being sexually abused or exploited. In view of recent high profile cases of child sexual exploitation, it is now recommended that, for under-16s, a risk assessment is performed to flag up any vulnerabilities or indicators of risk. 'Spotting the signs' is a national *pro forma* developed by BASHH and the young people's sexual health charity Brook. It provides a framework to help professionals to identify and assess risk and vulnerabilities and can be used in young people up to aged 18 years.

The presence of an STI may be a marker of child sexual abuse and, if sexual abuse is suspected, screening for STIs should be considered. If infection is found in a child aged <3 years for chlamydia and <1 years for gonorrhoea, vertical transmission from the mother is possible so she should be offered STI screening. This may be extended to the siblings and others in the household.

When prepubertal children present, they should be seen in a designated SARC, together with a consultant paediatrician who may be trained in forensic examination or who will work together with a forensics examiner. The paediatrician will usually be the lead for child protection and have links to safeguarding teams in the local area. A colposcope or other equipment for photo documentation of findings should be available. Post-pubertal children who are under 16 may be seen in dedicated children's services or, if they prefer, in an adult SARC or GUM/ISH clinic. Young people aged 16–18 are seen in an adult SARC or a GUM/ISH clinic.

All GUM / ISH clinics should have:
- Guidelines for the management of children.
- A nominated consultant physician to take the lead for children as part of a multidisciplinary team with access to formal child protection training.

- Details of local child protection policies and procedures.
- Chain of evidence procedures (➲ Chapter 6, 'Investigations', p. 107).
- Regular audit of adherence to child protection guidelines.

Consent to examination

If the child is under 13, they cannot consent to examination or treatment; written consent must be sought from a person with parental responsibility. If the child is between 13 and 16, ideally, they should be accompanied by a person with parental responsibility; they should sign the written consent together. If the child does not want a parent to be involved, an advocate over the age of 18 should be with them to witness consent.

Sexually transmitted infections

STI transmission, pathogenesis, presentation, and treatment depends upon the child's age and hormonal status. In view of positive and negative predictive values, the significance of an STI in children requires careful interpretation. It may be used as corroborative evidence to indicate sexual abuse and if there may be medico-legal proceedings, a 'chain of evidence' should be in place, so that a sample can be accounted for from the time it is taken until the result is known. If infection is found, test and treat any consensual or non-consensual sexual contacts (with consent), and test (and treat if appropriate) parents when there is a chance of vertical transmission.

STI testing

This should be performed at baseline, with tests for gonorrhoea and chlamydia repeated 2 weeks after the last penetrative contact (if necessary), and baseline serology for HIV, syphilis, and hepatitis B and C with repeat testing after 12 weeks. If high risk of exposure to hepatitis B or C, repeat serology after 6 months is advised.

NAATs are generally accepted as the gold standard for chlamydia, although they are unlicensed for oropharyngeal, rectal, and urogenital specimens in children. A positive result should be confirmed by a second NAAT (although culture is considered to be the most specific test for chlamydia, it is rarely available). Culture for gonorrhoea is required for legal purposes, although NAAT is more sensitive. Any positive NAAT should be confirmed by culture, where possible.

When testing prepubertal girls (usually <11 years) introital swabs should be used from inside the labia minora, but avoiding the hymen. A trans-hymenal swab (ear, nose and throat swabs are smaller) may be used if the hymenal orifice is large enough to allow the passage of a swab without distress. FVU for chlamydia and gonorrhoea NAAT should be undertaken in boys (and girls if other tests are not feasible).

Physician-taken or self-taken vulvovaginal swabs are sufficiently sensitive for NAAT. Self-sampling can be considered if age-appropriate, and depending on the wishes and understanding of the young person.

Sampling from all sites should be considered for any alleged sexual abuse in view of the fact that there may not be disclosure of all sites of sexual contact. For suspected abuse, decisions should be made on a case-by-case basis.

Samples

Table 6.4 Recommended samples after sexual assault

Girls: urogenital Essential	NAAT • *C. trachomatis* • *N. gonorrhoeae*	Vulvovaginal (post-pubertal), /trans-hymenal (prepubertal)
	Culture *N. gonorrhoeae*	NAAT for *N. gonorrhoeae* screening can be considered as highly sensitive, but should be confirmed by culture for medico-legal purposes.
	Microscopy	If symptomatic for *N. gonorrhoeae*
Girls: urogenital Optional	*Microscopy (if available)* • *T. vaginalis* • *Candida* spp. • Bacterial vaginosis	If discharge present

	Swab
	• (Amies medium)
	   • *T. vaginalis*
	   • *Candida* spp.
	• Culture and microscopy for clue cells.
	Swab for *T. vaginalis* NAAT if available	

	Urine NAAT for *C. trachomatis* and *N. gonorrhoeae*	Only if child/carer declines examination or if the vulvovaginal swab is self-taken
	Rectal swab: • NAAT for *C. trachomatis* and *N. gonorrhoeae* • Culture *N. gonorrhoeae*	If anal assault is alleged or suspected
	Pharyngeal swab NAAT for: • *C. trachomatis* and • *N. gonorrhoeae*	If oral assault is alleged or suspected
	Culture: • *N. gonorrhoeae*	
Boy: urogenital	• Microscopy for pus cells and Gram −ve intracellular diplococci • Culture for *N. gonorrhoeae*	If urethritis: • Meatal swab—prepubertal • Urethral swab—post-pubertal
	Urine for: • *C. trachomatis* • *N. gonorrhoeae*.	

Table 6.4 (Contd.)

	Rectal swab: • NAAT for *C. trachomatis* and *N. gonorrhoeae* • Culture *N. gonorrhoeae*	If anal assault is alleged or suspected
	Pharyngeal swab: • NAAT for *C. trachomatis* and *N. gonorrhoeae* • Culture *N. gonorrhoeae*	If oral assault is alleged or suspected
Anogenital blisters or ulcers	• Swab for HSV • NAAT • HSV serology for IgM and IgG (paired sera at 3-week interval) • Consider dark ground microscopy for *Treponema pallidum* • Swab for bacterial culture • Syphilis serology, repeated at 4-6 weeks and 12 weeks	
Anogenital warts		HPV typing of surgically removed warts is currently controversial. It may be considered in specific cases, but not justified for routine use.
Girls and boys	Serology: • HIV 4th generation test recommended (antibodies and p24 antigen)	Consider testing for HIV, syphilis, hepatitis B and C in all cases, depending on risk factors. • Check at presentation and 12 weeks after the assault. Repeat serology advised 6 months after the assault for hepatitis B and C if considered to be at high risk. • If blood-testing declined or not appropriate, saliva sampling, and POCT can be performed for HIV, repeated 12 weeks after sexual assault (role in children unknown.) If positive, requires confirmation with venous blood.

Management

Wherever possible treatment for children should be prescribed within the terms of the product licence. However, some conditions may require drugs not specifically licensed for paediatric use. If in doubt, discuss with local pharmacist.

Specific infections

Chlamydia

Can be found in the rectum, vagina, conjunctiva, or nasopharynx of children, and can be asymptomatic. The estimated risk of vertically acquired transmission is 50–70%, mostly conjunctivitis, but up to 15% have infection of the vagina and rectum (which can persist up to 3 years). The risk of chlamydia is 3–17% in sexually abused children and chlamydia was reported in 75–94% of 0–12-year-olds with a history of sexual abuse. Asymptomatic presentation is common, especially girls with cervico-vaginal infection. Sexual abuse is the most likely mode of transmission in a child with chlamydia and an urgent referral should be made to the safeguarding team.

Gonorrhoea

Gonorrhoea is uncommon in sexually abused children with a reported risk of 0–4% (0–2% in UK studies.) In children with non-conjunctival gonorrhoea, sexual abuse was reported in 36–83% of 0–12-year-olds and 90–100% of 5–12-year-olds had sexual contact. Estimated risk of perinatal transmission resulting in gonococcal ophthalmia is 30%.

Most common symptom is vaginal/urethral discharge, but ~45% is asymptomatic. Sexual abuse is the most likely mode of transmission in a child with gonorrhoea and an urgent referral should be made to the safeguarding team.

Herpes

Prevalence in prepubertal children is unknown, but is thought to be uncommon, reported in <1% of sexually abused children. Regardless of this, sexual abuse should always be considered in children with genital herpes. Auto-inoculation should also be considered. Although there are few published studies to inform whether sexual abuse is the likely mode of transmission in children with genital herpes, where infected children have been evaluated, 1 in 2, and 6 in 8 were found to have been abused. The diagnosis of genital herpes in a prepubertal child necessitates an urgent referral to the safeguarding team. A positive diagnosis of herpes in the mother does not exclude sexual abuse.

HIV

The risk of HIV acquisition in sexually abused children depends on the local prevalence. If vertical transmission or blood contamination is excluded, sexual abuse is the most likely source of HIV infection. Most children acquire HIV infection non-sexually, although transmission following assault has been reported. HIV infection in the mother of a child with HIV does not exclude the possibility of sexual abuse.

Syphilis

There is limited evidence on syphilis in sexually abused children. Although it is reported in less than 1% of sexually abused children between 0—12 years old, children presenting with 1° or 2° stages of syphilis should be considered to be victims of sexual abuse, where vertical perinatal or blood contamination has been excluded. Congenital syphilis is now uncommon in the UK, but this is likely to ↑ with the ↑ prevalence of syphilis.

The diagnosis of syphilis in a child under 13 years of age necessitates a referral to the safeguarding team, depending on the stage of infection and evidence of other modes of transmission. A positive diagnosis in the mother does not exclude sexual abuse.

Trichomoniasis

In girls with confirmed infection of *T. vaginalis*, sexual abuse is likely, although consensual sexual activity must be considered.

Although there is no evidence to inform at what age vertical transmission can be excluded, *T. vaginalis*, in girls younger than 2 months may be a result of perinatal infection, maintained by maternal oestrogen, although sexual abuse should still be considered.

If *T. vaginalis*, is diagnosed in a child between 6 weeks and 13 years old, an urgent referral should be made to the safeguarding team. In children over 13 years, it should be considered on a case-by-case basis.

Anogenital warts

Genital warts are more likely to indicate sexual abuse than previously thought and sexual abuse must always be considered in any child presenting with anogenital warts. In children with genital warts, sexual abuse was reported in 31–58% of 1–14 year olds. The diagnosis of anogenital warts in a child under 13 years of age necessitates an urgent referral to the safeguarding team.

HPV types 6 or 11 can cause genital warts in adults and children, but in children types 1 and 2 (cutaneous) are also found. Although sexual abuse must be considered, e.g. by touching, types 1 and 2 can also suggest possible non-sexual acquisition, including auto-inoculation. If HPV is vertically transmitted, genital warts may present months to years after birth. There is also a risk of laryngeal papillomatosis caused by peripartum transmission of HPV infection from the mother.

Bacterial vaginosis

The relevance of finding BV in children is unclear because BV is not classified as a STI. Variable rates of BV, from 7% to 34%, have been demonstrated in sexually abused girls. Although *Garderella vaginalis* has been isolated from the vagina in 4–14% (as for adults) and may be part of the normal flora, it has been shown to be related to an increase in sexual partners in sexually active girls.

Syphilis

Introduction *118*
Clinical features of acquired syphilis *120*
Pregnancy and congenital infection *123*
Diagnosis and investigation *125*
Management of syphilis *130*
Adverse treatment reactions *133*
Syphilis follow-up *134*
Partner notification and management *134*
Syphilis with HIV co-infection *135*

Introduction

The origins of syphilis are unclear, but it became an epidemic in Europe in the late 15th century, although skeletal evidence suggests earlier endemic infection. The name originates from a poem about the infected shepherd Syphilis written by Fracastoro in 1530.

Aetiology

Syphilis is caused by a delicate spirochaete, *Treponema pallidum* (TP). It has a cylindrical nucleus and cytoplasm contained within a cell wall and outer envelope with flagella in the periplasmic space, 6–20 μm × 0.1–0.18 μm in size. Micro-aerophilic, so can only be grown on tissue culture. It has limited viability outside its human host, so is usually transmitted sexually through micro-abrasions in mucosal skin.

Epidemiology and transmission

Currently high rates in Eastern Europe. In the UK, rates of transmission are highest amongst MSM, especially as outbreaks through anonymous sex in saunas, cruising sites, and geosocial networking apps, and in association with HIV infection. Entry site usually genital in heterosexuals, but often extra-genital (oral, anal, rectal) in MSM, via oro-genital, oro-anal, and anogenital contact.

Transmission routes are:
- *Sexual—only from early syphilis*: ~30–50% contacts are infected.
- *Accidental infection by inoculation*: e.g. healthcare professional.
- *Blood-borne*: needle sharing, blood transfusion (very rare as blood is screened and organisms die after 24–48 hours at 4°C.
- *Transplacental*: at any gestation. More common in early syphilis (80–90% risk) with RPR >1:8, rare after 4 years infection.

Natural history

➲ Chapter 7, 'Clinical features of acquired syphilis', pp. 120–2, for further details.

Acquired infection

Early syphilis

1°: chancre develops 9—90 days after infection (average 21 days), regional lymphadenopathy. Resolves by 3–8 weeks.
2°: dissemination of infection develops 6 weeks to 6 months after infection in 25% untreated. 25% relapse in first 2 years if untreated.

Latent syphilis

Asymptomatic infection. Early latent if infected <2 years. Late latent if > 2 years (</>1 year in USA), outcome in 2/3 untreated syphilis.

Late syphilis
- Occurs in 1/3 untreated.
- *Gummatous*: musculoskeletal (10%), viscera/mucosa (15%) can occur <2 years, but usually after ~15 years.
- *Cardiovascular (10%)*: occurs after 10–30 years.
- *Neurosyphilis (10%)*: meningovascular after 2–7 years; general paresis after 10–20 years; tabes dorsalis after15–25 years.

Congenital syphilis
Early congenital syphilis if <2 years old. Late congenital lesions usually develop after 2–3 years.

Frequently asked questions
Box 7.1 outlines questions patients frequently ask.

Box 7.1 Frequently asked questions

Can I catch syphilis from oral sex?
Yes, you can catch syphilis from unprotected oral sex.

When I have been treated am I immune?
No. Having been infected once does not protect you from re-infection.

My blood tests are still positive after treatment – do I still have syphilis?
No. After infection with syphilis your body produces antibodies, which will usually remain detectable for life, and will be positive on screening tests. They do not provide protection against future infection. It is important to measure their nadir levels after treatment, as re-infection would cause a rise in their levels.

Does my partner need treating?
Your partner will require testing, and be offered treatment, either epidemiologically or if test is positive. Previous partners may also require testing and treating depending on how long you are likely to have had syphilis, and when your last sexual relationship was.
- 1°: all sexual partners within the past 3 months should be tested +/− treated
- 2° or early latent: all sexual partners in past 2 years need testing/treating.
- *Late syphilis*: this depends on estimated duration of infection.

When can I have sex again?
Recommendation is to abstain from sex until signs of 1° syphilis have resolved and 2 weeks after completing treatment.

Clinical features of acquired syphilis

Early syphilis

Primary syphilis
- *Presentation*: classically initial painless papule at inoculation site, which expands and ulcerates producing a usually solitary painless round/oval chancre 1–2 cm in diameter with indurated margin and clear, moist base, and serous exudate on pressure (➔ Plate 7), but may be atypical or 'contemporary' (➔ Plate 8). Bilateral painless regional lymphadenopathy, e.g. inguinal if genital lesion. In recent years, it has become more common to find multiple painful ulcers with little induration, mimicking herpes infection. Oral sex is a significant route of transmission with subsequent oropharyngeal ulceration.
- *Chancre site*: Genital chancre may appear anywhere on genitals, but commonly on mucosal surfaces. Cervical lesions are usually asymptomatic and do not produce inguinal lymphadenopathy. Rarely intra-urethral chancres can present as urethritis. Balanitis has also been reported (rare, including balanitis of Follman). Extragenital chancres are common and have been reported on lips, tongue, tonsils, pharynx, anal margin (painful, resembling anal fissure), rectum, and rarely finger, hand/arm, nipple, eyelid, and supraclavicular.

Secondary syphilis
Symptoms are a result of haematogenous dissemination of infection.
- Constitutional symptoms of malaise, fever, headache, anorexia, myalgia.
- Skin lesions may be polymorphic (80%), pruritic (40%):
  - *Macular*—pink 1 cm diameter, mostly on trunk.
  - *Papular*—dull red with shiny surface or papulosquamous with surface scale, often extensive, affecting flexor surfaces, palms, and soles (firm non-prominent papules). (➔ Plate 9).
  - Pustular and hyper- or hypo-pigmented lesions also been seen.
- *Lympadenopathy*: 75% inguinal, 60% generalized, splenomegaly.
- *Mucous membrane lesions (30%) 'mucous patch'*: ulcer with white/grey border may coalesce or form snail track ulcer, found in oral cavity, larynx (sore throat, hoarse), nasal mucosa, genitalia, anus, rectum (diffuse distal proctitis).
- *Alopecia*: specific 'moth eaten' or non-specific diffuse telogen effluvium.
- *Musculoskeletal*: periostitis (25% pre-antibiotic era) causing bone pain, especially tibia, and bursitis (6%), causing arthralgia.
- *Hepatitis (20%)*: usually subclinical raised enzymes, mainly alkaline phosphatase.
- *Renal*: glomerulonephritis (rare), nephrotic syndrome. Both mild and self-limiting.
- *Neurological*: meningism (1–2%), transitory cerebrospinal fluid (CSF) white cell and protein ↑ (5–40%), rarely meningitis/meningovasculitis, nerve deafness, peripheral neuropathy.
- *Eyes*: iritis (<1%), anterior uveitis (↑ in HIV infection), choroidoretinitis, optic atrophy (usually asymptomatic).

Early latent
No signs/symptoms, but positive serology within 2 years of infection.

Differential diagnosis of secondary syphilis

Macular rash
- HIV seroconversion.
- Pityriasis rosea (has initial herald patch).
- Tinea/pityriasis versicolor (hypo- or hyperpigmented scaly, mostly over trunk. Culture scales for *Malassezia furfur*).
- Measles (oral Koplik spots).
- Rubella (posterior cervical lymphadenopathy).
- Infectious mononucleosis [may be associated with false positive VDRL/RPR (Venereal Disease Research Laboratory/rapid plasma reagin).
- Drug reaction (association with drug administration, pruritus).

Papular rash
- Psoriasis (extensor surfaces, knees, elbows, scalp, nail pitting).
- Lichen planus (oral lesions, Wickhams striae).

Late syphilis

Late latent
No signs or symptoms, but positive syphilis serology >2 years after acquisition. More common now as active late syphilis ↓ due to widespread use of antibiotics for other infections.

Gummatous syphilis
Gumma formation (syphilitic granulation tissue) is due to reactivation of residual treponemes in sensitized host. Gummata are nodules or nodulo-ulcers, indurated and indolent, single or few in number. They commonly heal with central scarring, while peripherally still active. Ulcers are described as 'punched out' with a basal 'wash leather' appearance due to slough. They are not contagious and resolve with treatment.

Sites
- *Skin*: especially below knee, buttocks, thighs, shoulders, scalp, face.
- *Bones*: gummatous periostitis (bony proliferation), e.g. sabre tibia; gummatous osteitis with bone destruction.
- *Mouth and throat*: palatal perforation; gumma of tongue or superficial glossitis, associated with leucoplakia and malignancy; epiglot-tis destruction and laryngeal infiltration causing hoarseness.
- *Other organs*: gummata of liver, testis, oesophagus, stomach, intestine, cerebrum, spinal cord, aortic wall, myocardium. Also reported in bronchi and lungs, kidney, bladder adrenal glands, and breast.

Cardiovascular syphilis
- *Conduction defects*: if gummatous involvement (e.g. Stokes–Adams syndrome).

- *Aortitis leading to*:
  - *Aortic aneurysm*—proximal ascending aorta, fusiform, or saccular, without dissection. Presents as chest pain or signs of compression of adjacent structures, e.g. hoarseness, dysphagia.
  - *Aortic regurgitation* (30% of those with cardiovascular syphilis)— insidious, so well compensated. Typical early diastolic murmur on forced expiration with patient inclined forward.
  - *Coronary ostia stenosis* leading to angina and heart failure.

Neurosyphilis

- *Asymptomatic*: just abnormal CSF findings. Found in up to 30% of 1° and 2° syphilis, and usually does not become clinically relevant. In the pre-antibiotic era 23–87% of cases progressed to clinical neuro-syphilis.
- *Meningovascular*: focal arteritis causing infarction and meningeal inflammation. Now the most common neurosyphilitic presentation. Consider if cerebrovascular accident in a young adult. Often sudden onset, preceded by prodromal headache, insomnia, emotional lability, and mental deterioration. Hemiplegia/paresis, aphasia, seizures are typical features, but ocular palsy and trigeminal neuralgia may occur.
- *Pupillary abnormalities* are frequent with a full Argyll Robertson pupil (constriction on accommodation, not to light) in 10%.
- *General paralysis*: cortical neuronal loss. Insidious, dulling of intellect, judgement, and insight. Memory loss, antisocial behaviour, grandiose delusions (rare), hand and facial tremor, depression, and dementia. Seizures and paresis (spastic) are late complications. Full Argyll Robertson pupil in 25%.
- *Tabes dorsalis*: selective inflammation and degeneration of the spinal dorsal columns and nerve roots. Lightning pains, paraesthesia, visceral crises (smooth muscle spasm), sensory ataxia with stamping gait, and positive Romberg sign. Diminished or absent reflexes, deep pain, vibration, and position sense. Trophic changes lead to neuropathic joints (Charcot) and painless perforating plantar ulcers. Optic atrophy and bilateral ptosis are common. Argyll Robertson pupil seen most commonly in tabes dorsalis, with at least 80% developing pupil abnormalities.

Pregnancy and congenital infection

Syphilis in pregnancy

All pregnant ♀ should be screened for syphilis at initial booking visit. If new risk factors or symptoms become apparent, tests should be repeated later in pregnancy, with referral to Sexual Health services. Syphilis can be transmitted at any stage of pregnancy, with foetal infection reported from 9th week of gestation. However, it is most likely to arise after the 18th week. It may result in polyhydramnios, preterm labour, hydrops, congenital syphilis, miscarriage, and stillbirth, with spontaneous abortion most commonly occurring in 2nd and early 3rd trimester. Outcome in untreated infection varies with stage.

- *1° or 2° syphilis*: up to 50% prematurity/perinatal death and 50% congenital infection.
- *Early latent syphilis*: up to 40% prematurity/perinatal death and 20% congenital infection.
- *Late latent syphilis*: up to 20% prematurity/perinatal death and 10% congenital infection.
- *Normal control*: 9% prematurity/perinatal death.

Despite treatment in early syphilis up to 14% may result in foetal death or congenital infection.

If untreated syphilis is detected, consideration should be given to testing children from earlier pregnancies.

Early congenital syphilis (within first 2 years of life)

Two-thirds are asymptomatic at birth, but most develop signs by 2–12 weeks after birth. Features include:

- failure to thrive
- *snuffles*: mucosal lesions with pharyngeal and nasal involvement progressing to local destruction and perforation
- *skin lesions*:
  - rashes similar to 2° syphilis, but prominent around the mouth and body orifices leading to scarring (rhagades)
  - blistering bullous eruption of palms and soles (syphilitic pemphigus)
  - condylomata lata around anus and genitalia (see Plate 10)
- sparse hair and brittle, atrophic nails
- hepatosplenomegaly and moderate generalized lymphadenopathy
- osteochondritis and later periostitis especially of the long bones (may present as pseudoparalysis)
- other features may include meningitis, nephrotic syndrome, choroidoretinitis, anaemia, thrombocytopenia.

Late congenital syphilis (after 2 years of age)

No clinical features in about 60% (diagnosed on serology). Otherwise, many features are similar to late-stage-acquired syphilis (although the cardiovascular system is usually spared) with clinical manifestations usually appearing around the time of puberty.

Inflammatory complications

Interstitial keratitis: most common late feature, 20–50%.

• Deafness 2° to otolabyrinthitis.
• *Clutton's joints*: bilateral painless effusion of the knee joints.
• Gummata of nasal septum, palate and throat; skin and bone.
• *Neurosyphilis*: seizures, mental deficiency, juvenile tabes dorsalis and general paralysis.
• Paroxysmal cold haemoglobinuria.

Malformations

• *Craniofacial*: frontal bossing; 'bulldog' appearance—hypoplastic maxilla, high-arched palate, and prominent mandible; 'saddle-nose'; rhagades (peri-oral fissures).
• *Dental*:
  • *Hutchinson's incisors (usually upper central)*—conical, tapered towards the apex and notched.
  • *Hutchinson's triad*—Hutchinson's incisors, interstitial keratitis, and nerve deafness.
  • *Mulberry molars*—1st lower molars dome-shaped with hypoplastic cusps.
• *Skeletal*: bony sclerosis (generalized) or nodules (localized). Long bones primarily affected, especially the tibia with anterior bowing ('sabre tibia').

Frequently asked questions

I am pregnant, is syphilis harmful to my baby?
Syphilis in pregnancy is associated with a high risk of spontaneous abortion, premature delivery, perinatal death, and congenital syphilis. Risks are greater with early syphilis. Despite treatment of early syphilis during pregnancy, up to 14% will have a foetal death or a baby with congenital syphilis. Early congenital syphilis occurs within the first 2 years of life, late congenital manifestations occur after 2 years of age.

Diagnosis and investigations

Microscopy

Dark ground microscopy

→ Chapter 5, 'Slide preparation', p. 70.

* *1° syphilis*: serum from chancres (79–86% sensitivity)—less reliable for non-genital lesions, especially oral, because of other treponemes.
* Aspiration of a regional lymph node (especially if the chancre is secondarily infected).
* *1° and early congenital syphilis*: serum from mucous patches, ulcers, and condylomata lata.
* Treponemes are very slender with tight spirals moving forwards and backwards, rotating about longitudinal axis and angulating to ~90°.
* If negative and there is clinical suspicion, send for syphilis PCR and early repeat serology.
* If 2° infection of ulcer, saline lavage or antibiotics inactive against *T. pallidum* to clear contaminants (e.g. co-trimoxazole, quinolones).

Serological tests

See Table 7.1.

Positive serology usually found 4 weeks after infection, but may take up to 3 months to develop. Negative in up to 15% of those with chancre. Similar response with endemic treponematoses (→ Chapter 19, 'Endemic syphilis (bejel, dichuchwa)', p. 258). Positive results should always be confirmed by testing a second sample.

Non-specific treponemal tests

Cardiolipin antigen tests (reagin)

E.g. VDRL test, RPR test. It is inexpensive, readily quantifiable, and useful in assessing serial titres, but has potential for biological false positives (Box 7.2), and poor sensitivity in late syphilis. Usually positive 4 weeks after infection. Prozone phenomenon (false-negative results from strongly positive samples due to blocking antibodies) is excluded by specimen dilution.

Box 7.2 Biological false-positive reactions

VDRL/RPR (biological) tests have false positive reaction in <1% of the general population.

* *Acute (lasting < 6 months)*: usually <30 years of age:
  * acute febrile illnesses (e.g. EBV, HIV, viral hepatitis).
  * vaccination
  * pregnancy.
* *Chronic (persists >6 months)*: usually >30 years of age:
  * chronic infections (e.g. leprosy)
  * autoimmune conditions (e.g. lupus erythematosus) injecting drug use.

Table 7.1 Syphilis serological response: confirm with second sample!

Stage	EIA	TPPA	VDRL/RPR	IgM
Primary	+ve (90%)	+ve (90–100%) Usual titre 80–320	+ve (60–90%) Usual titre Neat-1:16	+ve
Secondary	+ve	+ve High titres ~5120	+ve Usual titre 1:32–1:256	+ve
Early latent	+ve	+ve Titres still usually high	+ve Usual titre 1:16-1:64	Usually +ve
Late syphilis	+ve	+ve Low titres (80–640) unless active syphilis	+ve (50–65%)	Usually –ve
Old treated syphilis	Usually +ve	Usually +ve	Usually –ve or very low titre	–ve (unless recently treated)
Congenital syphilis	The demonstration of IgM is important as it does not cross the placenta and usually represents active infection. May take up to 3 months to appear.			

Specific anti-treponemal antibody tests
- *Agglutination*: T. pallidum particle assay (TPPA) is now recommended in preference to the TP haemagglutination assay (TPHA) or microhaemagglutination assay for TP (MHA-TP), as it is more sensitive in 1° infection. Titre does not correlate with disease activity or treatment response, but distinguishes weak from strong reactivity.
- *Enzyme immunoassay*: simple, can be automated, widely used for screening and confirmation. EIAs that detect both IgG (4–5 weeks post-infection) and immunoglobulin M (IgM; 2–3 weeks post-infection) recommended as more sensitive for 1° syphilis.
- *Specific antitreponemal IgM detection (EIA)*: usually first serological response. May remain reactive for 1–2 years. Important in diagnosing early congenital syphilis.
- *Immunoblot test (also known as Western blot)*: antibody detection by response to recombinant antigens. Used in cases with discrepant isolated EIA and TPPA results.
- *Fluorescent treponemal antibody absorbed (FTA abs) test*: previously used in cases of discrepant EIA and TPPA results. No longer recommended. Has been replaced by immunoblot.

Screening tests
- EIA (ideally IgM *plus* IgG) or TPPA recommended for routine screening.
- If ↑ syphilis risk (e.g. contact, suspicious oro-anogenital ulceration), request anti-treponemal IgM as well.
- Rapid POCTs (EIA +/− non-treponemal test) are available. Used in outreach projects or field conditions in developing countries.

Confirmatory tests
- Quantitative TPPA should be used to confirm +ve EIA.
- EIA should be used to confirm +ve TPPA.
- If discrepant results, test with IgG immunoblot.
- Quantitative VDRL/RPR testing and EIA IgM should be performed prior to treatment if screening tests positive.
- VDRL/RPR >1:16 suggests active syphilis.
- In patients previously treated for syphilis a 4-fold ↑ VDRL titre and/or confirmed change in IgM to +ve suggests reinfection/relapse.
FTA abs is not recommended, but sometimes used in specialist labs.

Treponema pallidum PCR

Can be performed on lesions of 1° or 2° syphilis, CSF, vitreous, blood. Most useful in assessing oral or other lesions, where contamination with commensal treponemes is likely (rendering dark ground microscopy unhelpful).
- *Sensitivities*: primary chancre 78%, plasma 39–55%, CSF 6–63%
- *Specificities*: primary chancre 96.6%, plasma 83–98%, CSF 85–96%
- Multiplex PCR has lower sensitivity and high HSV loads could lead to a false-negative PCR for T. pallidum.

Cerebrospinal fluid

- Recommended if neurosyphilis or treatment failure suspected.
- Serum RPR >1:32 after treatment predictive of neurosyphilis.
- CSF tests better at excluding than diagnosing.

- CT head if abnormal neurology or clinical evidence of ↑ intracranial pressure prior to lumbar puncture.
- CSF white cell count >5 × 10⁶/L in the majority of symptomatic neurosyphilis, or >20 if HIV+ or 6–20 if HIV+ on ART with VL<20 or CD4>200, supports a diagnosis of neurosyphilis.
- CSF protein >0.45 g/L usually seen in neurosyphilis.
- CSF VDRL/RPR (without blood contamination):
  - Sensitivity depends on stage and symptomatology—varies from10% (asymptomatic) to 90% (symptomatic).
  - Positive result in symptomatic patient considered diagnostic.
  - False negatives common.
- CSF treponemal tests have high specificity, but low sensitivity:
  - low specificity due to transudation from serum
  - highly sensitive, so negative test makes neurosyphilis unlikely
  - CSF TPPA >1:320 supports diagnosis of neurosyphilis.
  - PCR has poor sensitivity and specificity so is unhelpful.

See Table 7.2 for CSF results supporting neurosyphilis diagnosis.

Additional tests

- *Biopsy and histology*: for gummata, e.g. to exclude malignancy.
- *X-ray*: not recommended routinely, but as part of full assessment according to signs and symptoms:
  - *Cardiovascular*—aortic dilatation with linear 'egg-shell' calcification.
  - *Tabes dorsalis*—neuropathic joints (bone destruction, osteophytes).
  - *Bone gummata*—osteomyelitic lesions sometimes hidden by reactive osteosclerosis; periosteal thickening.
  - *Early congenital*—periostitis (new bone formation), metaphyseal calcification, dactylitis (spindle-shaped finger swelling).
- *CT angiography*: cardiovascular syphilis (level of ventricular reflux).
- *Ophthalmic slit lamp examination*: if eye pathology suspected.
- *Neurological imaging*: consider CT or MRI if neurological clinical features and certainly before lumbar puncture, if risk of ↑ intracranial pressure.
- *Ultrasonography*: to identify intrauterine congenital syphilis. Signs include hepatomegaly, splenomegaly, placentomegaly, scalp oedema, polyhydramnios.

Table 7.2 CSF results supporting diagnosis of neurosyphilis

CSF parameter	HIV –ve patients	HIV +ve patients
WBC	>5 µL	>20 µL or 6–20 µL if on ART/CD4 > 200 and VL < 20
Protein	>0.45 g/L	>0.45 g/L
RPR/VDRL	Positive	Positive
TPPA	>1:320	>1:320

Congenital infection and infants born to women with syphilis

All infants born to mothers with active syphilis during pregnancy require thorough clinical assessment with following investigations:

- *Dark ground microscopy*: e.g. from suspect lesions, nasal discharge.
- *Infant serum* (NB: not cord blood): should be tested for syphilis IgM and VDRL/RPR, in parallel with maternal serum if positive due to passive transfer of maternal treponemal IgG and non-treponemal antibodies, i.e. RPR/VDRL.
  - Positive IgM EIA test ± sustained VDRL/RPR titres >4 times maternal level diagnostic of congenital infection (confirmed on repeat testing). Further investigations should include full blood count (FBC), electrolytes, liver function tests (LFTs), long-bone X-rays, and ophthalmic assessment.
  - If IgM EIA –ve, VDRL/RPR titre <4 times maternal level, and no signs of congenital syphilis, repeat IgM and RPR/VDRL 3-monthly until –ve. No further follow-up once –ve.
  - RPR/VDRL usually –ve by 6–12 months.

Management of syphilis

General principles

Offer screening for other STIs, including HIV. Examine for signs of syphilis according to history. Give clear explanation of their diagnosis. Advise to abstain from sex until symptoms resolved or 2 weeks after treatment complete

Optimal treponemal antibody sensitivity occurs during bacterial division (every 33 hours). Penicillin (1st line treatment) levels must be >0.018 mg/L for 7–10 days for early syphilis and 14–21 days for late syphilis. Desensitization should be considered as an option in those with penicillin allergy. Antibiotic free time or suboptimal levels should not exceed 24–30 hours.

> **Top tips**
> - To reduce the pain associated with benzathine benzylpenicillin IM injections using 1% lidocaine as a diluent is recommended. Reconstitute vial of antibiotic with 8 mL of 1% lidocaine solution, divide resultant solution into two equal volumes, and administer by deep IM injection into two different sites, usually both gluteal muscles.
> - If drug administration is interrupted for more than 1 day at any point during treatment course, the entire course should be re-started.

Early syphilis

Benzathine benzylpenicillin 2.4 MU IM, single dose.

Alternatives (e.g. penicillin allergy/refusing parenteral treatment)
- Procaine benzylpenicillin 600,000 units IM daily for 10 days.
- Doxycycline 100 mg oral bd for 14 days.
- Ceftriaxone 500 mg IM daily for 10 days if no penicillin anaphylaxis.
- Amoxicillin 500 mg oral qds *plus* probenecid 500 mg oral qds for 14 days.
- Azithromycin 2 g od or 500 mg od for 10 days.
- Erythromycin 500 mg oral qds for 14 days (poor CSF and placental penetration).

▶ Treatment failure with macrolides reported so only use if no alternative, with close follow up.
▶ If ophthalmic involvement, treat as for neurosyphilis.

Late latent, cardiovascular, and gummatous syphilis

Benzathine benzylpenicillin 2.4 MU IM for 3 doses on days 1, 8, 15.
▶ For cardiovascular syphilis give 40–60 mg prednisolone daily for 3 days starting 24 hours before anti-treponemal antibiotics.

Alternatives
Doxycycline 100 mg oral bd for 28 days.
Amoxicillin 2 g oral tid *plus* probenecid 500 mg oral qds for 28 days

Neurosyphilis

Procaine benzylpenicillin 1.8–2.4 MU IM daily *plus* oral probenecid 500 mg qds for 14 days (Box 7.3).

Benzylpenicillin 1.8–2.4 g IV 4-hourly for 14 days.

▶ Prednisolone 40–60 mg daily for 3 days should be started 24 hours before initiation of anti-treponemal antibiotics for neurosyphilis

Alternatives

Doxycycline 200 mg oral bd for 28 days.

Amoxicillin 2 g oral tid *plus* probenecid 500 mg oral qds for 28 days

Ceftriaxone 2 g IV (diluted in water) or IM (diluted in lidocaine) daily for 10–14 days (if no penicillin anaphylaxis).

Unlicensed medications

Benzathine and procaine penicillins and probenecid are unlicensed in the UK. Practically, this means:

- use is justified by the clinical condition (recommended treatment)
- prescribers hold legal responsibility for the prescription
- the patient should be informed that the medication is unlicensed
- any adverse reactions should be reported via yellow card scheme.

Box 7.3 How to administer procaine benzylpenicillin

UK availability limited but may be imported as 1.2 MU/vial.

To produce standard dose of 1.8 MU:

- Obtain two 1.2 MU vials
- Reconstitute the powder in each vial with the 5 mL 1% lidocaine, making ~2 × 6mL = 2 × 1.2 MU procaine benzylpenicillin.
- After placing needle, aspirate to avoid inadvertent IV injection.

Inject 4.5 mL (0.9 MU) in each buttock =1.8 MU in total.

Management of positive syphilis serology in pregnancy

Timely referral to a sexual health physician is essential, with clear communication between sexual health, obstetrics, and midwifery, GP, paediatrics, and foetal medicine (if indicated), with consent.

- *Pro forma* for syphilis in pregnancy and birth plan are recommended.
- *Early syphilis*: as for non-pregnant in 1st and 2nd trimester with a second dose of benzathine benzylpenicillin a week later if treated after 28 weeks gestation (physiological changes in pregnancy alter drug concentrations). If second line treatment used, congenital infection has been reported with macrolides, so neonatal treatment is required after delivery. Doxycycline contra-indicated.
- *Late syphilis*: as for non-pregnant patients, except procaine benzylpenicillin 600,000 units IM daily for 10 days instead of doxycycline.
- *Previously treated syphilis*: consider retreatment if doubt about initial treatment, high re-infection risk, 4-fold drop in VDRL/RPR not achieved, serofast VDRL/RPR >1:8.

- Refer to foetal medicine if diagnosed after 26 weeks gestation for evaluation of foetal involvement and assessment of foetal distress during the first 24 hours (↑ if foetus has stigmata of congenital syphilis).
- Jarisch–Herxheimer reaction may cause uterine contractions, foetal distress, and preterm labour, especially if the foetus is infected. No evidence that steroid administration reduces these complications.
- Serological cure may take several months and may not be demonstrated prior to delivery. Repeat serology in third trimester to assess fall in titres gives some reassurance.

Neonates and congenital infection

- Treatment for congenital syphilis should be provided if:
  - suspected or serological evidence of congenital syphilis
  - mother has untreated syphilis
  - mother treated <4 weeks prior to delivery
  - mother treated with non-penicillin regimens
- Special care required if maternal serology remains serofast, especially if re-infection risk.
- *First-line treatment*: benzylpenicillin 30 mg/kg IV daily12-hourly in first 7 days of life, then 8-hourly, for a total of 10 days.
- *Alternative*: procaine benzylpenicillin 50,000 units/kg IM daily for 10 days.

Adverse treatment reactions

Patients should be warned about potential adverse side effects,

Penicillin allergy and anaphylactic shock

- Facilities to manage anaphylaxis should be available.
- Consider desensitization for those with history of penicillin allergy.

Jarisch–Herxheimer reaction

A febrile illness developing within 4 hours of antibiotic treatment and resolving within 24 hours. Most common in 2° (~75%) and 1° (~50%) syphilis. Rare in late syphilis, but potentially life-threatening if strategic sites involved (e.g. coronary ostia, larynx, nervous system).

- *Features*: myalgia, rigors/chills, flush/fever/hypotension/deterioration of clinical lesions (therapeutic paradox), then resolution.
- *Management*: warn and reassure, bed rest, aspirin/paracetamol. If involvement of coronary ostia, larynx, optic neuritis, uveitis, nerve deafness (severe deterioration), and pregnancy (especially if foetal infection) special care is required. Steroid therapy initiated 24 hours before anti-treponemal antibiotics in the following situations (see also 'Late latent, cardiovasular and gummatous syphilis', p. 130, 'Neurosyphilis', p. 131, 'Management of positive syphilis serology in pregnancy', pp. 131–2).
  - *interstitial keratitis*—0.1% betamethasone eye drops
  - *neurological involvement*—incl. optic atrophy, optic neuritis, 8th nerve deafness
  - *cardiac disease*—e.g. involvement of coronary ostia
  - *laryngeal involvement*—e.g. gumma
  - *if none of the above*—give reassurance, bed rest, and antipyretics.

Procaine reaction

Characterized by fear of impending death, hallucinations, or seizures, immediately following inadvertent IV injection of procaine benzylpenicillin. Lasts <20 minutes.

Syphilis follow-up

Follow-up is essential in order to assess serological response and detect recurrence or reinfection. Minimum serological review at 3, 6, and 12 months, or until serofast.

Treponemal antibody tests (except IgM) often remain +ve for life. It is important to communicate this to patients (as they may be tested elsewhere) and ensure that latest results and titres are clearly documented.

- Consider re-infection or relapse if VDRL/RPR antibody titres ↑ 4-fold (or greater), ideally compared with previous samples run in parallel or clinical evidence of infection.
- CSF analysis and re-treatment recommended if VDRL/RPR titres do not have 4-fold drop in 12 months.
- Lifelong annual syphilis serology recommended for people with HIV.

Partner notification and management

Early syphilis

- Primary syphilis: all sexual partners within previous 3 months.
- Secondary and early latent syphilis: consider all sexual contacts within previous 2 years, or 3 months prior to last negative screen.
- Asymptomatic contacts of early syphilis either epidemiological treatment or re-screen 12 weeks after last exposure.
- Epidemiological treatment is with benzathine benzylpenicillin 2.4MU IM single dose *or* doxycycline 100mg BD for 14 days *or* azithromycin 2g single dose
- 46-60% of contactable partners are infected.

Late syphilis

As index case is usually not sexually infectious at diagnosis an estimate of when the infection was acquired should be made (e.g. from previous negative serology) and contacts from within 2 years of this time notified. However, vertical infection, although most common in early syphilis, can occur for at least 10 years after infection. Therefore it is recommended that where prior serology is unavailable all children of women with late latent syphilis are screened.

Syphilis with HIV co-infection

- Temporary ↓ of CD4 count and ↑ viral load and shedding with new syphilis infection.
- ↑ risk of HIV acquisition with infectious syphilis 3–5-fold.
- Maternal co-infection with HIV may ↑ transmission risk of syphilis.
- Increased incidence of neurosyphilis in HIV-infected people
- CSF abnormalities ↑ in people with HIV especially if not using ART and CD4<200 or detectable VL even in absence of syphilis.
- Patients with CD4 <350 and VDRL/RPR >1:32 more likely to have clinical and CSF evidence of neurosyphilis.
- Careful neurological examination should be performed. Lumbar puncture only if neurological abnormality, with prior head CT/MRI.
- More rapid progression to gummatous syphilis.
- Syphilis serological response is usually normal, but rarely atypical reactions arise with a tendency for VDRL/RPR titres to be lower in 1° syphilis and higher in 2° syphilis.
- Prozone phenomenon is more likely.
- Testing and treatment should be as for HIV negative, but assess and monitor closely for signs of neurosyphilis or recurrence.
- Annual syphilis screening should be offered to all patients with HIV, or more often depending on sexual history.

Further information

British Association for Sexual Health and HIV Syphilis guideline ℔ https://www.bashh.org/guidelines

Gonorrhoea

Introduction *138*
Aetiology: *Neisseria gonorrhoeae* *138*
Epidemiology and transmission *139*
Clinical features *140*
Pregnancy and the neonate *143*
Diagnosis *145*
Management *147*

Introduction

Gonorrhoea—'flow of seed' as named by Galen, Greek physician, in the 2nd century AD—has probably been known to be sexually transmitted for several millennia, as shown by references in the Old Testament (*Leviticus* 15), and the attribution of 'strangury' to 'pleasures of Venus' by Hippocrates.

Aetiology: *Neisseria gonorrhoeae*

Gram −ve kidney-shaped cocci about 1 μm in diameter; appear in pairs (diplococci) with concave aspects facing each other, typically inside PMNLs.

Fastidious growth requirements: temperature 35–37°C, pH 6.5–7.5, atmosphere containing 5–7% carbon dioxide, selective and enriched culture media (e.g. Modified New York City) supplemented with iron, essential amino acids, glucose, and antimicrobials to inhibit other organisms.

Humans are the only natural host. Primarily infects the columnar epithelium of lower genital tract, rectum, pharynx, and conjunctiva with transluminal spread to epididymis and prostate in ♂ and endometrium and pelvic organs in ♀ with occasional haematogenous dissemination.

Epidemiology and transmission

WHO estimates 78 million cases annually worldwide. The UK incidence peaked around the early 1970s, followed by a marked ↓ between 1985 and 1995, coinciding with AIDS awareness campaigns. However, from 1997 to 2015 there has been a steady ↑ in incidence.

Highest incidence in the UK is in MSM, ages 15–29 years, urban and deprived populations, and black Carribeans. *N. gonorrhoeae* infection is regarded as a surrogate marker of high-risk sexual behaviour and is closely associated with other STIs, especially *Chlamydia trachomatis* (co-infection in up to 40% of ♀ and 25% of ♂ with gonorrhoea).

N. gonorrhoeae does not confer immunity as outer membrane proteins vary and re-infection is common.

Sexual and non-sexual transmission

- *Anogenital and pharyngeal infections:* almost exclusively sexually transmitted. Evidence of transmission from toilet seats is contentious, as the organism loses viability on drying. Fomite transmission is very unusual, but anecdotal cases have been reported following the shared use of a portable male urinal and inflatable sex doll.
- *Adult conjunctivitis:* often associated with anogenital infection due to auto-inoculation, but non-sexual transmission is possible as reported in sporadic epidemics and isolated cases attributed to poor hygiene, accidental inoculation, or irrigation with urine (folk remedy). Flies have been implicated as vectors in an Australian outbreak.
- *Neonatal infection:* vertical transmission due to exposure in birth canal.

Infectivity and clearance rates

- 60–80% transmission of gonorrhoea from ♂ to ♀ after one episode of sex. Risk reduced by ~40% with condom use.
- 20% transmission from ♀ to ♂ after one episode of sex. Risk reduced by 75% with condom use.
- Transmission from pharynx to urethra occurs in 26% of partners.
- 30% vertical transmission risk.
- Spontaneous clearance ~5% from pharynx in 10 days (no data for other sites of infection).

Clinical features

Sites of infection
See Table 8.1.

Table 8.1 Sites of infection. Infection commonly co-exists at several different sites

	Heterosexual ♂ (%)	MSM (%)	♀ (%)
Urethra	>90	60–70	65–75
Cervix	—	—	80–90
Pharynx + other site(s)	3–10	10–30	5–15
Pharynx only	<5	10–15	<5
Rectum + other site(s)	—	25–50	25–40
Rectum only	—	20–40	5

Male genital infection
Symptoms
- *Incubation period*: 2–5 days, range 1–14.
- Urethral discharge in 80% and/or dysuria in 50%. May be scanty and mucoid initially, but becomes profuse and purulent, yellow/green within 24 hours.
- Asymptomatic in 5–10%.

Signs
- Mucopurulent or purulent urethral discharge, typically profuse, but if scanty can be elicited by urethral massage.
- Erythema of the urethral meatus sometimes with oedema.
- Urine 'threads'—plugs of pus from urethral (Littré's) glands in FVU, indicating anterior urethritis.
- Rarely epididymal tenderness or balanitis.

Female genital infection
Symptoms
- Asymptomatic in ~50%. If symptomatic, may be due to co-infection.
- Symptoms, when present, appear within 10 days of infection.
- ↑ vaginal discharge in up to 50% (most common symptom).
- Lower abdominal pain in up to 25%.
- Dysuria without frequency ~12%.
- Intermenstrual bleeding or menorrhagia (unusual).

Signs
- Commonly no abnormal findings.
- Mucopurulent endocervical discharge and easily induced cervical bleeding (<50%).
- Pelvic/lower abdominal tenderness (<5%).

Extragenital infections in men and women

Rectal infection

Usually asymptomatic, but may cause anal discharge (12%), pain, discomfort, or pruritus (<7%), and less frequently rectal bleeding, tenesmus, and constipation. Proctoscopy may show mucoid or purulent discharge, erythema, oedema, and friability. In ♀, the positive correlation with duration of cervical infection suggests transmucosal spread of genital secretions into the anal canal as the main route, with anal intercourse implicated in ~10%.

Pharyngeal infection

Asymptomatic in >90%. Occasional mild pharyngitis and/or cervical lymphadenopathy. Almost 100% spontaneous clearance within 12 weeks; significant association with disseminated gonococcal infection.

Conjunctival infection

Adult infection, which is uncommon, presents with purulent discharge and inflammation affecting one or both eyes. If untreated, complications, such as keratitis and pan-ophthalmitis, can lead to blindness.

Prepubertal children

In girls, the vulval and vaginal epithelium are vulnerable to infection. Although, theoretically, infection may be acquired accidentally from infected secretions, especially with poor sanitation and hygiene, gonorrhoea is a strong indicator of sexual abuse. It usually presents as a purulent oedematous vulvovaginitis.

Gonococcal urethritis in boys, or pharyngeal and rectal infection in both sexes, is almost always the result of sexual abuse.

Complications

Complications are uncommon in both men and women.

Men

- *Infection of the median raphe*: linear erythematous swelling.
- *Tysonitis*: painful swelling of parafrenal gland.
- Meatal para-urethral gland abscess.
- *Peri-urethral cellulitis and abscess*: inflammation of Littré's glands with duct obstruction produces small cysts and abscesses causing tender swelling in fossa navicularis or bulb. Urine flow may be re-stricted. Painful erections +/− ventral angulation if corpus spongiosum is affected.
- Urethral strictures and fistulae: sequelae of peri-urethral abscess in untreated infection.
- *Cowperitis and abscess*: Cowper's (bulbo-urethral) glands at the base of the prostate are affected, causing fever, pain in perineum, particularly on defecation, and urinary frequency or retention.
  Abscesses usually point to one side of the perineum or are palpable rectally.
- *Prostatitis and seminal vesiculitis*: acute features include fever, malaise, perineal discomfort, tenesmus, suprapubic pain, urgency of micturition or retention, haematuria, and painful erections. Swollen prostate, tender on rectal examination. Chronic prostatitis may develop.
- *Epididymitis (<1%)*: ➔ Chapter 13, 'Epididymo-orchitis', pp. 193–200.

Women
- Inflammation of para-urethral (Skene's) glands.
- *Bartholinitis +/− Bartholin's abscess*: single or bilateral. Vulval pain and erythema with tender cystic swelling of the posterior half of the labium majora. Pus may be seen or expressed from the duct orifice.
- Pelvic inflammatory disease (PID ➜ Chapter 11, 'Pelvic inflammatory disease, pp. 169–79) may occur in 10–20% of untreated infections.

Systemic spread of infection

Perihepatitis (Fitz-Hugh–Curtis syndrome)
Usually found in ♀ with associated PID, suggesting intra-abdominal spread, but also rarely reported in ♂ implicating lymphatic or haematogenous dissemination (➜ Chapter 11, 'Complications and sequelae', p. 174).

Disseminated gonococcal infection (DGI)
- Occurs in <1% with mucosal infection.
- *Host factors*: 4-fold ↑ in ♀ (especially during or just after menstruation, or in pregnancy, particularly with pharyngeal infection). Complement deficiency predisposes to recurrent episodes in <10% with DGI.
- *Bacterial factors*:
  - serogroup IA-1(WI)
  - *auxotype AHU–* (arginine, hypoxanthine, and uracil dependent)
  - complement resistance
  - antibiotic resistance, which varies with time and region.

Clinical features
The preceding mucosal infection tends to be asymptomatic. Usually presents with mild fever, skin rash, and arthralgia +/− arthritis.
- *Skin (gonococcal dermatitis) in 67%*: initial macules develop into papules, vesicles with petechiae, and then typical necrotic pustules surrounded by erythema. Usually at extremities (especially hands).
- *Skeletal*: tenosynovitis (in ~33%) producing migratory arthralgia, mostly in wrists, fingers, toes, and ankles. Arthritis (single joint), in ~50%, with effusion typically involving the knee, wrist, or metacarpophalangeal joints.
- *Other sites (rare)*:
  - Endocarditis in 1–3% leading to aortic incompetence and cardiac failure; also pericarditis and myocarditis.
  - Hepatitis
  - Meningitis, similar to meningococcal (very rare).

Pregnancy and the neonate

Screening for gonorrhoea and chlamydia in 16–25-year-olds has become part of antenatal care in some areas, and is likely to reduce complications and adverse pregnancy outcomes due to both infections.

In pregnancy the proportion of pharyngeal infection is ↑ by 15–35%, presumably due to ↑ in oral sex. Genital infection is less likely to be complicated by PID (because of thickening of cervical mucus), but cases of salpingitis have been reported in the 1st trimester.

Adverse pregnancy outcomes

- Infection of chorio-amnion can cause septic abortion, but there is no consistent evidence for ↑ risk.
- Preterm delivery and low birth weight ↑ 3–6-fold.
- Premature rupture of membrane (PROM) is more frequent.
- Post-partum/intra-partum or post-abortal endometritis and pyrexia illness are ↑ 3-fold and occur in ~42% with gonorrhoea.
- Some studies suggest that risk of DGI is ↑, reflecting ↑ pharyngeal infection.
- Screening in pregnancy advisable in symptomatic women, PROM, septic abortion, intra/post-partum fever, or those at ↑ risk.

Neonatal gonococcal infection

Occurs because of exposure in birth canal during labour with ↑ risk if PROM or preterm delivery. Antenatal screening and treatment is the best way to prevent neonatal infection. The most severe manifestations are ophthalmia neonatorum and sepsis, with milder infections causing rhinitis, pharyngitis (in 33% with ophthalmia), vaginitis, urethritis, and infection at site of foetal monitoring. Meningitis is a rare complication.

Gonococcal ophthalmia neonatorum

A notifiable disease in the UK, defined as conjunctivitis with a purulent discharge in an infant arising within 21 days of birth. Occurs in 30–40% of those exposed. Typically develops within 2–5 days of delivery and presents with oedema of the conjunctiva and eyelids with profuse discharge. Without treatment infection may extend to sub-conjunctival connective tissue and the cornea leading to ulceration. If ulcers perforate, anterior synechiae formation or panophthalmitis may follow, which can result in blindness.

The rate of infection in at-risk infants is ↓ to 2–5% by prophylaxis with 0.5% erythromycin ointment applied once to both eyes soon after birth (other topical treatments are no longer recommended).

Gonococcal arthritis

Associated with vulvovaginitis, proctitis, or ophthalmia neonatorum. Usually polyarticular, presenting as pseudoparalysis and is rarely progressive.

Questions that are frequently asked by patients
See Box 8.1.

Box 8.1 Frequently asked questions

How long can I have had gonorrhoea for?
In ♂, urethral symptoms usually appear within 10 days of exposure to gonorrhoea, although 5–10% are asymptomatic when diagnosed. Symptoms are much less common with rectal and throat infection. Up to 70% of ♀ diagnosed with gonorrhoea are asymptomatic. Therefore, although most people are probably diagnosed shortly after being infected, it is possible that it may have been present for weeks or months.

Can it be cured?
Yes, gonorrhoea can be cured by antibiotics. When swabs are taken for gonorrhoea culture, the laboratory also tests for antibiotic sensitivities, so that the appropriate antibiotic is identified. It is recommended that, while awaiting these results, an antibiotic be used to which >95% of the local stains of *N. gonorrhoeae* are sensitive.

Will it have done any damage?
- *In ♀*: PID may occur in 10–20% of untreated cases of gonorrhoea. Infertility may occur as a result of PID.
- *In ♂*: urethral strictures and fistulae are sequelae of peri-urethral abscesses in untreated gonorrhoea and it may also cause epididymitis.

Do I need a test of cure?
Yes. With increasing emergence of antibiotic resistance it is important to have a test of cure about 2 weeks after treatment. Abstinence is advised until you and your partner(s) have a negative test of cure result.

Can I have caught this from a toilet seat?
Gonorrhoea can survive for up to 24 hours on surfaces such as toilet seats and there has been a report of acquisition by an 8-year-old girl from a dirty aeroplane toilet. However, it is very rare and, in children, infection should always raise concerns of sexual abuse.

I'm pregnant. Can it harm my baby?
There is a risk of neonatal infection due to exposure in the birth canal during labour. Gonococcal ophthalmia neonatorum is acquired by 30–40% of infants exposed to *N. gonorrhoeae*. Without treatment, there are ↑ risks of preterm delivery, low birth weight, premature rupture of membranes, and post-partum/post-abortion endometritis. Prompt treatment significantly reduces these risks and, if necessary, your baby will receive prophylaxis or treatment.

Diagnosis

Specimen collection

Asymptomatic screening

Sampling depends on sexual history. NAATs are recommended for screening as they have higher sensitivity than culture. If asymptomatic, but a contact of gonorrhoea infection, culture is also recommended.

- *Women*: health professional or self-taken vulvovaginal swab for NAAT testing. Consider pharyngeal and rectal swab depending on history.
- *Heterosexual ♂*: FVU (or urethral swab) for NAAT testing (pharyngeal swab not necessary, even if history of cunnilingus).
- *MSM*: FVU, pharyngeal and rectal swabs recommended for all (these can be self-taken). ~20% with rectal infection do not report receptive anal intercourse.

Testing symptomatic patients

Women

- *Endocervical*: microscopy. Culture if Gram −ve intracellular diplococci seen or gonorrhoea suspected (e.g. contact of gonorrhoea).
- *Vulvo-vagina*: NAAT.
- *Rectal*: depending on sexual history and symptoms, NAAT, microscopy of rectal slide if proctitis, consider culture if gonorrhoea suspected.
- Pharyngeal swab for NAAT depending on history (+/− culture).

Heterosexual men

Microscopy of urethral smear, FVU for NAAT, culture of urethral swab if gonorrhoea suspected.

MSM

- *Urethral sample*: microscopy if symptoms of urethritis, and culture of urethral swab if gonorrhoea suspected.
- Offer rectal NAAT for all (depending on history), with proctoscopy and microscopy if rectal symptoms and rectal gonorrhoea culture if gonorrhoea suspected.
- Pharyngeal swab for NAAT ± culture if gonorrhoea suspected.

Conjunctivitis

Swab from eyelid and test potential 1° infection sites with NAAT and culture.

Disseminated gonococcal infection

- Test potential 1° infection sites with NAAT and culture.
- Material from skin lesions and joint aspirate for NAAT and culture.
- Blood culture.

Microscopy

Microscopy (×1000) of Gram-stained genital specimens shows *N. gonorrhoeae* as Gram −ve diplococci within PMNLs (Plate 4). Smear sensitivity compared with culture:

- ♂: urethra 90–95% (symptomatic) and 50–75% (asymptomatic)
- ♀: cervix 37–50% and urethra 20%
- *rectum*: blind swab 40%, using proctoscope 70–80%.

Conjunctival specimens are suitable for Gram stain and microscopy, but pharyngeal specimens are not suitable as other neisserial commensals are commonly seen.

Laboratory detection of *N. gonorrhoeae*

Molecular detection

NAAT testing is the recommended first-line test for gonorrhoea and is widely available, commonly in combination with chlamydia NAAT. NAATs are significantly more sensitive from all sites compared with culture, with sensitivities >96% for both symptomatic and asymptomatic infection. They are suitable for ♂ urine, vulvo-vaginal (including self-collected), and endocervical samples (♀ urine sample has lower sensitivity). NAATs are recommended for rectal and pharyngeal testing as sensitivities are superior to culture, although they are unlicensed for testing at these sites, so local validation of testing platforms is required. Confirmatory testing of reactive NAAT using a second NAAT with a different target is required (unless already culture positive), where population prevalence is low and positive predictive value of reactive test is <90%.

Culture

Gonorrhoea culture less sensitive than NAAT, but is still required for detection of isolates with ↓ antimicrobial sensitivity (becoming an increasing concern). Sensitivity predicts success in >95% with intermediate sensitivity suggesting failure in 5–15%, although ↑ dosage may be effective. Resistance may be due to plasmids (circular DNA fragments independent of chromosome) or chromosomal mutation.

▶ Caution with lubricants during examination, as they may inhibit the growth of *N. gonorrhoeae*.

Specimens for culture may be directly inoculated onto culture medium and incubated, or transported in a non-nutrient medium (e.g. Amies, Stuart) or a CO_2-producing culture medium.

Transport media should be kept at 4°C after inoculation (check product information or with local lab). Provided that the material in the transport medium is processed within 48 hours, there is only ~5% loss in sensitivity compared with direct inoculation.

The culture medium is examined for growth at 24 and 48 hours. Presumptive identification is by positive cytochrome oxidase reaction and microscopy. Definitive identification by a combination of further tests, e.g. carbohydrate utilization (*N. gonorrhoeae* utilizes glucose only), monoclonal antibody test (e.g. Phadebact), and enzyme substrate degradation.

Further information

British Association for Sexual Health and HIV Gonorrhoea guideline ℘ https://www.bashh.org/guidelines

Management

▶ Advise avoidance of any sexual contact until patient and partner(s) have completed treatment, and received negative test of cure result.

▶ Offer full STI screen, including HIV. Repeat screening after the window periods should be recommended.

Treatment before antibiotic sensitivity is known should be with an antibiotic to which >95% of local strains are sensitive.

Uncomplicated anogenital and pharyngeal infections

Recommended

Ceftriaxone 1g IM single dose (NB Addition of azithromycin no longer recommended due to increasing resistance). Ciprofloxacin 500mg oral single dose if known to be sensitive. To treat gonococcal PID: Ceftriaxone 1g IM single dose plus chosen treatment regimen for PID (see Chapter 11). To treat gonococcal epididymo-orchitis: Ceftriaxone 1g IM single dose plus chosen treatment regimen for epididymo-orchitis (See Chapter 13)

Alternative (if regional prevalence of resistance <5%)

* Cefixime 400mg oral single dose plus azithromycin 2g oral single dose
* Gentamycin 240mg IM single dose plus azithromycin 2g oral single dose
* Spectinomycin 2g IM single dose plus azithromycin 2g oral single dose (not effective for treatment of pharyngeal infection)
* Azithromycin 2g oral single dose (high levels of resistance worldwide)

To treat PID ➔ Chapter 11, 'Pelvic inflammatory disease', pp. 169–79, and ➔ Chapter 13, 'Epididymo-orchitis' pp. 193–200.

Pregnancy and breastfeeding

❶ Quinolone and tetracycline antimicrobials are contraindicated:
* Ceftriaxone 1g IM single dose
* Spectinomycin 2g IM single dose
* Azithromycin 2g oral single dose

Adult gonococcal conjunctivitis

Systemic treatment for 3 days recommended in case of corneal involvement as the cornea is relatively avascular.
* *Recommended:* ceftriaxone 1g IM single dose
* *Alternative:* spectinomycin 2 g IM daily for 3 days or azithromycin 2 g oral single dose *plus* doxycycline 100 mg bd for 7 days *plus* ciprofloxacin 250 mg daily for 3 days

Disseminated gonococcal infection

Hospital admission is recommended. Assess for endocarditis or meningitis. Initial therapy should be parenteral:
* ceftriaxone 1 g IM/IV daily or cefotaxime 1 g IV 8-hourly *or*
* ciprofloxacin 500 mg IV 12-hourly *or*
* spectinomycin 2 g IM 12-hourly.

The parenteral antibiotic should be continued for 24–48 hours until improvement, and then replaced with one of the following oral antibiotics, to complete 7 days treatment: cefixime 400 mg; ciprofloxacin 500 mg; or ofloxacin 400 mg bd.

Top tip

Spectinomycin

Unlicensed in the UK (➔ Chapter 7, 'Unlicensed medications', p. 131). Guidelines advise as alternative treatment for uncomplicated anogenital and disseminated gonorrhoea infections.

Dosage and administration instructions

Reconstitute spectinomycin powder, 2 g with 3.2 mL of sterile water for injection, to make up 5 mL solution. Shake vigorously before drawing up into disposable syringe. Administer by injecting into the upper outer quadrant of the gluteal muscle using a 20 gauge needle.

Gonococcal meningitis and endocarditis

IV antibiotic for at least 2 weeks and 4 weeks, respectively, with ceftriaxone 2 g daily or 1 g 12-hourly *plus* single dose azithromycin 2 g oral. Seek specialist advice.

Gonococcal infection in neonates and prepubertal children.

- *Ophthalmia neonatorum*: single dose of ceftriaxone IV/IM 25–50 mg/kg up to a maximum of 125 mg.
- *Sepsis, scalp abscess, meningitis, or arthritis in neonate or prepubertal child <45 kg*: ceftriaxone 25–50 mg/kg daily IV/IM for 7–14 days.
- *Neonatal prophylaxis*: if mother is not treated before delivery, a single dose of ceftriaxone 25–50 mg/kg to a maximum of 125 mg.
- *For uncomplicated anogenital or pharyngeal infection if weight <45 kg*: single dose ceftriaxone 25–50 mg/kg IV/IM (max 125 mg).
- Treatment of children who weight >45 kg is as for adults.

Partner notification

PN is essential. Contact tracing period:

- *Men with symptomatic urethritis*: 2 weeks prior to onset of symptoms or until last sexual partner, if longer.
- *Asymptomatic men and women, or infection at other sites*: 3 months prior to diagnosis or until the last sexual partner.
- All sexual contacts should be offered full STI screen and epidemiological treatment. Similar principles should apply to the mother of a neonate with gonococcal infection and her sex partner(s).

Follow-up and test of cure (TOC)

TOC is recommended for all. If asymptomatic, a NAAT test should be performed >2 weeks after treatment. TOC is particularly important following treatment of pharyngeal infections, alternative treatment regimen or persisting symptoms. Culture (>72 hours after treatment complete) is recommended in addition if still symptomatic, alternative treatment regimen used or resistance detected on initial culture.

HIV infection

Gonorrhoea facilitates HIV transmission, producing ↑ in detectable virus in genital secretions. This is reversed following antibiotic treatment. Infection should be treated as for people without HIV infection.

Chlamydia

Introduction *150*
Aetiology *150*
Epidemiology and transmission *151*
Clinical features *152*
Pregnancy and the neonate *154*
Diagnosis *156*
Management *158*

Introduction

Although recognized since antiquity (description of trachoma in Egyptian papyri), the discovery of *Chlamydia trachomatis* as a cause of genital tract and ocular infections was only made in the early part of the 20th century.

Aetiology

The bacteria species *C. trachomatis* is divided into four biovars—LGV, trachoma, murine, and swine. These are subdivided into several serovars based on the major outer membrane protein (MOMP) antigens. Serovars D-K of the trachoma biovar are sexually transmissible, commonly referred to as 'chlamydia infection', while serovars L1–L3 cause LGV. Genotyping based on *MOMP* genes refines classification of the species and is a useful research tool.

C. trachomatis is an obligate intracellular pathogen, depending entirely on host cell adenosine triphosphate for its energy. Two distinct structures appear during its life cycle of 48–72 hours.

- *Elementary body (0.35 μm)*: infectious form, attaches to and enters host columnar or pseudostratified columnar cells. After 6–9 hours this transforms into a reticulate body.
- *Reticulate body (1 μm)*: non-infective replicative phase within intracellular endosomes. These fuse into an inclusion where reticulate bodies multiply for 24–48 hours. After maturation back into elementary bodies they are released.

Epidemiology and transmission

WHO estimated the annual worldwide incidence of new infections to be 131 million in 2012. Genital chlamydial infection is the most common bacterial STI in the UK, with the highest incidence amongst 15–24-year-olds, with an estimated prevalence of 1.5–10%. Risk factors for infection include having >1 sexual partner in past year and inconsistent condom use.

- *Transmissibility is high*: after a single act of unprotected penetrative sex ~10% transmission. Concordance between sexual partners is 75%. Correct use of condoms reduces the risk by ~40%.
- Spontaneous bacterial clearance is estimated to occur in ~20–28% within 3 months and 50% by 12 months. Persistence for up to 6 years has been reported and is believed to be longer in ♀ than ♂.
- Urogenital infection does not result in sustained immunity.

Clinical features

Sites of infection

- ♂: urethra (responsible for 35–50% of non-gonococcal urethritis (NGU)); epididymis; prostate (inconclusive evidence).
- ♀: cervix (75–85%); urethra (50–60% overall, 15–20% urethra only); Bartholin's gland; endometrium; fallopian tubes; vagina if prepubertal.
- *Extragenital*: conjunctiva; rectum (3–10% in MSM); pharynx (1–2%); hepatic capsule; synovium; rarely endocardium and meninges.

Male genital infection

Symptoms

Incubation period is 7–21 days. Up to 50% notice urethral discharge and/or dysuria, while the remainder are asymptomatic.

Signs

- About 60% of ♂ have signs.
- Usually mild to moderate opaque or clear urethral discharge.
- Sometimes oedema and erythema of the urethral meatus.
- Often urine 'threads': plugs of pus from urethral (Littré's) glands in FVU, indicating anterior urethritis.

Female genital infection

Symptoms

Asymptomatic in up to 80%; symptoms when present include:

- increased vaginal discharge
- dysuria without frequency
- inter-menstrual bleeding, menorrhagia, post-coital bleeding
- low abdominal pain.

Signs

- usually no abnormal findings
- mucopurulent cervicitis (~33% including asymptomatic): mucopurulent discharge, oedema, congestion, friable (bleeds easily)
- incidental finding on colposcopy of 'cobblestone' appearance of the cervix due to raised lymphoid follicles
- cervical ectopy is positively correlated with chlamydial infection.

Extragenital infections in men and women

Rectal infection

In MSM attending sexual health clinics

- ≤Up to 15% of those with proctitis caused by chlamydia (consider LGV ➲ Chapter 18 'Lymphogranuloma venereum', pp. 248–50).
- ≤Up to 10% + on routine screening (67% without urethral infection).
- Usually asymptomatic (>60%), but may cause anal discharge, pain, discomfort/pruritus, and less frequently rectal bleeding, severe anal pain, tenesmus, and constipation with overt proctitis.
- Occasionally external anal erythema or discharge. Proctoscopy may show mucoid or purulent discharge, erythema, oedema, or friability, even in those who are symptomatic. 'Cobblestone' appearance if magnified with a colposcope.

In women attending sexual health clinics
- Up to 5% prevalence (may occur without urogenital infection).
- May occur in women who do not report anal sex
- Usually asymptomatic but symptoms and signs as with ♂.

Pharyngeal infection
- MSM up to 2.3% carriage. Limited data for women.
- Usually asymptomatic, but occasionally mild pharyngeal symptoms.

Conjunctival infection
- Concomitant anogenital infection in 60–70%.
- *Partners*: ~50% ♀ and ~80% ♂ have chlamydia or NGU.

Uni- or bilateral follicular conjunctivitis presents 1–2 weeks after exposure with conjunctival irritation, discharge +/– photophobia/periorbital pain. Signs include conjunctival injection +/– chemosis and ulceration in severe cases, and hyperaemia with follicles 0.5–1 mm in diameter +/– palpebral conjunctival oedema. May cause conjunctival scarring. Epithelial keratitis (unusual) does not cause corneal scarring.

Prepubertal children

In girls, the vulval and vaginal epithelium are vulnerable to infection. Urethral, pharyngeal, and rectal infections may also occur. Prepubertal infection is a strong indicator of sexual abuse. ▶ However, perinatal *C. trachomatis* infection may persist for at least 3 years.

Complications

Men

⊃ Chapter 13, 'Epididymo-orchitis', pp. 193–200.
- Sexually acquired reactive arthritis (SARA) or Reiter's syndrome
  ⊃ Chapter 14, 'Sexually acquired reactive arthritis' pp. 201–12;
  polyarthritis affecting mostly weight-bearing joints, usually preceded by
  urethritis and conjunctivitis in <1% of chlamydial infections.
- Some evidence for association with male infertility.
- *Prostatitis and seminal vesiculitis*: evidence not well established.

Women

- Pelvic inflammatory disease (PID ⊃ Chapter 11, pp. 169–79) may occur
  in about 10–30% of untreated infections, with risk of ectopic pregnancy,
  infertility, and chronic pelvic pain.
- *Bartholinitis +/– Bartholin's abscess*: uni- or bilateral. Pain in vulva with
  tender cystic swelling of posterior labia majora with erythema. Pus may
  exude or be expressed from the duct orifice.
- *Endometritis*: may cause irregular vaginal bleeding.
- *Cervical neoplasia*: epidemiological and molecular studies show a
  correlation with chlamydial infection.
- *Perihepatitis (Fitz-Hugh–Curtis syndrome)*: usually found in ♀ with PID
  suggesting intra-abdominal spread, but also rarely in ♂, implicating
  lymphatic or haematogenous dissemination.
- SARA (⊃ 'Complications,' Men, above, p. 153).

Pregnancy and the neonate

Screening for gonorrhoea and chlamydia in 16–25-year-olds has become part of antenatal care in some areas, and is likely to reduce complications and adverse pregnancy outcomes due to both infections.

The infection rate in pregnancy varies from 2% to 30%. Genital infection is less likely to be complicated by PID (because of thick cervical mucus), but cases of salpingitis have been reported in the 1st trimester.

Adverse pregnancy outcomes of untreated chlamydia

Chlamydial infection in pregnancy may be associated with preterm delivery and low birth weight.

- Premature rupture of membrane (PROM) more frequent.
- *C. trachomatis* has been isolated from amniotic fluid.
- Intrapartum pyrexia and late post-partum endometritis ↑ by 20–25%.
- PID following abortion.

Neonatal chlamydial infection

Occurs because of exposure in birth canal during labour.

Chlamydial ophthalmia neonatorum

30–50% of exposed infants acquire chlamydial conjunctivitis, ↓ to 1–2% if mother treated before delivery. Incubation period 5–14 days (from delivery or PROM), but can be up to 2 months.

Conjunctivitis

Varies from mild (scant mucoid discharge) to severe (profuse discharge) with 67% bilateral involvement. Corneal scarring is rare.

Respiratory tract infection

- Nasopharyngeal infection occurs in 70–80% infected neonates, where it is usually asymptomatic.
- 30% with nasopharyngeal infection develop apyrexial pneumonia at 4–12 weeks of age with cough, tachypnoea, and crepitations on auscultation. Apnoeic episodes may occur. Long-term outcome includes impaired lung function and obstructive pulmonary disease.
- Investigations show hyperinflation on radiography, peripheral eosinophilia, and ↑ serum immunoglobulins.

Other sites of neonatal infection

- Otitis media complicating nasopharyngeal infection may become chronic if not treated early.
- Vaginal and rectal infection in 10–15% of exposed infants. Usually asymptomatic and may persist for at least 3 years.

Questions frequently asked by patients

See Box 9.1.

Box 9.1 Frequently asked questions

How long could I have had chlamydia for?
Up to 80% ♀ and 50% ♂ infected with chlamydia are asymptomatic. Therefore, it is possible to be infected for months and, in some cases, years before it is diagnosed.

Could I have caught if from a toilet seat?
No. There is no evidence for this.

Does my partner need to be seen?
Yes. There is a very high chance of infection. Screening for STIs is recommended, and treatment to cover chlamydial infection should be taken. It is important not to have sex with your partner until they have been tested/treated in order to prevent re-infection. Even if you use condoms this only reduces the risk of infection, but does not eliminate it. Your partner needs treatment and you need to be retreated.

How have I caught chlamydia when my only ever partner has tested negative?
Although tests for chlamydia are now very reliable, they are not 100% sensitive and, therefore, infection may be missed. In addition, your partner may have received antibiotics for something else or the infection may have cleared spontaneously. Despite conflicting results in a partnership, we recommend treatment for both of you.

Will it have affected my fertility?
Chlamydial infection is extremely common and does not appear to impair fertility in most people who are treated properly. Untreated chlamydia can lead to either symptomatic PID or silent episodes, which are associated with infertility. 90% of couples will conceive within 12 months of trying with regular unprotected intercourse. If you have concerns about your fertility in the future you should seek advice from your GP.

Do I need a test of cure?
Routine test of cure is not necessary following first-line treatment. If second-line therapy is used, e.g. due to allergy, a test of cure is recommended 3–5 weeks after completing treatment

Diagnosis

Investigations

Microscopy

Light microscopy (×1000) of Gram-stained smear does not show *C. trachomatis*, but can demonstrate PMNLs:

- *Urethral in ♂*: 5 PMNL/HPF in the absence of Gram –ve intracellular diplococci suggests NGU.
- *Cervical*: 30 PMNL/HPF suggests cervicitis.
- *Rectal*: 1 PMNL/HPF suggests proctitis.
- *Urine*: 10 PMNL/HPF in threads from first voided urine in ♂ suggests NGU.
- Sterile pyuria may be due to *C. trachomatis* infection.

Laboratory detection of Chlamydia trachomatis

Nucleic acid amplification tests

- NAATs are the current standard of care test for *C. trachomatis*. They have high specificity (98–100%) and sensitivity (urine: 85–>95%; cervical swabs: 88–>95%). Suitable for all sites, including self-collected vulvo-vaginal samples. Many assays are now validated for pharyngeal and rectal specimens. If delays >24 hours are anticipated, storage at 4°C is recommended to avoid sample degradation. Manufacturer's instructions should be followed.
- The most commonly used NAATs amplify by PCR, strand displacement amplification or transcription mediated amplification, using either cryptic plasmid or 23S rRNA.
- New variant *C. trachomatis*, reported in Scandinavia in 2006 had a deletion in the cryptic plasmid region used for amplification, leading to false negatives. Targets have since been re-designed to prevent evasion of these strains.
- Inhibitory controls are desirable in order to prevent false negatives.
- If the positive predictive value of a reactive result is >90% then confirmatory testing of reactive results is not required. This will depend on local prevalence, as well as sensitivity and specificity of the assay. If confirmatory testing is required, this can be done by repeating the test or by using a different target/platform.

Other methods of detection

EIA, direct fluorescent antibody (DFA), and cell culture have all be used for screening in the past, but are no longer recommended due to lower sensitivity and specificity, and poorer performance when compared with NAATs. Other DNA probe methods are now rarely used. Serum antibody tests, which use micro-immunofluorescence to detect species-specific antibody, are not routinely available and are of limited use as mucosal infections do not elicit a strong antibody response, and they are only useful for retrospective diagnosis. IgG titre >1:64 may indicate recent infection, IgA may indicate active infection and IgM may be useful in diagnosis of neonatal pneumonia.

Point of care tests

Not yet used as routine in most settings due to reduced sensitivity and specificity compared with laboratory-based methods. New EIA-based POCT have sensitivities up to 93% (aQcare Chlamydia TRF kit). NAAT-based POCTs are being developed for genital sampling and look promising.

Specimen collection

- Vulvo-vaginal swab (VVS), either self-taken or by HCW is the preferred method, with 96–98% sensitivity. Self-sampling reported higher acceptability than urine or cervical specimens.
- Endocervical specimens are less sensitive than VVS.
- FVU is less sensitive than VVS in women, but has equivalent sensitivity to urethral sampling and are preferred in men.
- Urethral swabs should be inserted 2–4 cm. Self-taken penile meatal swabs have shown good results, but are less acceptable.
- Extra-genital samples have variable sensitivities depending on the platform used:
  - rectal swabs can be taken blind, via proctoscopy or self-taken
  - pharyngeal swabs can be self-taken by HCW.
- Pooling of samples from different sites reduces costs. Local validation is required, as sensitivity may be reduced. The site of infection would not be known if the result was reactive.
- Men and women with proctitis, and all MSM with HIV and *C. trachomatis* at any site should have samples tested for LGV.

Medicolegal cases

NAAT is the recommended detection method. Chlamydia culture is no longer recommended. Samples should be taken from all sites of penetration. Reactive results should be confirmed using a different target.

Management

▶ Advise avoidance of any sexual contact, including with condoms, until the patient and partner(s) have completed treatment or 7 days after single dose azithromycin, and symptoms have resolved

▶ Patient should be given verbal and written information regarding natural history, transmission, treatment, and complications.

- All patients diagnosed with *C. trachomatis* should be offered screening for other STI.
- Retesting after window periods for bacterial and viral STI should be recommended.

For PID **⟶** Chapter 11, 'Pelvic inflammatory disease', pp. 169–79, and **⟶** Chapter 13, 'Epididymo-orchitis', pp. 193–200.

Uncomplicated genital and rectal infections

Recommended treatment regimens
- doxycycline 100 mg bd for 7 days (**do not use if pregnant**)

Alternative regimens
- azithromycin 1 g followed by 500 mg daily for further 2 days
- erythromycin 500 mg bd for 10–14 days *or*
- ofloxacin 200 mg bd or 400 mg od for 10–14 days.

Extra-genital infection

Rectal and pharyngeal infection
- *Recommended treatment*: doxycycline 100 mg bd for 7 days.
- *Alternative treatment (TOC recommended)*: azithromycin 1 g single dose, *or* ofloxacin (risk of *C. difficile* and tendon rupture), *or* erythromycin (↓ effective, ↑ side effects, ↑ daily dosing).

Adult conjunctival infection
Treat as for genital infection

Pregnancy and breastfeeding

❶ Tetracyclines, fluroquinolones, and co-trimoxazole are contraindi-cated, including doxycycline and ofloxacin.
- *Azithromycin*: 1 g followed by 500 mg daily for further 2 days. Adverse pregnancy outcomes unlikely but lack of data.
- *Erythromycin*: 500 mg bd 14 days or 4 times daily for 7 days.
- *Amoxicillin*: 500 mg tid for 7 days (better tolerated than erythromycin).
- Test of cure recommended for all women treated in pregnancy.

Infection in neonates and children

Neonatal testing
Infants born to mothers with untreated chlamydial infection should be moni-tored for signs of infection and/or given epidemiological treatment. Swabs should be taken for *C. trachomatis* NAAT testing from everted eyelids 5–10 days after birth, and nasopharynx if chlamydial pneumonia suspected.

Ophthalmia neonatorum and infant pneumonia
Recommended treatment
- *erythromycin*: 50 mg/kg oral daily divided into 4 doses for 14 days *or*
- *azithromycin*: 20 mg/kg oral daily in single dose for 3 days
- topical treatments are ineffective.

Infection in prepubertal children recommended treatment
- *erythromycin*: 50 mg/kg oral daily (up to 1 g) divided into 4 doses for 14 days *or*
- *if weight ≥45 kg*: azithromycin 1 g as a single dose *or*
- *if weight ≥45 kg and ≥8 years old*: doxycycline 100 mg bd for 7 days.

Partner notification

PN should be discussed with all index cases at the time of diagnosis.

All confirmed contacts should be offered full STI screen, including HIV, and offered epidemiological treatment.

Contact tracing period for the following index cases:
- *Men with symptomatic urethritis*: all contacts since onset and 4 weeks prior to onset of symptoms.
- *All others*: 6 months prior to presentation.

Similar principles should apply to the mother of neonate with chlamydial infection and her sex partner(s).

Follow-up

- Re-testing recommended after 3–6 months for patients <25 years old due to high re-infection rate.
- A test of cure following treatment of urogenital *C. trachomatis* infection, if not pregnant, is only recommended if not treated with doxycycline or azithromycin, symptoms persist, adherence issues.
- Repeat treatment if risk of re-infection from untreated partner.
- If persistent symptoms check compliance.
- Re-testing (if required) should be delayed until at least 3–5 weeks after the end of the treatment, to avoid false positive result

HIV infection

Chlamydial infection facilitates HIV transmission, producing ↑ in detectable virus in urethral/cervical secretions when infection is present. This is re-versed following antibiotic treatment.

LGV prevalence ↑ in this patient group, so all diagnosed with rectal chlamydia should either be tested for LGV, treated presumptively with 21 days doxycycline 100 mg bd, or have TOC.

Further information
British Association for Sexual Health and HIV Chlamydia guideline
൪ https://www.bashh.org/guidelines

Chapter 10

Non-gonococcal urethritis and mucopurulent cervicitis

Introduction 162
Aetiology 162
Clinical features 163
Diagnosis 164
Management 165

Introduction

Non-specific genital infection, NSU, and NGU are all terms that have been used to describe inflammation of the ♂ urethra in the absence of *Neisseria gonorrhoeae*; NGU is the preferred term. 11–50% of cases are caused by *Chlamydia trachomatis,* and *Mycoplasma genitalium* is increasingly being recognized with increasing access to standardized testing assays. The less well defined ♀ equivalent mucopurulent cervicitis (MPC) is more problematic to diagnose; 20–40% are caused by *C. trachomatis*.

Aetiology

Most commonly caused by *C. trachomatis* and *Mycoplasma genitalium*, especially in younger patients and those with urethral discharge or dysuria. *M. genitalium* may also be associated with balanoposthitis.

See Table 10.1.

- The rate of TV as a cause of NGU depends on prevalence in the community, and is more common in ♂ aged >30.
- *Adenovirus*; often with accompanying pharyngitis, conjunctivitis, and constitutional symptoms, probably transmitted via oral sex.
- EBV, *N. meningitidis, Candida* sp., *Haemophilus* sp. have also been reported causes.
- UTI found in up to 6%.
- BV is seen in 30% of ♀ partners.
- Organism negative NGU is poorly understood. Urethral strictures, urethral foreign body, trauma, manipulation, chemical irritation, allergens, and Stevens–Johnson syndrome have all been implicated.

Table 10.1 Non-gonococcal urethritis: commonest causative organisms

Chlamydia trachomatis	11–50%
Mycoplasma genitalium	6–50%
Ureaplasmas	5–26%
Trichomonas vaginalis	1–20%
Adenovirus	2–4%
Herpes simplex virus	2–3%

Clinical features

Symptoms and signs

See Table 10.2 for non-gonococcal urethritis.

Table 10.2 Symptoms and signs of non-gonococcal urethritis

Symptoms	Signs
• Urethral discharge	• Urethral discharge—varying amount, clear to yellow, spontaneous or expressed
• Dysuria	
• Penile irritation	• Balanoposthitis
• None	• None

Up to 20% of ♂ with observable discharge have no symptoms. NGU without symptoms and signs is less likely to be due to *C. trachomatis* or *M. genitalium*.

Mucopurulent cervicitis

• usually asymptomatic, but if severe may cause vaginal discharge and vulval irritation
• cervix appears inflamed, oedematous, and friable with an overlying mucopurulent discharge.

Complications

• epididymo-orchitis (➲ Chapter 13, 'Epididymo-orchitis', pp. 193–200)
• SARA/Reiter's syndrome, occurs in <1% (➲ Chapter 14, 'Sexually-acquired reactive arthritis', pp. 201–12)
• PID (➲ Chapter 11, 'Pelvic inflammatory disease', pp. 169–79)

Diagnosis

Only those with active symptoms or visible signs should be assessed for NGU/MPC.

Non-gonococcal urethritis

Urethral specimen, using a 5-mm plastic loop or cotton-tipped swab (after holding urine for 2–4 hours to improve sensitivity). If no urethral material, check FVU.

Urethritis diagnosed by high-power (×1000) microscopy of Gram-stained material and the presence of PMNLs, in the absence of intracellular gonococci:

- ≥5 PMNL/field of urethral smear in ≥5 fields
- ≥10 PMNL/field of threads or deposits from FVU.

Where microscopy is not available, diagnosis can be made based on:

- mucopurulent discharge on examination
- ≥1+ leucocyte esterase on FVU dipstick (poor sensitivity)
- presence of threads on FVU (may be physiological, e.g. semen).

Symptomatic ♂, without evidence of urethritis after holding urine for 2–4 hours, may be re-assessed after holding urine overnight.

Mucopurulent cervicitis

No definitive microscopic criteria for diagnosis as the number of cervical PMNLs varies physiologically. Diagnosis based on a friable cervix +/− mucopurulent cervical discharge on examination and microscopic finding of >30 PMNLs/HPF may be used.

Investigations

- *N .gonorrhoeae* and *C. trachomatis* NAAT as routine.
- MSSU to exclude UTI.
- *M. genitalium* NAAT if available, with macrolide resistance testing.
- Microscopy for TV and BV.

Management

- initiate treatment as soon as diagnosis made
- avoid sex until index patient and partner completed treatment
- give patient information regarding causes, health implications, treatment, importance of compliance, contact tracing, and treatment
- avoid over-examination/over-washing
- follow-up indicated if symptoms persist.

NGU

Both first line treatments are <85% effective. If infection is caused by *M. genitalium* treatment failures of <68% with doxycycline 100 mg bd for 7 days and <33% with azithromycin 1 g stat, although the latter is associated with inducing macrolide resistance mutations.

Recommended first line treatment of first episode NGU
Doxycycline 100 mg bd for 7 days

Alternative treatment
Azithromycin 1 g once followed by 500 mg od for next 2 days; *or* ofloxacin 200 mg bd or 400 mg od for 7 days

Persistent and recurrent NGU

Recurrent NGU (return of symptoms within 30–90 days) occurs in 10–20%. Re-infection should be considered.

Persistent NGU occurs in 15–25%, is multifactorial and is organism negative in >50%. In 20–40% of those treated with azithromycin 1 g stat *M. genitalium* is identified and in 10–20% *C. trachomatis* is found. TV and ureaplasmas may also play a role.

- ensure initial treatment complied with and reinfection considered
- only investigate if symptomatic or clinical evidence of urethritis
- consider TV and *M. genitalium* PCR testing if available.

Recommended treatment

- azithromycin 1 g once, followed by 500 mg od next 2 days (to be started within 2 weeks of doxycycline treatment) *plus* metronidazole 400 mg bd for 5 days.

Recommended treatment if azithromycin used first-line

- moxifloxacin 400 mg od for 10–14 days *plus* metronidazole 400 mg bd for 5 days.

❶ Risk of life-threatening liver reactions, Steven–Johnson syndrome, and haematological abnormalities with moxifloxacin.

Alternative treatment
doxycycline 100 mg bd *plus* metronidazole 400 mg bd 5 days.

Box 10.1 *Mycoplasma genitalium*

Mycoplasmas are the smallest free-living organisms. *M. genitalium* was isolated in 1980 from ♂ urethra. It is slow growing and difficult to isolate, preferentially colonizes the urethra, where it can invade epithelial cells.

Aetiology

Largely by genito-genital mucosal contact. Anogenital transmission can occur, but oro-genital transmission is unlikely to be significant as oral carriage is low. Prevalence 10–35% in ♂ with non-chlamydial NGU and 40% in ♂ with persistent NGU. Significant association between *M. genitalium* and cervicitis, ♀ urethritis, endometritis, PID, tubal infertility, and pre-term birth.

Clinical features

Up to 30% men and 75% women asymptomatic. In women dysuria, discharge, cervicitis, and rarely intermenstrual bleeding (IMB)/post-coital bleeding (PCB), low abdominal pain may be seen. In men, dysuria and urethral discharge, and in one study balano-posthitis may be present. Complications include SARA, epididimo-orchitis, PID, tubal infertility.

Diagnosis and management

Diagnosis is by NAAT, with macrolide resistance probe if positive. Intrinsic resistance to many antimicrobials. Sensitive to tetracyclines (except if *tetM* gene present), macrolides, and fluoroquinolones. Increasing resistance to macrolides due to widespread use of single dose azithromycin for treatment of NGU. Test for cure ≥3 weeks after treatment started.

Treatment of uncomplicated M. genitalium

Doxycycline 100 mg bd for 7 days followed by azithromycin 1 g once then 500 mg daily for next 2 days *or* moxifloxacin 400 mg daily 10days.

Persistent and macrolide resistant M. genitalium

Doxycycline 100 mg bd 7 days followed by pristinamycin 1 g qds 10 days *or* doxycycline 100 mg bd 14 days *or* pristinamycin 1 g qds 14 days *or* minocycline 100 mg bd 14 days.

Complicated (PID, epididymitis) M. genitalium infection

Moxifloxacin 400 mg od 14 days.

Treatment in pregnancy and breastfeeding

Azithromycin 1 g single dose followed by 500 mg daily for 2 days (in pregnancy and breastfeeding moxifloxacin is contraindicated, and doxycycline and pristinamycin not advised)

Continuing urethritis

- Limited evidence for management.
- Urological investigation recommended if urinary flow symptoms.
- Consider abacterial prostatitis, chronic pelvic pain syndrome, and psychosexual causes (➔ Chapter 12, 'Prostatitis/chronic pelvic pain syndrome in men, pp. 181–91).
- Consider retreatment of index and partner concurrently with same antimicrobials.
- Erythromycin 500 mg qds for 3 weeks or clarithromycin 500 mg bd for 3 weeks has been tried with success.

Mucopurulent cervicitis

If high risk of STI, presumptive treatment should be considered, alternatively awaiting results is an option. Follow-up to ensure resolution is advised.

Recommended treatment
Doxycycline 100 mg bd for 7 days.

Alternative treatment
Azithromycin 500 mg stat, then 250 mg daily for next 4 days.

Recurrent and persistent mucopurulent cervicitis

Management as for recurrent/persistent NGU.

Partner notification and epidemiological treatment

PN should be carried out with epidemiological treatment and testing for all contacts within the last 4 weeks of symptomatic patients with NGU and 8 weeks for contacts of MPC.

Recommended treatment for contacts of NGU and MPC
Provide epidemiological treatment with the same antimicrobials that resulted in cure in the index case.

Further information

British Association for Sexual Health and HIV guidelines for NGU and Mycoplasma Genitalium ℘ https://www.bashh.org/guidelines

Pelvic inflammatory disease

Introduction *170*
Aetiology *171*
Epidemiology *172*
Clinical features *173*
Complications and sequelae *174*
Investigations *175*
Diagnosis *176*
Management *178*

Introduction

PID refers to inflammation of the upper female genital tract (endometrium, fallopian tubes, and ovaries) and supporting structures (parametrium and pelvic peritoneum). It is usually a result of infection:

- ascending from the endocervix
- less commonly spread from other abdominal organs (e.g. appendicitis) or disseminated by blood.

Endometritis and endosalpingitis produce a purulent exudate that may escape into the recto-vaginal pouch, resulting in a pelvic abscess. Inflammation may spread to the ovaries (oophoritis), parametrium, and pelvic peritoneum (peritonitis).

Aetiology

Sexually transmitted infections

- *Chlamydia trachomatis* is the commonest cause in 14–35%. Induces Th-2 type immune response, damaging tubal epithelium.
- *Neisseria gonorrhoeae* produces complement-mediated necrosis of ciliated epithelial cells.
- *Mycoplasma genitalium* is also implicated as a cause of PID.

Worldwide data—wide ranges relate to variable infection rates and availability of reliable tests.

PID in 10–30% of untreated cervical chlamydial and gonococcal infections.

Other micro-organisms

- *BV associated organisms*: anaerobic bacilli (e.g. *Prevotella* and *Bacteroides* spp.), anaerobic cocci (e.g. *Peptostreptococcus* spp., *Gardenerella vaginalis*, *Mycoplasma hominis*, α and non-haemolytic streptococci). Recovered from fallopian tubes in up to 20% of ♀ with PID and 80% of endometrial samples in plasma cell endometritis (accompanying PID in ascending infection). Statistically significant association between BV and PID. Sialidase activity of *Prevotella* and *Bacteroides* spp., weakening cervical mucous barrier, possibly promotes ascending infection.
- Other organisms have also been recovered from the fallopian tubes: viridans group streptococci, group A–D streptococci, *Escherichia coli*, *Bacteroides fragilis*, *Haemophilis influenzae*, and coagulase –ve staphylococci.
- *Actinomyces israelii and related species*: occasionally cause a chronic pelvic abscess (<1 in 3000 cases of PID and 3% of all human actinomyces infections), usually in association with plastic IUDs and anaerobic co-infection.
- *Mycobacterium tuberculosis*: haematogenously disseminated; an important cause in areas of high prevalence.
- *Salmonella spp.*: rarely as a result of abdominal spread from an intestinal focus of infection in typhoid and paratyphoid.

Factors facilitating ascending infection

Physiological

- *Uterine contractions*: ↑ in the follicular phase until ovulation.
- Loss of cervical mucus plug (formed in the luteal phase) and retrograde flow during menstruation.
- Possible carriage of bacteria by spermatozoa.

Iatrogenic

- IUD insertion ↑ risk for 4–6 weeks after insertion.
- Uterine instrumentation.

Epidemiology

Estimated annual incidence in industrialized countries ~1/1000 in ♀ aged 15–34 years (1.5–2/1000 if 15–24) with wide geographical and temporal variations. Sexual transmission is the major aetiological factor.

Risk factors
See Box 11.1.

> ### Box 11.1 Factors that increase and decrease risk of PID
>
> *Factors increasing risk*
> - *Young age*: peak incidence in age group 15–24 years.
> - Multiple partners.
> - New partner within previous 3 months.
> - Frequency of sexual intercourse.
> - Past history of STI (patient or partner).
> - Past history of PID.
> - *Uterine instrumentation*:
>   - termination of pregnancy
>   - insertion of IUD within the previous 6 weeks (overall incidence of PID only 0.15%), but concomitant cervical chlamydial/gonococcal infection ↑ risk to 3–5%
>   - hysterosalpingography/hysteroscopy
>   - endometrial biopsy, curettage, and ablation
>   - *in vitro* fertilization procedure.
> - Post-partum endometritis.
> - Vaginal douching.
> - Cigarette smoking.
>
> *Factors reducing risk*
> - Hormonal contraception especially progesterone-only preparations (production of a 'luteal-type' cervical mucus plug and reduction in the tubal inflammatory response).
> - Consistent use of condom or diaphragm.
> - Spermicide.
> - *Pregnancy*: PID is uncommon because of thickened cervical mucus plug and only seen in early pregnancy as (after the first trimester) protection is afforded by the amniotic sac filling the uterine cavity.

Clinical features

Acute pelvic inflammatory disease (symptoms for <3 weeks)

Onset within 7 days of the 1st day of menstruation correlates with gono-coccal/chlamydial infection. Symptoms and signs tend to be more acute/intense in gonococcal than chlamydial PID.

Symptoms
- lower abdominal pain; usually subacute if mild and acute if severe
- deep dyspareunia, common
- menstrual irregularity in ~40%
- abnormal bleeding
- dysmenorrhoea
- vaginal discharge
- nausea +/− vomiting if severe.

Signs
- lower abdominal tenderness with guarding; rebound if severe
- adnexal and cervical motion (excitation) tenderness
- fever (>38°C) in ~50%; more likely in severe or gonococcal PID
- adnexal mass in 50% of ♀ with gonococcal PID
- abdominal distension due to paralytic ileus if very severe (~1%)

Chronic pelvic inflammatory disease ('silent PID')

May be asymptomatic and discovered only on investigation of infertility. Symptoms include constant or intermittent pain/discomfort in lower abdomen, groin or back, dyspareunia, malaise, and frequent/heavy menstrual periods. Usually, no appreciable signs, but thickening of tubes and/or fixed retroverted uterus may be palpable.

Complications and sequelae

Tubo-ovarian and pelvic abscess

Late complication, likely to be associated with anaerobic bacteria.

Peri-appendicitis

Direct spread of infection from the right fallopian tube to the appendiceal serosa may produce external inflammation (serositis) without mucosal involvement. Tubo-appendiceal mass develops. 2–10% of acute appendicitis in ♀ may be due to peri-appendicitis, 25–50% of which may be linked to tubal inflammation.

Infertility

Occurs in 8%, 20%, and 40% after 1, 2, and 3 episodes of PID, respectively. Due to tubal occlusion and peritubal adhesions. The more severe the episode, the higher the incidence of infertility. Conflicting evidence on risk ↓ with treatment of PID.

Ectopic pregnancy

Seven-fold ↑ in risk of ectopic pregnancy (9% compared with 1.3% in the absence of PID). Risk ↑ directly with PID severity and number of episodes.

Chronic pelvic pain

Incidence 12%, 33%, and 66% after 1, 2, and 3 episodes of PID, respectively. Due to pelvic adhesions that form after the initial or recurrent episodes. Affects psychosocial functioning and quality of life.

Perihepatitis (Fitz-Hugh–Curtis syndrome)

Inflammation of the hepatic capsule with 'violin string' adhesions between anterior surface of liver and abdominal wall. Results from peritoneal or lymphatic spread (haematogenous spread may be possible) of pelvic gonococcal/chlamydial infection. Occurs in 10–20% with PID.

Symptoms and signs of PID are not always present, but a past history of PID or lower genital infection may be obtained. Typical presentation is acute, often severe, with right upper quadrant pain radiating to the back and shoulder tip, made worse by deep inspiration and movement. Examination demonstrates tenderness and guarding in the right upper abdominal quadrant. Hepatic rub may be heard on auscultation. Pyrexia in ~50%.

Differential diagnosis: acute cholecystitis, biliary colic, pleurisy, pneumonia, or pulmonary embolism.

Investigations

Routine

- Lower genital tract swabs for *N. gonorrhoeae, C. trachomatis* and *M. genitalium*.
- *Gram-stained smear of cervical material*: may provide presumptive diagnosis of gonorrhoea. PMNLs are non-specific (positive predictive value only 17%), but useful for exclusion of PID (negative predictive value 95%).
- *Peripheral blood white blood cell (WBC) count*: ↑ in ~50%.
- *Erythrocyte sedimentation rate (ESR)*: ↑ in ~75%.
- *C-reactive protein (CRP)*: ↑ in ~75%, level reflects severity.
- *Chlamydial antibody*: only provides retrospective or inconclusive evidence; hence, of limited value in acute PID. However, in ♀ investigated for infertility antibody, especially at high level, correlates closely with frequency and severity of tubal damage, and adverse pregnancy outcome. Therefore, useful as a screening test to determine the likelihood of tubal damage and need for early laparoscopy.
- ▶ *Pregnancy test (urine or plasma βhCG)*: essential for acute pelvic pain in all ♀ of childbearing age.
- Urine analysis +/− MSSU if urinary tract infection is suspected.

Specialized

Endometrial histology/microbiology

Sensitivity ~70%, specificity ~90%.

Pelvic imaging

Abdominal ultrasound useful for detection of pelvic abscess. Transvaginal ultrasonography reported to have ~80% sensitivity and specificity (compared with laparoscopy/endometrial biopsy). May be necessary for differential diagnosis, particularly ectopic gestation.

Laparoscopy

Regarded as the gold standard, but not routinely performed (time/cost/complication risk). Allows diagnosis of acute PID by identifying:

- Pronounced hyperaemia of tubal surface
- Oedema of tubal wall
- Sticky exudate from fimbriae.
- Collection of laboratory specimens from affected sites.
- Identification of other causes (e.g. ectopic gestation, appendicitis, endometriosis) or complications (e.g. abscess, pelvic adhesions, 'violin string adhesions' of perihepatitis).

May fail to identify endosalpingitis/endometritis in early/mild infection.

Diagnosis

Clinical diagnosis of PID, based on signs and symptoms has positive predictive value of 65–90% compared with laparoscopy. In routine clinical practice, a lower threshold is often applied for prompt antibiotic treatment. Table 11.1 lists symptoms and signs suggestive of PID.

Table 11.1 Diagnostic criteria

Main	Additional
Low abdominal or pelvic pain	Temperature >38°C
Deep dyspareunia, cervical motion tenderness/adnexal tenderness on examination.	↑ CRP/ESR WBC >10 × 10⁹
Abnormal bleeding; intermenstrual, post coital, ↑ menstrual bleeding	Adnexal mass
Abnormal vaginal discharge	PMNLs in cervical/vaginal Gram-stained smears (positive predictive value 17%). Absence of endocervical or vaginal PMNLs has 95% negative predictive value

Differential diagnosis

Box 11.2 Differential diagnosis of PID includes

Acute/subacute

- *Ectopic pregnancy*: in ruptured ectopic pregnancy sudden onset of iliac fossa or hypogastric pain often associated with syncope. Vaginal spotting in early stages. Shoulder tip pain if blood tracked into abdominal cavity. Shock with intra-abdominal haemorrhage.
- *Acute appendicitis*: initial peri-umbilical pain later localizing to right iliac fossa with pronounced nausea and vomiting.
- *Ruptured ovarian or endometriotic cyst*: sudden onset of perimenstrual lower abdominal pain, usually afebrile.
- Complications of ovarian neoplasms.
- *Acute pyelonephritis*: pyrexia of sudden onset, rigors, loin/iliac fossa pain, urinary symptoms.
- Mesenteric lymphadenitis, inflammatory bowel disease.
- Adnexal torsion.

Chronic/recurrent

- Endometriosis.
- Pelvic congestion syndrome.
- Ovarian cysts.
- Ovarian and uterine neoplasms.
- Interstitial cystitis.
- Urethral syndrome.
- Irritable bowel syndrome.
- Inflammatory bowel disease.
- Previous surgery, leading to pelvic adhesions or nerve entrapment.
- Myofascial pain syndrome.
- *Psychosocial causes*: depression, previous physical and sexual abuse/trauma, leading to somatization disorder.

Management

General principles

Detailed explanation of condition and implications for long-term health of them and their partner(s), with provision of information leaflet.

▶ Advise avoidance of sexual intercourse until the patient and partner(s) have completed treatment and symptoms resolved.

To minimize sequelae, commence treatment promptly (even before definitive diagnosis). Hospital admission if:
* systemic disturbance is severe
* surgical/gynaecological emergency cannot be excluded
* patient is pregnant or immunocompromised
* tubo-ovarian or pelvic abscess is detected or suspected
* failure of oral therapy, or unable to tolerate oral treatment.

Monitor response with inflammatory and clinical markers. If failure of initial treatment, perform imaging to excluded tubo-ovarian abscess. Prescribe rest and adequate analgesia.

IUD removal should be considered in severe PID, if no improvement after 72 hours of treatment, if actinomycosis present, or patient requests. Offer emergency contraception on removal if pregnancy risk within preceding 7 days.

Treatment regimens

When choosing antibiotic regimen consider:
* severity and systemic disturbance—may need parenteral treatment
* optimal duration 10–14 days
* no difference in efficacy between the recommended regimens
* where antibiotic regimens below are not available antibiotics should cover *C. trachomatis, N. gonorrhoeae*, and anaerobes.
* in women with *M. genitalium* infection, moxifloxacin is recommended.

> Initial regimens may need to be altered when antibiotic sensitivities are available

Out-patient
* Ceftriaxone 500 mg IM single dose *plus* doxycycline 100 mg oral bd for 14 days *plus* metronidazole 400 mg bd for 7–14 days.
* Ofloxacin 400 mg bd for 14 days *plus* metronidazole 400 mg bd for 14 days.
* Moxifloxacin 400 mg daily for 14 days ❶ ↑ risk of life-threatening liver reactions, cardiac arrhythmias with QTc prolongation, rhabdomyolysis, and tendon rupture.

In-patient
Continue IV therapy until 24 hours after clinical improvement, then switch to oral treatment to complete 14 days total.
* Ceftriaxone 1 g IV/IM od *plus* doxycycline 100 mg oral (or IV if oral not tolerated) bd. Followed by oral doxycycline 100 mg bd *plus* metronidazole 500 mg bd to complete 14 days.

- Clindamycin IV 900 mg tid *plus* gentamicin 3–6 mg/kg IV or IM od with renal monitoring. Followed by *either* (clindamycin 450 mg oral qds) *or* (doxycycline 100 mg bd *plus* metronidazole 400 mg bd) to complete 14 days.

Alternative regimens
- Ofloxacin 400 mg IV bd *plus* metronidazole 500 mg IV tid for 14 days.
- Ceftriaxone 500 mg IM single dose *plus* azithromycin 1 g single dose followed by a second dose after 1 week.

Treatment in pregnancy
Parenteral treatment advisable. Replace doxycycline with erythromycin 50 mg/kg daily IV *plus* metronidazole 400 mg oral/IV tid or 1 g pre-rectum tid

HIV infection
- ↓ Production of interferon-γ may ↑ susceptibility to PID.
- Tubo-ovarian abscess formation more likely if immunocompromised.
- Symptoms may be more severe, but respond well to standard antibiotic regimens, although parenteral antibiotics may be required.

Treatment of actinomyces-like organisms

If a woman has actinomycoces-like organisms (ALOs) identified, pelvic pain, and an IUD *in situ* consider removal. (If ALOs are identified in an asymptomatic woman with an IUD, it can remain *in situ* and probably represents colonization, rather than infection.) Appropriate antibiotics will need to be continued for at least 8 weeks, and choice of antibiotic and route will depend on the clinical picture. Consult a local microbiologist. Benzylpenicillin 18–24 MU (10.8–14.4 g) IV daily as infusion (or 4-hourly injections) and metronidazole 500 mg IV 8-hourly is effective, with doxycycline, erythromycin, and clindamycin as alternatives to benzylpenicillin.

Partner notification

Sexual partner/s within a 6-month period of onset of symptoms should be contacted and offered screening for STIs (or according to sexual history). Any detected infections should be treated appropriately. Consider empirical broad spectrum treatment to cover other organisms implicated in PID, e.g. doxycycline 100 mg bd for 7 days. Avoid unprotected sex until they and their partner completed treatment.

Follow-up

Review those with moderate or severe symptoms after 72 hours. Failure to improve should prompt further investigations.

Further information

British Association for Sexual Health and HIV Pelvic inflammatory disease guideline ℘ https://www.bashh.org/guidelines

Prostatitis/chronic pelvic pain syndrome in men

Introduction *182*
Acute bacterial prostatitis (ABP) *183*
Chronic bacterial prostatitis (CBP) *185*
Chronic prostatitis/chronic pelvic pain syndrome (CPPS) *187*
Asymptomatic inflammatory prostatitis *191*
Other rare causes of prostatitis *191*
Sexually transmitted infections *191*
Prostatitis and HIV infection *191*

Introduction

Prostatitis affects up to 50% of men at some time in their lives, with a prevalence of 8.2% of prostatic symptoms, similar to prevalence of chronic pelvic pain in women and chronic asthma. The National Institutes of Health produced a classification following two consensus conferences in 1995 and 1998, which is now widely used:

- *Category I*: acute bacterial prostatitis.
- *Category II*: chronic bacterial prostatitis.
- *Category III*: chronic (non-bacterial) prostatitis/chronic pelvic pain syndrome (CP/CPPS). Subgroups of this class are (A) inflammatory and (B) non-inflammatory (previously prostatodynia).
- *Category IV*: asymptomatic inflammatory prostatitis.

The majority of cases are chronic and probably 90–95% of these are abacterial. Diagnosis is largely based on symptoms, as signs and objective clinical data may be inconclusive or lacking. Symptoms that may be attributed to prostatitis/chronic pelvic pain syndrome in men are outlined in Table 12.1.

Table 12.1 Symptoms that may indicate prostatitis or chronic pelvic pain syndrome in men

Urogenital pain	*Lower urinary tract symptoms (LUTS)*
• Perineum	• Frequency/nocturia
• Low abdomen/suprapubic	• Urgency
• Penis (especially tip)	• Incomplete voiding
• Testes	• Abnormal flow
• Rectum	• Urethral discharge
• Retropubis and upper thighs	• Haematospermia
• Low back/coccyx	
• Urethra	
Sexual dysfunction	*Psychological*
• Pain with/after ejaculation	• Reduced quality of life
• Low libido	• Depression
• Erectile dysfunction	• Anxiety

Acute bacterial prostatitis (ABP)

Uncommon, but clearly identifiable, and easiest to diagnose and treat effectively. Should be considered as a complication of acute lower urinary tract infection (LUTI), caused by urinary pathogens especially *Escherichia coli*. There may be an underlying structural abnormality of the urinary tract, which should be investigated after resolution of the acute episode.

Symptoms
- *Prostatitis*: perineal prostatic pain.
- *Those of a LUTI*: dysuria, frequency, urgency, incomplete bladder emptying (➔ Chapter 21, 'Urinary tract infection', pp. 267–76).
- *Bacteraemia*: pyrexia, rigors, myalgia, arthralgia.
- *Abscess (rare complication)*: intense pain and acute urinary retention. In the pre-antibiotic era, gonorrhoea was a frequent cause of a prostatic abscess.

Diagnosis
- *Gentle digital rectal examination*: prostate enlarged, tender, warm, and/or boggy. Prostatic massage contraindicated in ABP as it may precipitate bacteraemia.
- Midstream sample of urine (MSSU).
- STI screening.
- Exclude sepsis (BP, pulse, temperature, respiratory rate, FBC, CRP, blood glucose, renal function). If concerned, admit for further assessment in Emergency Department (blood cultures, arterial blood gases, lactate).
- Discuss with Urology.
- Urology may undertake additional investigations. Transrectal ultrasound (also useful to exclude prostatic abscess). Residual bladder ultrasound to check for urinary retention.

Management
- *ABP is a serious infection*: start antibiotics immediately. Oral fluoroquinolone (e.g. ciprofloxacin 500 mg bd or ofloxacin 200 mg bd). Trimethoprim 200 mg bd (if fluoroquinolone intolerant or allergic). All for 28 days. Review in 24–48 hours to check response; review with results.
- *Provide analgesia*: paracetamol and ibuprofen regularly combined. Stronger codeine-based analgesia if not helped.
- Admit to hospital if severely ill, unable to take oral antibiotics, urinary retention (seen in ~10%). Management as in-patient may include initial parenteral broad-spectrum cephalosporin (e.g. cefuroxime) plus gentamicin then switch to oral regimen once clinically stable. IV fluids and urinary drainage (if retention) may also be required. If abscess present that fails to respond to antibiotics—transurethral resection with drainage.

Causes of haematospermia
- *Trauma* (most common cause in young ♂): generally mild, often isolated episodes; usually self-limiting.
- *Inflammation*: prostatitis, seminal vesiculitis, urethritis, epididymitis.
- *Obstruction/dilatation of urogenital ducts*: prostatic cysts, urethral strictures, ejaculatory duct cysts, and strictures.
- *Vascular abnormalities*: arteriovenous malformations, venous malformations, haemangiomata.
- *Systemic disorders*:
  - severe hypertension
  - *haematological disorders*—coagulation disorders, leukaemia
  - cirrhosis.
- *Drugs*: e.g. warfarin.
- *Tumours*:
  - *Benign*—polyps, warts, benign prostatic hyperplasia
  - *Malignant*—carcinoma of genital tract

Chronic bacterial prostatitis (CBP)

Unusual, accounting for ~2–5% of prostatitis cases. Recurrent or persistent prostate infection usually due to *E. coli* (~80%). Patients experience recurrent UTIs with the prostate gland as the infection source, warranting urological referral. In addition, there may be obstructive urinary symptoms, perineal prostatic pain, and possibly sexual dysfunction, but unlike ABP, no systemic symptoms.

Diagnosis

- Consider if recurrent UTIs.
- Digital rectal *examination*: normal, hypertrophied, and/or tender prostate.
- *Evidence of prostatic infection*: bacterial colony count in expressed prostatic secretions or post-prostate massage urine specimen (Box 12.1) at least ×10 greater than FVU or MSSU.

Management

Antibiotics for 4–8 weeks according to antimicrobial sensitivity, preferably a fluoroquinolone (high relative concentration in prostate tissue, 2–3× serum levels), e.g. ciprofloxacin, ofloxacin. Levofloxacin plus azithromycin is an alternative. Trimethoprim, which also has good prostate penetration, can be considered as second-line treatment. If symptoms persist following infection clearance undertake management of CP/CPPS.

Box 12.1 Prostatic assessment for inflammation and infection

Prostatic massage
- Patient should not have:
  - taken antibiotics within previous 4 weeks
  - ejaculated within previous 48 hours
  - evidence of urethritis or UTI (exclude prior to prostatic massage).
- Obtain FVU (urethral) and MSSU (bladder) prior to massage.
- Place patient in left lateral position and ensure that he is breathing easily through his mouth (to avoid valsalva manoeuvre).
- With lubricated forefinger in rectum gently press on right and left lateral aspects of prostate gland in turn and move finger to the midline. Repeat 3–4 times.
- Press on superior aspect of prostate gland in midline and move finger to its lower pole. Repeat 2–3 times.
- Prostatic fluid should appear at the urethral meatus, although sometimes gentle milking of the urethra is required.
- If this fails, the process can be repeated. However, a dry massage is fairly common.
- Obtain FVU after massage.

Expressed prostatic secretions (EPS)
- pH8 suggestive, but not diagnostic of prostatitis.
- Bacterial colony count in the EPS and post-prostate massage urine sample must be at least ×10 greater than FVU and pre-massage MSSU to diagnose chronic bacterial prostatitis.
- ≥10 PMNL/HPF is considered diagnostic of inflammation. If dry massage, look for PMNLs 10/HPF greater in post-massage urine than FVU and MSSU. EPS PMNLs may be absent in cases of inflammation with infection and also 10/HPF found in up to 6% of healthy controls; therefore, unreliable in subclassifying CPPS into inflammatory and non-inflammatory categories.

Chronic prostatitis/chronic pelvic pain syndrome (CPPS)

The most common form of prostatitis (>90% of all cases). Understanding of the causes of this syndrome is limited and other organs (including pelvic floor, bladder, and seminal vesicles) may be involved.

↑ Genital tract post-inflammatory cytokines, possibly suggesting auto-immunity, post-infective triggers, or neurogenic inflammation. Genital or pelvic pain is required in its diagnosis, and exclusion criteria include urethritis, urogenital cancer, urinary tract disease, functionally relevant urethral stricture, or bladder neurological disease.

Subclassified as inflammatory if PMNLs found in EPS (Box 12.1), semen, or post-prostate massage urine. Patients with the non-inflammatory subtype have no evidence of inflammation. In practical terms, this differentiation is of little value as the clinical presentation and response to treatment are almost identical.

CPPS may present as chronic unilateral testicular pain, which may be provoked by coitus. This is usually idiopathic but may follow acute epididymitis, vasectomy, previous trauma, or be associated with a varicocele, hydrocele, or sexual dysfunction.

Symptoms

Quantitative assessment of severity of prostatitis useful in temporal review or in gauging therapeutic response using the Chronic Prostatitis Symptom Index (Box 12.2).

Diagnosis

- By exclusion of other causes, including bladder or prostate infection, urinary obstruction, testicular cancer, genitourinary tract calculi, hernias, radiculopathies, other chronic pain syndromes.
- *Digital rectal examination*: prostate gland usually feels normal with variable degrees of tenderness (local, diffuse) or none.
- Urinalysis and MSU.
- *STI screening*: Chlamydia, Gonorrhoea, Trichomonas, Ureaplasma and Mycoplasma where available.
- Consider TB, tropical infection in those at risk
- Microscopy of any discharge/threads
- *Prostatic specific antigen (PSA)*: request if abnormal prostate, patient concerns, symptoms of bladder outflow obstruction. Beware falsely high readings following digital rectal examination and other causes.
- *Urology opinion*: cystoscopy, urodynamic studies, prostatic biopsy.
- *Colorectal opinion*: if any concerns of bowel pathology, including rectal malignancy.
- *Magnetic resonance imaging (MRI) pelvis/lumbar spine*: history of lower back ache, injury, possible prostatic abscess. Discuss with multi-disciplinary team (MDT).
- *Psychological screening*: various tools available including Chronic Prostatitis Symptom Index (Box 12.2).

Box 12.2 Chronic Prostatitis Symptom Index

Pain or discomfort in the last week
1. Have you experienced any pain or discomfort in the following areas?
- Perineum (i.e. from rectum to testicles)
  - Yes (1)/No (0)
- Testicles
  - Yes (1)/No (0)
- Penile tip (unrelated to urination)
  - Yes (1)/No (0)
- Below waist (pubic/bladder area)
  - Yes (1)/No (0)
2. Have you experienced?
- Pain/burning during micturition
  - Yes (1)/No (0)
- Pain/discomfort during/after ejaculation
  - Yes (1)/No (0)
3. How often have you had pain or discomfort in any of these areas?
- Never (0)
- Rarely (1)
- Sometimes (2)
- Often (3)
- Usually (4)
- Always (5)
4. Which number describes your average pain/discomfort on the days you had it on a 0–10 point scale?
- 'No pain' (0) to 'Pain as bad as you can imagine' (10)

Urination over the last week
5. How often have you sensed incomplete bladder emptying?
- Never (0)
- <1 in 5 (1)
- <Half (2)
- About half (3)
- >Half (4)
- Almost always (5)
6. How often have you had to repeat urination within <2 hours?
- Never (0)
- <1 in 5 (1)
- <Half (2)
- About half (3)
- >Half (4)
- Almost always (5)

Impact of symptoms over the last week
7. How much have the symptoms restricted you from doing things?
- None (0)
- Only a little (1)
- Some (2)
- A lot (3)

(Continued)

Box 12.2 *(Contd.)*

8. How much have you thought about your symptoms?
- None (0)
- Only a little (1)
- Some (2)
- A lot (3)

Quality of life based on your symptoms over the past week
9. How would you feel if they persisted for the rest of your life?
- Delighted (0)
- Pleased (1)
- Mostly satisfied (2)
- Mixed (3)
- Mostly dissatisfied (4)
- Unhappy (5)
- Terrible (6)

Scoring
- *Calculate and report 3 separate scores*: pain (1–4), urinary symptoms (5 and 6), and impact of symptoms/quality of life (7–9).
- *Calculate and report a pain and urinary score (range 0–31) referred to as the 'symptom scale score'*:
  - Mild = 0–9
  - Moderate = 10–18
  - Severe = 19–31

Calculate and report total score (range 0–43), referred to as the 'total score'. Assess at baseline and follow over time (and treatment) using each patient as his own control. Can also be used to compare with established and published 'norms'.

Reproduced from Litwin M, McNaughton-Collins M., Floyd K. et. al. (1999) The National Institutes of Health Chronic Prostatitis Symptom Index: Development and Validation of a New Outcome Measure. J Urol **162**(2): 369–375, © American Urological Association, Inc. with permission from Elsevier.

Management

Investigations and management should be undertaken as part of a coordinated MDT to avoid delay, repetition, and improve the patient journey. Specialties involved may include: GUM, Urology, Colorectal, Pain team, Clinical psychology, Physiotherapy, and Psychosexual therapy, with advice from Microbiology and Radiology. A Biopsychosocial model of care should be provided.

In view of the lack of understanding and imprecision in diagnosis, it is difficult to evaluate treatments properly. No therapy has been demonstrated to be absolutely effective.

- *Antibiotics*: provide first line CBP regimen; only give a second line course if improvement of symptoms or proven infection. There is no benefit in giving further courses of antibiotics unless infection is isolated. Depending on presence/severity of symptoms can add in another agent to initial antibiotics. If not resolved after antibiotics, refer from sexual health based on local arrangements for further management.
- *Alpha-blocking drugs (e.g. tamulosin)*: relax the bladder neck and prostate gland. Give for 4–6 weeks and if no benefit stop. Particularly useful if lower urinary tract symptoms are present.
- Pain management: same principles as that of chronic pain (➔ Chapter 31, 'Management', pp. 368–71). Options include:
  - *non-steroidal anti-inflammatory drugs (NSAIDs)*—stop at 6 weeks if no benefit
  - *topical lidocaine*—can be applied to penile tip, perineum.
  - *neuropathic pain medication*—tricyclic antidepressants (e.g. amitriptyline) or anticonvulsants (gabapentin).
  - *pain team*—advice on prescribing, consideration of blocks, carbamazepine, opioids, specific pain psychology, and education of patient on pain theory.
- *Psychological treatment*: assessment required if depressed or distressed. Mindfulness and cognitive behavioural therapy can help with chronic pain management.
- *Physiotherapy*: assess and manage pelvic hypertonia, desensitization techniques, transcutaneous electrical nerve stimulation (TENS).
- *5-alpha reductase inhibitors (e.g. finasteride)*: if LUTS and benign prostatic enlargement present. No benefit seen in using alone.
- Surgery without evidence of pathology present is not recommended. (e.g. orchidectomy).

Asymptomatic inflammatory prostatitis

Usually an incidental finding arising during the investigation of the genitourinary tract for other reasons (e.g. prostate biopsy for possible prostate cancer because of an elevated serum prostate specific antigen test or infertility investigations). The patient has no symptoms, but excess leucocytes in the seminal fluid are common findings. STI screening should be undertaken and treated accordingly. Consider tuberculosis (TB).

Other rare causes of prostatitis

- *Mycobacterium tuberculosis* and other atypical mycobacteria: granulomatous prostatitis
- *Parasites*: e.g. *Trichomonas vaginalis, Schistosoma haematobium*.
- Viruses: e.g. HSV and cytomegalovirus (CMV) in immunocompromised patients. May also present acutely.
- *Mycoses*: e.g. coccidioidomycosis, blastomycosis, cryptococcosis, histoplasmosis, candidiasis. More common in immunosuppressed people causing a granulomatous reaction.

Sexually transmitted infections

Chlamydia trachomatis, Ureaplasma urealyticum, Mycoplasma genitalium, and *Mycoplasma hominis* have been implicated in chronic prostatitis. Their nucleotide sequences have been reported in up to 10% of cases from prostatic secretions or semen without associated demonstrable urethral infection. However, there is no clear consistent evidence to support a causative role. If found, they should be treated.

Prostatitis and HIV infection

↑ risk of prostatic abscess in those immunosuppressed with acute prostatitis.

Further information
http://uroweb.org/wp-content/uploads/EAU-Extended-Guidelines-2015-Edn..pdf
https://www.bashhguidelines.org/media/1065/bju-prostatitis-2015.pdf

Epididymo-orchitis

Aetiology *194*
Clinical features *196*
Complications *196*
Investigations *197*
Diagnosis *198*
Management *200*

Aetiology

Inflammation of the epididymis (epididymitis), the testicle (orchitis), or both (epididymo-orchitis) may be caused by the spread of infection, or less commonly, other agents, from:
- the urethra or bladder through the ejaculatory duct, seminal vesicle, and vas deferens
- distant sites through the lymphatic or blood vessels.

Genital infection

- *Chlamydia trachomatis* and/or *Neisseria gonorrhoeae* cause ~70% of acute epididymitis in sexually active ♂ aged <35 years and 5–30% in older ♂. Up to 30% of untreated urethral infections may lead to acute epididymitis, usually unilateral.
- Coliform enteric bacteria (acquired through insertive anal sex) in up to 65% of MSM with non-gonococcal non-chlamydial epididymitis.
- There is limited data suggesting *M. genitalium* as a causative agent
- *Treponema pallidum* is a rare cause of diffuse chronic interstitial inflammation of the testis in late benign syphilis, which may lead to a gumma (or atrophy).
- Evidence supporting *Ureaplasma urealyticum* as a cause is lacking.

Urinary tract infection

- Coliform bacteria (*Escherichia coli*, *Klebsiella* spp., and *Proteus* spp.) and *Pseudomonas aeroginosa* cause up to 80% of acute epididymitis in ♂ aged 35. May be associated with an underlying urological abnormality, e.g. obstruction, calculus, chronic bacterial prostatitis. Urethral instrumentation (e.g. catheterization) is a predisposing factor.
- *Mycobacterium tuberculosis*, associated with renal, prostatic, or seminal vesicle infection is an uncommon cause with usually insidious, occasionally acute, onset. 75% of ♂ with renal tuberculosis have associated epididymitis, 65% of which is bilateral.

Other micro-organisms

- *Mycobacterium leprae* commonly involves the testes +/– epididymis causing atrophy.
- *Mumps*: epididymo-orchitis in 20% of cases in adult ♂, 16% bilateral.
- *Brucella* spp. (*Br. melitensis* ×5 more than *Br. abortus*) may cause orchitis in 5–18% of cases (epididymitis less evident).
- Coxsackie virus B infections may include orchitis in up to 1/3 cases.
- Systemic fungal and yeast infections (e.g. cryptococcosis, histoplasmosis, coccidioidomycosis, and blastomycosis) may produce orchitis.
- Filarial organisms, *Wuchereria bancrofti* and *Wuchereria pacifica*, and less commonly *Brugia malayi*. If present in inguinal lymph nodes may cause chronic allergic lymphangitis of the spermatic cord and testis. This produces chronic epididymitis and orchitis with profuse effusion within the tunica vaginalis leading to scrotal oedema and elephantiasis.
- *Streptococcus pneumoniae*, *Nocardia* spp., *Haemophilus parainfluenzae*, group B *Salmonella* spp., *Neisseria meningitidis*, *Schistosoma haematobium*, and cytomegalovirus have been reported as probable causes.

Non-infective causes

- *Spermatic granuloma*: extravasation of spermatozoa into adjacent tissue inducing autoimmune granulomatous epididymitis (a cellular reaction) leading to fibrosis.
- *Granulomatous orchitis*: idiopathic or ♂ to systemic granulomatous disorders.
- *Behçet's disease*: epididymo-orchitis in up to 20% of ♂.
- *Amiodarone*: side-effects in up to 11% of ♂. Causes lymphocytic infiltration and fibrosis, usually bilateral.
- *Sarcoidosis*: may rarely cause non-caseating granulomatous epididymo-orchitis.
- Idiopathic lymphocytic orchitis.

Clinical features

Acute

- typically unilateral scrotal pain and swelling
- pyrexia may be present
- symptoms and/or signs of urethritis if sexually acquired
- symptoms of UTI may be present
- scrotal erythema
- tenderness and palpable swelling of the epididymis
- development of oedema and formation of a hydrocele may lead to a grossly enlarged scrotum
- haematospermia (rarely)
- in mumps orchitis the onset is usually within a week of parotid enlargement, but sometimes follows resolution of parotitis.

Chronic

- symptoms are of >3 months duration
- pain is of variable intensity
- epididymal and testicular swelling is gradual and depends on the underlying cause.

Complications

- Hydrocele in ~10% (usually resolves with antibiotics).
- Abscess in up to 3% of cases.
- Infarction of the testicle in <1% (due to compression of the swollen spermatic cord at the external inguinal ring).
- Recurrence due to lack of adequate treatment, re-infection, or chronic inflammation. High recurrence rates in MSM (coliform infection).
- Chronic epididymitis follows ~15% of acute episodes.
- *Infertility due to:*
  - occlusion of vasa deferentia (following bilateral epididymitis)
  - impaired spermatogenesis (following bilateral orchitis).
  - possibility of infertility after unilateral epididymitis +/− orchitis due to sperm agglutinins (suggested, but unproven).
- Chronic prostatitis (unusual).

Investigations

Initial investigations

Microscopy
- *May show urethritis*: i.e. 5PMNL/HPF +/− Gram −ve intracellular diplococci.
- *FVU*: for threads containing 10 PMNL/HPF (if no urethral material).

Urinalysis
MSSU: dipstick test (➲ Chapter 21, 'Urinary tract infection', pp. 267–76).

Laboratory investigations
- FVU or urethral swab for *C. trachomatis*, *N. gonorrhoeae*, and *M. genitalium* NAAT testing
- MSSU for microsopy and culture
- urethral swab for *N. gonorrhoeae* culture
- raised CRP can support a diagnosis of epididymo-orchitis
- if sexually transmitted epididymo-orchitis is suspected or confirmed, screening for other STIs, including blood borne viruses is important.

Ultrasonography
- *Doppler ultrasonography*: useful in the differential diagnosis of acute scrotal pain and swelling. Acute epididymitis/orchitis ⇄ blood flow, but normal findings cannot exclude the condition.
- *Real-time ultrasonography*: of great value in the differential diagnosis of scrotal swellings, particularly when malignancy or complications of acute epididymitis, requiring surgical intervention, are suspected.

Additional investigations
- epididymal aspiration for microbiological specimens (usually during surgical exploration)
- MRI when diagnosis is unclear despite ultrasonography
- further urological investigations (e.g. urethrocystoscopy and excretion urogram) if underlying urological abnormality is likely.

Diagnosis

Diagnosis is based on clinical findings, including symptoms, signs, age, sexual history, urethral Gram stain, and urine examination are important in establishing a diagnosis, supported by specialized investigations if indicated (Boxes 13.1 and 13.2). It is essential to exclude testicular torsion in acute presentation (requires emergency surgical intervention).

In the differential diagnosis of non-acute scrotal pain and swelling (Table 13.1), clinical assessment should attempt to identify if the lesion is within the body of the testis (malignancy more likely).

Box 13.1 Causes of scrotal mass/pain

- Trauma.
- Hydrocele.
- Epididymo-orchitis.
- Testicular torsion.
- Torsion of testicular appendix (in 6–12-year-old children).
- Spermatocele.
- Epididymal cyst.
- Varicocele.
- Hernia.
- *Testicular tumour*:
  - germ cell tumours—seminoma and malignant teratoma
  - lymphoma and other malignancies.
- Epididymal and non-testicular neoplasms.
- Fournier's gangrene.
- *Vasculitis*: Henoch–Schönlein purpura and Kawasaki disease (<15 years), Buerger's disease (adults).

Box 13.2 Three clues to diagnosis of scrotal mass

Clinical assessment should aim to answer three important questions in diagnosing the cause of scrotal mass.

- Is the mass intrascrotal ('get above the swelling')? Hernia extends above the scrotum.
- Is the mass cystic? Cystic mass (e.g. hydrocele) is usually transilluminable.
- Is the mass an integral part of the testis? Solid testicular mass should be regarded as malignant until proven otherwise, and urgent investigations should be arranged.

Table 13.1 Main differential diagnosis

	Testicular torsion	Epididymitis	Testicular cancer
Age range (years)	Most common 12–18 years Less common 18–30 years	Most common 19–40 years Less common <18 and >40years	Peak incidence ages 25–35. 74% in 20–49-year-olds
Pain	Sudden onset. 50% report previous short episodes of pain resolving spontaneously	Onset over 24–48 hours	Typically painless, but diffuse pain or dragging sensation/ ache in 730%; 5–15% present with acute pain
Urinary symptoms	90% normal urinalysis 4% ↑ frequency	Dysuria, frequency or urgency. Urethritis (smear/FVU) or pyuria	No association
GI symptoms	~33% nausea and vomiting. 20–30% abdominal pain	Nausea and vomiting if acute orchitis develops	May be due to metastases
Pyrexia	Usually absent	May be low grade. >40°C in acute orchitis	Usually absent
Inspection and palpation	Oedema and erythema of affected side Enlarged and exquisitely tender testis, high in scrotum Transverse lie and anterior epididymis on unaffected side	Oedema and erythema of affected side. Epididymis distinguishable from testis unless very advanced or scrotum grossly enlarged	Testicle enlarged, 15% with inflammation Solid lump not separated from testis
Cremastric reflex	Absent	Present	Present
Ultrasono-graphy	↓ Blood flow	↓ Blood flow	Hypo-echoic mass within the testis

Further information
British Association for Sexual Health and HIV Epididymo-orchitis guideline ℛ https://www.bashh.org/guidelines

Management

General

- scrotal support and analgesia (NSAID)
- avoid sexual intercourse until both patient and partner (if appropriate) are treated and follow-up is complete.

Treatment

Empirical therapy should be commenced immediately, taking into consideration the likely cause and local antibiotic sensitivities, and altered if necessary when laboratory results are available.

Sexually transmitted organism suspected/confirmed

- *Recommended*: doxycycline 100 mg bd for 14 days plus ceftriaxone 500 mg IM once.
- *Alternative*: (If gonorrhoea unlikely) ofloxacin 200 mg oral bd for 14 days or levofloxacin 500 mg od for 10 days:
  - ▶ where enteric organisms +/− STI suspected ceftriaxone 500 mg IM once *plus* levofloxacin 500 mg od for 10 days, or ofloxacin 200 mg bd for 14 days should be considered
  - ▶ where gonorrhoea is a likely cause, it is recommended to add azithromycin 1 g stat in addition to ceftriaxone and doxycycline
  - ▶ where *M. genitalium* confirmed/suspected moxifloxacin 400 mg od for 14 days is recommended

Non-STI enteric organism suspected/confirmed

- ofloxacin 200 mg oral bd for 14 days *or*
- levofloxacin 500 mg oral od for 10 days.

Partner notification

If the cause is or likely to be sexually transmitted, sexual contacts should be offered screening and epidemiological treatment. Contacts should be provided with treatment for uncomplicated chlamydia *and* treatment for gonorrhoea or *M. genitalium*, if identified in index patient. Recommended look-back periods are 6 months if *C. trachomatis* identified, 60 days for *N. gonorrhoeae* and 90 days for *M. genitalium*, for unidentified suspected sexually transmitted organism 60 days look-back is suggested.

Follow-up

If no improvement after 3 days review diagnosis and management. Reassess if swelling and tenderness persist after antimicrobial therapy is completed (swelling may take several weeks to resolve).

Test of cure by NAAT 4 weeks after treatment complete if *C. trachomatis* or *M. genitalium* confirmed, or 2 weeks after for *N. gonorrhoeae*.

If symptoms persist or diagnosis uncertain, further investigations, including scrotal ultrasound should be performed.

▶ If urinary tract pathogen is confirmed, refer to urology for investigation of possible urinary tract abnormality/obstruction.

HIV infection

- Case reports of poor response to standard treatment in people living with HIV infection.
- Unusual causes more common (CMV, *M. tuberculosis*, *H. influenzae*, *Nocardia asterioides*, *Candida* spp., and *Cryptococcus neoformans*).

Sexually acquired reactive arthritis

Introduction *202*
Aetiology *203*
Associations *204*
Clinical features *205*
Natural history *207*
Diagnosis *208*
Management *210*
HIV infection *212*

Introduction

Reactive (or post-infectious) arthritis (ReA) is a seronegative sterile inflammation of the synovial membrane (usually together with associated tendons and fascia) initiated by an external stimulant, usually an enteric or STI. Estimated prevalence is 30–40/100,000 adults).

When ReA is associated with both urethritis and conjunctivitis (a minority of cases), it is commonly referred to as Reiter's syndrome (after Hans Reiter who described a case preceded by dysentery in 1916).

As Reiter's syndrome may be incomplete and other clinical features may be present, the term sexually acquired ReA (SARA) is commonly used when the main component, arthritis, follows an STI. The manifestations of post-enteric ReA are similar.

Aetiology

Although an infective urethritis or enteritis commonly triggers ReA its multisystem involvement and potential for relapse/remission (similar to other seronegative spondylo-arthropathies) imply an underlying reactive aetiology. However, the detection of bacterial antigen or sensitized CD4 cells in inflamed synovial material from organisms that may provoke SARA, may suggest a more direct relationship. Other infections and conditions may be associated with rea (e.g. rheumatic fever), but have different clinical features. In ~25% of cases, no trigger can be identified.

Sexually acquired infection

SARA typically presents in ♂ 2–4 weeks after lower genital tract infection usually NGU. Although found in ♀ it is much more likely to be unrecognized as it is associated with cervicitis, usually latent. Most organisms associated with urethritis/cervicitis are linked to SARA. Their role is unclear and SARA may arise without any demonstrable bacterial infection.

Pathogens

0.8–4 % of those with lower genital tract infections develop SARA.

- *Chlamydia trachomatis*: the only urogenital pathogen consistently implicated in sporadic SARA. Chlamydia-like particles, seen by electron microscopy, and chlamydial DNA, using NAATs, have been identified from synovial fluid of some patients with SARA. Associated urogenital infection has been found by non-NAATs in 30–70%.
- *Ureaplasma urealyticum*: ↑ urogenital detection rate in some with SARA without evidence of chlamydial or enteric infection. DNA from synovial fluid has been reported in those with SARA (using NAAT).
- *Mycoplasma genitalium*: DNA found in synovial fluid (using NAAT).
- *Neisseria gonorrhoeae* has been implicated in up to 14–16% of cases of SARA, distinct from its association with septic arthritis.

Enteric infection (frequency of ReA 1–4%)

- *Shigella* spp.
- *Salmonella* spp.
- *Campylobacter* spp.
- *Yersinia enterocolitica* and *Yersinia pseudotuberculosis*.
- *Clostridium difficile*.

Other factors

Urethral or bowel trauma (e.g. catheterization, surgery). Unusual, but may precipitate recurrence.

Associations

- *Gender*:
  - SARA ~98% in ♂ (falsely high as undoubtedly under-diagnosed in ♀)
  - enteric ReA ~90% in ♂.
- *Age*: usually young adults.
- *Geography*: urethritis appears to precede ReA more commonly in the UK and USA, whereas an initial dysenteric illness has been reported more frequently in studies from continental Europe.
- *Human leucocyte antigen B27 (HLA-B27) positivity*: however, an association has only been established with the following infections: *Chlamydia, Campylobacter, Clostridium, Salmonella, Shigella,* and *Yersinia*.
- Diagnostic relevance dubious, although HLA-B27 may be associated with ↑ risk of chronicity and recurrence:
  - 30–90% of those with SARA
  - 50–80% with ReA following enteric infection.
- *Controls*:
  - northern Scandinavians: 26–50%
  - most Europeans: 7–10%
  - black people: <2%.
- *Genetic predisposition*: may be a family history of:
  - SARA
  - other seronegative spondylo-arthropathy (e.g. associated with ankylosing spondylitis, inflammatory bowel disease, psoriasis)
  - iritis.

Clinical features

The onset of arthritis is usually within 30 days of sexual contact, with a mean interval of 14 days between onset of genital symptoms and arthritis. ~10% do not have a preceding symptomatic infection.

Urogenital

Men

Urethritis (usually NGU): discharge/dysuria in ~80% with SARA. May be asymptomatic, but discharge present. NGU in ~60% of cases of recurrent SARA, which may be associated with a new infection or may arise spontaneously (a new infection does not necessarily trigger a recurrence).

Women

- urethritis (dysuria/discharge) uncommon (short urethra)
- cervicitis usually asymptomatic, but may be visible on examination
- salpingo-oophoritis (rarely).

Bladder and upper urinary tract

Mild sterile (by conventional culture) cystitis found in 20%, although severe haemorrhagic manifestations have been reported. Proteinuria and microscopic haematuria are common. Glomerulonephritis and IgA nephropathy rarely associated.

Musculoskeletal

- *Arthritis*: asymmetrical polyarthritis (>95%) predominantly affecting the lower limbs, usually involving 1–5 joints. Low back pain common (~50%) with sacroiliitis in 10%. Joints not involved simultaneously, but overall severity peaks ~14 days after the onset of the arthritis. Rapid muscle wasting in relation to joints involved is common.
- *Enthesitis (inflammation at insertion point of ligaments, tendons, and capsules) and tenosynovitis*:
  - plantar fasciitis in ~20%, may be associated with calcaneal enthesitis
  - Achilles tendonitis in 10–15%
  - dactylitis 'sausage digits'.

Contributes to painful feet and difficulty walking. Enthesitis may also be found at insertion points around the pelvis and ribs.

Ophthalmic

- Irritable sensation in eyes, potentially without redness is common
- *Conjunctivitis*: usually bilateral. Found in 20–50% of cases of SARA. Generally mild and self-limiting. Typically develops after the appearance of symptoms from the provoking infection and the onset of arthritis.
- *Iritis (acute anterior uveitis)*: late manifestation of an initial episode or recurrence in 2–11%. Usually unilateral, presenting as a painful eye with blurred vision and inflammation at the margins of the cornea. Associated with sacroiliitis. Slit lamp examination is needed to differentiate from conjunctivitis.
- *Episcleritis*: keratitis and corneal ulceration have also been reported.

Dermatological (skin manifestations commonly occur together)

- *Keratoderma blennorrhagica (KB)*: identical to pustular psoriasis and found in up to 33%, although may be greater as often asymptomatic. Most commonly found on the soles of the feet (often the only site involved), although other sites may be affected (e.g. penis, especially if circumcised, palms, toes, scalp, scrotum, and sometimes a generalized rash). The lesions, which may exhibit the Koebner phenomenon, typically appear as hard parakeratotic nodules or soft limpet-like patches, usually brown in colour and becoming pustular.
- *Erythema nodosum*: rarely reported with *Yersinia* infection.
- *Nails*: ~10% of patients develop thickening and ridging of the nails which may progress to subungual abscess formation with shedding. Pitting is not a feature.
- *Genital lesions*: balanitis (often asymptomatic) is found in 20–40% and is an early finding. If circumcised, the psoriatic lesions are elevated, dry, and scaly (as KB). In the uncircumcised, erythematous confluent patches appear circumscribed by a well-defined pale margin, creating a geographical appearance and referred to as circinate balanitis. May be found in ♂ presenting with urethritis and no other clinical features. Circinate vulvitis has also been reported in ♀. Lesions usually resolve spontaneously within 4 weeks.
- *Oral lesions*: found in 10–16% (although under-diagnosed as asymptomatic). The palate, buccal mucosa, gingiva, and tongue may show erythematous or circinate lesions and ulceration. Patchy loss of papillae can appear over the tongue (geographical tongue).

Other manifestations

- *Constitutional symptoms*: malaise and fever in ~10%.
- *Cardiovascular system*:
  - thrombophlebitis (deep leg veins) in ~3% (symptoms may resemble a ruptured knee joint capsule, a rare complication of arthritis)
  - myocarditis
  - electrocardiogram (ECG) abnormalities documented in 5–14%
  - pericarditis—rare
  - aortitis with aortic incompetence—very rare.
- *Respiratory system*: pleurisy in up to 8%.
- *Nervous system*: <2%—meningoencephalitis, peripheral neuropathies, amyotrophic lateral sclerosis.
- *Enteric*: non-specific mucous enterocolitis may occasionally appear at onset of symptoms.
- *Amyloidosis*: very rare.

Natural history

Self-limiting for the majority of patients. Most initial episodes resolve within 2–6 months, although they may extend to >1 year. 15–30% may develop progressive chronic arthritis, sacroiliitis, and dactylitis. Recurrences occur in ~50% with an annual risk of ~15%. Chronicity, aggressive arthritis, and recurrences more common if HLA-B27 +ve.

Without treatment urethritis and conjunctivitis usually resolve in up to 4 weeks. The dermatological manifestations also generally settle within 4 weeks, although KB may persist for 2–3 months or longer.

Iritis is liable to recur, especially if associated with sacroiliitis. Inadequately treated anterior uveitis may lead rapidly to cataract formation.

Diagnosis

▶ *Clinical*: there is no simple diagnostic test for SARA and Reiter's syndrome. Diagnosis is made on clinical grounds, although it may be supported by the following investigations:

- Screen for STIs (including rectal gonorrhoea and chlamydial infection if indicated by the sexual history and HIV).
- Stool cultures and *Yersinia* spp. serology if enteric infection suspected.
- *FBC*:
  - normochromic normocytic anaemia in severe cases
  - polymorphonuclear leucocytosis in up to 30%.
- *ESR/CRP*: elevated in >90% with SARA. Level gives an indication of disease activity.
- *Urinalysis*: proteinuria, microscopic haematuria, pyuria in up to 50%.
- *Radiology (affected and sacro-iliac joints)*: early SARA—no findings. In progressive disease:
  - periostitis (tibia, fibula, hands, and feet)
  - articular erosions with joint narrowing (hands, feet, posterior aspect of calcaneous)
  - periosteal reaction at sites of tendon insertion producing 'spurs' especially calcaneum (>50% of chronic cases)
  - sacroiliitis in 50% with severe chronic disease.
- *Slit-lamp examination*: suspected iritis.
- Electrocardiography (variable degrees of heart block) and echocardiography if suspected cardiac involvement.
- *Synovial fluid*: polymorphs in acute disease followed by lymphocytes. Sterile culture and no crystals.
- *Synovial biopsy*: polymorph infiltrate as with other rheumatic disease.
- *HLA-B27 test*: debatable value. It has low diagnostic predictive value, but may be of value in determining management and prognosis.
- *Negative/normal findings*:
  - antistreptolysin O titre
  - rheumatoid factor (although 4% positivity rate in normal population)
  - antinuclear antibody test
  - uric acid levels
  - chest X-ray and serum ACE

The most common differential diagnosis (Box 14.1) is gonococcal arthritis, especially if SARA presents as a monoarthritis (3–7% of cases). Culture of synovial fluid is usually negative and, as gonorrhoea, may also trigger SARA; if in doubt treatment should be given to cover disseminated gonococcal infection (➔ Chapter 8, 'Disseminated gonococcal infection (DGI)', p. 142), which unlike SARA, should show rapid improvement.

Box 14.1 Other causes of acute painful swollen joint(s)

Direct infection
- Acute septic arthritis (~80% due to Gram +ve aerobes).
- TB.
- *Fungal infections*: unusual (e.g. blastomycosis, *Candida* spp.).

Direct infection and/or reactive arthritis
- Gonococcal arthritis (usually monoarthritis).
- Meningococcal arthritis.
- Reaction to streptococcal infection (e.g. rheumatic fever).
- Bacterial endocarditis.
- Syphilis.
- Viral infections (including HIV, hepatitis B, HSV, and parvovirus).
- Lyme disease.
- Cat-scratch disease (atypical presentation).
- Brucellosis.
- Leptospirosis.

Others
- Trauma and foreign body reaction (also exacerbation of osteoarthritis).
- Seronegative HLA-B27 associated spondylo-arthropathies.
- Rheumatoid arthritis (RA) and other seropositive connective tissue diseases.
- Still's disease (juvenile RA, seronegative).
- Erythema multiforme and Stevens–Johnson syndrome.
- Reaction to drugs and vaccines.
- Behçet's.
- Gout/pseudogout.
- Haemochromatosis.
- Sarcoidosis.
- Haemophilia and other clotting deficiencies.
- Acute leukaemia.

Management

General

Full information on SARA and its clinical course should be provided with advice on the avoidance of future potential triggers. PN (with epidemiological treatment) may be required, depending on the initial provoking infection.

Management should be multidisciplinary. ▶ Liaise with or refer to the appropriate specialty for extra-genital manifestations, especially if severe.

Antibiotics

SARA

The provoking infection in acute SARA (usually NGU) should be treated as for an uncomplicated infection (➲ Chapter 10, 'Management', pp. 165–7). Treatment of the triggering infection does not appear to affect the course of any established skeletal, skin, or ophthalmic manifestations. Short-term antibiotics are not advised unless the triggering infection is still active.

Early treatment of urogenital infection may ↓ risk of relapsing arthritis in those with a history of ReA.

Enteric

Short-term antibiotics for the underlying enteric infection do not appear to alter the course of rea or Reiter's syndrome. Any associated urethritis should be treated as above.

Prolonged treatment for 4–6 weeks may be of benefit for arthritis triggered by *Yersinia enterocolitica*.

Ophthalmic

- *Conjunctivitis*: usually no treatment required.
- *Iritis*: mydriatics and topical steroids.

Arthritis and enthesitis

- Rest, avoidance of weight-bearing, passive muscle exercises to limit wasting.
- NSAIDs with dosage at night to reduce morning stiffness. If at high risk of upper gastrointestinal (GI) complications (e.g. GI bleeding) consider:
  - a cyclo-oxygenase 2 (COX-2) selective NSAID *or*
  - the addition of gastroprotective agents (e.g. misoprostol, histamine-2 blockers and a proton pump inhibitor)
  - in view of possible long-term increased cardiovascular risks, renal and GI toxicity; treatment duration should be kept as brief as possible.
- *Corticosteroids*:
  - systemic prednisolone only rarely indicated if severe polyarthritis with other systemic symptoms—local injection at tendon insertion or into a severely swollen knee joint following aspiration may be of value.
- Options for chronic disabling arthritis (persistence for 3 months or erosive joint damage) include:
  - sulfasalazine
  - methotrexate
  - azathioprine
  - gold salts.

- Tumour necrosis factor alpha (TNF-α) blocking agents are highly effective in treatment of other spondylo-arthropathies. Potential for short-term effectiveness in ReA, although drugs may re-activate the infective trigger.

Skin

Manifestations are self-limiting and, unless unusually severe, treatment is not required. However, topical corticosteroids may be indicated for severe circinate balanitis and KB with the options of topical calcipotriol, systemic methotrexate, and retinoid for intractable cases.

Pregnancy

- *Antibiotics*: for STIs as indicated (**➔** Chapter 8, 'Pregnancy and breastfeeding', p. 147; Chapter 9, 'Pregnancy and breastfeeding', p. 158; Chapter 10, 'Mycoplasma genitalium', p. 166).
- *NSAIDs*: may produce premature closure of the foetal ductus arteriosus, oligohydramnios, and delayed onset and ↑ duration of labour.
- *Corticosteroids*: low risk, but may cause growth restriction and foetal adrenal suppression.
- *Sulfasalazine*: small theoretical risk, so use with caution.
- *Azathioprine*: appears to be safe.
- Methotrexate, gold salts, and TNF-α blockers should be avoided.

HIV infection

Rising incidence in association with HIV in sub-Saharan Africa (up to 11%), but not in Caucasian populations. Musculoskeletal features are similar to those in non-HIV patients, but cutaneous manifestations and urethritis are common and more severe. White patients are usually HLA-B27 +ve, whereas non-white people are generally −ve.

Frequency of spondylo-arthropathies is unchanged with anti-retroviral treatment, although cutaneous lesions are less severe. Otherwise, management is similar to non-HIV-infected cases, with sulfasalazine beneficial in long-standing cases.

Further information
British Association for Sexual Health and HIV Chlamydia guideline
ℛ https://www.bashh.org/guidelines

Bacterial vaginosis and anaerobic balanitis

Introduction *214*
Aetiology *215*
Clinical features *217*
Associations *217*
Complications *218*
Diagnosis *220*
Management *222*
Anaerobic and *G. vaginalis*-associated
    balanitis/balanoposthitis *224*
HIV infection *224*

Introduction

First described as 'non-specific vaginitis' in 1955 by Gardner and Dukes, with the term 'bacterial vaginosis' (BV) formally introduced in 1984.

Characterized by bacteriological imbalance of vaginal flora with the overgrowth of characteristic commensal bacteria replacing normally predominant *Lactobacillus* spp. and producing an altered vaginal discharge. Most common cause of abnormal discharge in women of childbearing age. Prevalence is probably around 5–10%, but may be as high as 50% in ♀ from some ethnic groups.

Aetiology

Vaginal hydrogen peroxide, H_2O_2-producing lactobacilli, ~60% of vaginal lactobacilli strains (especially *Lactobacillus crispatus* and *Lactobacillus jensenii*), appear to be protective as the prevalence of BV is only 4% compared with 32% in those with non-H_2O_2-producing organisms.

Biofilms

Developing BV is now recognized to involve the presence of a dense, structured, and polymicrobial biofilm. Biofilms are communities of micro-organisms attached to a surface and encased in a polymeric matrix of polysaccharides, proteins, and nucleic acids. In the case of BV, clusters of *Gardnerella vaginalis* produce the matrix and other bacteria then attach. The biofilm is also strongly adherent to the vaginal epithelium.

Due to the fact that bacteria within biofilms are not effectively eliminated by the immune system or fully destroyed by antibiotics; biofilm-related infections tend to persist and, not surprisingly, BV tends to have a high rate of relapse and recurrence.

The *G. vaginalis* biofilm *in vitro* displays high resistance to the protective mechanisms of normal vaginal microflora (H_2O_2 and lactic acid produced by lactobacilli), as well as an increased tolerance to antibiotics.

Organisms

- *G. vaginalis*: facultative anaerobic small Gram −ve bacillus (often stains Gram +ve). Found in high concentrations (>×100 normal) in up to 95% of BV, but can be isolated in up to 58% of those with normal discharge. Vaginal carriage is associated with oral sex and hand-to-genital non-penetrative contact in ♀ who have never had penetrative vaginal sex.
- *Anaerobic bacteria in high concentrations*:
  - *Mobiluncus* spp.: sickle-shaped rods displaying vigorous motility, including corkscrew motion, in vaginal wet mounts. Cultured in 14–96% ♀ with BV (<6% without) and seen on microscopy in up to 77%. *Mobiluncus mulieris*—long, Gram −ve. *Mobiluncus curtisii*—short, Gram variable, but usually stain positive.
  - *Prevotella* spp. (e.g. *P. bivia*).
  - *Prophyromonas* spp.
  - Peptostreptococci (e.g. *Streptococcus intermedius*).
  - *Fusobacterium* spp.
  - *Bacteroides* spp.
- *Aerobic bacteria*: e.g. streptococci, coliforms.
- *Mycoplasma hominis*: found in 24–75% ♀ with BV (13–22% without BV).
- *More recently described bacteria*:
  - *Atopobium vaginae*—a metronidazole-resistant Gram +ve anaerobe frequently demonstrated in BV and may be responsible for metronidazole treatment failure.
  - *Leptotrichia/Sneathia*, *Eggerthella*-like bacterium, *Megasphaera* spp.—three novel bacteria (BV-associated bacteria 1–3) in the order *Clostridiales*.

Risk factors
- Non-white ethnicity.
- *Hormonal contraception*: combined oestrogen/progesterone associated with a ↓ risk, probably related to oestradiol levels, but shift to anaerobic predominance aided by progesterone injection.
- *IUD*: variable data, but possibly ↑ risk.
- *Vaginal douching*: although only apparently associated with BV if flora already imbalanced.
- *Diet*: BV has been shown to be associated with ↑ consumption of fat and severe vaginosis is associated with both saturated and mono-unsaturated fat. Increased intakes of folate, vitamin E, and calcium reduce the risk of severe vaginosis.
- *Cigarette smoking*: ↑ risk of BV possibly due to anti-oestrogenic effect.
- There is debate around whether purely an imbalance in vaginal flora or initiated as an STI. The following features suggest a sexual link:
  • Lower mean age of coitarche.
  • New sexual partner within previous 30 days, multiple sexual partners, unprotected heterosexual intercourse with associated anal sex.
  • Associated with *Neisseria gonorrhoeae* and *Chlamydia trachomatis*.
  • BV discharge (but not *G. vaginalis* in pure culture) inoculated into healthy vagina can induce BV in recipient
  • Women who have sex with women—2.5-fold ↑ rate compared with heterosexual ♀. Prevalence up to 25–52% with 20-fold ↑ if ♀ partner has BV. Apparent association with recent partner change, multiple concurrent partners, and receiving oral sex, but no other practices (including the shared use of dildos and anal penetration with fingers.)
- *Against sexual transmission*;
  • *Comparative study*—BV found in similar proportion of virginal and sexually active adolescents (12% and 15%, respectively).
  • Although *G. vaginalis* is isolated from the urethra in up to 80% of ♂ partners of ♀ with BV, their concurrent treatment does not ↓ ♀ recurrence rate.
- There is conflicting information regarding the circumcision status of ♂ partners.

Clinical features

- *Asymptomatic*: ~50%.
- *Vaginal discharge*: symptom in 49% (20% without BV), sign in 69% (3% without BV):
  - *volume*—usually moderate (varies from scanty to profuse)
  - *colour*— grey > white > yellow
  - *nature*—homogeneous vaginal discharge adhering to vaginal walls as a thin film). Frothy in 27–80% (1–18% normal ♀).
- *Malodorous*: fishy ammoniacal smell spontaneously reported in 20–49%, but probably higher (smell also reported in 20% without BV). Smell enhanced when vaginal pH ↑ (e.g. during menstruation and following contact with alkaline prostatic fluid after intercourse), releasing volatile amines.
- *Mild irritation*: a non-inflammatory process so soreness and itching absent in most cases.

Associations

- *N. gonorrhoeae* and *C. trachomatis*: 3.8-fold risk of *N. gonorrhoeae* or *C. trachomatis* in ♀ with symptomatic BV.
- Cervicitis (with risk factors distinct from gonococcal and chlamydial infections), may be related to absence of H_2O_2-producing lactobacilli.
- Non-specific urethritis (NSU) in ♂ partner.
- *Trichomoniasis*: bacterial overgrowth as BV, but purulent discharge.
- HSV-2 infection and viral shedding.
- CMV infection and replication.

Complications

- Persistence (11–29%) and recurrence (72% by 7 months). Thought to be due to the inability of antibiotics to fully eradicate BV vaginal biofilm-associated bacteria.
- Post-hysterectomy vaginal cuff cellulitis.
- Post-abortion PID.
- Possibly contributes to spontaneous PID and STI (including HIV) acquisition.
- *In pregnancy*: increased bacterial production of cytokines and prostaglandins and amniotic fluid/chorio-amniotic infection leading to:
  - chorioamnionitis
  - low birth weight
  - preterm birth (relative risk 1.5–2.3); history of previous premature delivery ↑ risk of further preterm birth 7-fold with BV.
  - 2nd trimester miscarriage (up to 3–6-fold risk)
  - endometritis (pre/post-delivery, including caesarean section).

Frequently asked questions

What is bacterial vaginosis?
It is a condition caused by the overgrowth of normal vaginal bacteria causing an imbalance and an altered vaginal discharge.

Is it sexually transmitted?
It is not thought to be sexually transmitted, and so partners of ♀ with BV are not routinely treated.

Is it like thrush?
Thrush (candidiasis) is caused by a yeast, usually *Candida albicans* (90%). BV is due to an imbalance of normal vaginal flora, with a loss or reduction in lactobacilli and an overgrowth of largely anaerobic bacteria, especially *Gardnerella vaginalis*.

  Thrush usually causes a thick white vaginal discharge, itching, and soreness. BV is usually associated with a thin white/grey discharge and an offensive fishy smell.

  Both thrush and BV have the potential to recur.

Is it treated with anti-thrush preparations?
No. Thrush is treated with topical azoles (pessaries/creams) or oral azoles. BV is treated with metronidazole or clindamycin either topically or orally.

Can my partner catch it from me?
It is not sexually transmitted. ♂ may occasionally develop balanitis with bacteria similar to those found with BV, but it does not appear to be related to intercourse with a partner who has BV. However, the increased incidence of BV in lesbian couples suggests a sexual link.

Does my partner who has no symptoms need treatment?
No. Treating an asymptomatic partner does not make any difference to recurrence rate.

Will I ever get rid of it?
Overall cure rate is 95%. Recurrence rate is about 15–30% with the majority recurring within 7 months of treatment.

Can I prevent it from coming back?
♀ who suffer from recurrent BV can be treated with episodic, anticipatory, or cyclical metronidazole or clindamycin. As BV is associated with a high vaginal pH, it is advisable to try to keep it low to prevent recurrences. This can be done by decreasing menstruation, e.g. with medroxyprogesterone acetate or using acidic vaginal gels. If a ♀ has an IUD and suffers from recurrent or persistent BV, it may be advisable to remove the IUD and try another method of contraception.

Is it harmful in pregnancy?
BV is associated with an increased risk of preterm delivery. Therefore, it is recommended that in ♀ with a history of a preterm delivery screening for BV is considered during pregnancy and treated if positive. It is not recommended that all pregnant ♀ are screened for BV. However, if a pregnant ♀ is found to have BV during routine testing (e.g. for a symptomatic discharge), she should be treated. Metronidazole is safe in pregnancy in all trimesters, although large doses are best avoided.

Diagnosis

Detection of *G. vaginalis* by culture cannot be used to diagnose BV as it can be isolated in >50% of ♀ with normal vaginal flora.

Gram stain

Simple, fast, and accurate way to diagnose BV. Typical appearance is substantial reduction or absence of lactobacilli (Gram-positive rods) replaced by small Gram-variable bacilli (*G. vaginalis*) adhering to shed epithelial ('clue') cells without polymorphs (Plate 2). Other small Gram-negative bacilli (e.g. *Bacteroides* spp.), Gram-positive cocci (e.g. peptostreptococci), Gram-variable sickle-shaped rods (*Mobiluncus* spp.) may be found. The last of these are seen more easily as motile organisms on a wet mount which may also show long thin pointed rods (fusiform bacilli).

Hay–Ison Gram-stain method

Simple qualitative method grading smears as follows:
- *grade 0*: epithelial cells/no bacteria
- *grade I* (normal): lactobacilli only
- *grade II* (intermediate): reduced lactobacilli/mixed bacteria, not found in BV as diagnosed by Amsel's criteria
- *grade III* (consistent with BV as diagnosed by Amsel's criteria), mixed bacteria with few or absent lactobacilli
- *grade IV*: epithelial cells covered with Gram +ve cocci only.

Nugent Gram-stain method

Although sensitive, this method is too complex and time-consuming for routine clinical use. It is based on the quantitative scoring of *Lactobacillus, G. vaginalis, Bacteroides* morphotypes, and *Mobiluncus* spp. on a Gram-stained vaginal smear. High scores (>6) equate to BV, medium scores (4–6) intermediate, and 0–3 normal.

Amsel's criteria (regarded as 'gold standard' for research)

Three of four criteria to be fulfilled:
- Characteristic discharge.
- *Positive amine ('sniff' or 'whiff') test*: drop of 10% potassium hydroxide on vaginal fluid releases 'fishy' smelling amines (avoid semen, which may give false-positive result). No longer recommended for safety reasons.
- pH >4.5 (avoiding cervical mucus (pH 7.0), blood, and seminal fluid).
- Vaginal 'clue' cells on wet-mount microscopy.
- Sensitivities and specificities of the separate components are shown in Table 15.1.

Other

- *Home tests* are available in some areas. These rely on a combination of vaginal pH and symptom scoring to enable women to differentiate between thrush, BV, or TV, as the potential cause of their symptoms.
- *POCT (chromogenic enzyme activity test)*: detecting elevated vaginal sialidase (enzyme produced by *G. vaginalis* and other BV associated bacteria) and reporting sensitivities of 93% and specificities of 98% when compared with Gram stain.

Table 15.1 Sensitivity and specificity of Amsel criteria

	Sensitivity (%)	Specificity (%)
Amsel criteria		
Atypical discharge	52–69	78–97
pH >4.5*	97	53
Amine test*	43–80	99
Clue cells	80–90	94

*Provided that sample is not contaminated with blood or seminal fluid.

Management

Offer an STI screen as standard. Variations in vaginal bacterial flora are common and BV-type features are often transient and self-limiting. Treatment is recommended for those with symptoms, those with clear signs of BV (who may report improvement after treatment), and those under-going certain surgical procedures, but otherwise not for asymptomatic BV or *G. vaginalis* colonization. The use of a soap substitute can be advocated.

- *Metronidazole*:
  - *oral*—400 mg bd for 5–7 days (or 2 g as a single-dose, but higher failure rates have been reported)
  - *intravaginal*—0.75% gel once daily (usually at night) for 5 days
- *Clindamycin*:
  - *oral*—300 mg bd for 7 days
  - *intravaginal*—2% cream od for 7 days (can weaken condoms).
- *Tinidazole (oral)*: 1 g daily for 5 days, 2 g daily for 2 days, or 2 g as a single dose.

Studies show that 7 days of oral metronidazole are as effective as 5 days of vaginal gel (symptomatic and microbiological cure rates of about 80% and 70%, respectively, at 1 month) and similar to clindamycin cream.

Cautions

⚠ Alcohol produces a disulfiram-like reaction in some people when taken with metronidazole, and possibly tinidazole, and should be avoided. No data are available on intravaginal preparations, but alcohol ingestion is not recommended. Both oral and topical clindamycin have been associated with pseudomembranous colitis.

Partners

No evidence of ↓ relapse rate if male partners are treated epidemiologically, but male condom may reduce the BV recurrence rate up to 5-fold. No data available on the value of treating female partners concurrently.

Pregnancy

Caution is advised in the use of metronidazole during pregnancy and breastfeeding, and high-dose regimens should be avoided. However, meta-analyses have shown no evidence linking birth defects to the use of metronidazole in early pregnancy. Antibiotic treatment can eradicate BV in pregnancy and it is advised for those with symptoms.

Data has been conflicting on whether screening and treating is beneficial. Evidence to support screening and treating all pregnant ♀ with asymptomatic BV in order to prevent preterm birth and its consequences is lacking even for women with recurrent or persistent BV. There is some suggestion that treatment before 20 weeks' gestation may ↓ risk of preterm birth. It may be therefore that consideration of other risk factors for preterm birth be taken into account when deciding on screening and treating individual women.

Breastfeeding

As both systemic metronidazole (alters the taste) and clindamycin enter the breast milk, intravaginal treatment should be considered.

Termination of pregnancy

Based on three independent studies, screening for and treating BV with metronidazole or clindamycin cream prior to TOP should be considered to ↓ the incidence of subsequent endometritis and PID.

Persisting or recurrent BV

Eliminate possible factors that may influence the microbiological flora (e.g. douching, shampoos, spermicides, smoking). Lack of evidence, but consider the following;

- *Persistent*:
  - change treatment (metronidazole to clindamycin, or vice versa)
  - consider removing IUD if *in situ*
  - oral co-amoxiclav (amoxicillin 250mg + clavulanic acid 125mg) 375mg 3 times a day for 7 days, as possibility of resistance or metronidazole de-activation by other vaginal bacteria. May also be considered initially if metronidazole and clindamycin cannot be used.
- *Recurrent*: following initial treatment mildly abnormal microscopy or elevated pH may be found suggesting relapse, rather than a new episode. If relevant, consider stopping menstrual flow (contraception) to maintain low pH. Ten days of induction therapy with vaginal metronidazole followed by twice weekly gel for 16 weeks can establish clinical cure of 75% at 16 weeks and 50% at 28 weeks. Other strategies include episodic, anticipatory, pulse, suppressive (e.g. twice weekly for 4–6 months using metronidazole gel 0.75% or clindamycin cream), or cyclical (e.g. oral metronidazole 400 mg bd for 3 days at the start and end of menstruation) treatment regimens.
- *Other approaches* (with the aim of disrupting biofilm formation):
  - *probiotics*—oral/vaginal lactobacillus replacement (limited data, but no conclusive evidence of benefit)
  - agents lowering vaginal pH (e.g. lactic or acetic acid gel)—suggested in those with recurrent BV (used as maintenance treatment) or in situations that raise pH, such as seminal fluid or menstrual blood in the vagina (e.g. for 3 days post-menstruation).

Anaerobic and *G. vaginalis*-associated balanitis/balanoposthitis

Male partners of ♀ with BV are usually asymptomatic and unlikely to develop balanitis/balanoposthitis.

Prevalence of *G. vaginalis* in men is 5-fold higher in heterosexual men than MSM.

G. vaginalis can be found in 31% of those with a non-candidal balanoposthitis. Usually mild, but may be foul smelling in association with anaerobes, especially *Bacteroides* spp. (commonly *B. melaninogenicus*). Normally found in those with underlying phimosis and poor hygiene. An offensive sub-preputial discharge may occur with erosions and preputial oedema. Usually resolves with advice on hygiene and the use of saline lavage, although oral metronidazole is sometimes required. Clindamycin cream 2% bd or oral co-amoxiclav 375 mg 3× a day for 1 week may also be used.

HIV infection

- Acquisition and transmission of HIV is ↑ with BV 2–5-fold.
- The acquisition of H_2O_2-producing lactobacilli significantly reduces HIV RNA in female genital secretions, while their loss ↑ these levels compared with stable colonization.
- The presence of BV has been shown to reduce the efficacy of tenofovir (TDF) containing vaginal PrEP, but further studies in relation to this are needed.

Further information
✒ https://www.bashhguidelines.org/media/1041/bv-2012.pdf
✒ https://www.bashhguidelines.org/media/1077/2062.pdf

Trichomoniasis

Aetiology 226
Epidemiology and transmission 227
Clinical features 228
Diagnosis 229
Management 230
Trichomoniasis and HIV infection 232

Aetiology

Trichomonas vaginalis (TV) was first described by Donné in 1836. A flagellated protozoan of the order Trichomonadida, which is parasitic to the human genitourinary tract (Fig. 16.1 and Plate 5). TV is usually oval and measures up to 15 µm in length *in vivo* (the size of a leucocyte). It is propelled by four anterior flagella arising from an anterior kinetosomal complex. An additional fifth flagellum is attached to an undulating membrane that extends halfway down the organism and an axostyle projects from the end of the body. Trichomonads lack mitochondria, but contain hydrogenosomes, large cytoplasmic granules involved in catabolism. It grows in a moist environment at 35–37°C and pH 4.9–7.5 (similar to bacterial vaginosis). Multiplication is by mitosis, occurring optimally every 8–12 hours.

Trichomonads infected by double-stranded RNA viruses have been identified, and are termed type II in contrast with virus-negative organisms designated type I. In a small comparative study type II isolates were found proportionately more commonly in ♀, especially older ♀.

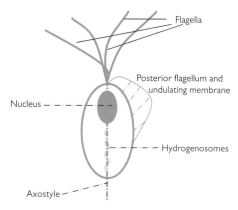

Fig. 16.1 Trichomonas vaginalis.

Epidemiology and transmission

Common worldwide, but steady decline in developed countries over the past 20 years. Reason is unclear, but may relate to standard cervical cytology screening, which can also detect TV. Almost exclusively sexually transmitted from infected genital secretions.

The parasite can be found in:
- ♀: vagina, cervix, urethra, bladder, and the ducts of Bartholin's and Skene's glands.
- ♂: anterior urethra, sub-preputial sac, glans penis, prostate, epididymis, and semen.

Sexual transmission
- Most commonly found in ♀ during the most sexually active years (16–35 years) and in those more sexually active (change in partner, intercourse twice weekly or more, 3 partners in past month).
- Recognized association with other STIs (e.g. gonorrhoea).
- High rate of re-infection unless ♂ partners are treated.
- Detection rates in ♂ contacts of infected ♀:
  - sex within previous 48 hours—70%
  - previous 5 days—40%
  - after 14 days—33%
  - after 21 days—12%.

Detection rates in ♀ contacts of infected ♂: 67–100%. ♀ to ♀ sexual transmission well recognized; may relate to the shared use of sex toys.

Non-sexual transmission

Protozoa may survive up to 45 minutes on toilet seats and for several hours in moist clothes, although transmission is unlikely.

Neonatal vulvovaginitis arising from infection acquired at delivery may arise, but is rare (5% of those born to mothers with TV). Commonly asymptomatic and usually spontaneously clears in 3–6 weeks as maternal oestrogen level falls.

Frequently asked questions

Is it always sexually transmitted?
Generally, yes, although it has been suggested that transmission could occur through moist flannels that are shared.

How long has it been present?
Symptoms usually develop within a month of acquiring infection, although up to 50% of ♀ are diagnosed without symptoms.

Does my male partner require treatment?
Yes. ♂ commonly carry *T. vaginalis* without any symptoms. Unless treated there is a high rate of re-infection.

Clinical features

Women

Incubation period (before symptoms develop): 4–28 days.

Symptoms
- 10–50% asymptomatic (depending on criteria).
- *Vaginal discharge*: 56%.
- *Dysuria*: 18%.
- *Low abdominal pain* (probably related to vaginitis): up to 12%.
- Vulval discomfort or itch.
- *Vaginal malodour*: ~50%, associated with concurrent anaerobic bacterial overgrowth.
- Vulval ulceration (rare).

Signs
- Altered vaginal discharge in up to 70%, frothy yellow in 10–30%.
- Vulvovaginitis.
- *'Strawberry cervix'* (colpitis macularis): small punctate cervical haemorrhages with ulceration found in 2–5%.
- *Urethritis*: 25%.
- *No signs*: 5–15%.
- Isolated case reports of detection from fallopian tubes (in salpingitis) and peritoneal fluid.

Pregnancy
- Independent association in pregnancy with premature rupture of membranes, preterm delivery, and low birth weight. Not proven to be causal.
- Although treatment of symptomatic ♀ is advocated, the risk of preterm birth is not ↓ with metronidazole treatment. One study of asymptomatic ♀ treated with metronidazole was stopped as there was an association with ↑ risk of preterm birth. Routine screening in pregnancy is not advised.

Complications
Association with cervical carcinoma reported, but uncontrolled for other genital pathogens (e.g. HPV); therefore, no proven causal relationship.

Men
- 75% asymptomatic.
- *Most common sign*: small to moderate urethral discharge—NGU. Trichomonal infection may be the cause in up to 15% of cases in high-prevalence areas. May present with dysuria.
- *Balanoposthitis*: 4–11% (rarely with ulceration).
- Reports of prostatitis, epididymitis, cystitis, penile ulceration, and median raphe suppuration.

Diagnosis

Test women presenting with vulvitis and/or vaginitis (swab from posterior fornix, self-taken vaginal swab, consider urine) and men who are either TV contacts or present with persistent urethritis (urethral specimen and/or urine).

Direct microscopy

Vaginal discharge examined as an isotonic saline suspension by phase contrast or dark ground microscopy. Slides must be read within 10 minutes as motility of the protozoa quickly declines and identification becomes harder. Readily recognizable motile protozoa propelled by flagella and undulating membrane are seen at ×400 magnification. (Fig. 16.1 and Plate 5). ♂ urethral discharge and sub-preputial material can be examined in a similar fashion. Alternatively, dried smears can be stained with acridine orange and viewed using fluorescent microscopy. This is more sensitive than wet preparations, but rarely used.

Compared with culture, the overall sensitivity of microscopy in ♀ is 40–80%, but in ♂ it is only ~30%, although the specificity is high.

Gram-stained vaginal smears typically show polymorphonuclear leucocytes, reduced or absent lactobacilli, and a mixed bacterial flora, as with BV. However, there is considerable variability.

Polymerase chain reaction

PCR should now be the test of choice where resources allow. The sensitivity of culture compared with PCR is poor, ranging from 34% to 59%, although its specificity is high at ~100%. TV PCR tests have sensitivities of 88–97% and specificities of 98–99%.

Culture

As well as vaginal, urethral, and sub-preputial samples, a centrifuged deposit of first morning urine can also be tested by culture (especially useful for ♂). Ideally, specimens should be placed in culture medium (e.g. Feinberg–Whittington). Otherwise, forward in transport medium (e.g. Amies or Stuart) and inoculate in growth medium within 24 hours. Microscopy is then carried out in the laboratory daily for 5 days. Culture is under partial or complete anaerobic conditions.

Point of care tests

Detect TV antigen. Have advantage over culture or PCR of giving a result within 15 minutes and have greater sensitivity (80–94%) than microscopy. Caution if using in a low prevalence population due to risk of false positives.

Cervical smears

TV is sometimes reported on cervical cytology. Sensitivity varies (60–80% compared with culture), but specificity is reported as over 98% with liquid-based cytology. The gold standard would be to confirm positive cases by microscopy ± culture. If unconfirmed the sensitivity and specificity of the tests, together with history and examination findings should allow a clinical decision to be made.

Management

- Sexual partners should be treated simultaneously, and sexual intercourse avoided until treatment has been completed.
- If ♂ contacts present with NGU, it is reasonable to treat initially as TV infection and review after treatment.
- Screening for other STIs for patients and their contacts is advised.
- Treatment should be systemic in view of the high rates of urethral and para-urethral gland involvement.
- Spontaneous resolution is estimated at around 20–25% in women.

Treatment

The only effective agents are the 5-nitroimidazoles (overall cure rates ~95%). There are no reliable alternative antibiotics.

Oral metronidazole

400–500 mg bd for 5–7 days or 2g in a single dose. If allergy reported consider metronidazole desensitization. Single dose has the advantage of ↑ adherence but has lower cure rate (by 6–12%), especially if partner(s) not treated simultaneously. ❶ Patients should be advised to avoid alcohol while taking treatment and for 48 hours thereafter, because of a possible disulfiram-like (Antabuse®) reaction (similar reaction possible with tinidazole). Vaginal metronidazole cream is not advised as cure rates only ~20% probably because of poor absorption and failure to penetrate infected Bartholin's and Skene's glands, and urethra. Plasma levels achieved when administered rectally or vaginally are only 50% and 20%, respectively, of those of oral metronidazole (although this varies with the formulation). Body weight plays a role in drug excretion; therefore, some fixed-dose regimens may not be appropriate for all patients. Although caution is advised in the use of metronidazole during pregnancy the manufacturers only warn against high-dose regimens; should also be avoided during breastfeeding.

Tinidazole

2 g in a single dose is an alternative. It is unknown whether there is cross-reactivity between metronidazole and tinidazole, therefore, it cannot be considered safe in cases of metronidazole allergy.

Tinidazole should be avoided in pregnancy.

Treatment failure is due to inadequate therapy (check adherence, vomiting), re-infection or resistance:

- *Low plasma zinc may contribute to treatment failure (unusual)*: provide oral zinc supplement.
- *5-nitroimidazole deactivation by vaginal bacteria*: no evidence to support this, but theoretically, aerobes and anaerobes, including β-haemolytic streptococci, could be implicated. Consider concurrent treatment with amoxicillin or erythromycin.
- *Resistance*: 5% of all clinical strains estimated to have at least some metronidazole resistance. Generally aerobic, but anaerobic resistance has also been reported. Resistance testing should be conducted in aerobic conditions, but is not readily available. Although

metronidazole-resistant strains show ↓ susceptibility to oral tinidazole, the minimal inhibitory concentration is likely to be significantly ↓. Tinidazole has a longer half-life, good tissue penetration, and lower levels of resistance, and should, therefore, be considered in this scenario.

Treatment options to consider in refractory cases

- 40% will respond to a repeat (7-day) course of standard therapy.
- If no response, then 70% of those remaining will respond if given a higher dose course (metronidazole or tinidazole 2 g daily for 5–7 days or metronidazole 800 mg tid for 7 days).
- If treatment failure follows and resistance testing is unavailable, very high dose tinidazole (1 g bd or tid or 2 g bd for 14 days) can be used. Consider the addition of intravaginal tinidazole 500 mg bd alongside this. 90–92% of those who failed the previous regimens respond to this.
- Intravaginal paromomycin or intravaginal furazolidone or acetarsol pessaries or nonoxynol-9 pessaries are all unlicensed preparations reported to have some success.

Test of cure

Consider if the patient remains symptomatic following treatment, or if symptoms recur.

Contact tracing

Current partners and sexual contacts from the preceding 4 weeks should be offered a full STI screen, including a test for TV, but offered treatment irrespective of the result. If urethritis is present in this scenario, this should be treated as TV first line.

Trichomoniasis and HIV infection

- TV may enhance HIV transmission (probably related to genital inflammation) Successful treatment of trichomonal urethritis in men ↓ levels of HIV RNA.
- There may be an increased risk of TV infection in those who have HIV.
- Single, high-dose metronidazole is possibly less effective in those with HIV. Consider a 7-day course.

Further information
⊗ https://www.bashhguidelines.org/media/1042/tv_2014-ijstda.pdf

Genital candidiasis

Introduction *234*
Aetiology *234*
Epidemiology and transmission *235*
Predisposing factors *236*
Clinical features *237*
Diagnosis *239*
Management *241*
Candidiasis and HIV infection *244*

Introduction

Also referred to as candidosis, moniliasis, or thrush. It is considered to be pathogenic activity by commensal yeasts in individuals with reduced local or systemic resistance. Association with vaginitis first described in 1849, although oral thrush was recognized in the 4th century BC.

Aetiology

Candida spp., especially *Candida albicans*, responsible for 85–90% of infections and *Candida glabrata* responsible for 3–15%. Other yeasts rarely implicated include *C. tropicalis* (~4%), *C. parapsilosis* (~4%), *C. krusei* (~2%), *C. stellatoidea*, and *C. gulliermondi*. Occasional cases of vaginitis reported include *Saccharomyces cerevisiae*, a yeast from the family Cryptococcaceae (to which *Candida* also belongs) and *C. dubliniensis*.

All pathogenic *Candida* spp. multiply by the production of buds from a blastospore (yeast cell), approximately 1–5.0 μm in diameter.

C. albicans produces:
- *Hyphae*: long tubes made up of multiple cell units divided by septa arising from blastospores or as branches of existing hyphae.
- *Pseudohyphae*: single elongated cells from blastospore buds with constrictions instead of septa. Each generation remains attached to its parent.
- *Chlamydospores*: large refractory bodies, with double-layered cell walls (probably a dormant phase).

The mycelium is the entire yeast aggregate (spores, hyphae, and branches).
- *C. glabrata* does not produce hyphae or pseudohyphae.
- *Candida* spp. contain their own set of virulence factors, which may contribute to their ability to cause infection. They include surface molecules that facilitate mucosal adherence, proteases when there is mucositis, and the ability to convert into a hyphal form. *C. albicans* has the greatest ability to adhere to and invade the mucosa, enhanced by the production of germ tubes (also useful in species identification), where it may form a reservoir for recurrences.

Epidemiology and transmission

75% of ♀ have at least one episode of genital candidiasis with 40–50% having multiple episodes. It is much less common for ♂ to present with symptomatic infection.

Candida spp. can be found anywhere on the body, but most commonly in the mouth (30–55% of young adults), vagina (8–32% of young ♀, 40% if pregnant), and anorectal canal (40–65%). C. albicans accounts for 80–90% of genital yeast isolates and 60–80% of oral carriage, although is seldom recovered from normal skin (C. parapsilosis and C. gulliermondi are more prevalent there).

Although peno-vaginal intercourse is a factor in the direct transmission of yeast infection, its role is unclear. However, it is generally accepted that, without predisposing factors, ♂ usually acquire infection sexually. In ♀, it seems that coitus is more likely to act as a trigger by introducing perineal organisms and causing microtrauma, which breaches mucosal integrity. Hypothetically, vaginal intercourse following anal penetration is more likely to introduce infection, although there are no data to support this. However, there does seem to be an association with recent receptive oral sex in ♀. This may be by direct transmission, with saliva promoting pathogenesis by moistening and irritating the vulval mucosa and altering the local immunity. Non-specific genital infection and other STIs have been shown to be associated with yeast infection in 39% of ♀ and 29% of ♂.

Frequently asked questions

What is thrush?

Thrush is an infection caused by a yeast, usually *Candida albicans*. *Candida* spp. commonly live in small numbers in and around the genitals, especially the vagina. People are asymptomatic until candida multiplies and penetrates the mucosal surface.

Is thrush sexually transmitted?

Usually not, especially in women. Partners do not need any treatment unless they have symptoms and signs of thrush themselves.

Predisposing factors

Reduction in local mucosal resistance
- Sexual contact causing microfissures.
- Inflammation (e.g. eczema related to contact irritants, other dermatoses, tight/non-absorbent clothing, although evidence is inconclusive).

Diabetes mellitus
Produces a glucose-rich environment, ideal for the growth of yeasts, especially in poorly controlled diabetes. Associated with a 20% ↑ in oral colonization by *Candida* spp.

Hormonal factors
- *Physiological*: oestrogen raises the amount of glycogen in the vagina and ↓ cell-mediated immunity. Progesterone is also immunosuppressive and stimulates germ tube formation. Therefore, symptomatic candidiasis is uncommon before menarche and after the menopause. It is most commonly found in the child-bearing years:
  - in the luteal phase of the menstrual cycle
  - during pregnancy, especially the 3rd trimester (↑ vaginal glycogen and immunological factors)—a large proportion of ♀ who subsequently present with recurrent vulvo-vaginal candidiasis (RVVC), first present with infection during pregnancy.
- *Combined oral contraceptives*: only clearly associated with high-dose oestrogen (50 mcg) preparations.
- *Oestrogen replacement treatment*: probable relative ↑.

Impaired immunity
Includes HIV and drugs (e.g. corticosteroids, chemotherapy).

Broad-spectrum antibiotics
↑ Vaginal yeast carriage by 10–30%. Although there is an association with candidiasis, it is small, and the vast majority of ♀ on antibiotic treatment are unaffected.

Other contraceptives
Conflicting evidence of an association with the use of spermicides (cidal effect on lactobacilli), diaphragms, and caps (causing re-infection) and IUDs. More likely to be carriage, rather than disease.

Local factors
Lack of consistent evidence relating intimate hygiene practices or menstrual sanitation (use of external towels or pads) with genital candidiasis. Vaginal deodorants, disinfectants, and perfumed products may exacerbate candidiasis by causing dermatitis. No evidence to support re-infection by fomites such as underwear.

Clinical features

Acute vulvo-vaginitis

Accounts for 90% presentations in ♀. There is significant clinical overlap with other conditions, particularly vulval dermatoses and, as candida is commonly isolated from reproductive-age women (colonization rate is 10–20%), attention must be paid to whether it is the cause of, contributing to, or a concurrent finding in relation to symptoms.

Symptoms
Vulval pruritus and burning, with external dysuria and dyspareunia being common. Usually starts or worsens from mid-menstrual cycle, often improving with menstruation.

Signs
Vulval erythema with fissuring is the most common finding. Usually localized to the vulval mucocutaneous margins, but can spread to involve the labia majora, perineum, and perigenital skin where satellite lesions (small areas of erythema adjacent to but separate from the main body of inflammation) may be seen. Vaginal erythema seen in 20%, with a thick white curdy adherent discharge in 20% (70% if pregnant) forming plaques on the vagina, cervix, and vulva. Discharge may, however, also be purulent or watery.

Recurrent vulvovaginal candidiasis (RVVC)

Definition
Four or more episodes of symptomatic candidiasis annually with at least partial resolution of symptoms between episodes with positive microscopy or culture on at least 2 occasions when symptomatic.

Frequency
Occurs in ~5% of ♀. Thought to be due to incomplete elimination of infection or inadequate treatment with a change in the protective vaginal mucosa cell-mediated host defence mechanisms, leading to relapses.

Other factors
- *Hypersensitivity*: probably important as shown by associations with perennial allergic rhinitis and a family history of allergies. Compared with ♀ with isolated episodes, ♀ with RVVC cannot tolerate small numbers of yeast organisms.
- *Sex*: positive association between the monthly frequency of sexual intercourse and the incidence of RVVC. Asymptomatic penile colonization with *Candida* spp. occurs ×4 more commonly in partners of ♀ with RVVC.

Clinical features
Vulval pruritus with burning common, but signs (erythema, oedema, fissures, white curdy discharge) are found less commonly than in acute cases.

Chronic persistent candidiasis
Vulval lichenification and local oedema; more commonly found in older obese diabetics.

Men

In colonized ♂ most common symptom is post-coital itching or burning.

Clinical presentation

- Direct infection with inflammation of glans (balanitis) and/or prepuce (posthitis). More common in the uncircumcised, presenting as a glazed erythematous rash, sometimes with white papules/discharge and, if severe, fissuring, oedema, and phimosis.
- Contact hypersensitivity reaction.
- Usually mild to moderate balanoposthitis within 24 hours of contact with vaginal candidiasis. Yeasts are often not detected from the penis.

~20% of ♂ contacts of ♀ with RVVC complain of soreness and irritation lasting for 24–48 hours starting shortly after intercourse and penile colonization with candida occurs in ~20% of the uncircumcised partners of ♀ with RVVC, usually with identical strains, but this is often asymptomatic.

Rarely occurs as non-gonococcal urethritis.

Chronic mucocutaneous candidiasis

Characteristically involves skin-folds, nails, skin in and around the mouth, and vulva/vagina. If present consider:

- Anaemia.
- Autoimmune conditions, e.g.
  - Addison's disease
  - hypothyroidism
  - hypoparathyroidism
- Thymomas

These conditions are not associated with simple genital candidiasis.

Diagnosis

Patient's self-assessment is not a reliable method of diagnosing candidiasis. Only pruritus and objectively gauged signs are reliable clinical indicators. Microscopy and culture are the standard of care.

Sampling

- *Women*: specimens should be taken of vaginal discharge and also from the lateral vaginal walls, using a plastic loop or swab. Material can also be taken from inflamed areas on vulva or surrounding skin.
- *Men*: sampling for microscopy is more difficult and a variety of methods are used including dry or moistened swabs, plastic loops (which may also be moistened with normal saline), skin scrapings, or a dry slide pressed against the penis.

Laboratory culture

This is the gold standard. Genital specimens are usually sent in transport medium (e.g. Amies, Feinberg–Whittington) and cultured on growth medium (e.g. Sabouraud). Culture allows speciation and sensitivity testing which may be important in the patient's management. Germ tube formation is used in the presumptive identification of *C. albicans* with an accuracy of 95–100%.

Direct microscopy

Hyphae, pseudohyphae, spores (*C. glabrata* only produces spores) may be seen in vulvo-vaginal saline suspensions viewed as wet-mount preparations in 40–60% of women with symptomatic candidiasis. If 10–20% potassium hydroxide is used in the wet mount to lyse epithelial and blood cells, sensitivity improves by ~10%. Alternatively, vulvovaginal material examined by Gram-stain detects infection in ~65% of symptomatic cases (spores and hyphae staining Gram +ve; Plate 3).

Other investigations

- *Latex agglutination test*: limited use—sensitivity 75%, specificity 97%.
- *PCR*: not routinely available, doubts over sensitivity and specificity.
- *Vaginal pH*: remains normal at 4.0–4.5. pH >5 may suggest BV. *C. glabrata* grows at a higher pH than *C. albicans* and may be associated with BV.
- Home testing kits use either a combination of vaginal pH testing and symptom review or antigen testing to provide a 'diagnosis'. Sensitivity and specificity will vary depending on the patient and the test.
- *Urinalysis*: for sugar to exclude diabetes (especially if recurrent).

Recurrent vulvo-vaginal candidiasis

Requires clinical examination, culture with speciation (as *C. glabrata* and *C. krusei* are more resistant to azoles), consideration of underlying disease. Important to exclude pregnancy, diabetes, and other risk factors (e.g. immunodeficiency, repeated antibiotic or corticosteroid use).

Sensitivity testing is important as *C. albicans* can be fluconazole-resistant. It should also be remembered that different *Candida* spp. can co-exist and dominant species only may be reported on the culture.

Frequently asked questions

Why do I keep getting it?

Treatment of candidiasis may not eliminate it entirely from the vagina, so remaining spores/hyphae may multiply again when the conditions are right, producing a recurrent attack of thrush. Certain situations make thrush more likely (e.g. pregnancy, diabetes, immunosuppression, antibiotics). Avoid precipitants and irritants, such as bubble baths, perfumed soaps, vaginal douching, and tight-fitting synthetic underwear. About 5–10% of cases are due to *C. glabrata*, which may be more resistant to azoles.

Is there anything that I can take to prevent it from coming back?

Recurrent thrush is defined as four or more symptomatic episodes in a year. Some people seem to go through phases of recurrence, which is probably because of incomplete eradication. A longer course of topical or oral therapy may help. Women with frequent episodes can try prophylactic treatment such as a clotrimazole 500 mg pessary weekly or oral fluconazole 150 mg weekly for up to 6 months. Thrush is associated with recently receiving oral sex in women, therefore, avoidance may prevent recurrence.

Does my Pill make my thrush worse?

The usual type of combined contraceptive pill prescribed contains low levels of oestrogen and is not related to increased rates of thrush, but it may have an effect of recurrent episodes. The progesterone-only pill may be helpful in some women.

Do I need to go on a yeast-free diet?

There is no evidence that yeast-free diets make any difference to vaginal thrush infections. Studies to eliminate *Candida* spp. from the gut using long-term oral medication have shown that recurrent vaginal thrush is not prevented.

I am pregnant. Is thrush harmful to my baby?

Thrush is more common in pregnancy. Asymptomatic colonization rates are higher and symptomatic episodes more common in pregnancy. Thrush can be treated with topical azoles in pregnancy, but oral preparations are contraindicated. There is no evidence that colonization with candida in pregnancy affects pregnancy outcome.

Does yoghurt help?

Probably not, but we're not sure. Intravaginal use (by applicator or on a tampon) has been tried with varying degrees of success, although it may just sooth irritation. Daily oral ingestion of 8 ounces of active yoghurt has, in one study, been shown to decrease both candidal colonization and infection, but this has not been confirmed in other studies.

Management

As yeasts are commensals, treatment is not required unless clinically indicated. Routine use of an emollient as a moisturizer and soap substitute, as well as avoiding tight fitting synthetic clothing and local irritants is advised.

Acute vulvovaginitis: principles

See Box 17.1 for drugs.

- Bathing in saline or sodium bicarbonate may provide symptomatic relief and if severe, analgesics (e.g. NSAIDs) are beneficial.
- Little difference in efficacy between the drugs available and their route of administration (short-duration treatments improve adherence and so are favoured). Azole therapies are the mainstay of treatment with a 80–95% clinical and mycological cure rate in acute candidiasis (if non-pregnant) with no difference between topical and oral preparations. Cure rates for nystatin are slightly lower (70–90%). Oral treatments are contraindicated if pregnant or breast feeding. If severe, creams may be preferred as they are more soothing than pessaries and may produce more prompt relief of symptoms than oral treatment (however, conversely, in some may produce local irritation.) Nystatin stains the underwear yellow. Although candidal vulvitis can be treated locally with cream, it is almost always associated with vaginal infection, which should also be treated.
- Topical preparations may damage latex in condoms or diaphragms.
- If the candidiasis is a result of dermatitis or there appears to be a hypersensitivity reaction, an antimycotic–hydrocortisone combination should be considered.
- Unless symptomatic, no action is required for ♂ partners.

Balanoposthitis: principles

See Box 17.1 for drugs.

- Mild cases will respond to simple saline lavage. Moderate or severe inflammation usually requires antimycotic treatment, commonly prescribed as a cream, although similar results are achieved with oral azoles. Consider hydrocortisone-containing topical combinations if underlying dermatitis or hypersensitivity.
- ♀ Sexual partners can be offered screening +/– epidemiological treatment.

Drug resistance

~50% of all *C. glabrata* strains have ↓ sensitivity to azoles and there are higher levels of resistance with *C. cerevisiae* and *C. krusei* (intrinsic resistance to fluconazole). Polyene antifungal resistance is rare.

Persistent infection

- Confirm candida present (including typing and sensitivity testing)
- Consider an alternative from Box 17.1.

Box 17.1 Standard antimycotics for acute genital candidiasis

Azoles

Intravaginal
- Clotrimazole:
  - *pessary*—500 mg single dose, 200 mg for 3 nights, 100 mg for 6 nights
  - *cream*—10% as a single 5 g intravaginal dose.
- Econazole: pessary—150 mg single dose or 150 mg for 3 nights.
- Miconazole:
  - *pessary*—100 mg for 14 nights (or 200 mg for 7 nights)
  - *ovule*—1.2 g single dose.
- Fenticonazole: pessary—200 mg for 3 nights (or 600 mg single dose).

External
- Clotrimazole cream: 1% or 2% 2–3 times daily
- Econazole nitrate cream: 1% bd
- Ketoconazole cream: 2% once or bd
- Miconazole nitrate cream: 2% bd

Oral
- ❶ Avoid in pregnancy and breastfeeding.
- Fluconazole: 150 mg as a single dose.
- Itraconazole: 200 mg bd for 1 day.

Polyenes

Intravaginal nystatin
- Pessaries: 1000,000 units 1 or 2 for 14 nights .
- Cream: 100,000 units 4 g for 14 nights.

Topical combinations with hydrocortisone
- Canesten HC®: clotrimazole 1% + hydrocortisone 1% cream
- Daktacort®: miconazole nitrate 2% + hydrocortisone 1% cream
- Econacort®: econazole nitrate 1% + hydrocortisone 1% cream
- Nystaform-HC®: nystatin 100,000U + hydrocortisone 0.5% cream

Azoles not available in the UK
- Butaconazole: 2% cream—5 g daily for 3 days, intravaginal
- Terconazole:
  - *0.4% cream*—5 g for 7 days, intravaginal
  - *0.8% cream*—5 g for 3 days intravaginal
  - *pessary*—80 mg pessary for 3 nights
- Tioconazole: 6.5% ointment—5 g single dose, intravaginal.

Recurrent vulvovaginal candidiasis

Induction followed by maintenance
- Fluconazole 150 mg every 72 hours × 3 doses followed by 150 mg weekly for 6 months.
- Alternatives can be use of a topical imidazole for 10–14 days as induction, followed by clotrimazole pessary 500 mg once a week or itraconazole 50–100 mg daily or ketoconazole 100 mg daily.
- If relapse occurs in between doses using the first regimen; consider fluconazole 150 mg twice weekly or 50 mg daily.

❶ Oral azoles carry a low risk of idiosyncratic hepatitis and, remember, these regimens may fall outside of the product license.

During maintenance 90% ♀ remain free from symptomatic recurrences. However, they may occur in 30–40% of ♀ after cessation.

No evidence of ↓ recurrences by:
- routinely treating asymptomatic ♂ partners; however, limited data suggest treatment benefit if ♂ are colonized (systemic treatment because of the possibility of oral reservoir)
- reducing intestinal colonization (e.g. with oral nystatin)
- zinc supplements (no evidence of association with zinc deficiency)
- special cleaning of underwear.

Non-albicans species
Show higher rates of fluconazole resistance than *C. albicans* and higher MIC for oral azoles so consider higher doses. Alternative treatments (all unlicensed):
- Nystatin pessaries.
- Voriconazole.
- *Boric acid*: 600 mg vaginally as a gelatin capsule od or bd for 10–14 days has shown promising results with mycological cure rates of around 75% for *C. glabrata*. A 300 mg dose is suggested if mucositis develops. Contraindicated in pregnancy. Although maintenance has been used (twice a week or for 5 days during menstruation), data limited; because of potential toxicity nystatin pessaries advocated.
- Flucytosine cream or pessary and/or amphotericin in cream or K-Y Jelly⁽ⁿ⁾ for vaginal insertion

Other approaches
- *Self-help measures*: avoid products that may cause vulval irritation (e.g. vaginal deodorants, perfumed preparations) and wear loose cotton underwear. Avoid douching.
- *Desensitization*: studies have shown a significant reduction in the frequency of RVVC following immunotherapy with *C. albicans* extract. There are also limited data suggesting that zafirlukast (a leukotriene receptor antagonist) may be beneficial.
- *Switch combined to progesterone-only contraception*: limited data.
- Consider antihisthamine for symptomatic relief

Candidiasis and HIV infection

- Carriage rates high; *C .albicans*—vagina (75–85%), oropharynx (90–95%).
- Although vaginitis due to *Candida* spp. is more common and persistent in ♀ with HIV infection, it is clinically similar to that found in HIV-negative ♀ and can be treated with conventional therapy.
- Recurrent genital infection is not in itself an indicator of HIV infection. Oral candidiasis, however, is.
- In AIDS, colonization with fluconazole-resistant *Candida* spp. is more common.

Further information
℘ https://www.bashhguidelines.org/media/1155/united-kingdom-national-guideline-on-the-management-of-vulvovaginal-candidiasis.pdf

Tropical genital and sexually acquired infections

Chancroid 246
Lymphogranuloma venereum 248
Granuloma inguinale (Donovanosis) 251
Other genital infections 253

Chancroid

Aetiology: *Haemophilus ducreyi*

Small Gram –ve anaerobic coccobacillus occurring in chains. Culture requires blood-enriched medium incubated in an atmosphere of 5–10% carbon dioxide. Most clinical isolates are β-lactamase producers.

Epidemiology and transmission

Cases are now only diagnosed sporadically, even where there was a significant prevalence, such as tropical and subtropical countries (especially Africa, south-west Asia, South America, and the Caribbean). Genital ulcer disease (GUD) in these countries is commonly caused by HSV-2. Co-infections of *H. ducreyi* with *Treponema pallidum* and HSV infection found in over 10% in African studies. In UK, the majority of cases are either acquired abroad or from a partner who has been abroad. A few sporadic outbreaks were previously reported in Europe and the USA

Sexually transmitted (including oral sex), but also auto-inoculated, especially by fingers. Infection rate following single exposure from male to female ≈60%. Carriage of *H. ducreyi* without symptoms or signs has been reported in sex workers, who may be an important infection reservoir. No evidence of congenital or perinatal transmission.

Associated with the prepuce (the uncircumcised twice as susceptible), sex work, crack cocaine use (in USA), HIV infection (GUD enhances the transmission of HIV).

Clinical features

- *Incubation period*: 4–7 days (range 1–14 days).
- Initial tender red papule, which progresses to a pustule then an ulcer after 2–3 days. Ulcers can be single or multiple (Plate 12), and are painful. Multiple ulcers may be facilitated by auto-inoculation—'kissing' lesions. Usually 1–2 cm in diameter, irregular margins, bleed on touch, non-indurated (soft chancre or sore). May coalesce into giant ulcers.
- *Main features*:
  - *Males*—prepuce (may cause phimosis), coronal sulcus, frenulum and anus (MSM)
  - *Females*—labia minora, fourchette, and rarely vagina, cervix, and perianal region
  - *Extragenital*—very unusual (fingers, breasts, conjunctivae)
  - *Inguinal lymphadenopathy*—usually unilateral occurring in ≈50% as a tender swelling, which may develop into a unilocular abscess (bubo) in 25%.
- Disseminated infection not reported.

Complications

Bacterial superinfection with tissue destruction (phagedenic chancroid); chronic suppurative inguinal sinuses.

Diagnosis

Polymerase chain reaction (pcr)

Most sensitive technique: 95% sensitive compared with culture (due to presence of polymerase inhibitors). Multiplex PCR test is available and detects *H. ducreyi*, *T. pallidum*, and HSV simultaneously.

Culture

Material obtained from ulcer base (remove superficial pus) or pus aspirated from the bubo. Many culture media are available and the use of more than one increases sensitivity to up to 80%. In endemic areas, positive culture is achievable in 60–80% of those clinically considered to have chancroid.

Microscopy

Low sensitivity and not recommended as a diagnostic test. Smear from cleaned ulcer or pus aspirate from bubo by rolling the swab through 180° on the slide and stain with Gram stain. Typically, small Gram +ve rods running in parallel and forming chains; 'shoals of fish' seen (unreliable due to bacterial contamination).

Serology

Only useful for epidemiological studies.

Management

- Oral azithromycin 1g single dose.
- Oral ciprofloxacin 500 mg bd for 3 days (no effect against treponemes; therefore, will not mask developing syphilis).
- IM ceftriaxone 250 mg single dose.
- Oral erythromycin 500 mg qds for 7 days.

Ciprofloxacin and erythromycin are recommended for HIV +ve individuals.

Fluctuant buboes should be aspirated (by needle) from adjacent healthy skin under antibiotic cover. Patients should be re-examined 3–7 days after treatment to ensure symptomatic improvement. Re-epithelization occurs within 7 days of the onset of therapy. Resolution of fluctuant lymphadenopathy is slower than that of ulcers and may require repeated needle aspiration.

Partner notification

Sexual contacts within 10 days of disease onset should be examined and given epidemiological treatment as for a clinical case.

Lymphogranuloma venereum

Aetiology

L1, L2, L3 serovars of *Chlamydia trachomatis,* a primitive obligatory intracellular bacterium (➲ Chapter 9, 'Aetiology', p. 150).

Epidemiology and transmission

Classical areas

Africa, India, Caribbean, central America, south-east Asia. However, since 2003 outbreaks and epidemics in the UK, Western Europe and America in MSM. New cases peaked in the UK in 2005, but are maintained at an endemic level (UK has highest rates in Europe).

Traditionally sexually acquired in tropical and subtropical areas. Highest rates in the 20–30-year age group and associated with sex work, multiple sexual partners, other STIs, and social deprivation. Congenital infection does not occur, but perinatal infection may be acquired from birth canal.

Western European/American cases almost entirely MSM, with high levels of co-infection with HIV (up to 80%) and other STIs, although heterosexual and female cases have been reported. Cases caused by the L2 serovar. Most infections have been acquired following local sexual contact, and factors implicated include MSM having sex at sex-on-premises venues or sex parties, Internet dating, unprotected anal sex, fisting, and use of enemas and sex toys. Mode of transmission unclear in view of the overwhelming predominance of rectal infection. Recent data indicate that new index cases report significantly fewer sexual partners, suggesting that LGV may be moving into MSM with lower risk status. In the UK, this is currently being monitored by Public Health England as an enhanced surveillance programme.

Clinical features

Primary LGV

Incubation period: 3–30 days. Small painless papule at site of infection progressing to a pustule and asymptomatic ulcer that heals without scarring. Primary lesion reported by only 20–50% of men. Some ulcers in the recent MSM outbreak are indurated and painful, and durations lasting for weeks. Sites involved include coronal sulcus, prepuce, glans, scrotum, vulva, vagina, cervix (cervicitis). Extra-genital lesions such as perianal ulcers, lip and oral cavity lesions have been reported.

Secondary lgv (inguinal syndrome)

LGV serovars are lymphotropic infecting lymphocytes and macrophages. The pathological process is thrombolymphangitis and perilymphangitis. Lymphadenopathy follows the primary lesion by 10–30 days, rarely months. In men, usual presentation is unilateral lymphadenopathy (≈70%). Only 20–30% of women with LGV develop inguinal lymphadenopathy as lesions from the posterior vulva, anus, and vagina drain to the perirectal or pelvic nodes. Femoral nodes may also be involved (20%) and the 'groove sign' (enlargement of nodes above and below the inguinal ligament) is found in 15–33% (see Plate 14). Lymphadenopathy progressing to multilocular abscesses (buboes), which may rupture producing sinuses, occurs in ≈33%. Otherwise, they involve, forming firm inguinal masses. Constitutional features include fever, arthritis, aseptic meningitis, hepatitis, perihepatitis, pneumonia, erythema multiforme, and erythema nodosum.

Tertiary LGV (anorectal syndrome)

Majority of patients recover after the secondary stage. In a few patients, infection persists or progresses in anogenital tissues leading to chronic inflammatory response with tissue destruction, manifesting as proctitis, proctocolitis mimicking Crohn's disease, fistulae, strictures, and disfiguring fibrosis and scarring of the vulva with esthiomene (Greek word meaning 'eating away'). In men, penile and scrotal oedema may develop causing distortion, which may produce the 'saxophone penis".

Tertiary complications of anorectal LGV have rarely been observed in the MSM outbreak.

LGV proctitis in MSM

Asymptomatic infection is uncommon. Most cases present with haemorrhagic proctitis following direct transmission to the rectal mucosa. Symptoms include rectal pain, anorectal bleeding, rectal discharge, tenesmus, constipation, and other symptoms of lower GI inflammation. About 25% have systemic symptoms. Genital ulcers and inguinal symptoms are rare (~2%).

Pharyngeal LGV have been reported causing ulcers and pharyngitis.

Complications

Genital lymphoedema (elephantiasis), suppurative fistulae and sinuses, rectal strictures leading to intestinal obstruction, rectal carcinoma.

Diagnosis

Obtain samples containing cellular material from ulcer base exudate, rectal swabs and pharyngeal swabs, aspirated pus from lymph nodes or buboes and urethral swab/first catch urine. Test using:

- Nucleic acid amplification tests: If *C. trachomatis* detected, the specimen is tested for LGV-specific DNA.
- Cell culture from suspected LGV lesions: sensitivity ≈80% from ulcer, ≈30% bubo pus. Not appropriate for urine testing.
- *Serology*: less value and limited availability. Four techniques are used: complement fixation test (CFT), single L-type immunofluorescence test, micro-immunofluorescence (micro-IF) and anti-MOMP IgA assay. A 4-fold antibody rise or single-point titres of >1:64 or >1:128 for the micro-IF is considered positive as only invasive infection, such as that caused by LGV would achieve these levels. All serological tests have low sensitivities and specificities, and cannot distinguish past from current LGV infection.
- *Other tests*: patients must be tested for other STIs, including IHV and HCV.

Management
- *Oral doxycycline*: 100 mg bd for 3 weeks
- *Erythromycin*: 500mg 4 times a day for 3 weeks
- *Alternative regimens*:
  - Azithromycin 1 g stat and 1 g weekly for 3 weeks for rectal LGV in MSM
  - Ofloxacin or Moxifloxacin for 2 weeks, expected to be effective and may be give if clinically necessary with test of cure 2 weeks after completion of therapy
- Repeat needle aspiration of buboes may be required.

As buboes are multilocular, surgical incision of fluctuant glands is contraindicated. Surgery may be required for late manifestations.

PN: sexual contacts within 30 days before the onset of symptoms or the last 3 months if asymptomatic LGV, they should be examined, tested for rectal, urethral, and cervical and pharyngeal chlamydial infection. They should receive epidemiological treatment with 3 weeks doxycycline 100 mg bd or an alternative regimen for the same duration.

Granuloma inguinale (Donovanosis)

Aetiology: *Klebsiella*

- Formerly called *Calymmatobacterium granulomatis*.
- Human parasite (no animal model). Gram –ve pleomorphic bacterium with a well-defined capsule 1–1.5 µm long and 0.6 µm wide.

Epidemiology and transmission

Main areas

Papua New Guinea, South Africa, Southern India, and Brazil. Infection routes are unclear. Sexual transmission, especially anal intercourse, most likely, but accidental inoculation from skin contact and faecal contamination possible. Mother-to-child transmission at birth.

In support of STI origin

- Most commonly affects sexually active adults aged <30 years
- Genital infection usual (including cervix as sole site, anus with receptive intercourse)
- Associated with concurrent STIs, including HIV.

Against STI origin

- Occurs in young children (allegedly from sitting on lap of infected adult) and the sexually inactive
- Relatively uncommon in sex workers
- Rare in partners of those with open lesions
- An outbreak has been linked to a HCP.

Clinical features

Incubation period: uncertain (1–360 days), probably ≈50 days. The genitals are affected in 90% and inguinal area in 10%. Extra-genital in 6%, including lips, cheek, palate, and pharynx. Lymphadenitis is uncommon. Haematogenous spread to bone, liver, and spleen rare.

Four types described

- *Ulcerogranulomatous*: the most common. Single or multiple, non-tender, fleshy, exuberant, beefy red ulcers that bleed easily when touched (Plate 13).
- *Hypertrophic or verrucous type*: an ulcer or growth with raised irregular edge, sometimes with a walnut appearance.
- Necrotic, usually deep foul smelling ulcer causing tissue destruction.
- Sclerotic with extensive scarring.

Complications

Include lymphatic genital oedema (elephantiasis) in 15–20%, stenosis (anus, urethra, vagina), and local skin malignancy.

Diagnosis

- *Direct microscopy*: tissue smear or biopsy from lesion stained with Giemsa stain. Donovan bodies (bipolar, resembling 'closed safety-pins') within mononuclear leucocytes.
- *Histological examination*: Donovan bodies and chronic inflammatory picture.
- PCR and culture are not routinely available.

Management

- *Recommended*: oral azithromycin 1 g weekly or 500 mg od for 3 weeks, or until lesions healed completely.
- *Alternative*: oral co-trimoxazole 960 mg bd, doxycycline 100 mg bd, erythromycin 500 mg ×4 daily (all for 3 weeks or until lesions healed).
- *Pregnancy*: oral erythromycin 500 mg ×4 daily (minimum 3 weeks or until lesions healed) and Caesarean section if active cervical lesions (which may complicate delivery).
- *PN*: all sexual contacts in the last 6 months should have clinical examination for lesions.

Other genital infections

Other non-sexually transmitted infections (mostly tropical) which may affect the genitalia

- *Schistosomiasis (Schistosoma haematobium)*: from swimming in freshwater lakes in Africa (e.g. Lake Malawi). Usual urinary symptoms include dysuria and haematuria. Other features:
  - urethritis, lumpy semen, haematospermia
  - friable polyps and ulcers of cervix, vagina, and vulva; groin/scrotal cutanea tarda.
- *Bancroftian filariasis (E. Africa)*: spermatic cord inflammation (funiculitis), hydrocele, scrotal, and vulval elephantiasis.
- *Onchocerciasis (tropical Africa, Central and South America)*: itchy papules and nodules around genitalia similar to scabies.
- *Guinea worm infestation (dracunculiasis)*: remote parts of Africa, especially South Sudan; presents as a blister from which the worm's head protrudes. Usually affects lower limbs, but may involve the scrotum.
- *Amoebiasis (Entamoeba histolytica)*: especially Africa, Asia, Central and South America; peri-anal, cervical, and penile ulceration especially in MSM.
- *Leishmaniasis (Middle East, Indian subcontinent)*: genital ulceration and annular perigenital skin lesions.
- *Cutaneous larva migrans (Ancyclostoma caninum, dog hookworm), tropical and subtropical countries*: usually acquired from bare skin contact (e.g. nude sunbathing) with infected tropical beaches. Pruritic erythematous papules or tracts moving several millimetres a day may be seen affecting the glutei and genitalia.
- *Myiasis (Central and South America)*: infestation by the larvae of certain fly species, e.g. *Dermatobia hominis* (botfly); may rarely affect healthy external genital tissue, especially the scrotum. Presents as a nodular inflammatory lesion.

Further information

British Association for Sexual Health and HIV guidelines for Chancroid, Donovanosis and LGV ⬥ https://www.bashh.org/guidelines

Endemic treponematoses

Introduction 256
Yaws (framboesia, pian, buba) 257
Pinta 257
Endemic syphilis (bejel, dichuchwa) 258
Management of endemic treponematoses 258

Introduction

Important differential diagnosis of reactive syphilis serology in those coming from countries where such infections are found. Currently available tests cannot distinguish them easily from venereal syphilis. Molecular identification assays to distinguish between the different *Treponemal* species are not widely available. Identification of scars from old healed lesions may aid diagnosis. However, if there is doubt about the possibility of underlying syphilis or active non-venereal treponematosis, the patient should be fully treated for syphilis.

Endemic treponematoses share similarities in pathogenesis and natural history. All are transmitted by direct contact with infectious lesions and manifest in multiple stages involving the skin. All except pinta can progress to cause serious and destructive lesions of skin, bone, and cartilage. As in venereal syphilis, the clinical manifestations of endemic treponematoses are commonly divided into an early stage (encompassing primary and secondary) and a late stage. Early-stage lesions are highly infectious and can persist for weeks to months, or even years. Once the early manifestations spontaneously regress due to the host's immune responses, the patient enters a state of latency that, in many cases, lasts for life. In a relatively small percentage of cases, the infection may progress from latency to tertiary disease, characterized by destruction of tissues.

Endemic treponematoses are found in remote areas with limited healthcare and associated with poor hygiene. Worldwide prevalence ↓ by 95% between 1950 and 1970 with global control programmes, but changes in administration and delivery of these programmes resulted in re-emergence. In 2012, the World Health Organization (WHO) officially set a goal for yaws eradication by 2020.

Yaws (framboesia, pian, buba)

- *Causative organism: Treponema pertenue.*
- *Areas found*: warm humid tropical areas of Africa, South America, the Caribbean, Southeast Asia, and some Pacific islands.
- *Transmission*: direct contact with infectious lesions, especially in children. Spread by flies (*Hippelates pallipes*) has been suggested. Not vertically transmitted.
- *Clinical features*:
  - 1° proliferative papilloma, often ulcerating, at site of infection, after an incubation period of 10–45 days or longer. Usually heals after 3–6 months with a scar; found most commonly on legs.
  - 2° rashes and mucosal lesions similar to secondary syphilis. First crop may appear before primary lesion has healed, but take 1–2 years to develop. Often, multiple lesions, including macules, papules, nodules, hyperkeratosis, and ulcerations. Tender lymphadenitis may occur proximal to lesions. Lesions on the soles of the feet may become hyperkeratotic, cracked, discoloured, or secondarily infected. They can be very painful and result in a crab-like gait. Relapses common in first 5 years, but skin lesions heal without scarring. Painful (especially at night) osteoperiostitis with development of sabre tibia.
  - *Late*—gummatous skin lesions, hyperkeratosis, juxta-articular nodules, and nasal and palatal collapse from underlying tissue destruction (gangosa). No cardiovascular and neurological sequelae.

Pinta

- *Causative organism: Treponema carateum.*
- *Areas found*: warm semi arid areas of central and northern South America.
- *Transmission*: direct skin contact, especially in children. No vertical transmission.
- *Clinical features (only involves the skin)*:
  - 1°—initial papule that may form a plaque, especially affecting limbs, with local lymphadenopathy.
  - 2°—widespread coloured skin rashes and papules with generalized lymphadenopathy, sometimes persisting for years.
  - *Late*—patchy altered skin pigmentation (hyperpigmentation and leukoderma) with pruritus and skin atrophy. No neurological or cardiovascular involvement.

Endemic syphilis (bejel, dichuchwa)

- *Causative organism: Treponema endemicum.*
- *Areas found*: hot dry countries (e.g. Arabian Peninsula and Saharan/sub-Saharan Africa).
- *Transmission*: skin contact, the use of shared eating and drinking utensils, especially in children. No vertical transmission.
- *Clinical features*:
  - 1°—rarely seen (mucous patches in mouth most common site).
  - 2°—Mucocutaneous papules around mouth and genitalia, condylomata lata (may persist for years), painful osteoperiostitis.
  - *Late*—nasal and palate collapse because of underlying bone and cartilage destruction (gangosa), skin gummata, periostitis. No neurological or cardiovascular involvement.

Management of endemic treponematoses

Single dose IM benzathine benzylpenicillin 1.2 g (or 600 mg if <10 years old) is curative, although scars may remain. Azithromycin is equally effective. The WHO considers azithromycin (30 mg/kg, not to exceed 2 g) as the drug of first choice due ease of administration and low cost. Alternatives include doxycycline, other penicillins, cephalosporins, and macrolides. Contacts should be treated similarly.

Proctocolitis and enteric sexually acquired infections

Introduction 260
Sexually transmitted causes and clinical features 261
No infection demonstrable 263
Infections usually sexually transmitted 263
Infections not usually sexually transmitted 264

Introduction

Proctitis is inflammation of the rectal mucosa; proctocolitis is inflammation extending >15 cm into the sigmoid colon.

Related to penetrative anorectal intercourse and analingus. Rarely found in ♀, most arise in MSM. Proctitis increases transmission of HIV.

Sexually transmitted causes and clinical features

Symptoms

Symptoms depend on site. HSV and syphilis infect anal verge and perianal area, and may be painful. Chlamydia and gonorrhoea infect rectum and thus may be less painful (85% can be asymptomatic).

Proctitis

- *Rectal inflammation: Neisseria gonorrhoeae, Chlamydia trachomatis* genotypes (D-K and LGV genotypes), *Treponema pallidum,* HSV, syphilis, possibly *Mycoplasma genitalium* (limited evidence).
- *Acute:*
  - feeling of rectal fullness or incomplete defaecation, leading to urge to defecate (most common)
  - mucopurulent anal discharge
  - rectal bleeding
  - constipation
  - tenesmus.
- *Mild/chronic:*
  - mucus streaking of stool
  - constipation
  - feeling of incomplete defaecation (sometimes).

Acute proctocolitis

- *Shigella* spp., *Campylobacter* spp., *Salmonella* spp., *Entamoeba histolytica, Cryptosporidium* spp., CMV
- As with proctitis
- small-volume diarrhoea
- lower abdominal pain
- abdominal tenderness
- bloating
- rectal bleeding
- feeling of incomplete defaecation.

Enteritis

- *inflammation of the small intestine: Giardia duodenalis, Cryptosporidium* spp.
- large-volume watery diarrhoea
- mid-abdominal cramps
- bloating and flatulence
- nausea > vomiting
- malaise
- weight loss

Pruritus ani

- *Anal irritation: Enterobius vermicularis*
- *Anal itching,* especially at night

Signs
- *Distal proctitis* (i.e. distal 12–15 cm of the rectum):
  - mucopus in rectal lumen
  - loss of normal vascular pattern (although may not be evident in distal 10 cm of normal rectum)
  - mucosal oedema
  - contact bleeding
  - ulceration (sometimes)
  - inflammatory mass (sometimes, e.g. with syphilis and LGV).
- *Proctocolitis*: as for distal proctitis, but changes beyond rectosigmoid junction.
- *Enteritis*: normal rectal mucosa unless concurrent infection with organisms causing proctitis.

No infection demonstrable

- Acute anorectal symptoms related to peno-anal intercourse or the insertion of a fist, forearm, or foreign body. May lead to:
  - prolapsed haemorrhoids
  - fissures, ulcers, tears, and rectal perforation
  - retained foreign bodies.
- *Chronic symptoms* (non-specific proctitis): possibly related to recurrent trauma associated with rectal coitus and associated with an 8-fold ↑ in HIV infection.

Infections usually sexually transmitted

- *Neisseria gonorrhoeae* (⊃ Chapter 8, 'Clinical features', pp. 140–2).
- *Chlamydia trachomatis* (⊃ Chapter 9, 'Clinical features', pp. 152–3).
- *Treponema pallidum* (⊃ Chapter 7, 'Clinical features of acquired syphilis', pp. 120–2).
- HSV (⊃ Chapter 22, 'Clinical features', pp. 280–1).
- *Tropical STIs*: chancroid, LGV (current epidemics and endemic outbreaks in MSM in Western Europe and America), and granuloma inguinale (⊃ Chapter 18, 'Tropical genital and sexually acquired infections', pp. 245–53).
- HIV infection (⊃ Chapter 42, 'Enteric disease', pp. 495–500, and 'Anal disease', pp. 501–2).
- *Mycoplasma genitalium* (limited evidence for causative association; ⊃ Chapter 10, Box 10.1, p. 166).

Investigations

If altered bowel habits, take stool samples for culture and microscopy for ova, cysts, and parasites. Proctoscopy, swabs for *C. trachomatis* (including LGV), *N. gonorrhoeae*, +/− *M. genitalium*. Syphilis serology, HIV serology.

Empiric treatment

Consider empiric treatment of proctitis for *N. gonorrhoeae* and *C. trachomatis*.

Infections not usually sexually transmitted

Bacteria

Bacillary dysentery: Shigella spp. (usually S. sonnei and S. flexneri)

- *Usual spread*: hand to mouth, fomites, water, and food. Outbreaks reported in MSM.
- *Incubation period 2–7 days*: apyrexial; frequent loose stools usually resolving in a week. Occasionally, chronic proctocolitis develops. Reactive arthritis may complicate. Prepubertal ♀ may develop vaginitis, especially with *S. flexneri*.
- Diagnosed by stool culture.
- Treated conservatively with bed rest, fluid replacement, and anti-motility drugs if necessary. Unless severe or patient has AIDS, antibiotics should be avoided to ↓ risk of resistance, normally self-limiting. If required, drug choice informed by local antimicrobial resistance pattern.

Typhoid. Salmonella enterica serotype typhi

- *Usual spread*: food or water contaminated with faecal material, but clusters reported amongst MSM, considered to have been spread sexually. Non-*typhi* serotypes have not been recognized as sexually transmitted, despite their importance as a cause of bloodstream infection in those with HIV infection.
- Patient may be systemically unwell with fever.
- Diagnosed by stool culture and/or blood culture.
- Should be treated with antibiotics, depending on antimicrobial sensitivity.

Campylobacter infection: Campylobacter spp. (usually C. jejuni)

- *Usual spread*: contaminated water, food, and milk. In MSM sporadic case reports and higher rates in those with proctocolitis (compared with asymptomatic controls).
- *Incubation period up to 10 days*: sudden diarrhoea with abdominal pain, malaise, pyrexia, muscle, and joint pains. Usually resolves in 10 days. Reactive arthritis rarely.
- Diagnosed by stool culture and serology.
- No treatment unless severe; antibiotics guided by sensitivity pattern.

Helicobacter pylori infection

It has been suggested that *H. pylori* may be transmitted by the ingestion of infected vomit and regurgitated food during sexual contact, although there is no firm evidence.

Virus

Cytomegalovirus

Only in severely immunocompromised patients in the context of HIV infection with CD4 counts <100/mm^3.

Protozoa

Cryptosporidiosis: Cryptosporidium spp. (usually C. parvum)

- *Usual spread*: oral–faecal (in poor social conditions), by water or animal contact. Symptomatic disease more commonly associated with HIV infection, where outbreaks occur. Sporadic cases in immunocompetent MSM, associated with multiple contacts (especially at sex-on-premises venues) and anal sex.
- Offensive watery diarrhoea with abdominal pain, low-grade pyrexia, anorexia, and vomiting, which spontaneously resolves in 1–3 weeks.
- *Diagnosed by*:
  - detecting oocysts in faecal samples
  - jejunal, colonic, rectal biopsies showing various stages of the organism within enterocytes
  - cryptosporidial antigen detection using enzyme immuno-assay or direct immunofluorescence tests
  - PCR for cryptosporidium is developed.
- *Treatment*: no specific treatment, but anti-motility drugs as required. Where severe and intractable, particularly in HIV, nitazoxanide or paromomycin may be used.

Giardiasis: Giardia duodenalis

- *Usual spread*: water or food contaminated with faecal material. Sexual transmission recognized, especially in MSM.
- *Incubation period 1–14 days*: sudden onset of foul-smelling diarrhoea, abdominal pain, and distension. Stools float due to steatorrhoea with malabsorption contributing to weight loss. Symptoms resolve in 2–6 weeks and by 3 months in most.
- *Diagnosed by*:
  - microscopy of fluid stool samples for trophozoites and cysts, or solid samples for cysts—repeated examinations (at least 3) are often required
  - jejunal biopsy if clinical suspicion and negative stools
  - antigen detection tests (available and more sensitive than single-specimen microscopy, but at least two samples should be submitted).
- *Treatment*: oral metronidazole 2 g daily for 3 days, or 400 mg tid for 5 days or tinidazole 2 g orally as a single dose.

Amoebiasis: Entamoeba histolytica

- *Usual spread*: from faecally contaminated water and food (infecting about 10% of the world's population). The non-pathogenic strain, reclassified as *Entamoeba dispar*, is commonly found in faeces of MSM.
- >90% are asymptomatic. Symptoms include bloody diarrhoea, abdominal discomfort, weight loss, and fever with colitis in >20%. Invasive disease includes hepatic abscess and granulating ulceration around the anus and genitalia, but is rare in MSM.
- *Diagnosed by*:
  - detecting trophozoites on diarrhoeal stool samples, rectal exudate, or scrapings from rectal ulcers by microscopy as *E. histolytica* if trophozoites contain red blood cells
  - detecting cysts in diarrhoeal or formed stools by microscopy, differentiating between *E. histolytica* and the non-pathogenic *E. dispar* by PCR
  - serology (for invasive disease).

- *Treatment*:
  - oral metronidazole 800mg 3 times a day or tinidazole 2g daily, both for 5-8 days (for trophozoites)
  - simultaneous oral diloxanide furoate 500 mg tid for 10 days (to eliminate all bowel infection)
  - hepatic abscesses may require aspiration if large or close to liver capsule.

Nematodes

Threadworms: Enterobius vermicularis

- *Usual spread*: by food or fomites contaminated by ova (especially in children). Associated with analingus in MSM.
- Rarely causes vaginal infection in prepubertal girls. Cause pruritus ani (or vulvo-vaginitis in young girls).
- Diagnosed by seeing the adult worm in the anal canal or detecting ova from the peri-anal skin by microscopy using material collected on transparent adhesive tape.
- *Treatment*: oral mebendazole single 100 mg dose, or oral piperazine single 4 g dose repeated in 14 days. Neither treatment is advised in pregnancy.

Strongyloides stercoralis infection

Reports of detection in faeces of MSM STI clinic attenders (rarely sexually transmitted).

Urinary tract infection

Aetiology 268
Women 269
Men 272
Diagnostic tests 273
Management 275

Aetiology

Considerable geographical variation in cause, but predominant organism is *E. coli* in 80% of confirmed infections.

Other community-acquired organisms include:

- *Staphylococcus saprophyticus*: 10% overall, 15–30% of sexually active young ♀.
- *Proteus mirabilis*.
- Enterococci.
- *Klebsiella* and *Enterobacter* spp.

Bacterial factors

For the urinary tract to become infected, bacteria must gain entry to the tract, avoid being flushed away, adhere to the epithelial surface, and multiply.

Some strains develop uropathogenic properties, including adhesins (e.g. type 1 pili adhesive organelles), serum resistance, and cytotoxins (e.g. haemolysins). These are important in overcoming host resistance in uncomplicated UTIs, and uropathogenic bacteria have been shown to remain in the bladder epithelium for weeks.

Resistance

In England, non-susceptibility to amoxicillin of urinary *E. coli* isolates is so common that the empirical use of this antibiotic for the treatment of UTI is strongly discouraged. With regards to other antimicrobials, data from 2016 reports: 33% of urinary *E. coli* isolates test non-susceptible to trimethoprim; 16.4% test non-susceptible to co-amoxiclav, 10.5% test non-susceptible to ciprofloxacin, 9.6% test non-susceptible to cephalexin; 6.8% test non-susceptible to pivmecillinam and 2.5% test non-susceptible to nitrofurantoin. Resistance patterns vary significantly with geography. Before prescribing, check local sensitivity patterns and treatment guidelines (e.g. for co-amoxiclav, 24.9% of urinary *E. coli* isolates in Anglia and Essex test non-susceptible, compared with the national average of 16.4%.)

Women

- Common; 1/3 ♀ will have had a UTI by age 24 and 1/2 ♀ will be treated for a symptomatic UTI during their lifetime.
- Most UTIs in ♀ are not associated with a risk factor.

Risk factors for those with recurrent UTIs

- Maternal history of UTI.
- Use of spermicides (↑ risk ×2–3) often in ♀ using diaphragm for contraception.
- Shorter distance between urethra and anus, but on average only 0.2cm shorter than controls.
- Atrophic urethritis and vaginitis (post-menopausal).
- Abnormalities of urinary tract (e.g. in-dwelling catheter, anatomical abnormalities, previous urinary tract surgery).
- Incomplete bladder emptying.
- UTI before the age of 15 years.
- Sexual activity (coitus >4 times a month, new sexual partner during the past year). Relative odds of UTI increases by a factor of 60 during the 48 hours following intercourse.
- Diabetes mellitus.
- Pregnancy (pyelonephritis most common at end of 2nd trimester).

There is no consistent evidence that following factors are implicated:
- Voiding habits (e.g. pre- and post-coital micturition).
- Lifetime number of sexual partners.
- Sexually transmitted infections.
- Personal hygiene (e.g. wiping back to front, tampon use, douching, use of panty liners type of underwear).
- BV.

Clinical features

A definitive diagnosis of a UTI requires microbiological confirmation of bacteria in the urine. The clinical diagnosis of UTI in otherwise healthy, non-pregnant, non-catheterized adult ♀ aged <65 is, however, based primarily on symptoms and signs. Routine urine culture is not required to appropriately manage LUTI in these women. Culture is recommended if impaired renal function, an abnormal renal tract or immunosuppression.

Specific clinical scenarios

LUTI

LUTI = infection of the bladder. Dysuria, frequency (in particular nocturia), suprapubic tenderness, urgency, polyuria, haematuria. If symptoms severe or ≥3 present (and in the absence of vaginal discharge or irritation), empirical antibiotics are recommended. If dysuria and frequency are both present, then the probability of UTI is increased to >90%. If vaginal discharge is present, the probability reduces and STIs (e.g. *Chlamydia trachomatis, Neisseria gonorrhoeae,* HSV) and vulvo-vaginitis (e.g. *Candida* spp., *Trichomonas vaginalis,* vulval dermatitis, atrophy) should be explored as alternative diagnoses.

Near patient tests for LUTI

Urine turbidity and dipstick testing may be reserved to help guide treatment decisions in otherwise healthy women aged <65, presenting with mild, or 2 or fewer symptoms of a UTI (where the diagnosis is unclear). They are not recommended to inform a diagnosis in women with moderate/severe symptoms

Urine dipstick testing

- If positive for nitrite +/− leucocyte +/− blood [positive predictive value (PPV) 92% if all 3], UTI probable so treat.
- If negative nitrite and positive leucocyte, UTI or other diagnoses are equally likely; consider delayed antibiotics and urine culture.
- If negative for nitrites, leucocytes, and blood [negative predictive value (NPV) 76%], UTI is unlikely.

Upper UTI (UUTI)

UUTI = pyelonephritis. May be accompanied by bacteraemia, making it life threatening. Diagnosis is based on evidence of a UTI in a person with loin pain and/or a temperature >38°C. Always send a urine culture.

Asymptomatic bacteriuria

The count of bacteria in the urine exceeds the threshold for diagnosing infection, but there are no symptoms or signs of infection. Risk factors include sexual activity, comorbid diabetes, institutionalization, catheterization. Prevalence increases with age and non-pregnant women of any age should not routinely be treated with an antibiotic.

Pregnancy

2–9% Pregnant women are bacteriuric in first trimester (similar to age-matched non-pregnant women) 10–40% of these women develop UUTI in 2nd or 3rd trimester if untreated. Bacteriuria is also linked to preterm delivery. All pregnant women should be screened for bacteriuria with urine culture at their first antenatal visit. The presence of asymptomatic bacteriuria should be confirmed with a second urine culture and if present treated. All pregnant women presenting with symptoms of a UTI should have a urine sample sent for culture prior to consideration of empirical antibiotics.

Catheterized patients

Change catheter before starting antibiotics. Send urine for culture. Do not treat asymptomatic bacteriuria (all people with long-term in-dwelling catheters will have bacteriuria for this reason intermittent catheterization is preferred if appropriate and practical.)

Haematuria

Should not persist after infection has been treated. Urine should be sent for culture to confirm infection for anyone with symptoms of a UTI associated with macro or microscopic haematuria, but not to confirm the presence of blood (laboratory microscopy for red cells is less sensitive than dipstick.) If frank haematuria persists after UTI is treated, urological cancer should be excluded.

If there is persistent microscopic haematuria and aged >50 years; suspect urological cancer. If <50 years and proteinuria +/− ↑ creatinine; suspect renal disease. If <50 years with no proteinuria and creatinine normal; suspect non-malignant urological disease, e.g. renal calculi. (Overlap between these age groups and diagnoses should always be borne in mind, and an urgent referral to urology sought if suspicion of urological cancer)

Elderly patients

Typical features may be absent. The presence of one of—new costovertebral tenderness, rigors, new onset delirium or fever (>37.9°C or 1.5°C above baseline) suggests a UTI.

Other

Urethral syndrome

Cystitis symptoms, but no underlying infection on urine culture (occurs in ~25%). May be caused by *C. trachomatis*, low count bacterial urinary pathogens, vulvo-vaginal inflammation/atrophy, previous urogenital trauma (e.g. following obstetric procedures).

Interstitial cystitis

Frequency, urgency, suprapubic pain without a diagnosable cause. Bladder histology shows chronic inflammation, commonly with mast cell infiltration, which may progress to bladder contracture.

Drug-induced cystitis

Allopurinol, cyclophosphamide, danazol, tiaprofenic acid.

Threadworms

Urination causes discomfort outside of the bladder and urethra with perianal/perivaginal itch.

Men

- UTIs uncommon in ♂ <50 years old, but ↑ thereafter as a result of incomplete bladder emptying 2° to prostatism or catheterization.
- In younger ♂, possible underlying urological abnormality, but uncomplicated infection probably related to uropathogenic strains of *E. coli*. May present as an acute urethritis (purulent urethral discharge and dysuria). Differential diagnosis includes prostatitis, urethritis, epididymitis.
- *Risk factors include:*
  - calculi and other foreign bodies
  - non-circumcision (enhanced colonization of the glans and subpreputial sac by *E. coli*)
  - bacterial prostatitis, prostatic calcification
  - reflux nephropathy.
- Others that have been suggested include:
  - anal sex and urethral exposure to coliforms
  - sexual partner with vagina colonized by uropathogens.

All men presenting with symptoms of a UTI should have a urine sample sent for culture prior to empirical antibiotics.

At least 50% of men with recurrent UTI and >90% of men with febrile UTI have prostatic involvement. Complications can include prostatic abscess or chronic bacterial prostatitis; ➔ Chapter 12, 'Symptoms', p. 183).

Consider urology referral for men if they have symptoms of UUTI, fail to respond to appropriate antibiotics or have recurrent UTI.

Diagnostic tests

- *Urine appearance*: often turbid (cloudy), but this may be produced by amorphous phosphate crystals, which clear on acidification (addition of 5% acetic acid to an aliquot of the specimen). Persisting turbidity has 66.4% specificity and 90.4% sensitivity for predicting symptomatic bacteriuria. Small numbers of bacteria and white cells will not alter turbidity. A fishy-smelling urine is highly suggestive of infection, but is unusual.
- *Urine dipstick testing*:
  - *leucocyte esterase* (enzyme from neutrophil granules)—72–97% sensitivity and may be more accurate than microscopy as enzyme activity is retained after white cells have disintegrated
  - *nitrate reductase* (enzyme reducing nitrate to nitrite)—present in coliforms, but not other bacteria (e.g. *Staph. saprophyticus* and enterococci); sensitivity 35–85%, high specificity, when combined with leucocyte esterase, sensitivity ↑ to 70–100% with only small ↓ in specificity
  - *protein*—poor indicator of infection with high rate of false positives and negatives
  - *haemoglobin*—poor specificity and ascorbic acid may produce false negatives.
- *Laboratory culture* (midstream sample of urine): studies conducted in the 1950s remain the basis for interpreting urine culture results. Bacterial counts >= 10^5 cfu/mL are indicative of an infection and counts below this usually indicate contamination (for alternatives, see Box 21.1). Clinical context (symptoms, signs, risk factors), within which the specimen is being sent, specimen quality, the presence or absence of pyuria, and the organism isolated are all hugely relevant to the interpretation of a culture result.
- *Collection*: peri-urethral area should be cleaned, and then around 10 mL of urine collected mid-stream (without interrupting the urine flow to start or stop the collection) into a sterile container.
- *Containers*: transfer urine from any collecting vessel, to a sterile specimen bottle within 30 minutes of collection. If the bottle contains boric acid as a preservative fill to the marked line (low volume of urine can create a concentration of boric acid high enough to be bactericidal)
- *Storage*: refrigerate at 4°C while awaiting processing. Urine stored for 48 hours is suitable for culture. Urine preserved with boric acid may be stored for up to 96 hours.

Box 21.1 Pyuria with no or low bacterial counts

Consider the following:

- Prior antibiotics.
- Incorrect sampling (disinfectant contamination).
- Urine acidification or alkalinization.
- Bacterial infection not growing on standard medium (e.g. *C. trachomatis, N. gonorrhoeae, Mycobacterium tuberculosis*).
- Genital tract infection/inflammation (including prostatitis).
- Renal tract neoplasia.
- Foreign body (also important to consider in recurrent UTI):
  - *Indigenous*—calculi, penetration from GI tract into bladder (chicken/fish bones, swallowed needles and pins)
  - *iatrogenic*—catheterization, objects inserted into the lower urinary tract for sexual stimulation (more commonly ♂; reports include needles, screws, wire, pencils, pens, ink cartridges, insects, grasses, wood), and rarely into the bladder via the vagina
  - *invasive*—parasites (the parasitic catfish *Vandellia cirrhosa*, found in the River Amazon, is said to penetrate the urethra of bathers, especially if they urinate in the water, and cling to the urethral wall by spines from the gills and jaw).

Management

- Encourage fluids.
- Acute uncomplicated LUTI can be a self-limiting benign condition that usually resolves within a few days. In women with at least moderately severe symptoms the average number of days to symptom resolution; 3.32 for women treated with an antibiotic to which the pathogen is sensitive, 4.73 if the pathogen is resistant to the antibiotic chosen, 4.94 if no antibiotic given. Main complication of conservative management is ascending infection.
- Treat non-pregnant women of any age with acute LUTI with a 3 day course of a narrow spectrum antibiotic such as trimethoprim or nitrofurantoin. Choice should be informed by local resistance patterns. Nitrofurantoin should be used with particular caution in the elderly and is contraindicated in renal impairment and with concurrent use of alkalinizing agents. Broad spectrum antibiotics should be avoided as they increase the risk of *Clostridium difficile*, MRSA and resistant UTIs. Second line treatment (following treatment failure) should be guided by urine culture result.
- Treat non-pregnant women with symptoms or signs of acute UUTI with a course of ciprofloxacin (7 days) or co-amoxiclav (14 days). Where the organism is known to be sensitive; a 14 day course of trimethoprim can be used. Admission to hospital is recommended where there is no response to antibiotics within 24 hours or if severe systemic upset present.
- For pregnant women with asymptomatic bacteriuria or acute LUTI a 7 day course of treatment is normally sufficient, with a urine culture taken 7 days after completion of treatment as a test of cure. Antibiotic choice should be advised by local guidance and is a balance between potential drug toxicity and antimicrobial activity. Specific examples for consideration with individual antibiotics; amoxicillin (deemed safe but only if sensitivities known, high resistance), nitrofurantoin (not in late pregnancy; risk of haemolytic anaemia in neonate), trimethoprim (not if established folate deficiency, low dietary folate intake or those taking concurrent folate antagonists - ensure high dose folate supplements are given concurrently in the first trimester), cefalexin (safe but broad spectrum) Always inform the antenatal team if *Streptococcus agalactiae* is isolated. (➔ Chapter 32 'Group B β- haemolytic streptococci (GBS): *Streptococcus agalactiae*', pp. 374–5)
- Treat catheterized women with a 7 day course of antibiotics.
- Longer courses of antibiotics (5-10 days) may be advisable for women with complicated LUTI i.e. when one or more factors are present that predispose to persistent infection, recurrent infection or treatment failure e.g. impaired renal function, an abnormal urological tract, impaired immunity or a particularly virulent organism (e.g. *S. aureus*)
- Treat men with uncomplicated LUTI with a 7 day course of a narrow spectrum antibiotic. Treat men with LUTI and symptoms suggestive of prostatitis with a 4 week course of a quinolone. Quinolones have superior penetration of prostatic fluid, compared to nitrofurantoin or cephalosporins.

- For recurrent UTI options include:
  - Daily prophylactic low-dose antibiotic for 6–12 months e.g. trimethoprim 100mg, nitrofurantoin 50mg (not MR version). Weak evidence to support this.
  - Post-coital antibiotics (if related to intercourse) e.g. single-dose trimethoprim 100mg taken within 2 hours of intercourse
  - Standby short-course antibiotics
  - Cranberry juice is no longer recommended for the prevention of recurrent cystitis (although cranberry proanthocyanidins have been shown to reduce the adherence of *E.coli* to cultured bladder epithelial cells and vaginal epithelial cells, there is an inadequate evidence base to advocate this routinely)

Urology referral

Urgent referral if urological cancer is suspected. Consider routine referral if other concerns e.g. suspicion of an abnormality of the urological tract, immunocompromise, diabetes mellitus, poor response to preventative measures.

Anogenital herpes

Introduction 278
Aetiology 278
Terminology 278
Epidemiology and transmission 279
Clinical features 280
Diagnosis 282
Management: discussion and support 283
Management: treatment 284
Pregnancy and neonatal infection 286
Herpes and HIV 289

Introduction

'Herpes' is named from ancient Greek, 'to creep or crawl', with the typical spreading skin lesions described by Hippocrates.

Aetiology

HSV types 1 and 2 is a neurotropic virus, with a central DNA core with outer icosahedral capsid and enveloped in a lipid membrane derived from the host cell. There are two viral types—HSV-1 (most commonly affecting orolabial mucosa) and HSV-2 (usually transmitted by contact with infected genital mucosa sexually or at delivery). HSV is readily inactivated at room temperature and by drying; therefore, fomite and aerosol spread are unusual. Previous oral HSV-1 infection protects against genital HSV-1, but not HSV-2 disease, although it reduces severity of first episode genital herpes and makes asymptomatic seroconversion more likely.

Terminology

- 1° *infection*: first exposure to any HSV.
- *Initial infection*: 1st infection by HSV. Either 1° (~50%) or non-1°, if there has been exposure to other viral type, which may be detected serologically. Generally, ↓ severity if non-1°.
- *Latency*: dormant HSV in sensory (dorsal root) ganglia of nerves serving affected sites—sacral ganglia (S2–S5) for anogenital herpes (AGH).
- *Reactivation*: process unclear, but precipitating factors include local nerve stimulation (e.g. by trauma, ultraviolet light) and immunosuppression by other infections, such as HIV, drugs, and malignancy. Persistent stress implicated. Association with menstruation unclear.
- *Recurrence*: latent virus reactivates, causing peripheral lesions to appear.
- *Asymptomatic viral shedding*: reactivated HSV at nerve periphery without visible lesions. Viral shedding more common with HSV-2 (18–55%) than HSV-1 (10–29%). Most common in first 6 months after infection (during a mean 6% of days), diminishing thereafter, and falling by at least 66% after 10 years. Oral HSV-2 shedding is infrequent and usually asymptomatic.

Epidemiology and transmission

HSV-1 antibodies ↑ with age up to ~80%, more common in low socio-economic groups. ↑ Prevalence rate at adolescence suggests transmission by sexual contact. HSV-2 antibodies (usually indicating anogenital infection) appear at puberty and correlate with sexual activity, with a lifetime sero-prevalence rate of 10–80%, ↑ in ♀. Only 5–20% of those with HSV-2 antibodies recollect previous symptoms. Over the past 20 years, there has been a disproportionate ↑ in HSV-1 as a cause of initial AGH, especially in young ♀, now with up to 80% affected, but lower rates are found (35–45%) in ♂. HSV-2 sexual transmission rate between discordant couples is about 15–20% per year (↑ from ♀ to ♂). Transmission follows direct skin contact. In ♀ hormonal contraceptive use, BV, and high-density vaginal group B streptococcal infection have been reported as risk factors for genital HSV-2 shedding. Male circumcision may provide weak protection against HSV-2 infection.

Frequently asked questions

How have I caught it if my partner does not have symptoms?
It is possible to be infected with HSV without knowing. Two-thirds of people who contract the virus, catch it from someone who is asymptomatic. People who have recurrent symptoms may occasionally shed virus asymptomatically, as may those who have never had symptoms. Also commonly acquired from the lips through oral sex.

Can I catch herpes from a toilet seat?
HSV can only survive a short time away from the body. It may live for a short time on a wet towel and theoretically be passed on this way. It is not thought possible to catch herpes from a toilet seat.

How often will I get an attack?
Some people have no further episodes after their initial attack, a few get frequent recurrences (i.e. >6 episodes per year). With HSV-2 90% have a recurrence within the 1st year. The frequency of attacks is often related to the severity of the initial infection. Frequency of attacks tends to decrease after the 1st year. With HSV-1, 60% will have a recurrence in the 1st year, but only rarely after 1st year.

What brings on an attack?
A recurrence occurs when latent virus is reactivated, causing a peripheral lesion to appear. It is not clear why, but precipitating factors have been recognized. Local nerve stimulation (e.g. local trauma or UV light); immunosuppression (e.g. HIV, drugs, or malignancies); and persistent stress have been implicated. The association with menstruation is unclear.

Will all the attacks be this painful?
The first symptomatic attack of herpes is usually the worst. Subsequent attacks tend to be shorter and less painful. Patients are advised to use painkillers and salt baths. Urinating into a bath may be more comfortable, particularly ♀ with painful vulval/urethral sores.

Clinical features

Initial infection

~70% of new infections acquired from asymptomatic partners. 25% of those presenting with a first clinical HSV-2 episode have HSV-2 antibodies, indicating previous asymptomatic acquisition (pre-existing genital herpes). Over 60% of newly acquired HSV-2 infections are asymptomatic (↑ in ♂). In those with symptoms, 13% have atypical clinical features.

Incubation period is variable, but typically 3–14 days. Clinical features, and course of HSV-1 and HSV-2 AGH are similar, although severity of symptoms (systemic and local) and complications ↑ in ♀.

Constitutional symptoms occur within 1st week in >50% (fever, headache, malaise, and myalgia). Non-1° infections are less likely to have constitutional or severe symptoms.

Local symptoms include pain, irritation, regional tender lymphadenopathy, and vaginal/urethral discharge (~33% of ♂ with 1° HSV-2). Typically, vesicles appear over a local area of erythema and may become pustular before breaking down to form multiple tender ulcers, commonly with local oedema (Plate 11). Persists for 4–15 days before being followed by crusting (if keratinized skin) and re-epithelialization. New lesions during the episode occur in 75%, usually within first 10 days. Resolution time without treatment 17–20 days (unusually *up to* 6 weeks) and viral shedding time ~12 days.

Problems with micturition, including urine retention, more common in ♀ than in ♂. Cervicitis occurs in 70–90% (with HSV-2). ♂ may develop 2° phimosis.

Anal infection, usually related to anal sexual contact; if symptomatic, presents with pain, irritation, discharge, tenesmus, and sacral autonomic dysfunction. External peri anal lesions only seen in ~50%.

Extra-anogenital lesions occur around groin, buttocks, lips, fingers (whitlow), and eyes (keratoconjunctivitis), and by infecting eczematous skin (eczema herpeticum).

Complications

- Associated HSV pharyngitis (both HSV-1 and HSV-2). Occurs in ~10% with HSV-2 AGH.
- 2° Bacterial and yeast infection.
- Adhesions (especially labial in ♀).
- Aseptic meningitis (symptoms/signs of meningeal involvement in 36% ♀ and 13% ♂ with 1° HSV-2 AGH).
- *Sacral radiculopathy*: urinary retention, constipation, sacral anaesthesia (~1% with HSV-2 AGH).
- *Disseminated infection*: very rare, but more common in the immunosuppressed and pregnant.
- *Psychological*: including denial, anger, anxiety, loneliness, fear, poor self-image.
- HSV-2 infection associated with occurrence of bacterial vaginosis.

Recurrent infection

Following initial AGH:

- *HSV-2*: 90% of patients (↑ ♂) have recurrences in 1st year (median 0.33/month). Frequency of recurrences related to severity of initial infection. Significant reduction in second year and thereafter, though marked variability.
- *HSV-1*: 60% clinical recurrence in 1st year (median 0.11/month). Recurrences are unusual beyond 1st year.
- Factors that ↑ risk of symptomatic recurrences include severe initial episode, and immunodeficiency (e.g. HIV infection).

Signs and symptoms are confined to affected anogenital site. Prodrome (local skin tingling, sciatic nerve pain) occurs up to 48 hours before appearance of lesions in ~50%. Although symptomatic recurrences are more common in ♂, severity ↑ in ♀. Lesions similar to initial infection, but area of skin involvement one-tenth and re-epithelialization occurs in 6–10 days with viral shedding about 4 days. Cervical infection only found in 15–30% ♀.

Main complication is psychological, especially if recurrences are frequent, and include shame, frustration, depression, and withdrawal from social and sexual interaction.

Rarely erythema multiforme.

Recurrent rectal/peri-rectal herpes in men more likely to be HSV-1.

Atypical anogenital Herpes

Very common, especially when recurrent. May present as non-specific erythema, erosions, fissures, and even frenal tear.

Causes of anogenital ulceration

- Trauma.
- STIs:
  - anogenital herpes
  - 1° or 2° syphilis
  - chancroid
  - lymphogranuloma venereum
  - granuloma inguinale
- Herpes zoster.
- Aphthosis.
- Behçet's disease.
- *Drugs*: fixed drug eruptions; nicorandil—anal ulceration.
- Erythema multiforme.
- Pyoderma gangrenosum.
- Inflammatory bowel disease.
- Cicatricial pemphigoid.
- Lichen planus.
- Lichen sclerosis.
- Basal cell carcinoma.
- Squamous cell carcinoma.
- Melanoma.

Diagnosis

- Confirmation and typing should directly identify HSV-1 or HSV-2 virus from anogenital or rectal lesions.
- *Clinical presentation*: important for early initiation of treatment. However, sensitivity 40%, specificity 99%, and false-positive 20%.
- *Real time PCR*: swabs from lesions, including vesicle fluid. Preferred diagnostic method. Most sensitive method (detects 3–5 times more cases than culture), rapid, and highly specific. Other NAATS have shown similar results to PCR. In-house PCR tests must be appropriately validated.
- *Viral cell culture*: swabs from lesions including vesicle fluid (best source—sensitivity up to 90%, falling to 70% for ulcers, and 25% for crusted lesions). 1° lesions twice as likely to yield positive cultures than recurrences. Standard transport medium should be retained at 4°C, but systems not requiring refrigeration are commercially available. 30% ↓ sensitive compared with PCR testing.
- *Immunofluorescent antigen detection*: smears from lesions. Quick result, but ↓ sensitivity.
- *Antibodies*: usually appear within 2–3 weeks of infection.
  - Type specific serology can indicate infection with HSV 1 or 2 at some time in the past
  - IgM detection is unreliable and it is, therefore, not possible to say if the infection is recent. May be possible to demonstrate seroconversion (1° infection) with samples taken a few weeks apart
  - *Type-specific serology (Western blot)*—response may take 8–12 weeks to develop. Not widely available. Care with interpretation as HSV-1 and 2 are not site specific, and there is extensive cross-reactivity between the two antibodies. HSV-2 serology has sensitivity and specificity of 91–99% and 92–98%, respectively, which limits value in low prevalence populations.
- Type specific serology may be useful to identify recurrent genital ulcer disease of unknown aetiology, to investigate asymptomatic partners to aid counselling in discordant couples.
- *Cervical cytology (multinucleate giant cells)*: sensitivity ~60% compared with culture.

Management: discussion and support

For many patients, diagnosis of AGH infection and implications of recurrence can provoke severe emotions often fuelled by misinformation. Although chronic psychological morbidity may have an adverse effect, acute anxiety situations, and everyday stresses do not ↑ recurrences. Time spent discussing AGH and its implications is important in its management. Points to consider include accurate information on natural course of infection, recurrences (recognition of prodrome); management and implications of current episode and future recurrences, the avoidance of sexual contact until a week after the lesions disappear; in future recurrences, from the onset of the prodrome (to cover the period of highest risk of viral shedding), relevance of infection to current and potential future relationships, balanced consideration of potential to transmit infection, both with and without symptoms (understood by the patient and clearly documented), safe sex issues and condom information, and issues relating to pregnancy.

Information received initially may not be retained, so an information leaflet containing key points should be supplied.

Herpes Viruses Association (ℜ www.herpes.org.uk).

Frequently asked questions

Do I need to treat each attack?
Treatment of subsequent attacks has little influence on symptoms or duration. Symptomatic treatment is advised, e.g. saline baths and simple painkillers. Episodic treatment may be considered if someone has warning (prodromal) symptoms before an attack. Patients with symptomatic attacks >6 times a year may be offered suppressive treatment.

How do I tell a new partner that I have herpes?
Informing a new partner about having herpes is strongly encouraged, as there is a small risk of transmitting herpes even without lesions being present. Some people find it easier to practice safer sex and disclose when the relationship has strengthened.

Will I give it to a new partner?
Sexual transmission between discordant couples is about 10–15% a year. Risk of transmission is ↓ by avoiding sex when lesions are present, but asymptomatic shedding may occur with subsequent risk of transmission. Consistent condom use can ↓ transmission by 50%.

Should my partner be seen?
Your partner should be seen if they have symptoms, would like testing for other STIs or has questions about genital herpes.

Management: treatment

Initial anogenital herpes

General advice

- Saline washes to reduce risk of superinfection.
- Urinate in bath/use water jug to rinse to reduce dysuria in women.
- Drink plenty to keep urine dilute.
- *Analgesia*:
  - *oral*—e.g. codeine phosphate 30–60 mg 4–6 hourly as required
  - *topical*—e.g. 5% lidocaine ointment (do small test area initially)
  - rarely, hospital admission may be required for urinary retention (suprapubic catheterization), meningitis, or other severe symptoms.
- *Antiviral management*:
  - start within 5 days of onset or while new lesions are appearing
  - always use systemic treatment (usually oral)
  - 5 days treatment adequate unless new lesions still appearing
  - duration of symptoms ↓ by 50% and viral shedding ↓ by ~60%
  - antiviral treatment does not influence recurrence rate
  - intravenous therapy may occasionally be necessary if unable to swallow or frequent vomiting.
- *Oral antiviral drugs, all 5-day courses*:
  - aciclovir 400 mg tid (or 200 mg ×5 daily)
  - valaciclovir 500 mg bd
  - famciclovir 250 mg tid.

Recurrent anogenital herpes

Typically, mild and self-limiting. Unless unusually severe, antiviral treatment is of limited benefit in reducing duration and viral shedding. General advice and support are often adequate

Regular recurrences

Episodic treatment

May be considered for infrequent but regular recurrences. Treatment should be commenced as early as possible, ideally at prodrome, by providing the patient with medication in anticipation, to reduce duration by a median of 1–2 days. Treatment regimens are same as for initial herpes except that famciclovir is reduced to 125 mg bd. Short treatments have also shown to be effective, i.e. aciclovir 800 mg tid for 2 days, famciclovir 1g bd for 1 day, or valaciclovir 500 mg bd for 3 days. These treatments and regimens are all equivalent; however, the prodrugs (valaciclovir and famciclovir) allow bd dosing

Suppressive treatment

Usually considered for >6 recurrences a year. Provide continuous treatment for 6–12 months, then discontinue for reassessment. If recurrences resume at a high level, further suppressive treatment may be required. >90% have a significant reduction in recurrences (mean recurrence rates of 12.8/year pretreatment falling to 1.8 during treatment). ~20% experience a reduction in frequency of recurrences after completion. Daily suppressive treatment with valaciclovir has been shown to reduce HSV-2 transmission among HSV-2 discordant couples by 75% for clinical disease and reduced acquisition (measured by serology) by 48%.

- *Aciclovir*: 400 mg bd or 200 mg × 4 times daily.
- *Famciclovir*: 250 mg bd.
- *Valaciclovir*: 500 mg daily.
- If break through recurrences occur while taking suppressive treatment, the daily dose should be increased, e.g. aciclovir increased to 400 mg tid.
- Aciclovir been used >20 years no adverse effects; no monitoring recommended in previously well patients. Dose adjustment if severe renal disease.

Aciclovir resistance

Rarely found in immunocompetent patients, but reported in ~6% of those with immunosuppression, including HIV infection. Resistant strains can be treated with foscarnet and cidofovir.

Herbal treatment

Extract from the plant *Echinacea purpura* has been advocated in treatment of genital herpes, but a double-blind trial in recurrent AGH showed no significant benefit when compared with placebo.

Transmission prevention

- *Condoms*: laboratory experiments indicate that latex is impervious to HSV-2. Data on effectiveness is conflicting, with only some evidence of partial prevention from infected ♂ to their ♀ sex partners. Studies of HSV-2 serodiscordant couples or those with four sex partners support condom use, but other studies of sex workers, their clients, and male heterosexual attenders at GUM clinics recorded no evidence of protection. One study reported female condoms as effective as male condoms in preventing genital ulcer disease.
- *Antiviral drugs*: all ↓ asymptomatic shedding by 80–90% with small studies showing ↑ suppression with aciclovir (400 mg bd) and valaciclovir (1 g daily) compared with famciclovir. In serodiscordant couples suppressive valaciclovir has been shown to ↓ risk of acquiring symptomatic infection by 75%, although ~60 people require treatment to prevent one transmission.
- *Circumcision*: circumcised ♂ have 25% ↓ risk of HSV-2 infection and wives of circumcised ♂ have ↓ risk of genital ulcer disease (generally herpes).

Pregnancy and neonatal infection

Clinical aspects

- *Epidemiology*: incidence of new HSV-1 or HSV-2 infection during pregnancy ~2%, relatively evenly distributed by trimester. About 10% ♀ HSV-2 seronegative have seropositive partners.
- *Woman*: clinical course of AGH in pregnancy, similar to non-pregnant, with most new infections asymptomatic, except disseminated infection (visceral) more common with recurrences more frequent and severe. If ♀ have recurrent AGH, ~75% can expect one recurrence during pregnancy with ~14% having prodromal symptoms or clinical recurrence at delivery.
- *Pregnancy*: there is no evidence of increased risk of miscarriage with primary genital herpes in the first trimester. There is limited evidence showing increased risk of preterm labour and low birth weight in third trimester acquisition. There is no evidence that HSV acquired in pregnancy is associated with an increased incidence of congenital abnormalities Complications do not usually arise from recurrent herpes. Although the propensity for HSV-1 reactivation is substantially less, when it does occur during delivery it is much more likely to be transmitted to the neonate (relative risk ~60)
- *Neonate incidence of neonatal infection*: in UK 1.65/100,000 live births annually from 1986–91; USA estimated average incidence is 1/15,000 with ~30–50% due to HSV-1. 80% of infected infants born to mothers with no history of AGH. Maternal neutralizing antibodies protect neonate, so the highest risk of transmitting HSV is when acquisition occurs at or near labour. Risk of neonatal herpes with 1° AGH at term delivered vaginally from five studies is 41% falling to ~20% for initial HSV-2 infection with previous HSV-1 infection. Rate of neonatal transmission with maternal recurrent herpes is estimated at <1%. Transmission rate for ♀ with recurrent AGH and no visible lesions at delivery estimated to be 2/10,000. In 85% of cases, neonatal infection occurs at delivery, 10% post-partum (from family or carers), and only 5% antepartum.
- *Clinical features of neonatal herpes infection and natural course (without treatment)*: signs usually start towards end of the 1st week of life (up to 3 weeks) and infections classified as:
  - superficial (45%)—skin (vesicular) lesions (often protracted), conjunctivitis, and gingivostomatitis—low mortality
  - central nervous system (CNS) disease (30%)—4% mortality
  - disseminated (25%)—multi-organ especially CNS, liver, lung, and superficial sites—30% mortality.

Overall mortality has substantially ↓ in past 20 years but still ~20% of survivors have long-term neurological sequelae.

Diagnosis

- *Pregnancy*: as above. No value in taking serial swabs in late pregnancy from ♀ with recurrent herpes to detect viral shedding.
- *Infant*: if infection is suspected, or for babies born to ♀ with initial genital herpes test for HSV PCR—urine, stool, oropharyngeal, and conjunctival swabs, skin vesicle fluid.

Management

Consult local guidelines (which may vary).

Prevention

Avoid intercourse during partner's recurrences and during last 6 weeks of pregnancy. Advise about risk of acquiring HSV-1 through cunnilingus. Advise use of condoms during pregnancy and particularly in last trimester. Routine HSV screening of pregnant ♀ and routine ante-partum HSV swabs in those with a history of AGH are not recommended.

All women should have thorough inspection of vulva at time of delivery for herpetic lesions. Anyone with herpetic whitlows or oral herpetic lesions should be advised to have no direct contact with neonate.

Consider type-specific serology if:

- ♂ partner has herpes and ♀ has no history (suppressive antiviral treatment is an option if pregnant partner is discordant)
- first episode in pregnancy, especially in final trimester
- suggestive clinical features and negative PCR or culture
- HIV seropositivity.

Invasive procedures in labour should be avoided or minimized for ♀ with recurrent AGH.

Treatment

Aciclovir is well tolerated and has been shown to be safe in pregnancy (from Pregnancy Registry data up to 1999), but its use is not currently licensed. Therefore, although it is widely prescribed, this must be discussed with the patient and documented. Oral aciclovir should be prescribed as indicated for initial episodes, and IV aciclovir for severe genital or disseminated infection with case reports demonstrating significantly improved survival. It is rarely indicated for the treatment of recurrences during pregnancy. There are no documented adverse foetal effects because of medication exposure. There are insufficient data for the use of valaciclovir and famciclovir in pregnancy.

UK guidelines

First or second trimester acquisition

Treat with standard doses as for non-pregnant women: aciclovir 400 mg tid for 5 days followed by daily suppressive aciclovir treatment 400 mg tid from 36 weeks gestation until delivery. Treatment from 36 weeks gestation reduces HSV lesions at term and decreases asymptomatic viral shedding. A systematic review of suppressive aciclovir prescribed in pregnancy (after 36 weeks of gestation) demonstrated a 75% ↓ in recurrences at delivery and a 40% ↓ in Caesarean section rate for recurrent AGH. Viral detection at delivery was reduced by 90%, although shedding was not completely eliminated, and there were no cases of neonatal infection.

Third trimester acquisition

Treat with standard doses: aciclovir 400 mg tid until delivery.

Recurrent herpes

Advise that the risk of transmission is low even if lesions present at delivery (0–3% for vaginal delivery).

May only need symptomatic treatment, e.g. saline bathing and paracetamol for recurrences during pregnancy. Daily suppressive aciclovir 400 mg tid should be considered from 36 weeks gestation until delivery as may reduce shedding and recurrences at time of delivery. Discuss with women who have a history of herpes.

Primary lesions present at onset of labour

If primary lesions are present, the risk of transmission to the neonate is up to 41% with a vaginal delivery. Caesarean section is, therefore, routinely advised to all women with primary lesions at time of delivery or within 6 weeks of expected delivery date. If vaginal delivery is unavoidable, the mother and baby should be treated with aciclovir and invasive procedures, e.g. foetal scalp electrodes should be avoided.

Recurrent lesions present at onset of labour

Risk of transmission is 0–3% for vaginal delivery

Evidence from Netherlands indicates vaginal deliveries in presence of recurrent lesions were not associated with an ↑ neonatal HSV cases. However, in a large study of ♀ with recurrence at delivery, neonatal herpes occurred in 1.2% infants delivered by Caesarean section compared with 7.7% delivered vaginally. US guidance recommends Caesarean section if prodromal symptoms or active lesions at delivery.

Offer vaginal delivery to women with active recurrences at onset of labour. Can consider Caesarean section, but need to balance obstetric risks to mother against low risk of neonatal HSV transmission.

Caesarean section not advised for ♀ with history of AGH, but no active genital lesions at delivery.

Infant with HSV infection

IV aciclovir 20 mg/kg body weight 8-hourly for 10 days.

Frequently asked questions

Is herpes dangerous in pregnancy?

1° herpes in the last 6 weeks of pregnancy it is associated with ↑ risk of neonatal herpes, in which case the woman should be treated with aciclovir and delivered by Caesarean section. If ♀ has never had herpes, but her partner has, they should use condoms for intercourse throughout pregnancy. The ♂ partner can be offered suppressive treatment for the duration of the pregnancy to ↓ risk of a 1° attack of herpes in the ♀ in pregnancy. Recurrent attacks of herpes in pregnancy are treated as for non-pregnant ♀. There is now evidence that Caesarean section is not necessary for a non-1° attacks in pregnancy, even if the attack is in the last 6 weeks of pregnancy.

Herpes and HIV

- Strong association between HSV-2 and HIV infection, increasing transmission of both, with prevalent HSV-2 infection associated with a 3-fold risk of HIV acquisition among both ♂ and ♀.
- Atypical lesions if immunosuppressed, e.g. extensive persistent ulceration, herpes vegetans (proliferative, verrucous), hyperkeratotic lesions.
- Viral shedding ↑ with low cd4 counts.
- Enhanced antiviral treatment is recommended, especially if immunodeficient.
- *Initial*:
  - *aciclovir*—400 mg 5 times daily for 7–10 days
  - *valaciclovir*—500 mg to 1 g bd for 10 days
  - *famciclovir*—250–500 mg tid for 10 days.
- *Episodic*:
  - If no sign of immune failure use standard doses for 5 days.
  - If advanced disease double dose and use beyond 5 days:
    - — aciclovir 800 mg tid for 5–10 days
    - — famciclovir 250 mg bd for 5–10 days
    - — valaciclovir 1 g bd for 5–10 days.
- *Suppressive*:
  - *aciclovir*—400 mg 2 or 3 times daily
  - *valaciclovir*—500 mg bd
  - if above treatments do not control disease try doubling dose, and if still no control try famciclovir 500 mg bd.
- In pregnancy, ♀ are at increased risk of more frequent and severe AGH recurrences with increased replication of both viruses. Therefore, genital reactivation of HSV may increase the risk of perinatal transmission of both HIV and HSV. Women who are HIV +ve with a history of recurrent herpes should be offered suppressive aciclovir 400 mg tid from 32 weeks gestation to reduce risk of HIV transmission.
- Aciclovir resistance (>1–3 mg/L for inhibition). Found in 5–7% isolates from AGH lesions of those with HIV infection, usually due to thymidine kinase deficiency. Partially resistant strains may respond to high-dose IV antiviral treatment, but fully aciclovir-resistant strains are also resistant to valaciclovir and ganciclovir, and most are resistant to famciclovir. Alternative treatments demonstrating benefit:
  - *foscarnet*—1% cream; 40 mg/kg body weight IV every 8 hours until resolution
  - *cidofovir*—1% gel; 5 mg/kg body weight IV weekly infusion with oral probenecid until resolution.

Further information

British Association for Sexual Health and HIV Herpes guideline ℘ https://www.bashh.org/guidelines

Anogenital warts

Introduction 292
Aetiology 292
Epidemiology and natural history 293
Transmission 293
Clinical features 294
Diagnosis 295
Pregnancy and infection in neonate and children 296
Management 297
HPV and HIV 304

Introduction

References to anogenital warts date back to Roman and Hellenic periods, with Celsus observing, in the 1st century AD, that anal warts resulted from sexual intercourse.

Aetiology

HPV is in the family of papilloma viruses with a double-stranded DNA structure. It infects the mucosa of the anogenital tract, upper respiratory tract, and surface of the skin. The virion is 55 nm in diameter. The capsid (envelope) comprising 72 capsomeres has an icosahedral symmetry. Hybrid capture II and PCR are highly sensitive in detecting HPV.

HPV is classified by the nucleotide sequence of the major capsid gene *L1* into >100 types, which are identified by a number and are usually site specific (Table 23.1). Types frequently detected in anogenital squamous cell carcinomas (SCC) are described as oncogenic ('high risk') and the remainder as non-oncogenic ('low risk'). 'Low-risk' types HPV6 and HPV11 account for ~90% of anogenital warts; 'high-risk' HPV is found in >95% of cervical squamous cell carcinomas. 80–85% of anal carcinomas, 50% of penile carcinomas, 40–70% vulval and vaginal carcinomas, and 70% of oropharyngeal carcinomas. HPV 16 is most commonly implicated in high grade neoplasias. Infection begins in the basal stem cells of the epithelium. Active viral replication occurs in the well-differentiated layers near the surface. Virions are then released from desquamating cells.

Table 23.1 HPV types in lesions

Lesion	HPV types (more common types in bold)
Skin warts	**1, 2, 3**, 4, **7, 10**, 26, 28, 29, 41, 49, 57, 60, 63, 65
Anogenital warts	**6, 11**, 16, 40, 41, 42, 43, 44, 55, 61, 72, 73, 81
Squamous intra-epithelial lesions*	**6, 11, 16, 18**, 30, **31**, 33, 34, 35, **52**, 56, 57, 58, 59, 62, 64, 67, 68, 69, 70
Anogenital squamous cell carcinoma	**16, 18, 31, 33**, 35, 39, **45**, 51, **52**, 56, **58**, 59, 68
Oral warts	2, **6, 11, 16** (7, 13, 18, 32 in HIV +ve)
Laryngeal papilloma	**6, 11**
Head and neck carcinoma	**16**, 18, 33, 57

*Cervical, vaginal, vulval, anal, or penile intra-epithelial neoplasia.

Epidemiology and natural history

With the introduction from 2008 of national HPV vaccination for girls in the UK, the incidence rates of genital warts in ♀ and heterosexual ♂ aged 16–25 years has fallen steadily. However, genital warts remain one of the most common STIs and accounted for 16% of new diagnoses in GUM clinics in 2015. In MSM and unvaccinated heterosexuals genital tract HPV DNA is found in 10–40% of those aged 15–49 years. It is estimated that the majority of the sexually active population will have HPV infection at some time. However, <10% have clinically apparent lesions. The peak age of prevalence is 20–24 years in ♂ and 16–24 years in ♀. The infection rate ↑ in smokers (>5-fold).

The incubation period of genital warts is usually 3–8 months, but can be much longer. In the immunocompetent, 70% of warts regress within 1 year and 90% within 2 years. Immune response to E6 antigen leads to clearance, but E7 results in persistent or relapsing infection, which in high risk types may lead to development of squamous cell carcinoma. Following visible regression HPV may still be present, but in ~95% can no longer be detected 2 years after infection.

Transmission

Transmission is through contact with apparent or subclinical epithelial lesions and/or genital fluids containing infective virus, usually during sexual intercourse (including non-penetrative contact). Resultant micro-abrasions enable viral inoculation into the basal layers of the epithelium. Occasional reports of anogenital types at other sites (e.g. fingers) and non-anogenital types on anogenital skin suggest digital–genital transmission (including auto-inoculation). This may explain the absence of a history of genital–genital/anal or oro-genital–anal sexual contact reported in ~1% of ♀ with anogenital warts (no data available for ♂). The finding of oral, laryngeal, conjunctival, and nasal lesions in those with anogenital warts (~5%), with the same HPV type, suggests oro-genital transmission.

Mother-to-child transmission may occur during vaginal delivery, with a 10–70% rate of neonatal infection, and has also been reported following Caesarean section. In prepubertal children digital warts may be transmitted to anogenital regions, up to 20% of which may be due to skin types.

Clinical features

Symptoms

Usually little physical discomfort, but disfiguring lesions may lead to psychological distress. Peri-anal or large growths may cause irritation and soreness. Urethral, anal, and cervical warts may cause bleeding, and urethral warts may distort the urinary stream.

Signs

Plate 15.

Warts (usually multiple) appear most commonly at sites likely to be traumatized during sexual intercourse with HPV detectable in apparently normal surrounding skin. Peri-anal and anal warts (almost always below the pectinate line) may occur in both ♂ and ♀, more commonly, but not only with receptive anal sex. Warts may be found on the cervix, and in the vagina, anal canal, urethral meatus, with rare involvement of urethra and bladder (Table 23.2)

Lesions are either pedunculated or sessile and sometimes pigmented. They may be:

- *Condylomata acuminata*: soft/non-keratinized, 'cauliflower-like' in appearance, found on mucosae/warm moist non-hairy skin.
- *Keratinized*: resembling skin warts, usually on dry anogenital skin.
- Smooth papules on dry skin (e.g. penile shaft).

Subclinical infection may be detected as aceto-white patches with 5% acetic acid, better visualized through a colposcope (❶ low specificity). Atypical balanoposthitis/vulvitis may be associated with HPV 💣.

Giant condyloma of Buschke and Lowenstein

Usually associated with HPV6 and HPV11. Resembles a very large wart, but invades the dermis and underlying tissue (e.g. corpus cavernosum). Starts as a keratotic papule and grows into a large cauliflower-like lesion. Most commonly located on the glans penis, but may occur anywhere on the penis, scrotum, vulva, vagina, rectum, and bladder. Does not metastasize, but malignant transformation (verrucous carcinoma) develops in up to 50%. Diagnosed histologically. Liable to recur if not completely excised.

Table 23.2 Relative frequency (reported range) of location of genital warts

	% of cases (range)		% of cases (range)
Prepuce	**65** (49–80)	Posterior introitus	**73** (77–94)
Frenulum, corona and glans	**46** (22–70)	Labia, clitoris	32
Urethral meatus	**34** (24–45)	Cervix	**34** (6–64)
Penile shaft	**27** (16–55)	Vagina	**42** (32–52)
Scrotum	**23** (2–25)	Urethra	8
Peri-anal area	8 (3–15)	Perianal area	**18** (13–85)
		Perineum	23

Diagnosis

- Usually on clinical appearance.
- *Internal examination*:
  - speculum for vaginal/cervical warts
  - proctoscopy for anal warts if peri-anal lesions present
  - urethral meatoscopy (with an otoscope) if meatal warts.
- Biopsy under local anaesthetic if in doubt, or lesion atypical, or pigmented. This may be aided by the use of a colposcope.
- Routine DNA detection is unnecessary and is not cost effective.
- Differential diagnoses are outlined in Table 23.3.

Table 23.3 Differential diagnosis of external anogenital warts

Achrocordon (skin tag)	Molluscum contagiosum
Epidermal/melanocytic naevi	Condylomata lata (secondary syphilis)
Sebaceous glands	Seborrhoeic keratosis
Penile pearly papules	Dermatofibroma
Vulval papillae	Angiokeratoma
Ectopic sebaceous glands (Fordyce spots)	Epidermal cyst
Prominent hair follicles	Lichen planus
Nabothian follicles (cervix)	Psoriasis
	Penile/anal intra-epithelial neoplasia
	Giant condyloma of Buschke and Lowenstein
	Squamous cell carcinoma
	Basal cell carcinoma

Pregnancy and infection in the neonate and children

Warts may rapidly enlarge with pronounced vascularity during pregnancy (probably as a result of altered immunocompetence or ↑ oestrogen/progesterone) and regress in the puerperium, often with complete resolution. Warts do not usually obstruct vaginal delivery.

Neonatal infection commonly clears within 6 weeks. Persistence is usually subclinical, but may lead to recurrent respiratory papillomatosis, or ano- or extra-genital warts. Recurrent respiratory papillomatosis incidence is 0.25% in children (3 months–5 years of age) born to mothers with warts. Mainly caused by HPV6 and HPV11. Usually located on the vocal cords and epiglottis (laryngeal papillomas), rarely on the entire larynx, tracheobronchial tree, or even the lungs.

Perinatal infection is the usual cause of anogenital warts in children up to 3 years of age. However, sexual abuse and non-sexual transmission should be considered in older children.

Management

General principles

The aim of treatment is essentially cosmetic or for symptomatic relief. Systematic reviews of RCTs of all treatment modalities show a lack of high quality comparative studies. No method can be recommended as superior to another. Therapy aims to reduce visible warts, but does not necessarily effect eradication of HPV or reduce infectivity. Diagnosis of subclinical infection is of no practical benefit. In immunocompetent adults 40% warts resolve spontaneously within 4 months Treatment options, therefore, include no treatment at all.

Frequently asked questions

How have I caught them?

Genital warts are usually sexually transmitted by direct skin-to-skin contact. It is thought that ~90% of people who are infected with HPV have no visible warts. After infection, it takes a mean of 3 months for warts to develop, but may extend to months or years.

Will they go on their own?

Warts left untreated may disappear on their own (usually within 18 months), but they can also grow and spread, becoming unsightly and more difficult to treat.

Will I ever get rid of them?

When warts are treated they should clear, but HPV may persist, depending on the host's immunological response. Therefore, the patient should be warned that they may recur. Recurrences are more likely within 3 months of treatment. HPV usually clears within 24 months, although this may be longer, especially if the patient is immunocompromised.

Am I infectious?

Someone infected with HPV is infectious until it clears. The level of infection is probably greater when warts are present as viral shedding is likely to be greater.

Can I have sex?

It is recommended that if visible warts are present condoms should be used during sex—they do not completely prevent transmission of HPV, but do reduce the risk. Friction associated with coitus may spread warts. However, it is likely that the regular partner of someone who has warts will also be infected with the wart virus, whether they have visible warts or not.

Do warts cause cervical cancer?

There are many strains of HPV, but those causing genital warts are different from the types associated with cervical cancer. It is recommended that a ♀ attends for routine smear tests that will detect abnormalities associated with the HPV strains that may be related to cervical cancer. ♀ with warts do not need extra smears.

My partner does not have warts. Does he/she need to be seen?

Only if there are concerns about possible warts or other STIs.

The use of a clinical algorithm to direct treatment choice improves treatment outcome (Figs 23.1 and 23.2).

Treatment choice should encompass patient preference.

▶ Risk of scarring and pigment changes should be discussed before treatment.

Serial documentation of the number, size, appearance, and distribution of warts in genital maps gives a visual record of treatment response. If the wart area is >4 cm² treatment under direct supervision of clinical staff is recommended.

Consistent use of condoms reduces the acquisition of HPV infection and genital warts by 30–60%, and may also reduce the time to resolution of visible warts, when both partners are infected. Smoking cessation should be encouraged.

Psychological distress may require referral for counselling. The possibility of a long incubation period should be discussed, especially if there are concerns about infidelity.

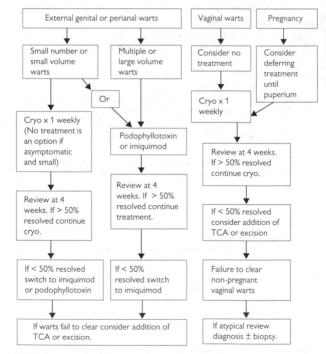

Fig 23.1 Treatment algorithm for genital warts in women

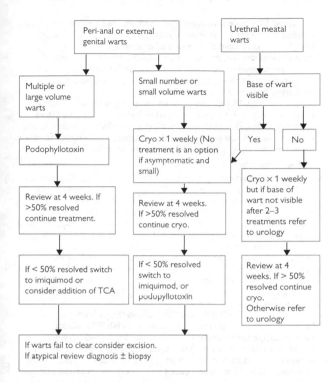

Fig 23.2 Treatment algorithm for genital warts in men

Scissor excision and electrosurgery have the best chance of complete clearance at first visit (approaching 100%) Clearance rates for other modalities vary and are roughly equivalent. Most warts respond to treatment within 3 months Recurrence following clearance with all therapies, particularly in the first 3 months is common. All methods may cause local skin inflammation, irritation, ulceration, and pain.

Specific treatments

Home-based therapies

- *Podophyllotoxin*: the active lignan ingredient of podophyllin resin and an antimitotic agent cause local tissue necrosis. Available as 0.5% solution or 0.15% cream. Should be applied bd for 3 consecutive days, repeated at weekly intervals for a total of up to 4–5 three-day treatments. Cream may be easier to apply. Repeat cycles, although not licensed, may be considered if warts are responding.

- *Imiquimod 5% cream*: stimulates innate and acquired immune responses. Applied ×3 a week on alternate nights and washed off 10–16 hours later, for up to 16 weeks. Generally takes longer to work than podophyllotoxin. Treatment may be extended beyond 16 weeks if warts are responding. Although some clinical trials have suggested a lower recurrence rate following treatment with imiquimod this is not supported by large comparative RCTs.
- *Sinecatechins 10–15% extract of green tea leaf* from *Camellia sinensis*. Catephen®10% ointment was licenced in the UK in 2015. The active ingredient is epigallocatechingallate. Mechanism of action is unclear and comparative trails are lacking, but efficacy appears to be similar to other topical modalities. It is applied ×3 a week for up to 16 weeks.

Clinic-based therapies
- *Cryotherapy*: liquid nitrogen spray (–180°C), swab (–20°C) or probe (–196°C), nitrous oxide probe (–75°C), or carbon dioxide snow (–79°C) may be used to freeze (for ~20–30 seconds) the wart(s) and a margin ('halo') of 1–3 mm of surrounding epithelium. The depth of freezing achieved is variable and operator-dependent. Local anaesthetic is not usually needed, but may be required depending on pain tolerance and extent of warts. Adequate cryotherapy causes immediate erythema followed in a few hours by blistering due to cytolysis of the epithelial cells. Healing takes 7–10 days with minimal scarring. If the treated area is large, severe ulceration may occur causing wound-care problems and scarring. Cryotherapy may be repeated at 1–2-week intervals.
- *Trichloroacetic acid (TCA)*: caustic agent causes chemical coagulation leading to necrosis. Applied once a week as an 80–90% solution (unlicensed), ensuring protection of surrounding epithelium with petroleum jelly. A neutralizing agent, e.g. sodium bicarbonate should be available. May be combined with cryotherapy and can be used in most anatomical sites. Treatment-induced pain, ulceration, irritation, and scarring limit its use. Not recommended for large volume warts.
- *Electrosurgery*: tissue destruction by electrically produced heat. Common methods include:
  - *electrocautery*—application of heat to warts and surrounding tissue under local anaesthesia
  - *hyfrecation*—high-frequency (0.5–3 MHz) low-power (1–30 W) electricity heats the tissue causing necrosis. Patient return electrode ('diathermy pad') is not needed since low power is used. Two techniques are used—electrofulguration (current sparks across an air gap) and electrodessication (electrode in contact with or penetrating warts). Requires local anaesthesia.
  - *surgical diathermy*—high-frequency (0.5–3 MHz) high-power (up to 400 W) electricity (requiring 'diathermy pad') to produce coagulation or cutting. More suitable for large warts. Requires general anaesthesia.
- *Excision*: using scalpel, curette, or scissors under local anaesthesia. Haemostasis can be achieved with electrosurgery or paste (e.g. ferric subsulfate–Monsels solution). Very effective and probably under-used treatment option.

- *Laser therapy*: vaporization of warts under local or general anaesthesia using CO_2 or diode laser. Particularly useful for treating warts in anatomically difficult sites, such as urethral meatus and anal canal. Also useful for large volume warts.
- *5-Fluorouracil 5% cream*: pyrimidine analogue inhibiting RNA/DNA synthesis. Associated with severe local reactions, including chronic neovascularization and vulval burning. It may also be teratogenic and is not recommended for routine management.
- *Interferons*: various regimens have been described using interferon α, β, or γ, as intralesional or systemic injection. Local use seems to be more effective than systemic. Use is limited by a variable response rate, systemic side-effects, and expense. Cyclical low-dose intralesional injections used as an adjunct to laser therapy have been reported to reduce relapse rate, although further research is required and interferons are not recommended for routine management.
- *Podophyllin resin 15–25%*: no longer a recommended treatment. It is less effective than podophyllotoxin and has a worse side effect profile.

Combination therapy

The use of clinic-based cryotherapy with home-based podophylotoxin or imiquimod is sometimes used. There is little evidence to support this. It may result in more rapid initial clearance of warts, but has not been shown to be superior with regards to long-term clearance rates.

Management: sexual partners

Current sexual partner(s) may benefit from assessment for undetected genital warts and other STIs, and there may be a need for explanation and advice about disease process.

Special situations

- *Pregnancy*: women with sub-clinical infection may develop warts in pregnancy. ↓ in wart volume at delivery is desirable to reduce the level of exposure of the neonate to HPV. However, eradication is difficult, due to the reduced immune response, and treatment may not be the best management option. Cryotherapy, TCA, excision, electrocautery, and laser vaporization are suitable options. Caesarean section is not indicated to prevent vertical transmission. Recurrent respiratory papillomatosis in the infant is a rare complication of maternal HPV infection. Very rarely Caesarean section may be indicated because of obstruction.
- ❶ Podophyllotoxin and 5-fluorouracil are contraindicated because of possible teratogenic effects. Imiquimod is not licensed for use in pregnancy as no safety data is available.
- *Vagina*: treatment may not be necessary, especially if warts are small or asymptomatic. Cryotherapy is the usual first-line therapy. Electrosurgery, TCA, podophyllotoxin (not licensed for internal use, total area treated <2 cm^2 weekly), or gynaecological referral are other options.

- *Cervix*:
  - Routine colposcopy in women with cervical warts is not recommended. If there is diagnostic uncertainty however colposcopy ± biopsy in women of any age is indicated to exclude cervical intra-epithelial neoplasia (CIN). Cryotherapy, electrosurgery, TCA, laser ablation or excision are options if required (no treatment is also an option).
  - *Cytology*—no changes to routine screening intervals necessary.
- *Urethral meatus*: if base of lesions seen, preferred treatment is cryotherapy or electrosurgery. Other options are podophyllotoxin or imiquimod, but use with caution. Deeper lesions require surgical ablation under direct vision.
- *Anal canal*: surgical excision or laser preferred. If small and accessible—cryotherapy, TCA, electrosurgery.
- *Immunosuppressed patients*: poor treatment response, ↑ relapse, and dysplasia more likely with ↓ cell-mediated immunity, e.g. following renal transplant or HIV infection. Careful follow-up required.

Vaccine

Virus-like particle (VLP), the capsid without dna, is immunogenic but non-infectious. Three vaccines using VLP to induce immunity have been shown by trials to be effective. Gardasil® is a quadrivalent vaccine licensed for use in ♂ and ♀ from age 9. It is 99% effective in preventing infection from HPV 6, 11, 16, and 18. It has been used in the UK since 2012 as part of the National HPV Immunization Programme for girls. In 2018 this was extended to include boys aged 12–13 years and MSM up to and including 45 years of age. Cervarix® is a bivalent vaccine providing protection against HPV 16 and

---

Frequently asked questions

Can I treat warts myself?

It is advisable not to treat warts at home with over-the-counter preparations. These preparations are designed for use on hands or feet, and may damage genital skin.

There are special prescription-only preparations (podophyllotoxin and imiquimod) for home use, although the treatments recommended depend on the position, number, and appearance of the warts.

Can I pass them to my children?

The HPV types that usually cause genital infection almost exclusively favour this site and so are sexually transmitted. However, occasionally, other types, such as those causing warts on the hands, can be spread to the genitals and have been found in children.

I am pregnant. Are the warts harmful to my baby?

Warts are common in pregnancy, often grow more quickly, and are more difficult to manage as certain treatments cannot be used. They often resolve spontaneously after the pregnancy is over. Although HPV can be transmitted to babies at delivery it is unusual. Treating the warts will not remove the underlying infection.

18 and was used in the UK vaccination programme 2008–2012. Gardasil9®
provides protection against HPV 6, 11, 16, 18, 31, 35, 45, 52, and 58, and
received a licence in Europe in 2015. In countries where the quadrivalent
vaccine has been used there have been large reductions in the rate of genital
wart diagnoses in the vaccinated population. In the UK, rates of first diagnosis of genital warts in 15–19-year-old females dropped by 38.9% between
2009 and 2015. Reductions were greatest among 15-year-old girls (83.2%)
who were largely offered Gardasil®. A reduction of 30.2% was also seen
in 15–19-year-old heterosexual males, illustrating herd immunity. Cervarix®
and, to a lesser degree, Gardasil® provide some cross-protection against
HPV types 31, 33, 45, and 58 (92%, 52%, 100%, and 65% with Cervarix®).
All 3 vaccines are licensed for the protection of individuals against genital
infection and associated disease related to HPV vaccine types. None of
the vaccines are licensed for treatment of existing HPV infection or HPV-
related disease. Studies to assess the effect of the vaccines in those already
sexually active or HPV-infected are being conducted. Following Gardasil®
vaccination, a retrospective pooled analysis of women with previously
treated warts showed disease recurrence. There is also evidence of regression of cervical intra-epithelial neoplasia (CIN)-related disease in young
vaccinated ♀.

HPV and HIV

- HPV infection has not been associated with ↑ risk of HIV acquisition.
- Those with HIV infection appear to be at greater risk of acquiring or reactivating HPV.
- Oral warts (due to HPV types 7, 13, 18, and 32) are more common in those with HIV infection.
- Duration and natural history of concurrent HPV infection may be altered, leading to ↑ incidence of cervical and anal neoplasia.

Futher information

British Association for Sexual Health and HIV guideline on Anogenital warts ℘ https://www.bashh.org/guidelines

Molluscum contagiosum

Introduction 306
Aetiology and epidemiology 306
Clinical features 306
Diagnosis 307
Management 307
HIV infection 308

Introduction

First described in 1817. Viral origin discovered by Juliusburg in 1907.

Aetiology and epidemiology

Benign skin eruption caused by replication of the large DNA virus Molluscum contagiosum virus (MCV) in epithelial cells. Family Poxviridae, genus Molluscipox; the 4 subtypes MCV 1–4 are clinically the same. MCV-1 is the commonest, MCV-2 commoner in the immunocompromised, and MCV3 and 4 rare.

Worldwide, more common in warm climates. Equal sex distribution. Transmitted by direct skin-to-skin contact. Microscopic abrasions and a warm moist environment facilitate transmission. Prone to koebnerization. The period of infectivity and viral shedding is thought to be equal to the duration of lesions.

Transmission can be by routine physical contact, commonly seen in:
• pre-adolescent children (90% attending GP are aged <15 years)
• individuals with impaired cellular immunity
• sports involving skin-to-skin contact
• those using gyms, swimming pools, and saunas (including fomites, e.g. shared towels).

If sexually acquired, lesions are often around the anogenital area in:
• sexually active adults aged 20–29 years
• those with a history or presence of other STIs
• those whose partner has molluscum contagiosum.

There are no documented cases of maternal–foetal transmission.

Clinical features

Incubation period usually 2–12 weeks, up to 6 months. Smooth pearly umbilicated lesions (Plate 16), growing over several weeks to a diameter of 2–6 mm, occasionally larger. In adults, when sexually acquired, found in pubic region, thighs, buttocks, lower abdomen, and less commonly, external genitalia sparing mucous membranes. Usually, 1–30 lesions unless immunosuppressed. May appear during pregnancy and generally resolve after delivery. Typically, asymptomatic, but may cause pruritus. 10% develop dermatitis around lesions. Auto-inoculation can occur through excoriation. In children, lesions are characteristic on face, upper limbs, and trunk, but 10–50% have genital lesions.

Spontaneous resolution within 2–3 months is common, but recurrences occur in 15–35% over 8–24 months.

Diagnosis

Diagnosis is by characteristic appearance of lesions. Atypical lesions may require biopsy. Histology shows enlarged epithelial cells with intra-cytoplasmic molluscum bodies. Molecular diagnostic methods are available, but not used in clinical practice.

Management

Advice regarding auto-inoculation, avoid shaving/waxing, avoid sharing towels. Squeezing can cause superinfection, and viral spread. Cover lesions when swimming, etc. A full STI screen is recommended in those presenting with genital lesions, at least an HIV test in those with facial lesions.

No treatment is advised for immunocompetent patients, as spontaneous resolution with no long-term sequelae is usual. Patients seeking treatment must consider the possible risk of post-treatment scarring. Some treatments may shorten disease course, but data on efficacy is limited. Options include:
- cryotherapy, curettage, electrocautery
- podophyllotoxin 0.5%
- imiquimod cream 5%.

Partner notification
- Unnecessary. No evidence that treating partner prevents re-infection.

Frequently asked questions

Where have I caught it?
Molluscum contagiosum is a viral infection spread by skin-to-skin contact. If lesions appear around the genitals has probably been sexually transmitted.

How long has the infection has been there and how long will the lesions stay?
Lesions usually appear after an incubation period of 3–12 weeks, although this can be longer, and usually disappear spontaneously within 2–3 months. Clearance depends on the body mounting a suitable immunological response against the causative poxvirus.

Does it need treating?
As molluscum resolves spontaneously, treatment is offered for cosmetic purposes only. Generally, people with genital lesions want them cleared up as soon as possible.

Can it be treated?
The usual treatment is by cryotherapy, but curettage, diathermy, and piercing with an orange stick followed by application of iodine or phenol have also been used. There are limited data on podophyllotoxin cream and imiquimod cream (currently unlicensed).

Will it recur?
33% of people will experience recurrences over the next 1–2 years.

HIV infection

Molluscum contagiosum is found in up to 20% of those with HIV. Lesions may become widespread in those with low CD4 counts, and often affect the face. Atypical hypertrophic lesions may be seen. Use of ART may lead to resolution of lesions, but conversely, may present following an immune reconstitution inflammatory syndrome (IRIS) (➔ Chapter 55, 'Immune reconstitution', p. 642). Topical cidofovir or IV cidofovir for extensive recalcitrant molluscum have been tried for non-genital lesions, but trial data available. Differential diagnosis for umbilicated lesions in immunocompromised patients includes cutaneous cryptococcal infection.

Further information

British Association for Sexual Health and HIV Molluscum contagiosum guideline ℜ https://www.bashh.org/guidelines

Sexually acquired viral hepatitis

Introduction *310*
Hepatitis A virus (HAV) infection *311*
Hepatitis B virus (HBV) infection *313*
Hepatitis C virus (HCV) infection *318*

Introduction

Viral hepatitis is responsible for over 1.34 million deaths worldwide; this is comparable to the number of deaths caused by HIV and TB. The majority of deaths arise from chronic infection with HCV or HBV, leading to end-stage liver disease or hepatocellular carcinoma.

The risk of sexual transmission of viruses causing hepatitis is very variable. In general, transmission is more likely through anal sex, traumatic sex, or with concommitent STI. Many of the viruses involved may cause little or no symptoms during seroconversion.

Hepatitis A virus (HAV) infection

Aetiology

A highly infectious RNA picornavirus. Identified in 1972, but condition had been known for a long time as epidemic jaundice, yellow jaundice, or infectious hepatitis.

Epidemiology and transmission

Humans are the only known natural reservoir. Common in developing countries (poor sanitation) and with close personal contact. 1.4 million symptomatic cases/year. Seroprevalence in USA and western Europe 10–33% (90% in developing world). Transmission usually faeco-oral (contaminated food/water). Associated with urine contamination and contact with infected urine (e.g. urophilia). Most commonly affects children, but outbreaks reported in MSM (faecal contact), people who inject drugs (PWIDs), and institutions. Patients are infectious for 2 weeks before and 1 week after the onset of jaundice. After infection, immunity is life-long.

Clinical features

Incubation period

Usually 2–6 weeks.

Symptoms

Most children and up to 50% of all adults are either asymptomatic or have mild non specific symptoms with no obvious jaundice. An icteric illness with jaundice, anorexia, nausea, diarrhoea and fatigue usually lasting 1–3 weeks (up to 12 weeks) is preceded by prodromal, flu-like symptoms (malaise, myalgia, fatigue, nausea) often with right upper abdominal pain lasting 3–10 days. Pyrexia usually disappears at the beginning of the icteric phase with symptomatic improvement at onset of jaundice.

Signs

Jaundice (hepatic and/or homeostatic), often with pale stools and dark urine. Liver tenderness and dehydration may occur.

Complications

Fulminant hepatitis in 0.4% (more common in those with hepatitis C). Up to 15% of symptomatic patients may require hospitalization with 25% having severe hepatitis. HAV-associated mortality very low (<0.2%). Chronic infection does not usually occur.

HAV in pregnancy

Associated with ↑ rate of premature labour and miscarriage proportional to severity of illness. Vertical transmission rarely reported.

Diagnosis and investigations

- *HAV-IgM*: positive within 5 days of illness (up to 6 months).
- *HAV-IgG*: indicates past exposure or response to vaccination.
- Alanine aminotransferase (ALT)/aspartate aminotransferase (AST) and bilirubin can ↑ to 10,000 IU/L and 500 µmol/L, respectively.
- Alkaline phosphatase (ALP) ↑ modestly, but higher with cholestasis.

- Prothrombin time prolongation of >5 seconds suggests decompensation.
- Screen for other hepatotropic infections and STIs if appropriate.

Management

Provision of information and advice (avoid alcohol, food handling, and unprotected sexual intercourse until non-infectious). Most cases managed on an outpatient basis. Follow-up only necessary for patients whose ALT or bilirubin does not settle within 4–8 weeks.

HAV infection is a notifiable disease with contacts requiring follow-up by public health authorities including PN for sexual partners. Human normal immunoglobulin (HNIG) or early HAV vaccine may be considered for non-immune close contacts including neonates. Breastfeeding can be continued.

Vaccination

Active vaccination recommended for travellers to endemic countries, and in outbreak situations (e.g. amongst MSM), chronic liver disease, PWIDs, and those with HIV infection.

Schedule: 2 doses at 0 and 6–12 months giving 95% protection for 5–10 years. Vaccination provides protection for up to 25 years. Combination vaccine with hepatitis B follows same schedule as hepatitis B vaccination. HAV vaccine response may be lower in HIV or immunocompromised patients.

Hepatitis B virus (HBV) infection

Hepatitis B Virus

Hepatitis B (HBV) was initially known as the Australia antigen, the virus was discovered in 1965 by Dr Blumberg and colleagues. HBV is a hepadnavirus and is a small partially double-stranded DNA virus. Structurally, a lipoprotein coat containing HBV surface antigen (HBsAg) surrounds a nucleocapsid made up of hepatitis B core antigen within which the HBV genome and DNA polymerase reside. Replication occurs within hepatocyte nuclei where HBV DNA is converted into covalently closed circular DNA (cccDNA). This is responsible for viral persistence and in patients with chronic infection is resistant to clearance by antivirals. Nuclear cccDNA results in infective virus particles and large amounts of non-infective HBsAg, both of which may be found in the serum of chronically infected patients

There are 6 genotypes A–F.

Epidemiology

About 257 million people or 5% of the world's population are HBsAg +ve and, therefore, have chronic HBV infection. The rate of carriage varies in the population from 0.1% in northern European countries to over 6% in the western Pacific and African regions; rates can be as high as 20%.

The main mode of transmission varies depending on rates of infection in the population. In areas of high endemicity vertical transmission is common, risk reducing through vaccination from 4.7% to 1.3% of new infection seen in under 5 years. In areas of low endemicity sexual transmission and blood-borne transmission more common.

Transmission occurs in 40% of non-immune heterosexual partners of patients with chronic HBV. In the UK, the incidence of acute HBV is 0.83 per 100,000 (2/3 men). Risk ↑ in MSM, >7 sexual partners, PWID.

Clinical features

Incubation period
Incubation 30–180 days.

Symptoms
- Infants and children usually have asymptomatic acute infection.
- 10–50% of adults are asymptomatic.
- Symptoms more likely if seroconversion.

Signs
- *Acute*: similar to HAV.
- *Chronic*: usually no physical signs. After many years, signs of chronic liver disease may emerge including spider naevi, finger clubbing, gynaecomastia, palmer erythema, and in end stage, disease jaundice, ascites, liver flap, and encephalopathy.

Complications
- *Acute infection*: mortality is <1% due to fulminant hepatitis.
- *Chronic infection*: defined as >6 months of HBsAg-positivity. In immunocompetent adults <5% develop chronic infection. Generally, asymptomatic. More common in HIV infection, chronic renal failure, the immunosuppressed, and >90% of vertically infected children.

May progress to cirrhosis (8–20% with active disease over 5 years) with attendant clinical features and the annual risk of hepatocellular carcinoma (HCC) is 2–5%. Decompensated liver disease occurs in 20% of those with cirrhosis over 5 years. Immunosuppression can also lead to HBV reactivation. Concurrent infection with HCV can lead to more progressive chronic liver disease. Co-infection with hepatitis D (Delta agent), usually seen in PWID, may lead to rapid deterioration and poor treatment response

- HCC may develop without cirrhosis. Risk of development of HCC is increased in patients with cirrhosis/necro-inflammation of liver, males, older age, African origin, smokers, diabetes/metabolic syndrome, alcohol excess, family history, high HBV/HBsAg levels, genotype C infection.

Diagnosis

Acute infection

- If suspected, check hepatitis B core antibody (HBcAb) and HBsAg. If HBsAg +ve in acute infection check HBeAg and hepatitis B IgM should be positive. HBV viral load will be high >1 million IU/mL. Acute hepatitis with ↑ ALT, bilirubin and alkaline phosphatase. If prothrombin time ↑ significantly, consider fulminant hepatitis. Clearance is suggested with loss of HBeAg and HBsAg at 6 months and development of eAb.

Chronic infection

- There are 4 phases of chronic infection (see Table 25.1).
- Patients should have fibrosis blood test or Fibroscan® (<6 kPa mild disease, >12 kPa severe disease/cirrhosis) to assess fibrosis. ↑ Fibroscan score with ALT>5ULN (upper limit of normal), food, steatosis, alcohol may artificially. Serum biomarkers may be helpful in addition. FIB-4 (platelets, AST and ALT) commonly used.
- Patients should have HCV, HIV, HDV tested. ALT, AST,

Management

- Information and advice, including avoiding unprotected sexual intercourse until non-infectious or partner successfully vaccinated.
- Stop or ↓ alcohol consumption.
- Refer to specialist unit if acute deteriorating liver disease.
- *Notifiable disease*: PN and screening of close family contacts are important with public health involvement for non-sexual contacts.

Treatment

Treatment options include directly acting antivirals (DAA); TDF, tenofovir alafenamide (TAF) or entecavir (ETV) or interferon; pegylated interferon alfa α (PegIFNα). Lamivudine, adefovir and telbivudine are not recommended.

Cleared infection (HBsAg –ve)

No treatment, but warn patient to inform doctor if going to be immunosupressed as reactivation possible and treatment with DAA may be required.

Acute infection

Treatment not recommended, as can ↑ risk of chronic infection, consider DAA if life threatening.

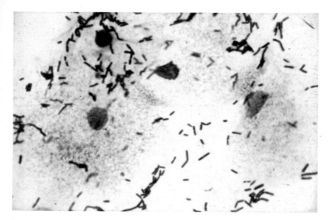

Plate 1 Gram stain lactobacilli (5).

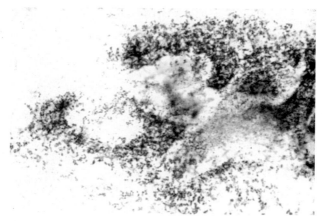

Plate 2 Gram stain BV (15).

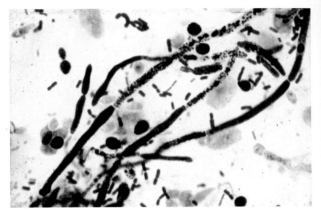

Plate 3 Gram stain candidiasis (17).

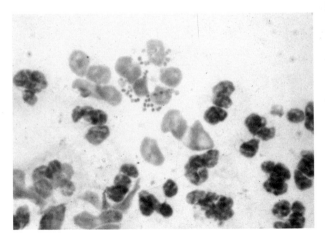

Plate 4 Gram stain gonorrhoea (8).

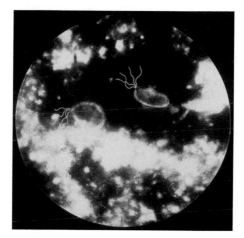

Plate 5 Dark-ground trichomonas vaginalis (16).

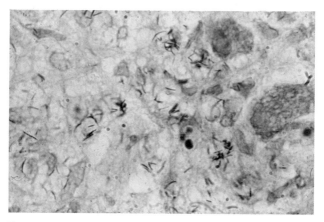

Plate 6 Ziehl–Nielsen stain Mycobacteria (48).

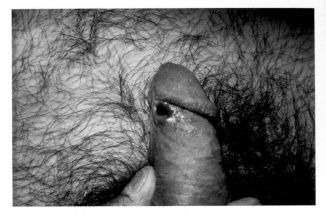

Plate 7 Classic chancre (7).

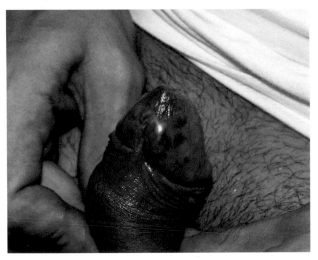

Plate 8 'Contemporary' chancre (7).

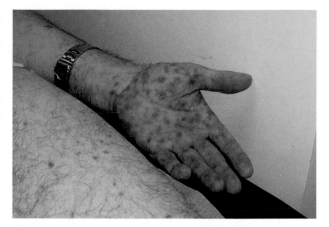

Plate 9 Secondary syphilis (7).

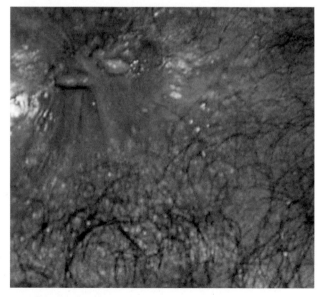

Plate 10 Condolymata lata (7).

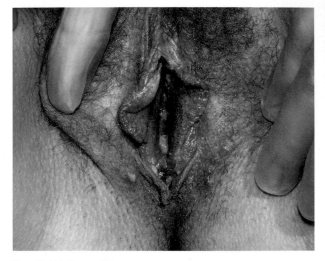

Plate 11 Vulval herpes (22).

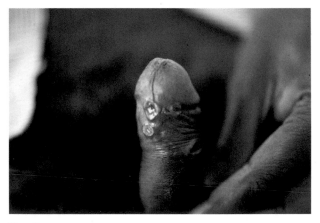

Plate 12 Chancroid (18).

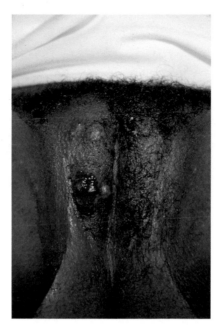

Plate 13 Granuloma inguinale (18).

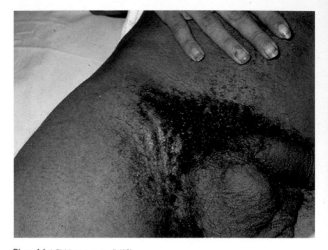

Plate 14 LGV "groove sign" (18).

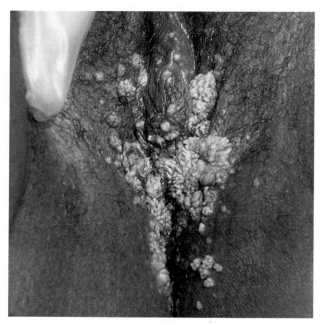

Plate 15 Anogenital warts (23).

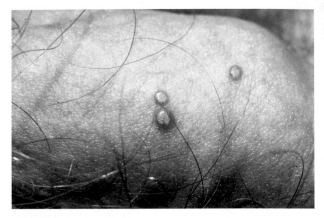

Plate 16 Molluscum contagiosum (24).

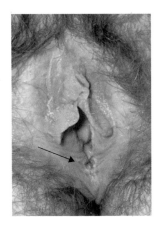

Plate 17 VIN (29).

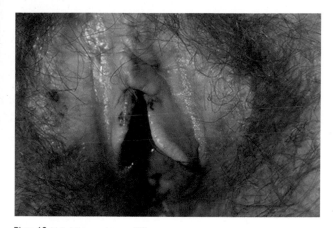

Plate 18 Vulval lichen sclerosus (29).

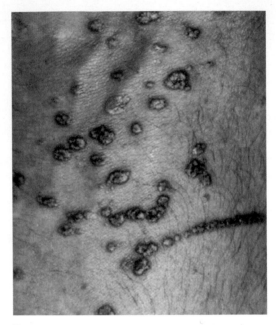

Plate 19 Lichen planus; purple papules with whickaam striae showing koebnerization (29).

Reprinted from Lewis-Jones S. (2010) *Paediatric Dermatology* (Oxford Specialist Handbooks in Paediatrics), with permission from Oxford University Press.

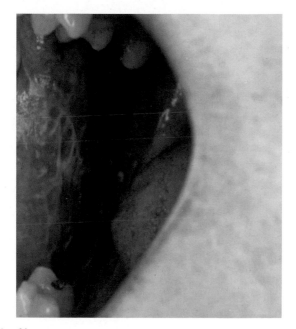

Plate 20 Lichen planus; hyperkeratosis on buccal mucosa (29).

Reprinted from Burge S., Matin R., and Wallis D. (2016) *Oxford Handbook of Medical Dermatology*, 2nd edn. with permission from Oxford University Press.

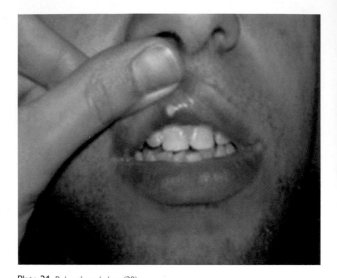

Plate 21 Behçet's oral ulcer (29).

Reprinted from Watts, R. et. al. (2013) *Oxford Textbook of Rheumatology*, 4th edn, with permission from Oxford University Press.

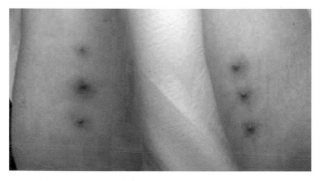

Plate 22 Pathergy reaction (29).

Reprinted from Watts, R. et. al. (2013) *Oxford Textbook of Rheumatology*, 4th edn, with permission from Oxford University Press.

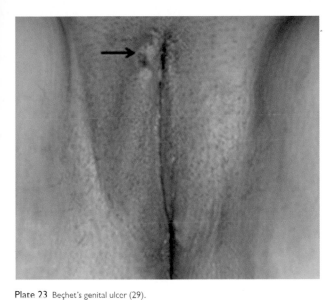

Plate 23 Beçhet's genital ulcer (29).

Reprinted from Watts, R. et. al. (2013) *Oxford Textbook of Rheumatology*, 4th edn, with permission from Oxford University Press.

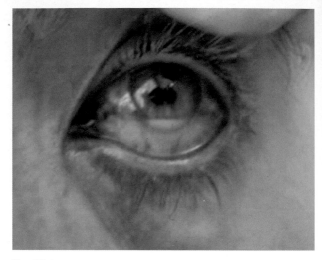

Plate 24 Anterior uveitis with hypopyon (29).

Reprinted from Watts, R. et. al. (2013) *Oxford Textbook of Rheumatology*, 4th edn, with permission from Oxford University Press.

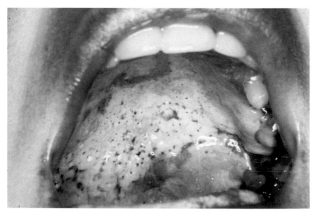

Plate 25 Oral candidiasis and HIV (42).

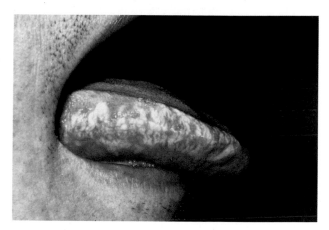

Plate 26 HIV: oral hairy leukoplakia (42).

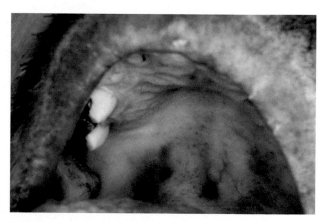

Plate 27 Oral Kaposi's sarcoma (42).

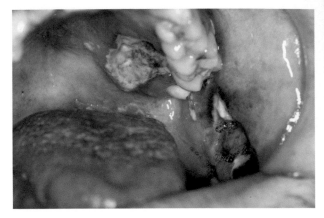

Plate 28 Oral lymphoma and HIV (42).

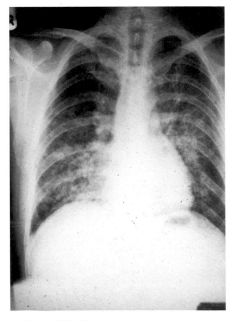

Plate 29 Chest X-ray—PCP (45).

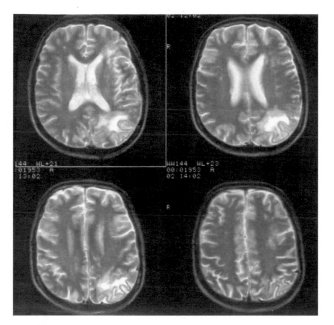

Plate 30 MRI—progressive multifocal leukoencephalopathy (46).

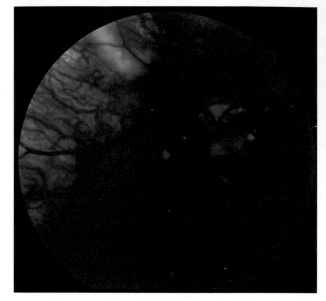

Plate 31 CMV retinitis (44).

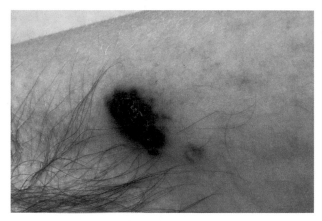

Plate 32 Cutaneous Kaposi's sarcoma (47).

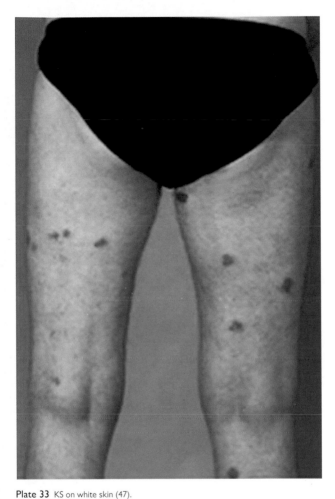

Plate 33 KS on white skin (47).

Reprinted from Warrell D., Cox T., and Firth J. (2010) *Oxford Textbook of Medicine*, © D A Warrell, with permission from Oxford University Press.

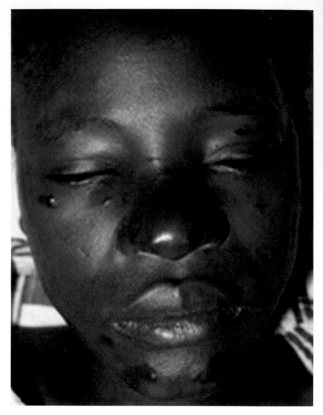

Plate 34 KS on the face (54).

Reprinted from Warrell D., Cox T., and Firth J. (2010) *Oxford Textbook of Medicine*, © D A Warrell with permission from Oxford University Press.

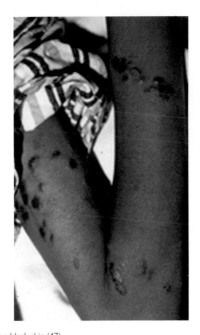

Plate 35 KS on black skin (47).

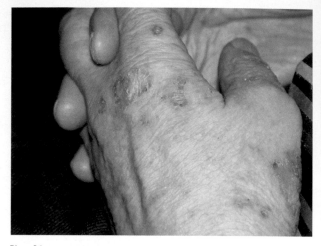

Plate 36 Crusted 'Norwegian' scabies (27).

Reprinted from Gosney M., Harper A., and Conroy, S. (2012) *Geriatric Medicine* (Oxford Desk Reference), with permission from Oxford University Press.

Table 25.1 Phases of chronic HBV infection

Phase I	• HBeAg +ve • HBV VL >10^7 IU/mL • HBsAg level high • ALT normal • No significant fibrosis	• Common in perinatal infection, once established rare to lose HBeAg • Highly infectious
Phase II	• HBeAg +ve • HBV VL 10^4 –10^7 IU/mL • HBsAg level high • ALT raised • Evidence of liver fibrosis	• Some patients may convert to HBeAb, although there is risk of progressive liver damage if this does not happen • Highly infectious
Phase III	• HBeAg –ve • HBV VL <2000 IU/mL (can be over, but normally <200000 IU/mL) • HBsAg low • ALT normal • Low levels of fibrosis	• Usually no progression, but may progress to phase 4 • 1–3% per annum lose HBsAg and develop HBsAb
Phase IV	• HBeAg –ve • HBV VL >2000 IU/mL • HBsAg intermediate • Intermittently raised ALT • Evidence of liver fibrosis	Pre-core mutation has allowed virus to replicate, unlikely to spontaneously lose HBsAg
Phase V	• HBsAg –ve • Undetectable HBV VL • Normal ALT	Cleared HBV, however, if immunosuppressed may reactivate and if cirrhotic at risk of HCC

Chronic infection
See Table 25.2.

Treatment should be considered for all severe liver disease, HCC, or cirrhotic, HBV DNA >2000 IU/mL and ALT >ULN and moderate fibrosis on liver Bx or Fibroscan (consider strongly if ALT normal and liver Bx moderate), HBV >20,000 IU/mL and ALT >2ULN can start treatment without biopsy.

Treatment with DAA vs PegIFNα depends on genotype (A>D/E with PegIFNα), age, severity of disease (PegIFNα contraindicated in decompensated liver disease), co-morbidities (PegIFNα use with caution in diabetics, vascular disease, or significant mental health problems).

In those not considering treatment monitor with ALT, HBV VL, HBsAg/eAg/eAb in those with eAg +ve <30 years monitor 3–6-monthly; HBeAg –ve, HBV VL <2000 IU/mL monitor every 6–12 months; HBeAg –ve HBV VL >2000 IU/mL monitor every 3 months for 1 year then 6-monthly.

Table 25.2 HBV treatment options

	Peg INFα	ETV, TDF, TAF
Route of administration	Weekly injection	Oral
Treatment duration	48weeks	Long-term or until HBeAg or sAg loss
Stopping rules	• Genotype B/C 12 weeks if HBsAg >20,000 IU/mL or no response • Genotype A/D >20,000 IU/mL at 24 weeks in all genotype	• HBeAg seroconversion • HBsAg loss
Efficacy eAg +ve	• HBeAg seroconversion 30% • ALT normalization 40% • HBV VL <60 IU/mL 10% • HBsAg loss 5%	• HBeAg seroconversion 10-20% • ALT normalization 70% • HBV VL <60 IU/mL 70% • HBsAg loss 1–3%
eAg -ve	• ALT normalization 60% • HBV VL <60 IU/mL 20% • HBsAg loss 2–4%	• ALT normalization 80% • HBV VL <60 IU/mL 90% • HBsAg loss 0%

Prevention

Horizontal transmission
If not vaccinated or HBsAb post-vaccination <10 IU/mL consider specific HBV immunoglobulin 500 U IM (ideally ≤48 hours or within 1 week) and rapid vaccination of recent sexual contacts.

Vertical transmission
Treat mother if HBV VL >200,000 IU/mL. Vaccination (rapid schedule) in all born to HBV +ve mothers and HBV specific immunoglobulin 200 U IM (all born to mothers HBeAg +ve, sAg +ve if eAb –ve, or HBV VL >10^6) ↓ vertical transmission by 90%. Breastfeeding can continue.

Vaccination
Apart from contacts, including household contacts, vaccination should be considered for those at ↑ risk, e.g. MSM, sex workers, association with endemic areas, prisoners, PWIDs, those sexually assaulted, occupational/needlestick risk, severe renal/liver disease. Protection of vaccinated patients is assessed by HBsAb level >100 mIU/mL is ideal, but levels >10 mIU/mL may be adequate, subsequent HBV infection is very rare. It has been suggested that memory cells provide protection as immunity appears to be maintained, even if HBsAb ↓ provided there has been a good initial response.

Engerix B®, HBvaxPRO® and Fendrix® are used. HBvaxPRO 40® is used in dialysis patients; may offer ↑ immunogenicity in immunocompromised as can Fendrix®. Twinrix® is combined HAV/HBV vaccines.

Active hepatitis A and B vaccines

Hepatitis A vaccine
Havrix monodose®: adult dose 1 mL with the deltoid region the preferred site (subcutaneous may be used in those with bleeding disorders).

Hepatitis B vaccine
Engerix B®, HBvaxPRO®, HBvaxPRO40®, Fendrix®: adult dose—1 mL (0.5 mL Fendrix®) with the deltoid region the preferred site (subcutaneous may be used in those with bleeding disorders). Should not be injected into the buttocks (efficacy reduced).

Combined hepatitis A and hepatitis B vaccine
Twinrix®: inactivated HAV and recombinant HBV surface antigen
Adult dose—1 mL with the deltoid region the preferred site (subcutaneous may be used in those with bleeding disorders, although immune response may be reduced). Should not be injected into the buttocks (efficacy reduced).

Schedules
- *Ultra-rapid course*: of recombinant vaccine schedule (Engerix B®) 3 doses and booster at 0, 7, 21/28 days plus 12-month booster.
- *Rapid* course schedule for post-exposure: 3 doses and booster at 0, 1, 2 months plus 12-month booster.

Note these schedules are not licensed for neonates.
- *Standard schedule*: 3 doses—0, 1, 6 months, booster dose at 12 months if protective antibody level <100 IU/mL.

Further 5-year booster recommended no need to recheck HBsAb level.

Protective antibody level in 80–95% after full course of vaccination, but lower response rates if aged >40 years or immunocompromised, e.g. HIV infection particularly if CD4 < 200 cells/μL, but even <500 cells/μL. High-dose vaccine HBvaxPRO 40®, Engerix® double dose or Fendrix® are more immunogenic in immunocompromised. If HBsAb <10 IU/mL should be considered non-immune, alternative vaccine can be considered and/or higher dose.

Hepatitis C virus (HCV) infection

RNA virus of the family Flaviviridae discovered in 1989. Six predominant genotypes. In the UK genotype 1 (G1) is most common (~50% of cases) followed by G3 (together 40–50%). G1 relatively more common in those infected through blood products and G3 in PWID.

HCV is a single strand +ve sense RNA virus. It exists as a lipo-viral particle in serum, thus escaping the immune system through association with apolipoprotein and multiple quasi-species. After entry into the liver cell via multiple receptors, replication occurs in cytoplasm. NS5B RNA dependent polymerase facilitates replication through synthesis of −ve strand RNA, which acts as a template for HCV polyprotein (cleaved by NS4A protease) and HCV +ve strand viral RNA to produce new virions.

Epidemiology and transmission

Worldwide 2.5% infected with HCV (177.5 million). UK has prevalence of around 0.5% with a higher prevalence in PWIDs (20–50% PWIDs). High prevalence in Egypt (40% in some areas), Mongolia, Eastern Europe, and some areas of SE Asia.

Transmission, mainly parenteral through shared needles, syringes, or equipment. Found in up to 1% of GUM patients <2% infection are sexually acquired. Sexual transmission very rare in heterosexuals 1:380,000 per sexual contact. Outbreaks described in HIV +ve MSM and ⇄ prevalence in ♀ sex workers. Vertical transmission occurs in 5–8%, ↑ with HIV co-infection, prematurity, HCV VL >10^6.

Clinical features

- *Incubation period*: 4–20 weeks.
- *Symptoms*: acute hepatitis occurs in 20% and is less likely to be followed by chronic infection.
- *Signs*: similar to HAV and HBV.
- *Complications*: acute fulminant hepatitis is rare, but can occur.
- *Natural history*:
  - >80% become chronically infected with HCV, most unaware.
  - high alcohol intake, co-existing HBV, HIV, and other chronic liver diseases can lead to a more rapid progression to cirrhosis and liver cancer
  - progression to cirrhosis in 10–20% after 20–30 years
  - thereafter, annual rate of developing cancer 1–5% and developing decompensation 3–6%. ALT may be normal, despite severe liver disease.

Diagnosis and investigations

Screening with HCV Ab should be offered to:
- all PWIDs (past and present)
- in the UK recipients of:
  - blood (prior to September 1991)
  - blood products pre-1986
  - tissues/organs before 1992

- regular sexual partners of those with HCV infection
- HCP exposure to blood/needlesticks
- those with HIV infection, particularly MSM
- people tattooed or with skin piercings, where poor infection control
- children of mothers with HCV infection.

Some groups with ongoing risk may need repeat screening. It may be advised for prisoners/ex-prisoners; those sexually assaulted or if outbreak identified.

- If HCV antibody (Ab) +ve confirmation by PCR test for viral RNA. Abs usually appear within 3 (rarely 6) months of infection. HCV Ab may be –ve in HIV or the immunocompromised.
- *Genotype testing*: influences choice of treatment.
- Liver function, clotting tests, and exclusion of other viral hepatotropic infections, HIV and liver-related diseases are helpful.
- FibroScan® can be used to assess for severe fibrosis (≥14 kPa cirrhosis, ≥9.6 kPa severe fibrosis) and APRI can help determine severe fibrosis.
- Abdominal ultrasound and α-fetoprotein recommended.

Management

A notifiable infection with partner notification and public health implications:
- Provide information and advice (PWID risk of sharing, risks of sexual transmission).
- Stop (or ↓) alcohol consumption.
- If patient amenable to further management, refer to specialist.

Acute infection

Monitor if still +ve at 6 months consider treatment with anti HCV DAA.

Chronic infection

- Based on genotype.
- DAA act on HCV protease (NS3/4A inhibitor) HCV RNA dependent polymerase (NS5B), modulator of NS5B (NS5A) see Table 25.3.
- Interferon no longer recommended.

Treatment combinations are outlined in Table 25.4. Drug interactions may be important (see Chapter 55, 'HIV: management', pp. 621–51).

Table 25.3 HCV Treatment classes

	NS3/4A inhibitors	NS5A inhibitors	NS5B inhibitors
HCV drugs	Glecaprevir	Daclatasvir	Sofosbuvir
	Grazoprevir	Elbasvir	Dasabuvir
	Paritaprevir	Ledipasvir	
	Voxilaprevir	Ombitasvir	
		Velpatasvir	
		Pibrentasvir	

Table 25.4 HCV treatment regimes

HCV GT	Treatment regime	Treatment duration		
		Non-cirrhotic	Compensated cirrhosis	Treatment experienced to DAA
1or 4	SOF/LDV	8–12 weeks	12 weeks	12 weeks +RBV
	SOF/VEL	12 weeks	12 weeks	12 weeks +/- RBV
	SOF/VEL + VOX[1]	8 weeks	12 weeks	12 weeks if DAA experienced
	SOF/DCV	12 weeks	12weeks + RBV	12 weeks +RBV
	OMB/PAT/r + DSV (not GT4)	1a–12 weeks with RBV 1b 12 weeks	1a–12 weeks with RBV 1b 12 weeks	24 weeks + RBV
	OMB/PAT/r + RBV (GT4)	12 weeks + RBV		
	EBR/GZR	GT1a or GT4 treatment experienced; 12 week if VL ≤800 000 IU/mL, Add RBV 12 weeks of VL >800 000 IU/mL GT1b or GT4 naïve; 12 weeks		
	GLE/PIB	8 weeks	12 weeks	12–16 weeks
2	SOF/DCV	12 weeks		
	SOF/VEL	12 weeks		
	GLE/PIB	8 weeks	12 weeks	8–12 weeks
3	SOF /DCV	12 weeks	12 weeks + RBV	24 weeks + RBV
	SOF/VEL	12 weeks	12 weeks + RBV	
	SOF/VEL/VOX	8 weeks		12 weeks
	GLE/PIB	8 weeks	12 weeks	16 weeks
5or 6	SOF/LDV	12 weeks	12 weeks + RBV	
	SOF/VEL	12 weeks		
	SOF/VEL/VOX	8 weeks	12 weeks	12 weeks + RBV
	SOF/DCV	12 weeks	12 weeks + RBV	
	GLE/PIB	8 weeks	12 weeks	8 weeks

DCV, daclatasvir; DSV, dasabuvir; EBR, elbasvir; GLE, glecaprevir; GZR, grazoprevir; LDV, ledipasvir; OMB, ombitasvir; PIB, pibrentasvir; PTV/r, paritaprevir/ritonavir; RBV, ribavirin; SOF, sofosbuvir; VEL, velpatasvir; VOX, voxilaprevir.

Resistance

NS5a RAS mutations may ↓ effectiveness of treatment, particularly G3 or G1a treatment experienced. Y93H is a key mutation. Testing should be considered in treatment experienced and, if +ve, add RBV/lengthen treatment. Consider in naïve G1a if using EBR/GZR or in 3a if using SOF/DCV, and adding RBV or using alternative agent.

Prevention and prophylaxis

No vaccine available. Currently, no treatment for needlestick injuries recommended.

Tests for HCA, HBV, and HCV

For different tests, see Table 25.5.

Table 25.5 Serological, virological, and liver enzyme tests in different stages of viral hepatitis A, B, C

	HAV	HBV	HCV
Acute infection	• HAV IgM +ve • ALT ↑ usually	• Usually HBsAg +ve • Anti HBc IgM +ve • ALT ↑ • HBV DNA present	• HCV IgG +/−ve • ALT ↑ often • HCVRNA +ve (usually)
Chronic infection	Does not usually occur	• HBsAg +ve • HBeAg +/−ve • HBc IgG +ve • ALT ↑ or ↔ • HBV-DNA +/−ve	• HCV IgG +ve • ALT ↑ or ↔ • HCV-RNA +ve
Recovered infection	• HAV IgG +ve • Normal ALT	• HBs IgG +ve • HBc IgG +ve • ALT normal	• HCV IgG +ve • HCVRNA −ve • ALT normal
Successful vaccination	HAV IgG +ve	• HBs IgG +ve • HBc IgG −ve	Not available

Other viral infections

Epstein–Barr virus *324*
Cytomegalovirus *326*
Other viruses *327*
Human T-cell lymphotropic virus 1 (HTLV-1) *328*
Human herpes virus-8 *329*

Epstein–Barr virus

Aetiology

A DNA herpes virus consisting of types EBV1 and EBV2. Infects >90% of humans, persisting for life. Probably evolved from a non-human primate virus.

Epidemiology and transmission

Virtually all children infected in developing countries (especially with socioeconomic deprivation).

In developed countries most infections are acquired by those aged 15–25 years. Characteristically spread by ingestion of infected saliva from a seropositive carrier during kissing. Although unproven, reports of EBV isolated from a vulval ulcer, semen, and cervical secretions, suggest the potential for sexual transmission.

Clinical features

Incubation period: 4–6 weeks. Infection in children usually asymptomatic. In adolescents and young adults >50% present with infectious mononucleosis (glandular fever):

- fever
- lymphadenopathy
- pharyngitis
- >10% develop hepatosplenomegaly and palatal petechiae (Forscheimer spots).

Other less common features include anaemia (haemolytic and aplastic), thrombocytopenia, myocarditis, hepatitis, genital ulcers, Guillain–Barré syndrome, encephalitis, and meningitis.

Non-specific diffuse central rashes may be found in up to 50% with an immune complex macular rash and in >70% of those taking ampicillin or amoxicillin.

Investigations

- *Haematology*: lymphocytosis with 20% of cells atypical. May also be thrombocytopenia.
- *Biochemistry*: elevated liver enzymes in up to 100%.
- *Antibody and PCR testing*:
  - *Monospot test*—heterophil antibodies; sensitivity ≈80% in adults
  - *EBV antibody tests*—IgM to viral capsid antigen (transient); most reliable test is paired IgG showing >4-fold titre rise; IgG to EBV nuclear antigen (EBNA) appears in convalescence, denotes past infection
  - EBV PCR can be used to detect virus in blood and/or CSF if significant complication.

Management

- Bed rest, analgesics, antipyretics.
- Antibiotics (not ampicillin/amoxicillin) if 2° bacterial infection.
- Steroids if airways obstruction.

Prognosis

Self-limiting, although associated with persisting tiredness and possible relapses during the first 6–12 months.

Other conditions associated with EBV

These include:
- Burkitt's and Hodgkin's lymphomas.
- Nasopharyngeal carcinoma.
- Lymphoproliferative disease.
- In HIV infection:
  - oral hairy leucoplakia
  - some non-Hodgkin's lymphomas.

Cytomegalovirus

The largest known DNA herpesvirus; host-specific, with four human/higher primate subtypes.

Epidemiology and horizontal transmission

Worldwide distribution favouring developing countries and low socioeconomic classes. Spread through contact with infected saliva (kissing), urine, genital fluids (cervical, vaginal seminal), breastmilk, and blood. Infection with multiple strains reported in sexually active individuals. ↑ rates found in those with history of STIs, BBV, seroprevalence proportional to number of lifetime partners. In STI clinics, prevalence of CMV antibodies in MSM is about 1.5 times that of heterosexual ♂.

Epidemiology and vertical/neonatal transmission

Most common vertically transmitted viral infection. Worldwide incidence of foetal CMV acquisition during pregnancy 0.8–4%. In UK ≈50% ♀ becoming pregnant are CMV seronegative, with ≈3% becoming infected during their pregnancy (largely from young children). 30–40% with 1° infection and about 1% with recurrent CMV will infect their foetus (overall congenital infection rate 0.5–1%).

Acquired by foetal ingestion of infected amniotic material, haematological transplacental spread, and lactation.

Clinical features

Horizontal transmission

- Generally causes asymptomatic infection unless immunosuppressed.
- Only 10% of 1° infections cause an infectious mononucleosis type illness, consisting of fever, myalgia, cervical lymphadenopathy, and less commonly pneumonitis and hepatitis.
- Illness self-limiting, although lifelong viral persistence, often with extended periods of asymptomatic viral shedding (e.g. during pregnancy).

Vertical transmission

Severity of neonatal symptoms/signs less if mother seropositive (neutralizing antibodies). Range from none (in about 80%) to the classical congenital syndrome—hepatosplenomegaly (with jaundice) and thrombocytopenia (with purpura), which are self-limiting. Less common, but permanent CNS features include microcephaly, chorioretinitis, a progressive sensorineuronal deafness.

Diagnosis

- *Immunocompetent adults*: serology; 4-fold ↑ in IgG CMV antibodies from paired blood samples taken 10–14 days apart or IgM from single specimen (persists up to 20 weeks).
- *Foetal infection*: CMV detection from amniotic fluid by PCR after 21 weeks gestation.
- *Congenital/neonatal infection*: cmv culture or pcr from urine and pharynx.

Management

Symptomatic treatment (as for EBV infection, see Chapter 26, 'Epstein–Barr virus', p. 324).

For CMV associated with HIV infection see Chapter 44, 'HIV: Disorders' of the eye', pp. 513–21.

Other viruses

A number of other viruses may be sexually transmitted, including Zika virus, Marburg haemorrhagic fever virus, Lassa virus, Ebola virus, and many of the other haemorrhagic fever viruses.

It is likely that other viruses will be found to have significant sexual transmission in the future. For highly significant viruses, such as the category 4 haemorrhagic fever viruses, that are known to be transmitted via seminal fluid, condoms should be used or abstinence should be practiced. Sexual transmission may occur months after the symptomatic phase is over (varying between viruses). Seminal fluid may be taken for PCR.

If PCR is negative on 2 separate occasions, it is thought that transmission is unlikely to occur. Specialist advice should be sought.

Zika

Zika virus is now endemic in many countries within the tropics. It is mainly transmitted through mosquito bite, but sexual transmission can occur.

If contracted during pregnancy, birth defects can occur, including microcephaly. It is advised that pregnant women consider carefully the risks of travelling to areas where Zika is endemic and, if travel is undertaken, avoid mosquito bites, where possible, with insect repellent and bed nets.

♀ should avoid becoming pregnant up to 8 weeks after travel and ♂ should use condoms for 6 months. Testing is available for symptomatic patients who are ill within 2 weeks of travel or during travel, and should be considered in those who have travelled and have become pregnant or whose partner has become pregnant within the above time periods (8 weeks for ♀ or 6 months for ♂).

Human T-cell lymphotropic virus 1 (HTLV-1)

Single-stranded RNA retrovirus.

Epidemiology and transmission

Endemic in Japan and parts of the Caribbean, South America, and sub-Saharan Africa. Main transmission routes are breastfeeding and sexual intercourse (mostly heterosexual), but also from blood products and sharing injecting drug equipment.

Diagnosis

Serology: enzyme immunoassay for HTLV antibody must be followed up by PCR or Western blot. HTLV testing is recommended in transplant for donor and recipient, blood transfusion, and in pregnant women from high-prevalence areas.

Clinical features

Most infected individuals remain healthy carriers adult T-cell leukaemia (ATL) or myelopathy (cumulative lifetime risk 1–4%).

ATL

Leukaemic involvement with wide-ranging skin lesions in ≈40%. Other manifestations include hepatosplenomegaly, lymphadenopathy, hypercalcaemia, and sometimes immunosuppression.

Myelopathy (tropical spastic paraparesis)

Demyelination of long motor neurons of spinal cord producing lower- extremity weakness, spasticity, urinary incontinence, and erectile dysfunction.

Management

ATL has poor prognosis (median survival without treatment <1 year). Besides conventional chemotherapy and allogeneic stem-cell transplantation, other therapeutic approaches include interferon alfa plus zidovudine, and retinoid derivatives. Mogamulizumab (monoclonal antibody against CCR4) may have activity by reducing proviral DNA and is under investigation in ATL and myelopathy.

Human herpes virus-8

Herpes virus with five major variants (A–E). Variants B and C predominate in Europe and the USA.

Transmission

Sexual contact, particularly oro-anal sex, and also mouth-to-mouth contact as HHV-8 is found in saliva. Implicated in close family contact in endemic areas (Africa), especially when associated with poor hygiene. In developed countries ↑ rates among MSM. Transmission does not appear to be related to pregnancy or breastfeeding.

Clinical features

- Associated with >95% of cases of Kaposi's sarcoma with immunosuppression an important co-factor, although now less common with use of antiretroviral treatment (Chapter 54, 'Kaposi's sarcoma', p. 596).
- Associated with Castleman's disease—of nearly all HIV cases (Chapter 54, 'Multicentric Castleman's disease', p. 617) and ~50% of non-HIV cases

Scabies

Introduction *332*
Aetiology *332*
Epidemiology *334*
Transmission *334*
Clinical features *335*
Diagnosis *337*
Management *338*

Introduction

Discovered in 1687 by Bonomo, arthropod class Arachnida, subclass Acari, family Sarcoptidae. In the human host, infestation is with *Sarcoptes scabiei* var *hominis*

Aetiology

A parasitic mite with no natural predator. The ♀ penetrates the stratum corneum constructing short burrows where she lays 1–3 eggs daily during a lifespan of 4–6 weeks. Eggs are oval and 0.1–0.15 mm long. Six-legged larvae hatch in 3–4 days, then moult to form an eight-legged nymph. After a further moult, the adult develops. The total time to maturity is 10 days with females becoming gravid within 14 days.

The adult is tortoise-like in shape with 8 legs (Fig. 27.1). The two sets of anterior legs end in stalked pulvilli (suckers), which allow the mite to grip the host's skin, aiding its movement. Spines and bristles cover the body. Mites are blind with no eyes. The adult female measures 0.4 mm across; the male is smaller and dies after mating. It has no spiracles, trachea, or body armour, and obtains its oxygen through its surface. Mites can move rapidly on warm skin at ~2.5 cm/min. Burrows are created at variable rates (0.5–5.0 mm/day) and are lined with scar tissue to prevent them collapsing, thus allowing the mite to breathe and larvae to escape. Mites feed on the lymph and lysed tissue. Survival of the mite away from its host is contentious, but is unlikely to be >48–72 hours and is probably much less.

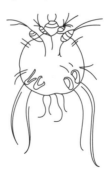

Fig. 27.1 Sarcoptes scabie*i*

Frequently asked questions

Is scabies always sexually transmitted?

No. The majority of cases are not sexually transmitted. It commonly occurs in people living closely together and is spread by prolonged skin contact, including holding hands.

Does anyone else require treatment?

Treatment is advised for current and recent sexual partners and intimate household contacts.

I finished the treatment 2 weeks ago, but still have some itching.
Do I need to repeat it again?

No, not if you have used it properly and not been re-infected. Symptoms often take 4–5 weeks to resolve as they are due to a hypersensitivity reaction stimulated by mite products. It usually takes this time for them to be expelled from the skin and for the reaction to settle. If relief is required, topical crotamiton or antihistamines should help.

Epidemiology

Appears as sporadic outbreaks, especially in families, schools, dormitories, institutions, and nurseries. Epidemics occur in 15–30 year cycles. Mammals such as domestic cats, dogs, pigs, and horses may be infected with other sarcoptidae (mange), which may be transferred to humans, resulting in irritation without infestation. These lesions are self-limiting. Treatment of mange is of the infested animal.

Transmission

Holding hands is the most likely route of transmission. The more parasites on a person, the greater the risk of transmission. Prolonged skin-to-skin contact is necessary; mites are transferred after about 10–20 minutes of close contact and can penetrate the epidermis within 30 minutes. The parasites may remain viable on inanimate objects for 2–3 days, but fomite transmission is uncommon.

May occur in those using a bed recently occupied by an infested person. More likely in crusted scabies due to the greater number of mites present. Not vectors of other infections.

Clinical features

Classical scabies

Patients may be asymptomatic for the first 4–6 weeks in first infection. Intense irritation occurs due to delayed Type IV hypersensitivity reaction to mites, their faeces, and eggs. In re-infestation, signs and symptoms become evident in 24–48 hours because of previous sensitization. Symmetrical polymorphic lesions appear, most commonly on hands (especially finger webs), wrists, axillae, genitals, buttocks, and extensor aspects of elbows (Fig. 27.2). Back relatively not involved, head spared (except in children). People are infectious before the rash develops. Rash is eczematous and associated with burrows (linear intraepidermal tunnels seen as fine short serpiginous grey channels 5–10 mm long, often with a small associated papule or vesicle). Nodules and papules seen on penis and scrotum. Urticarial lesions are rare. On average, 10–15 mites per host in primary infestations.

Crusted scabies (Norwegian scabies)

Found in the immunocompromised and elderly; may be related to failure of sensitization to mite antigen. For this reason itch less prominent. Highly contagious, with honeycombed cavities in the skin containing many thousands of mites. Extensive crusted lesions with thick hyperkeratotic scales ('breadcrumb') develop over the elbows, palms, knees, and soles of the feet, but can affect any part of the body including the face and scalp (see Plate 36). Scabies contracted by a healthy patient from a patient with crusted scabies is no different from classical scabies. Sepsis is a frequent complication.

Scabies in people with HIV

May be atypical. Crusted scabies or minimal pruritus (if immunosuppressed), papular lesions, psoriasiform lesions, and generalized pruritus (with few lesions) may all be seen.

Scabies incognito

Altered picture seen following topical steroids. Widespread atypical papular lesions that mimic eczema.

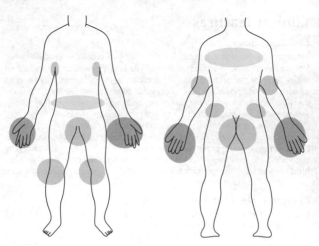

Fig. 27.2 Distribution of scabies

Diagnosis

Scabies should be suspected if history of itch, worse at night, affecting close contacts and classical skin rash (typical lesions, typical distribution). The diagnosis is usually clinical.

Definitive diagnosis is by microscopy.

Material can be obtained by;
- extraction of mites (or eggs) from their burrows with a needle
- scraping the skin using a scalpel blade, following local application of liquid paraffin.

Burrow ink test involves staining the suspected site with a washable felt-tip marker. After removal by washing, the ink will be found to have delineated the burrow (seen as a dark zigzag line running across and away from the lesion).

Mites can be recovered from the wrists (63%), extensor aspect of elbows (11%), feet and ankles (9%), genitals (9%), buttocks (4%), and axillae (2%).

Other possible methods of diagnosis (rarely used clinically) include; videodermatoscopy, epiluminescence microscopy, or skin biopsy. *S. scabei* DNA can be detected from skin scales using PCR.

Management

Irritation may last for several weeks following successful treatment (antigenic material in the dermis and epidermis). Suspect treatment failure if itch >2–4 weeks following last dose of scabicide. Sedative antihistamines, crotamiton 10% cream bd/tid, or calamine 15% lotion may give symptomatic relief. Potentially contaminated clothes or bed linen (anything used by infested person or their contacts in the 4 days before treatment) should be washed at >60°C and dried in a hot dryer or dry cleaned. Patients with crusted scabies should be isolated in hospital to prevent nosocomial spread.

Treatment

Permethrin 5% cream

First line of treatment. Apply to the whole body from chin and ears downwards. Consider application to face and scalp in very young or elderly. Apply to cool skin (not following a hot bath as this may remove it from its site of action by ↑ absorption into the bloodstream.) Allow to dry before dressing. Wash off after 8–12 hours. Reapply after 1 week. If hands are washed with soap within 8 hours, cream should be reapplied to hands.

Malathion 0.5% aqueous lotion

If permethrin not appropriate (e.g. if a person has an allergy to chrysanthemums.) Advice as above but should be left on body (including hands) for 24 hours before washing off.

Ivermectin

- 200 mcg/kg, 2 doses, 2 weeks apart if weight >15kg
- available on a named patient basis, if no response to topical treatments.

Crusted scabies

Topical permethrin od for 7 days, then twice weekly until cure, plus oral ivermectin on days 1, 2, 8, 9, and 15.

Pregnancy/breastfeeding

Permethrin is the treatment of choice. Malathion is an alternative. Remove cream or lotion from nipples before breastfeeding and reapply following.

Resistance

Has been reported to both permethrin and ivermectin.

Partner notification

Treat current sexual and household contacts at the same time. Contact tracing of partners from the previous 1 month is advised.

Further information

℘ https://www.bashhguidelines.org/media/1137/scabies-2016.pdf

Pediculosis pubis

Introduction *340*
Aetiology *341*
Epidemiology *343*
Transmission *343*
Clinical features *343*
Diagnosis *344*
Management *344*

Introduction

Pthiriasis (pediculosis) is an ancient disease. Nits (eggs of lice) have been discovered on the pubic hair of a 2000-year-old Chilean mummy, and also in fossilized form, dating back 10,000 years. Despite a rise in other STIs in recent years, it is now seen with less frequency in sexual health clinics. It has been suggested that the trend for pubic hair removal (through shaving, waxing, etc.) has resulted in the dramatic decline in the number of cases of pediculosis pubis recorded.

Aetiology

Belonging to the sub-order of Anoplura (sucking lice), the families of Pediculidae (body lice) and Pthiridae (pubic lice) are wingless insects unable to fly or jump. Humans are host to three species of lice. The pubic or crab louse, *Pthirus pubis* (Fig. 28.1), is classified as a species of the genus Pthirus. Head lice, *Pediculus humanus capitis*, and body lice, *Pediculus humanus* or *corporis*, are morphologically similar to each other and easily distinguished from pubic lice (which are smaller and squatter with thicker crab-like legs). The life-cycle of pubic lice is ~15–25 days occurring in three stages.

The nit

- white oval egg <0.8 mm attached to the hair base by a chitinous envelope
- encased by a proteinaceous sheath, except for the operculum, allowing ventilation
- appears to move up the hair and away from the skin as hair grows.

The nymph

- resembles a pubic louse, but is smaller
- hatches in 7 days by releasing itself from the egg with air expelled from its anus
- migrates back to the hair base to suck blood and mature.

The adult

- ~1–2 mm in length, dark grey to brown in colour. ♂ is smaller and has a more pointed tail.
- three distinct pairs of legs, each with claw-like appendages whose grasp is designed to match the diameter of pubic or axillary hair in contrast with the finer scalp hair. Can move ~10 cm/day.
- sensory antennae detect human smell and tactile hairs on its body determine surface type. Eyes are faceted; it is almost blind, but photophobic.
- buries sharp mouthpiece stylets inside a pubic hair follicle to obtain a constant blood supply. Ingests several times its own weight in blood during each feed. May feed at the same place for days.
- single pair of spiracles allow gaseous exchange and prevent dehydration.
- ♀ will lay 2–3 eggs during a 24-hour period and 15–50 eggs over a lifetime.

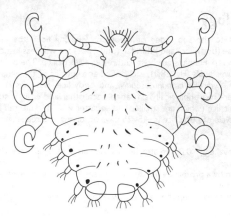

Fig. 28.1 Pthirus pubis

Frequently asked questions

How have I got them?

The crab louse is transmitted by close body contact and, hence, during sexual contact. More rarely, infestation can be spread through contact with an infested person's bed linen, towel, or clothes.

Will shaving get rid of the lice?

Lice are treated with topical preparations. All body hair needs to be treated, not just the pubic hair. Shaving is not, therefore, recommended as treatment.

Do I need to wash all my bedding?

Yes, it is recommended that all clothes and bed linen are machine washed on a hot water cycle.

Does my partner need treatment?

Yes, current sexual partners need treatment. Avoid close body contact until partner(s) have completed treatment. Contact tracing of all partners in the previous 3 months is recommended.

Pthirus or Phthirus?

Spelling varies, with both *Pthirus* and *Phthirus* widely used. Although the name is derived from the Greek *phtheir* (louse), the former spelling is used more widely.

Epidemiology

- Essentially a human parasite, although reported to infest higher apes.
- Does not occur in epidemics, although more common in the cooler months of the year (unlike body and head lice, which occur more often in the warmer months).
- Considered to be usually sexually transmitted because:
  - found most commonly in sexually active adults (aged 16–25 years)
  - associated with other STIs, especially chlamydia.
- Related to crowded living conditions, poor personal hygiene, and low socio-economic status.
- Infestation of the scalp is rare (about 1% of louse infestation), but occurs more often in red-headed people, who have fewer hairs per unit area than others.
- Rarely reported in the scalp and eyelashes of children. Acquisition from nipple hairs during breastfeeding has been reported and transmission through other close body contact is recognized. Sexual abuse should be considered.
- Can be used as a forensic tool. A mixed DNA profile of two hosts can be detectable in blood meals of the lice that have had close contact between an assailant and a victim.
- Not known to be vectors of human disease (unlike body and head lice, which may carry organisms responsible for epidemic or louse-borne typhus, trench fever, and louse-borne relapsing fever).

Transmission

- Usually by skin-to-skin contact with up to 95% of sexual contacts of an active carrier developing an infestation.
- Occasionally by clothing, bedding, or towels.
- It is unlikely that lice can survive for more than 24–48 hours if removed from the host.

Clinical features

Pediculosis pubis is the name of the condition caused by infestation of the pubic hair by *Pthirus pubis*. ~76% complain of intense irritation in the genital area because of hypersensitivity, with ~40% of patients experiencing erythema. In the hirsute, infestation may spread to the thighs, perineum, trunk, abdomen, or axillary hair.

Pediculosis ciliaris or pthiriasis palpebrarum is infestation of the eyelashes by the pubic louse, where it can be responsible for a severe blepharoconjunctivitis. Eyebrows may also be infested. Headlice are very rarely responsible for eyelash infestation.

Blue macules (maculae cerulae) caused by an enzyme secreted from the salivary glands of the lice may be visible at feeding sites. They are 2–3 mm in diameter, with an irregular outline, painless, do not disappear on pressure, and appear to be in the deeper tissues. They become apparent some hours after the louse has fed, and last for several days. 'Black spots' on underwear or in the genital area usually indicate insect faecal matter or blood spots.

Concomitant STIs are present in ~30% of those infested.

Diagnosis

Identify lice, eggs, or maculae ceruleae with the naked eye. Low-power microscopy of the louse may show movement, sucking pumps in the head, and a blood-filled oesophagus.

Management

Offer full screening for STIs and advise avoidance of close body contact until patient and partner(s) complete treatment. Clothes and bed linen should be washed at 50°C or dry-cleaned.

Because of the delicate nature of the genital skin, aqueous, rather than alcohol-based preparations are recommended. Lotions are more effective than shampoos. All body hair should be treated (to include genital and anal areas, thighs, trunk, axillae, moustache and beard areas) and left on as per manufacturer's instructions. A second treatment after 7 days is advisable to kill lice emerging from any surviving nits. Dead nits may continue to adhere to hairs for several weeks following treatment and can be removed with a fine-tooth comb.

Suggested insecticide treatments

- Permethrin 5% dermal cream (a pyrethoid).
- Malathion 0.5% aqueous lotion (an organophosphate).

Alternatives

- Phenothrin 0.2% (a pyrethoid) only available as an alcoholic preparation and, therefore, more irritant. Same type of insecticide as permethrin; therefore, confers no advantage in cases of suspected permethrin resistance.
- Ivermectin (po) can be considered in resistant cases.

Eyelashes

Eyes must be kept closed throughout. Insecticide should be applied for 5–10 minutes and then rinsed off thoroughly. Treatment should be repeated after 7 days:

- Permethrin, 1% cream rinse, ensuring patient keeps eyes closed throughout the procedure and for the following 10 minutes.
- Malathion, 1% cream shampoo (unlicensed for eyelashes and cannot be prescribed on the NHS, but can be bought over the counter).
- Application of yellow soft paraffin or white soft paraffin, which suffocates and kills the lice by occluding their spiracles. This should be done bd for 8–10 days.
- Removal of lice with forceps.

Partner notification

Sexual partners within the previous 3 months should be advised to seek screening and treatment. Those sharing the same bedding may also require treatment.

Further information

℘ https://www.bashhguidelines.org/media/1074/28.pdf

Anogenital dermatoses

Common benign lesions/anomalies 346
Degenerative condition 347
Infective conditions 347
Inflammatory conditions 348
Ulcerative conditions 352
Premalignant conditions 354
Malignant conditions 356
Topical treatments 356

Common benign lesions/anomalies

- *Angiokeratomas*: purple/dark red papules on labia majora, scrotum, and penile shaft. Benign hyperkeratosis with dilated capillaries. Rarely associated with Anderson–Fabry disease.
- *Ectopic sebaceous glands (Fordyce spots)*: tiny yellow grouped papules. Occasionally, form larger nodules. Usually found on the mucosal surface of the prepuce and inner labia minora.
- *Epidermoid cysts*: white or creamy coloured nodules commonly found over scrotum and labia majora. Hair follicles blocked with keratin and filled with sebaceous matter. Can be removed surgically.
- *Epidermal naevi*: epidermal outgrowths present at birth (50%) or developing during childhood.
- *Haemangioma*: red macule up to 3–5 mm in diameter on glans penis or vulval mucosa.
- *Idiopathic calcinosis of the scrotum with multiple nodules*: starts in the teens and may be mistaken for cysts. Surgery may be necessary for troublesome lesions, but should be avoided if possible.
- *Melanocytic naevi (moles)*: genital lesions (keratinized skin) are found in 15% of the population.
- *Nabothian follicles*: bluish or yellow coloured translucent lumps on cervix. Retention cysts from cervical 'glands'.
- *Pearly penile papules*: white dome-shaped papules found at the corona and adjacent to the frenulum. Sometimes confused with warts. Reported in 20–50%, usually <1 mm in size, may extend to 3 mm. Consists of connective tissue core with central, thinned epidermis. Removal generally not recommended, but clearance possible with cryosurgery and CO_2 laser ablation.
- *Pigmentary changes*:
  - *vitiligo*—depigmentation (may also affect hair); association with autoimmunity, especially thyroiditis
  - *mucosal melanosis* (genital lentiginosis)—although unlikely to be malignant, all cases of vulval melanosis should be biopsied.
- *Prominent hair follicles*: found on penile shaft, scrotum, labia majora.
- *Seborrhoeic keratosis*: domed, often pigmented, papules. Commonly found on mons pubis, penile shaft, labia majora (usually in those aged >50 years). If removal required, cryosurgery or curettage.
- *Skin tags (achrocordon)*: common around the groin and thighs, especially in those aged >50 years; more common if obese.
- *Vulval papillae*: fleshy filiform papules, commonly found within the labia minora and often confused with warts. Typically, soft, symmetrical, linear, and pink with separate bases.

Degenerative condition

Ovarian failure, usually ↓ to the menopause, leads to urogenital atrophy, symptomatic in >50%. Symptoms include vulvo-vaginal dryness with discomfort, irritation, and dyspareunia. Often associated with other systemic symptoms, which may influence management. Treat with oestrogen-based hormone replacement therapy, which can be administered by various routes (oral, transdermal, vaginal). Urogenital symptoms may take some months to respond.

Infective conditions

Tinea cruris

Dermatophytic fungal infection commonly due to *Trichophyton rubrum* or *Epidermophyton floccosum*. Found in those sharing communal facilities (e.g. towels) and auto-inoculation from tinea pedis. Pruritic plaques in the groin, spreading out to the thigh, with well-defined erythematous scaly edge and central clearing.

Diagnosis

Appearance, scraping from margins for microscopy (dekeratinize with potassium hydroxide), and culture.

Management

Topical imidazoles bd for 2 weeks or topical terbinafine for 1–2 weeks; oral terbinafine 250 mg daily for 2–4 weeks or itraconazole 100 mg daily for 15 days or 200 mg daily for 7 days.

Erythrasma

Chronic infection of crural folds (especially axilla and groin) caused by *Corynebacterium minutissimum*. Associated with hyperhidrosis, diabetes mellitus, and living in crowded conditions. Dull red or brownish uniform scaly patch with little or no pruritus.

Diagnosis

Coral-pink fluorescence with Wood's light makes culture of scale unnecessary.

Management

Topical imidazoles for 2 weeks are usually effective. Sodium fusidate ointment 2%, topical erythromycin gel 2% bd for 2 weeks, or oral erythromycin are alternatives.

Inflammatory conditions

Irritant and contact dermatitis

See Box 29.1.
- *Irritant*: direct response to noxious agent, e.g. urine, chemicals, soaps, disinfectants.
- *Allergic*: idiosyncratic hypersensitivity reaction, e.g. spermicides, semen, or its contents (e.g. antibiotics), local anaesthetics, latex, deodorants, fragrances, lubricants, and body lotions containing propylene glycol or glycerin, anti-mycotic creams, or other topical medications.

Erythema, excoriation, pruritus
Thin mucosal skin is more prone to react to contact agents. May become chronic (lichen simplex chronicus) with excoriation producing lichenification and erythema, or hyperpigmentation.

Diagnosis
History, appearance, exclude infection. For contact dermatitis, patch testing can be considered, although positive results are often not relevant. Radio-allergosorbent and skin-prick tests can be performed for suspected Type I immediate hypersensitivity.

Management
Advise on avoiding irritants. If moderate to severe, low-potency topical steroids. If lichenified or failure to respond, moderate-potency topical steroids.

Seborrhoeic dermatitis

Scaly inflammation of sebaceous skin. More common with HIV infection. Presents as dry erythema with yellow scale (labia minora, sub-preputial sac, and glans penis).

Diagnosis
Appearance of erythematous lesions covered with greasy yellowish scales at other typical sites (scalp, eyebrows, nasolabial folds, sternum, axillae, umbilicus, natal cleft).

Box 29.1 Genital allergic contact hypersensitivity
- *Seminal fluid or its contents* (e.g. antibiotics): often associated with systemic symptoms.
- Spermicides and lubricants (may cause irritant or contact dermatitis).
- Latex or products used in condom manufacturing (e.g. carbamates).
- Topical skin preparations or chemicals (e.g. steroid preparations, anaesthetics, imidazoles). May cause irritant or allergic contact dermatitis.
- *Perfumes and cosmetic preparations*:
  - female hygiene sprays or wipes
  - bubble baths, scented soaps, hair shampoos
  - sanitary pads and towels (may be chemically treated).

Management

Combined imidazole plus hydrocortisone cream, ketoconazole shampoo (can use as shower gel), low-potency topical steroids and oral itraconazole if severe and extensive.

Fixed drug eruption

Reaction at the same site in an individual to repeated use of a systemic agent. Over 500 drugs implicated, including tetracyclines, barbiturates, phenolphthalein (chocolate laxative), sulfonamides, paracetamol. Preferentially affects genitals (especially glans penis). Sudden onset of erythematous macule or bulla with irritation or pain.

Diagnosis

History and appearance.

Management

Stop drug. Spontaneously resolves, but may leave hyperpigmentation.

Psoriasis

Affects ~2% of UK population, 30% familial incidence, increased severity with HIV infection. Anogenital/perigenital lesions common, which may be:
- *Well-demarcated erythematous scaly papules or plaques*: usually found on skin around genitalia, labia majora, scrotum, penile shaft, and occasionally glans penis.
- *Flexural*: macular erythematous non-scaly moist patches arising in perigenital flexures, peri-anal, labia minora, sub-preputial sac, and glans penis.

Diagnosis

Appearance: lesions in more classic sites (knees, elbows, scalp, nails with pitting), and histology.

Management

Moderate-potency topical corticosteroids, coal tar preparations. Systemic treatment (methotrexate, acitretin, ciclosporin,) may be necessary if disease is severe or extensive. Increasingly, biological agents such as etanercept are being used.

Lichen planus

Polygonal violaceous papules (2–10 mm) or annular lesions, which may be covered by white streaks (Wickham's striae). Usually found around flexor aspect of wrists, but genital involvement common and may cause erosions on mucous epithelium (See Plates 19 and 20) May lead to scarring with narrowing of introitus. Reticulate network over the buccal mucosa is characteristic. Itchy on skin; may be painful on mucous membranes. Has been associated with the development of squamous cell carcinoma (SCC) of the vulva.

Diagnosis

Appearance, classic sites, and histology (showing a band-like lymphohistiocytic infiltrate in the upper dermis, cytoid bodies, and basal cell hydropic degeneration.)

Management

Potent topical corticosteroids. Topical tacrolimus has been shown to be of benefit. This is an unlicensed indication and as the risk of malignancy is unknown, tacrolimus is not recommended as a first line agent.

Plasma cell balanitis (of Zoon)

Condition of middle-aged/older uncircumcised men. Moist shiny area of speckled erythema on glans or mucosal aspect of prepuce and often on adjacent surfaces. Half of cases have multiple lesions. Relatively asymptomatic despite striking appearance.

Diagnosis

Histology with heavy plasma cell infiltration; lozenge-shaped keratinocytes.

Management

Topical corticosteroids often combined with antimicrobials, e.g. Trimovate®, Betnovate C®. Persistent cases respond well to circumcision.

Plasma cell vulvitis

Similar histopathological features, but more symptomatic. Clinically resembles erosive lichen planus. Often associated with other dermatoses, such as lichen sclerosus, lichen planus, vulval and penile intraepithelial neoplasia.

Lichen sclerosus (LS)

Associated with autoimmune conditions, especially thyroid abnormalities in women and with trauma (Koebner phenomenon). Anogenital skin involvement common, but may also occur in extragenital sites. May be asymptomatic or cause pruritus, discomfort, and painful intercourse and defaecation.

Although there may be signs of acute inflammation, typical finding is ivory-white appearance associated with atrophy, purpura, erosions, or lichenification (see Plate 18). Men may develop phimosis and meatal strictures. Women may develop labial adhesions with fusion and anal fissuring, or stenosis and a loss of clitoral architecture. LS may simulate signs of sexual abuse in prepubertal girls, although abuse causing trauma may also predispose. May also cause phimosis in prepubertal boys.

▶ Penile carcinoma rarely reported with LS, but up to 5% ♀ with LS develop SCC of the vulva.

Diagnosis

Histology shows atrophic epidermis, hyalinization of the upper dermis, and a lymphohistiocytic infiltrate.

Management

If active, potent or very potent topical corticosteroids for 3 months then ↓ frequency of application, titrating against response. Topical tacrolimus has been helpful in some cases, but should be used cautiously due to risk of malignancy. Lubricants may help with intercourse. Acitretin has been shown to be of benefit, but is rarely necessary. UVA1 phototherapy has been used with some success. Surgical intervention may be required for urethral stenosis and circumcision for phimosis. Circumcision may be curative in men.

Hidradenitis suppurativa

Chronic inflammatory disorder of apocrine glands. Associated with acne, obesity, familial predisposition. Painful nodules, which may progress to abscesses, sinuses, fistulae, and scarring. Found in axillae, groin, buttocks, peri-anal skin.

Diagnosis

Clinical appearance. Exclude Crohn's disease.

Management

Weight reduction, chlorhexidine wash, topical clindamycin, long-term tetracyclines, other antibiotics used for acne, local or systemic steroids, and surgery for severe disease. A non-controlled study of oral clindamycin combined with rifampicin showed benefit. Biological drugs, including infliximab and etanercept, have been used with benefit in severe cases.

Ulcerative conditions

Aphthous ulcers

Common condition of unknown aetiology. Recurrent oral ulcers, rarely genital (especially vulva and scrotum). May be familial. Shallow painful ulcers about 1–10 mm in diameter with no systemic symptoms.

Diagnosis

Clinical features. Exclude HSV infection and Behçet's disease.

Management

Local anaesthetic gel, very potent topical steroids (if severe).

Lipschutz ulcers

Rapid onset, painful ulcers affecting vulva (typically labia minora) or lower vagina in young women. Often preceded by glandular fever type illness (has been associated with EBV, and other viral and bacterial infections).

Diagnosis

Classical history. Often a diagnosis of exclusion.

Management

Supportive (self-limiting, heal without scarring), pain relief (topical anaesthetics). Consider topical or short course oral steroids.

Behçet's disease

Multisystem disease of unknown aetiology, but more commonly found in the Middle and Far East (Silk Route). Associated with certain HLA types, especially B51.

Diagnosis

Based on defined clinical features according to the International Study Group for Behçet's disease (see Plates 21–24).
- Recurrent oral ulceration (as aphthosis) at least three times a year and two of the following:
  - genital ulcers (including epididymitis)
  - eye lesions (iritis, uveitis, cells in vitreous on slit-lamp examination, retinal vasculitis)
  - skin lesions (erythema nodosum, folliculitis, or papulopustular lesions, acneiform nodules in post-adolescents not on corticosteroids)
  - positive pathergy test (papule/pustule over 2 mm developing at site of hypodermic needle puncture; read at 24–48 hours).
- Neurological (meningoencephalitis, nerve palsies, brainstem, and spinal cord lesions), psychiatric changes, arthritis, thrombophlebitis and gastrointestinal features (diarrhoea, abdominal pain) may appear.

Management

Local topical steroids. Severe disease—systemic steroids, azathioprine, colchicine, dapsone, thalidomide. Anti-TNF therapy shows promise.

Erythema multiforme (EM) and Stevens–Johnson syndrome (SJS)

Acute skin reaction of unknown aetiology, but precipitated by infection (e.g. herpes simplex virus, *Mycoplasma pneumoniae*, *Histoplasma capsulatum*), drugs (e.g. sulfonamides, phenytoin, penicillin), autoimmune diseases (e.g. polyarteritis nodosa), sarcoidosis, malignancy, ↑ frequency of SJS with HIV infection. Non-pruritic maculopapular circular lesions with a deep red centre (may form bullae), and erythema producing target or iris lesions, typically found around the hands and feet. The severe bullous form (SJS) includes orogenital bullae with ulceration, urethritis, conjunctivitis and keratitis, pyrexia, and multisystem disease. Secondary infection and death may occur.

Diagnosis

Clinical features and histopathological changes with necrotic epidermal cells.

Management

EM resolves without scarring in 2–3 weeks. Currently, no active therapeutic regimen with unequivocal benefit exists for SJS, although a number of agents including systemic steroids, IV immunoglobulin, and ciclosporin have been tried.

Pyoderma gangrenosum

Associated with many conditions, particularly inflammatory bowel disease, seropositive and seronegative arthritis, and blood dyscrasias. Initial pustule progressing to a painful necrotic ulcer, occasionally affecting the vulva, penis, or scrotum.

Diagnosis

Appearance of ulcer with black undermined edge and associated pathology. Histology usually non-specific.

Management

Treat underlying condition. Topical or systemic corticosteroids, topical tacrolimus, ciclosporin. There are case reports of other immunomodulatory agents and biological drugs including infliximab and adalumimab being of value in treatment.

Pemphigus vulgaris

Most common type of pemphigus. Autoimmune condition. Age group 50–60 years usually affected. Cutaneous lesions appear as flaccid bullae, which burst to form erosions or ulcers. The mucosae, especially the mouth, are commonly involved. Genital ulcers are slow to heal, but only occasionally scar. Finger pressure on skin may cause epidermis to separate because of its poor attachment.

Diagnosis

Histology with direct or immunofluorescence to show intercellular deposits of IgG, and complement and serology to show circulating anti-epidermal antibodies.

Management

Local or systemic corticosteroids, tetracyclines, immunosuppressants (dapsone, azathioprine, mycophenolate mofetil). Biological drugs, especially rituximab, look promising in refractory cases.

Premalignant conditions

Extra-mammary Paget's disease

Most commonly found around anus and genitals, especially labia majora, typically presenting as well-defined erythematous scaly plaques, which may be itchy. May be associated with underlying adnexal carcinoma, possibly of sweat glands. A significant proportion have a primary carcinoma of other organs, particularly rectum, urethra, cervix, or breast.

Diagnosis

Histology shows typical large clear Paget cells in the epidermis.

Management

Excision where possible, but recurrence is common, as it is often multifocal. Topical imiquimod and photodynamic therapy have been reported to be helpful. Patients should be investigated for other carcinomas as above.

High-grade squamous intraepithelial lesions (HSIL) and low-grade squamous intraepithelial lesions (LSIL) of the genital tract

These pathological descriptive names encompass and replace other terms used to describe dysplasia and squamous cell carcinoma *in situ*, including Bowen's disease, bowenoid papulosis, and erythroplasia of Queyrat. Intra-epithelial neoplasia (IN) is commonly associated with LS, high-risk HPV in-fection and risk of IN elsewhere and is also found more frequently in those who are immunosuppressed (including with HIV infection). In 2004, the International Society for the Study of Vulvovaginal Diseases suggested only HSIL be classified as VIN, which was subdivided into usual type (associated with carcinogenic genotypes of HPV, smoking, and immunocompromised states) and differentiated type (associated with dermatological conditions such as LS). In 2015, a further reclassification was suggested, in which HSIL is analogous to usual type VIN and differentiated VIN remains the same. Flat lesions associated with basal cell atypia and koilocytic changes (formerly termed VIN1) are considered LSIL.

Vulval lesions

Usually ♀ aged 30–40 years, 70% current or past cigarette smokers, 50–90% association with HPV (especially type 16). Clinical appearance varies, but often presents as white plaques or nodular lesions, which may be pig-mented, with multifocal involvement (see Plate 17).

Penile lesions

Associated with HPV (especially type 16), smoking, and possibly agricultural chemicals. High-grade lesions found most commonly in the 6th decade. Usually presents as multiple lesions which may be:
- flat (grey/red, well demarcated with increased vascularity)
- small plaques of leukoplakia (hyperkeratinized)
- papular and pigmented.

In addition, usually in older uncircumcised ♂, there may be mucosal erythroplastic lesions (shiny friable moist red lesions on glans penis or mu-cosal surface of prepuce).

Anal lesions

Found most commonly in MSM, especially those with HIV infection, and in ♀ with a history of anal sex. Human papilloma virus 16 is associated with anal SCC.

Management of external anogenital IN

There is little evidence-based data on the management of this group of conditions. Current practice depends on the grading and extent of the pathology, influenced by clinical factors, such as appearance and symptoms. Patients should be screened for HIV infection. If HIV +ve, review should be maintained indefinitely. HSIL carries a 5–10% risk of subsequent SCC; therefore, treatment is usually advised. This includes topical imiquimod, surgical excision, and destructive methods including laser and electrodessication. Review after treatment required as ~30% recur within 5 years.

Malignant conditions

Rarely seen in the GUM clinic, but require urgent referral elsewhere.
- *SCC*: associated with IN and LS.
- *Melanoma*: rare on penis, but genital lesions reported to account for 2–3% of melanomas in ♀.
- *Basal cell carcinoma*: rare on surfaces not commonly exposed to the sun. However, genital lesions have been reported, especially scrotal.

Topical treatments

Emollients

Oil-based emollients are preferable to water-based emollients as they are better absorbed and contain fewer preservatives, which can be potentially irritant or sensitizing.

It may be helpful to give patients a selection of emollient samples so that they can choose their favourite and, therefore, improve adherence.

Aqueous cream should only be used as a soap substitute. It is not suitable as a 'leave-on' product, as it contains sodium lauryl sulphate.

Spray emollients can be useful as they are easy to apply and can reduce 'drag' on delicate, inflamed skin/genital mucosa.

Steroids

See Table 29.1.

Table 29.1 Topical steroid preparations

Strength	Name
Mild	Hydrocortisone 0.1–2.5%
	Mild with antimicrobials: e.g. Canesten HC®
Moderate	*Betamethasone valerate 0.025%*: e.g. Betnovate-RD®
	Clobetasone butyrate 0.05%: e.g. Eumovate®
	Moderate with antimicrobials: e.g. Trimovate®
Potent	*Beclomethasone diproprionate 0.025%*: e.g. Betnovate®
	Hydrocortisone butyrate 0.1%: e.g. Locoid®
	Potent with antimicrobials: e.g. Betnovate-C®
Very potent	*Clobetasol propionate 0.05%*: e.g. Dermovate®
	Diflucortolone valerate 0.3%: e.g. Nerisone Forte®
	Very potent with antimicrobials: e.g. clobetasol with neomycin and nystatin 'Dermovate® NN'

Chapter 30

Cervical neoplasia

Introduction 358
Histology of the normal cervix 358
Risk factors 359
Clinical features 359
Screening 360
Diagnosis 362
Management 363
Primary prevention 363
Pregnancy 364
HIV 364

Introduction

Cervical cancer is a malignant neoplasm of the uterine cervix and the 4th most common cancer in ♀ worldwide. 85% of cases occur in developing countries. An estimated 266,000 deaths from cervical cancer occurred worldwide in 2012, which accounts for 7.5% of ♀ cancer deaths. Cervical screening and treatment of high-grade cervical intraepithelial neoplasia HGCIN aims to prevent development of invasive cervical cancer (ICC).

Histology of the normal cervix

The vagina and ectocervix are lined with stratified squamous epithelium, and the endocervix with columnar epithelium. The position of the squamo-columnar junction (SCJ) varies throughout life. Hormonal changes (puberty, pregnancy) lead to enlarging of the cervix and eversion of the endocervical columnar epithelium, moving the SCJ distally. This is counterbalanced by squamous metaplasia (the normal process of reversion to squamous epithelium). The area between the original and receding SCJ is known as the transformation zone (TZ), which is susceptible to malignant change when exposed to oncogenic stimuli.

Terminology

- *Atypia*: epithelial cells showing nuclear or cytoplasmic abnormalities that are not considered to be malignant or premalignant. Koilocytic atypia describes atypical cells with a perinuclear halo associated with HPV infection.
- *Dyskaryosis*: nuclear abnormality of cervical epithelial cells, graded as low or high grade. This is examined for during cytological cervical screening programmes.
- *CIN*: squamous cell premalignant lesion (also known as dysplasia). Architectural and cytological changes in squamous epithelial cells; a histological diagnosis. Grades of CIN are based on depth of epithelial involvement. The basement membrane is always intact.
  - *CIN1*—lowest 1/3 only (mild dysplasia)
  - *CIN2*—lower 2/3 (moderate dysplasia)
  - *CIN3*—>2/3 of epithelial cells abnormal (severe dysplasia).
- *Cervical glandular intra-epithelial neoplasia (CGIN)*: columnar cell premalignant lesion, less common than CIN; also a histological diagnosis. Nuclear, nucleolar, and glandular structural abnormalities are seen in columnar epithelial cells. Low-grade (LCGIN) is also known as endocervical gland dysplasia. HCGIN is also known as adenocarcinoma *in situ*.
- *ICC*: penetration of basement membrane by malignant epithelial cells.

Risk factors

- *HPV* (➲ Chapter 23, 'Aetiology', p. 292): High risk HPV (HR-HPV) is implicated in both SCC and adenocarcinoma, although only a small number of ♀ infected with HR-HPV develop cervical cancer. HPV DNA is detected in 95% of cervical cancer precursors. HPV 16 and 18 have been associated with around 70% of cervical cancers.
- *CIN*: has the potential to develop into cervical cancer, but may regress or persist as CIN. The oncogenic potential of the HPV type and environmental factors (e.g. smoking, immunosuppression) will influence risk of progression, as well as histological grade of CIN. Estimates of progression from CIN 3 to ICC range 12–40%.
- *CGIN*: pre-invasive stage of adenocarcinoma.
- *Other STIs*: may ↑ risk of progression of HPV infection to dyskaryosis, probably 2° to cervicitis.
- *Sexual activity*: relative risk 2.5 if coitarche <18 years compared with >21 years. ≥5 lifetime partners confers a relative risk of 2.8.
- *Parity and age at first pregnancy*: ↑ risk with ↑ parity, independent of other risk factors. ↑ risk with ↓ age at 1st pregnancy.
- *Smoking*: appears to ↑ risk of ICC two-fold.
- *Lower socioeconomic class*: linked to ↑ risk of ICC.
- *Combined oral contraception*: long-term use (>10 years).
- *Immunosuppression*: ↑ persistence of HPV infection.

Clinical features

- CIN is typically asymptomatic, but should be considered in those with PCB or IMB.
- ICC can have a variety of clinical presentations. Women may be asymptomatic, present with irregular vaginal bleeding or, if advanced, with symptoms of a mass or metastatic disease.
- If ICC presents with symptoms, it is usually more advanced so signs are often evident, e.g. fixed uterus and parametrial/posterior pelvic induration, hepatosplenomegaly or inguinal/supraclavicular lymph node enlargement. Subtle signs of early stages of ICC may be missed, e.g. pronounced cervical contact bleeding, hard or irregular and enlarged or ulcerated cervix, profuse offensive vaginal discharge.

Screening

Cytological screening involves collection, staining, and microscopic examination of epithelial cells from the cervix, looking for dyskaryosis

Liquid-based cytology

- The newer technique of liquid-based cytology (LBC) has replaced Papinacolaou smears (see Box 30.1).
- Advantages include less unsatisfactory samples, easier analysis, and the ability for the sample to be tested for HPV DNA and other biomarkers.
- 'Unsatisfactory' results (usually <2%) are due to insufficient epithelial cells, or the presence of blood or pus cells.
- False-negative results may be found in established ICC because of cell necrosis.
- Closer correlation between cytological and histological findings occurs with higher degrees of abnormality.
- Cytology laboratories will advise on the correct management and follow-up of abnormal cytology. (See Box 30.2 for English guidance).
- Coincidental findings (including *Trichomonas vaginalis* (TV), *Candida* spp., *Neisseria gonorrhoeae*, genital herpes, and *Actinomyces*-like organisms) may be seen during microscopy. Most would require clinical evaluation and confirmation before treatment. It should be noted, however, that the specificity for the finding of TV probably exceeds 98% on LBC samples.

Classification

The British Association for Cytopathology (BAC)/NHS Cervical Screening Program (NHSCSP) 2013 classification of cervical cytology is used in the UK, and the Bethesda system is used more widely worldwide (Tables 30.1 and 30.2).

HPV DNA triage and primary screening

The NHSCSP has introduced HPV triage to discriminate between ♀ at increased risk of high-grade CIN requiring colposcopic diagnosis and low risk ♀, who may return to routine screening (➔ Chapter 30, 'Cytological indications for colposcopy', p. 362).

Trans people

Any trans person with a cervix should be offered cervical screening. This may fall outside of the national call/recall system if their gender identity on their NHS records is male. A local arrangement for reminders may need to be sought. (➔ Chapter 3, 'Other issues', p. 46).

> **Box 30.1 Cervical cytology technique**
> - Take cervical smear before cleaning the cervix and taking any endocervical swabs.
> - Note macroscopic appearance of the cervix. Defer cytology if marked cervicitis.
> - Sweep 360° around the cervix ×5 in a clockwise direction, ensuring TZ sampling.
> - For LBC, the end of the sampling brush is rinsed or broken off into the preservative medium.

Box 30.2 Cervical cytology guidance in England

A computerized call–recall system invites ♀ registered with a GP for screening:

- 3-yearly aged 25–49.
- 5-yearly aged 50–64.
- ♀ aged 65+, only if not screened since age 50 or a recent abnormality).

Screening can be done in GUM, sexual health, and primary care. A copy of the result should go to the patient's GP. In the UK, screening commences at age 25. Below this age, most low-grade abnormalities due to HR-HPV resolves spontaneously and, where identified, may result in over-investigation and/or treatment with potential adverse reproductive outcomes. Furthermore, the rate of cervical cancer is extremely low, with cytology screening not having any impact.

Table 30.1 Classification of CIN: squamous lesions

BAC/NHSCSP (2013)	Bethesda system (2015)	
Cytology		Histology
Borderline changes in squamous cells	Atypical squamous cells of uncertain significance (ASCUS)	HPV
	Atypical squamous cells cannot exclude HSIL	
Low-grade dyskaryosis	LSIL	CIN1
High-grade dyskaryosis (moderate)	HSIL	CIN2
High-grade dyskaryosis (severe)	HSIL	CIN3
High-grade dyskaryosis/ invasive SCC	HSIL SCC	SCC

Data from: NHS Cervical Screening Programme (2013) Achievable standards, benchmarks for reporting, and criteria for evaluating cervical cytopathology, and Nayar and Wilbur (2015) *The Bethesda System for Reporting Cervical Cytology.* Berlin, Springer.

Table 30.2 Classification of glandular lesions

BAC/NHSCSP (2013)	Bethesda system (2015)
Borderline nuclear changes, endocervical	Atypical glandular cells (endocervical/endometrial/glandular)
Glandular neoplasia of endocervical type or glandular neoplasia of non-cervical type	Atypical glandular cells (endocervical/glandular) favour neoplastic
	Endocervical adenocarcinoma *in situ*
	Adenocarcinoma (endocervical, endometrial, extra-uterine, other)

Data from: NHS Cervical Screening Programme (2013) Achievable standards, Benchmarks for reporting, and Criteria for evaluating cervical cytopathology, and Nayar and Wilbur (2015) *The Bethesda System for Reporting Cervical Cytology.* Berlin: Springer.

Diagnosis

Colposcopy is an investigation of cervical premalignancy. It uses up to ×40 magnification and acetic acid +/− iodine, to visually grade CIN, and highlight optimal sites for biopsy for histopathological assessment.

The entire SCJ should be visualized and abnormalities graded by:

- appearances of acetowhite epithelium
- iodine negativity
- vascular pattern, e.g. mosaicism, punctuation.

CIN

Cytological indications for colposcopy

- *suspected ICC or glandular neoplasia*: urgent
- high grade dyskaryosis (moderate or severe)
- low grade dyskaryosis/borderline nuclear changes if the sample is HR-HPV positive or if ♀ is HIV positive
- *unsatisfactory/inadequate samples*: indicated if three consecutive unsatisfactory smears (taken at 3-monthly intervals).

Clinical indications for colposcopy or gynaecological assessment

Symptoms raising suspicion of cancer after excluding infection (e.g. persistent vaginal discharge, IMB, PCB in ♀ >40 years, post-menopausal bleeding).

CGIN

Atypical glandular cytology may indicate invasive cervical adenocarcinoma, CGIN, CIN, or endometrial pathology. Endometrial cells on cytology in post-menopausal ♀ raises suspicion of endometrial disease and should be investigated. If borderline glandular cells are present, colposcopy is recommended for cervical biopsies and endometrial sampling. Punch biopsy not reliable for atypical glandular cytology. Excisional conization for diagnosis +/− treatment is recommended.

ICC

A suspicious-looking cervix may warrant further investigation. Speculum examination may reveal an obvious cervical tumour, requiring biopsy to confirm the diagnosis.

Management

Management of CIN and CGIN

Aims of treatment are to eradicate intraepithelial lesions, while minimizing associated morbidity and adverse reproductive outcomes.

CIN is managed by accredited colposcopists and ♀ should receive clear information and have access to appropriate counselling.

Options include:

- *Ablation*: by cryotherapy (only for small size CIN1) or laser vaporization (unless suspected invasion, glandular disease, SCJ not visualized, or previous treatment for CIN).
- *Excision*: has largely replaced ablation because of better results, greater applicability, more rapid treatment with less bleeding, and lower cost of equipment.
- *Cone biopsy*: preferred method for adenocarcinoma *in situ*.

CGIN can be managed with local excision and surveillance if excision margins are free from disease. If family is complete, hysterectomy should be considered.

There is risk of residual or recurrent disease after CIN and CGIN treatment. HPV DNA as a 'test of cure' reduces the duration of surveillance following treatment by safely returning women who test negative to routine recall at an earlier date.

Management of cervical cancer

Histological diagnosis and clinical staging guide treatment decisions. Age, fertility requirements, and general fitness influence management. As for all cancer treatments, these may be curative or palliative.

Treatment options include cone biopsy/loop excision/trachelectomy (removal of cervix only), total/radical hysterectomy, radiotherapy, and chemotherapy.

The treatment of ICC and its associated effects include early menopause, loss of fertility, and vaginal stenosis causing dyspareunia.

Primary Prevention

HPV vaccination aims to prevent CIN, ICC and other HPV related disease. Both bivalent and quadrivalent vaccines have been shown in large randomized control trials to be highly efficacious at reducing CIN and also provide herd immunity against other HPV types.

Pregnancy

Routine cervical screening should be deferred if pregnant until postpartum unless the ♀ has missed or defaulted her appointment prior to pregnancy. Colposcopic assessment of the pregnant ♀ requires a high degree of skill. The aim is to exclude invasive disease and where possible to defer biopsy or treatment until postpartum.

HIV

Cervical cancer is ~5× more common in women living with HIV. Advanced HIV disease is the strongest independent risk factor for developing cervical abnormalities. All ♀ with a new HIV diagnosis should ideally have a baseline colposcopy and thereafter, annual cervical screening. Subsequent colposcopy should follow national screening guidance. The recommended age range for screening is the same as for all women (although clinicians may make local arrangements for younger women). Invasive cervical cancer is AIDS defining.

Vulval pain

Introduction 366
Aetiology 367
Clinical features 367
Management 368
Prognosis 372

Introduction

Vulval pain has many causes—inflammatory, infectious, and neoplastic. This chapter describes an approach to managing vulvodynia as a cause of vulval pain; however, pain management principles can be applied to other causes of vulval and pelvic pain, and apply to male urogenital pain.

Definition of vulvodynia

Vulvodynia is described as 'vulval discomfort, most often described as burning pain, occurring in the absence of relevant visible findings or a specific, clinically identifiable, neurological disorder' (International Society for the Study of Vulval Diseases).

Classification
- *provoked*: pain occurs on touch
- *spontaneous*: pain can occur at any time
- *mixed*: occurs on touch, but can also be spontaneous.

It is then subdivided into:
- *local*: an isolated area of pain (vestibulodynia)
- *generalized*: it is more widespread over the vulval area.

Vulvodynia is a clinical diagnosis without identifiable pathology. It is important not to diagnose someone with vulvodynia unless other causes of vulval pain are excluded; otherwise pathology and treatment options may be missed. Descriptions such as vestibulitis and vulval dysaesthesia should be avoided as they can lead to confusion.

It is not uncommon for ♀ to have experienced many years of symptoms before a diagnosis is reached. They have often self-treated for *Candida* infection or may have attributed their symptoms to other causes, such as the menopause. Recognition and appreciation of a defined clinical entity is important and reassures the patient.

Vulvodynia can be devastating for the ♀—it can affect intimate relationships, and lead to social isolation and depression. Both the physical pain and the psychosocial consequences of the pain need management.

Aetiology

About 50% will have a trigger factor, e.g. childbirth, chronic candida infection. The remaining cases develop gradually, with no identifiable provoking factor. Several aetiological factors have been proposed, including pelvic floor muscle hypertonicity, genetic factors, bacterial inflammatory processes, and altered CNS function. It is likely to be multifactorial. The European Association of Urologists Guidelines on chronic pelvic pain are updated annually and available online. The introduction contains details on aetiology and mechanism of pain.

Clinical features

Neuralgic type vulval discomfort is characterized usually by burning, stinging, irritation, and/or rawness. Symptoms may be described as hyperaesthesia (exaggerated pain response) or allodynia (when sensation differs to that applied, e.g. light touch can cause pain response).

For ♀ with unprovoked pain, symptoms can worsen while sitting and towards the end of the day. Provoked pain typically causes associated intolerance of tampon insertion because of local pain, and pain on touch or attempted vaginal entry (superficial dyspareunia).

Management

Management should be a team approach. Involve the GP, specialist physio-therapist, psychosexual therapist (if relevant), and pain team, in addition to the vulval specialist. The biopsychosocial approach to pain management should be followed.

History-taking

- Explore the site and extent of pain, psychosexual and relationship issues, and possible features of depression.
- Ask the patient what the pain prevents them from doing.
- Ask the patient to score the pain on a scale from 0 to 10 (where 10 is the worst pain imaginable).
- Check if pain is provoked by sitting and relieved by standing, which can be a sign of pudendal neuralgia (refer to pain team for assessment and pudendal nerve block).
- Is the pain intermittent lasting few days/weeks then resolving completely before next episode, or do exacerbations follow this pattern? Atypical herpes presentation could be considered, and trial of suppressive acyclovir prescribed.
- Do they experience pain elsewhere – bladder pain, bowel pain (irritable bowel syndrome), dysmenorrhoea, trigeminal neuralgia, fibromyalgia.
- Establish who they have seen and are currently under, and what investigations have been performed. Gain consent to communicate with all those involved in care to ensure team approach to pain management.

Examination and investigations

No visible signs usually, but can be associated with varying degree of ery-thema. However, a light touch with a cotton bud can produce pain that outweighs any mild erythema present. It can be useful to map out the area of pain experienced, to determine whether it is local or generalized.

- *Exclude other causes*: full STI screen (including tests for chlamydia, gonorrhoea, trichomonas, and candida, and microscopy.) Blind self-taken swabs should be considered if speculum not tolerated.
- Examine vulval skin for signs of genital dermatological conditions.
- In cases of diagnostic uncertainty, a second opinion may be helpful.
- Pelvic MRI for unprovoked pain is not routinely recommended. Consider imaging if associated back pain, unilateral pain, or history of trauma.
- Biopsy is not helpful unless a genital dermatosis suspected.

Patient information

- *Establish the diagnosis*: if it is uncertain diagnose 'vulval pain of unknown cause' until clear.
- Provide verbal and written advice on vulvodynia.
- Give details of Vulval Pain Society for further information and telephone advice (℘ www.vulvalpainsociety.org).
- Avoid skin allergens and advise washing with a soap substitute, such as epaderm ointment.
- Advise those who experience pain on sitting to purchase a doughnut-shaped cushion.

Topical treatment

- *5% lidocaine ointment* can be applied to site of pain if external for men and women. Takes 10 minutes to start taking effect.
- Always suggest small test area to genitals first, as some may experience burning. Advise the patient to wait for 10 minutes after applying and if the area is still burning, wash off the ointment thoroughly. Burning sensation usually subsides after a couple of minutes.
- Can be used 'as and when' (e.g. prior to sex, car journeys, or other provoking factors), or applied regularly qds.
- *If using for sex*: non-latex condoms need to be used to prevent lidocaine transferring on to partner. Lidocaine can affect the durability of latex condoms.
- Alternatively, place lidocaine on cotton wool pad/ball and apply to area of pain at night, wearing underwear to keep in place. Wash off next morning. If no adverse reaction, continue every night for 3–6 months (some evidence to support lasting analgesic effects.)

Oral treatments

- *Useful for managing unprovoked pain*: evidence for provoked pain less clear, but can be used when topical, physiotherapy, and psychological therapies are not resolving pain
- *Start dose low and build up gradually*: explain to patient that benefit might not be immediate or occur at low dose. Roughly 1 in 3 ♀ have to switch treatments due to side effects, and 1 in 3 ♀ do not gain relief from the chosen treatment and need to switch. Therefore, unusual to get a 'quick fix' and patients should be aware of this.
- Consider simple analgesia if they are providing partial benefit (paracetamol, NSAIDS, codeine phosphate), while awaiting effects from/in addition to other oral treatments listed below. Discontinue if ineffective or if side effects outweigh benefits.
- Once pain controlled, continue drug treatment for a period of stability (months). They should not be stopped suddenly, but withdrawn slowly (build-up in reverse), while assessing effect. If pain returns, continue drug in lowest effective dosage. Can be difficult to discontinue. Support and reassurance vital.
- *Things to consider when choosing drug options*:
  - drug interactions with other medications
  - check contraindications in BNF
  - previous treatments tried (what dose did they reach, why did they stop); often drugs stopped too soon or used incorrectly, and taken 'as and when', rather than daily. Consider retrying. Good practice to include detailed relevant drug history in correspondence
  - cost
  - *other symptoms*—depression, anxiety, urinary frequency (may be able to choose a drug that treats these symptoms, too)
  - drugs such as pregabalin have a 'street value'.
- *First line*: nortriptyline, amitriptyline, and/or gabapentin.
- *Second line*: pregabalin.
- *Third line*: duloxetine.

- *Nortriptyline/amitriptyline*: start at 10 mg and increase every 1–2 weeks by 10 mg to maximum of 75 mg. Amitriptyline cheaper than nortriptyline and often used first line, but if not tolerated, a direct switch at the same dose can be made between the two drugs. If unable to exclude arrhythmia/cardiac history, request ECG prior to starting nortriptyline. If dose not tolerated due to side effects consider:
  - switching amitriptyline to nortriptyline
  - switching nortriptyline to gabapentin.
- If benefiting from sedative effects, but not complete analgesic response, continue nortriptyline/amitriptyline, add gabapentin, and assess monthly for analgesic effect up to 2 months.
- *Gabapentin*: consider baseline FBC, urea & electrolytes (U&E), LFT (if normal no need for further monitoring, but if continuing long term, consider an annual check). See Table 31.1 for dose increases. If dose tolerated, continue to next step. If pain relief not achieved following 2 weeks of 900 mg tid, then unlikely to improve further. Swap gabapentin to pregabalin if side effects.
- *Pregabalin*: consider baseline FBC, U&E, LFT (if normal no need for further monitoring, but if continuing long term, consider an annual check). Remember cost of pregabalin is per tablet, not dose, therefore, do not prescribe 75 mg tablets for 300 mg dose as this is ×8 more expensive. This does not apply to gabapentin. If not helping, wean patient off and try something else. *Escalation steps*—every 3–7 days depending on tolerability (see Table 31.2).
- *Duloxetine*: this is more expensive so reserve for when other medication is contraindicated or fails to reduce pain. No blood monitoring needed. Suggest taking with food before bedtime. Start 30 mg for 2 weeks and increase to 60 mg from week 3 if needed.

Table 31.1 Gabapentin dose increases

Week	Dose am	Dose noon	Dose bedtime
1	0	0	300 mg
2	300 mg	0	300 mg
3	300 mg	300 mg	300 mg
4	300 mg	300 mg	600 mg
5	300 mg	600 mg	600 mg
6	600 mg	600 mg	600 mg
7	600 mg	600 mg	900 mg
8	600 mg	900 mg	900 mg
9	900 mg	900 mg	900 mg

Table 31.2 Pregabalin escalation steps

Escalation steps	Dose am	Dose bedtime
1	0	75 mg
2	75 mg	75 mg
3	75 mg	150 mg
4	150 mg	150 mg
5	150 mg	225 mg
6	225 mg	225 mg
7	225 mg	300 mg
8 onwards	300 mg	300 mg

Physiotherapy

- Pelvic hypertonia and vaginismus can be associated with any chronic cause of vulval pain. Use biofeedback technique to help relax pelvic floor to lessen pain (sensor is placed in vagina and contraction results in light change or computer image).
- Massage, TENS, and vaginal trainers can also be used.
- 70% of women have complete response or notice improvement for provoked pain.

Clinical psychology

Techniques such as mindfulness and cognitive behavioural therapy can be used to improve quality of life and improve pain-coping mechanisms.

Psychosexual therapy

Ideally, with their partner. Can help with 2° complications (e.g. vaginismus, loss of libido, anorgasmia, poor lubrication) and improving non-coital sexual contact.

Other treatments

- *Codeine, dihydrocodeine, tramadol (in addition to above drugs)*: only continue if analgesic, rather than sedative benefit, not recommended long term.
- *Strong opioids*: discuss with pain team.
- *Carbamazepine*: discuss with pain team.
- *Nerve blocks*: discuss with pain team.
- *Local excision*: for localized provoked pain—combine with psychotherapy and consider only if all other options unsuccessful. Always remember to reconsider the diagnosis if patient is unresponsive to treatment. Modified vestibulectomy works best, with 90% having complete or partial response. Vestibuloplasty and laser vaporization are not recommended.
- *Reduce urinary oxalate concentration*: low oxalate diet and calcium citrate without vitamin D. Evidence lacking, but some patients find it helpful.
- Apply white soft paraffin over vulva for swimming.
- *Antihistamines*: if patient has dermographism.
- *Acupuncture*: some women with unprovoked pain have had benefit.
- *Botox® injection into affected areas*: to date, use is limited, but looks promising.

Prognosis

At least partial relief of symptoms occurs in 40–50% of cases (regardless of approach). If triggered by an infection, prognosis is better.

Streptococcal and staphylococcal infections

Streptococcal infections 374
Staphylococcus aureus 376

Streptococcal infections

Group A β-haemolytic streptococci (GAS): *Streptococcus pyogenes*

- Infection control hazard organism (5–12% of severe infections are healthcare-associated).
- Significant cause of puerperal sepsis on maternity units.
- Transmission is mostly by direct contact (Semmelweis identified the importance of handwashing in the prevention of spread of infection).
- Recognized cause of acute vaginitis (including in pre-pubertal girls), purulent vaginal discharge and balanitis (e.g. pyoderma following receptive oral sex).
- Important cause of necrotizing fasciitis.

Management
Simple infections pending antibiotic sensitivities
- Amoxicillin 500 mg tid for 5 days, or phenoxymethylpenicillin (Penicillin V) 500 mg qds for 10 days.
- Azithromycin 500 mg od for 5 days, or clindamycin 300 mg qds for 10 days.

Group B β-haemolytic streptococci (GBS): *Streptococcus agalactiae*

- GBS is present in the bowel flora of 20–40% of adults (colonization).
- Usually not pathogenic (except in pregnancy).
- Diabetes, neurological impairment, and cirrhosis ↑ risk for invasive GBS disease.
- Skin, soft-tissue, and osteoarticular infections, and urosepsis are relatively common presentations.
- In men, GBS may cause mild balanitis, rarely progressing to cellulitis. In women, it can be associated with BV and rarely vaginitis.

Pregnancy
- Most frequent cause of severe early-onset (EO) infection in newborn infants.
- The incidence of EO GBS disease in the UK and Ireland in 2015 was 0.57/1000 births (517 cases).

Risk factors for neonatal infection include:
- Previous baby affected by GBS disease.
- GBS bacteriuria or vaginal swab positive for GBS.
- Preterm birth or prolonged rupture of membranes, or maternal temperature of 38°C or greater in labour, or chorioamnionitis.

Screening for GBS
- Universal bacteriological screening is not recommended by the Royal College of Obstetricians & Gynaecologists in the UK (Green-top Guideline no. 36)

- However, if the woman is found to be a carrier during the current pregnancy, intrapartum antibiotic prophylaxis (IAP) should be offered. Antenatal treatment is not recommended.
- A positive bacteriological test indicates an approximate risk of 1 in 400 for EO GBS in the newborn infant.

IAP

- Practice varies worldwide. Since 2002, US guidelines have advised that all pregnant women should be offered screening for GBS carriage at 35–37 weeks gestation, and those found to be colonized with GBS (or who go into labour before this time) should be offered IAP.
- The antibiotic regimen of choice will depend on local microbiology guidance.
- In the UK, most guidelines recommend benzylpenicillin, also known as penicillin G. Recommended regimen is IV benzylpenicillin 3 g at onset of labour, then 1.5 g six times daily until delivery (alternatively cefuroxime 1.5 g loading dose followed by 750 mg tid, or vancomycin 1 g bd).
- In case of maternal pyrexia or chorioamnionitis, the recommended regimen is IV amoxicillin 2 g qds (alternatively, cefuroxime 1.5 g qds).
- Clindamycin can no longer be recommended, as the current resistance rate in the UK is 16%.

Staphylococcus aureus

- Vaginal colonization is common (10–15% of women).
- Colonization of the nose and groin is even more common (approximately 30% of the adult population).
- Common cause of vaginitis in children.
- In adults, may cause folliculitis, balanitis, Bartholin's gland infections, as well as inguinal lymphadenopathy and soreness.
- Vulvo-vaginitis may be associated with poor hygiene, or skin irritation due to soaps.
- Post-partum endometritis is often polymicrobial, but may be caused by *S. aureus.*
- HIV infection predisposes to MRSA colonization.

Panton–Valentine Leucocidin-positive (PVL) S. aureus

- PVL is a toxin produced by certain types of *S. aureus,* which can kill WBC, and cause damage to skin and deeper tissues.
- The symptoms include recurrent and painful boils or red areas on the skin, often in more than one place, which do not get better, despite antibiotic treatment.
- *Risk factors ('5 C's'):* close contact; contaminated items (including razors); crowding; cuts and grazes; and cleanliness (poor hygiene conditions).

Toxic shock syndrome (TSS)

- An acute multi-system illness characterized by fever, hypotension, erythematous rash, diarrhoea, and desquamation of the skin upon recovery.
- In the appropriate clinical context, isolation of a toxin-producing *S. aureus* from a mucous membrane is strong support for a diagnosis of TSS.
- Risk factors for TSS include tampon use, childbirth or other surgical wound infection, contraceptive diaphragm use, and cervicovaginal colonization with *S. aureus.*
- Tampons should be changed regularly, and diaphragms should not be left *in situ* for longer than contraceptive need dictates.

Management

- Simple infections pending antibiotic sensitivities: flucloxacillin 500 mg qds for 5 days (alternatively clindamycin 300 mg qds for 5 days).
- In case of MRSA infection, seek antibiotic susceptibility data; MRSA is inherently resistant to flucloxacillin.
- *TSS:* supportive treatment (for shock), removal of retained tampon or diaphragm, and treatment with high-dose antibiotics. Also consider IV immunoglobulin.

Genital anomalies

Men *378*
Women *380*

Men

Epispadias

Absence of upper wall of urethra. Frequency 1 in 30,000. Urethra opens onto the dorsum of the glans penis or penile shaft as an epithelial-lined groove.

Hypospadias

Termination of urethra ventral and posterior to its normal opening. Frequency 1 in 160–1800. Orifice found anywhere from the glans to the perineum. Often associated with other local anomalies [under-developed foreskin, chordee (downward bending of penis), meatal stenosis].

Lymphocele

Non-tender cord-like firm swelling in coronal sulcus. Probably related to sexual trauma (prolonged or frequent intercourse). May be associated with preputial oedema. Self-limiting (usually within days, up to 3 weeks); just requires reassurance.

Paraphimosis

Strangulation of the glans penis by retracted prepuce. Usually results from partially phimotic prepuce, which has been retracted and cannot be reduced. However, may follow trauma with swelling of the glans (e.g. from vigorous sexual activity) with a retracted normal calibre prepuce. Requires urgent intervention either by manual reduction (using anaesthetic cream and ice to reduce oedema) or by surgical intervention to prevent infection and gangrene.

Peyronie's disease

Fibrous infiltration of the penile intracavernous septum. Leads to single plaque formation, causing curvature and angulation of the erect penis, pain and subsequent erectile dysfunction. Cause unknown, but associated with penile trauma, diabetes mellitus, and Dupuytren's contracture. May spontaneously resolve. If not, medical treatments (intralesional or systemic) or surgical options may be considered.

Phimosis

Tight constriction of the prepuce, preventing retraction over the glans penis. Aetiology includes;
- *Congenital*: physiological in 1st year of life.
- *Acute*: underlying infection, e.g. syphilis (sub-preputial chancre), genital herpes, candidiasis.
- *Chronic and progressive*: response to repeated trauma (physical, chemical, repeated infections), skin disorders (e.g. lichen sclerosus), local malignancy.

Surgical referral for circumcision may be required.

Priapism

Pathologically prolonged erection without libido. May be associated with blood disorders (e.g. sickle-cell disease, leukaemia), drugs used to manage erectile dysfunction, and rarely infection (e.g. gonorrhoea). ▶ Failure to achieve detumescence using ice packs requires urgent urological referral.

Spermatoceles and epididymal cysts

Commonly detected as incidental findings or raised by concerned patient, especially those aged >40 years. Usually <1 cm in diameter and filled with spermatozoa (spermatoceles) or serum (epididymal cysts); therefore, they transilluminate well. They arise from the epididymis (not testis) and generally reassurance can be given. If large or painful, they can be aspirated by needle, but surgical removal is not advised as there is a risk of sterility. Ultrasonography is recommended for intrascrotal lumps or swellings where malignancy is considered.

Urethral channels (accessory)

Open dorsal or ventral to urethra, and are usually rudimentary blind tracts, although they may terminate in bladder or posterior urethra. Accessory peri-urethral ducts are commonly found in ♂ opening into or around the meatus, and are blind tracts extending from 2 to 10 mm.

Varicocele

Dilatation and tortuosity of the veins of the scrotal pampiniform plexus (along the spermatic cord). 90% are left sided (due to difference in drainage routes of left versus right spermatic veins) 10–17% of young ♂ affected, with spontaneous regression common. Swollen veins within the scrotum are bluish and feel like a 'bag of worms'. Most commonly diagnosed because of infertility, but 67% of ♂ with varicoceles are fertile (infertility possibly results from impairing the mechanism that usually keeps scrotal temperature below body temperature, or because of impaired blood supply). Adolescents found to have a varicocele should have an annual assessment of ipsilateral testicular volume and be referred if there are concerns. Baseline investigations for an adult could include semen analysis, follicle-stimulating hormone (FSH) and serum testosterone. Abnormal sperm concentration or motility may identify those more likely to benefit from surgery. Generally, no treatment is required, although further assessment and surgical intervention should also be considered if any of the following occur: sudden onset and associated pain, varicocele does not drain when the patient is supine, solitary right-sided varicocele (to exclude a mass obstructing the downstream testicular vein)

Women

Bartholin gland cyst and abscess

Cysts arise following obstruction of the drainage duct, whereas abscesses are caused by local pathogens, most commonly *Neisseria gonorrhoeae* (up to 80% of abscesses) but also *Chlamydia trachomatis*, staphylococci, streptococci, and Gram −ve enteric bacteria. Found most commonly in ♀ aged 20–29 years with abscesses occurring about ×3 as commonly as cysts. Most small abscesses respond well to appropriate antibiotics, although needle aspiration may be required. Chronic or recurrent cysts may require duct catheterization or marsupialization. In ♀ >40 years, cyst edges should be examined histologically to exclude carcinoma. Recurrences may occur in up to 20%.

Cervical polyp

Often an incidental finding during routine examination but may present with post-coital or intermenstrual bleeding. Red fleshy cervical projections, ~1–2cm long, containing both squamous and columnar cell epithelium. Found more commonly in multiparous ♀ >20 years and may be associated with chronic local inflammation. 1.7% are malignant and 27% are associated with an endometrial polyp. Usually, removed by gently twisting the base, which should be sent for histology to exclude malignancy. Excision with basal electrocautery or laser vaporization may be required for larger lesions.

Mullerian duct anomalies (MDAs)

Most are associated with functioning ovaries and age-appropriate external genitalia, but also abnormalities of the renal and axial skeletal systems. Examples include vaginal agenesis, longitudinal or transverse vaginal septae, unicornuate uterus (1 hemi-uterus, ovary and fallopian tube), uterus didelphys (2 hemi-uteri, 2 cervices, 1 or 2 vaginas), bicornuate uterus (2 separate, but communicating endometrial cavities, 1 cervix and vagina) septate uterus (incomplete resorption of the fibromuscular uterine medial septum). Some may present in early adolescence (with cryptomenorrhoea, cyclical abdominal pain, and haematocolpos), but others may not present until a woman becomes sexually active, needs a vaginal speculum examination, or becomes pregnant.

Urethral caruncle

Seen primarily in post-menopausal women. Caused by eversion of a portion of the distal urethra (most commonly the posterior edge). Treatment is conservative (warm baths) or with hormone replacement therapy (HRT). Differential diagnosis includes urethral prolapse (circumferentially everted mucosa) or urethral malignancy.

Contraception, including contraception for women living with HIV

Introduction 382
Combined hormonal contraceptives (CHCs), including
     the combined pill, vaginal ring, and patch 384
Progestogen-only pill (POP) 388
Injectable contraception 391
Contraceptive implant 394
Levonorgestrel intra-uterine system 397
Copper intra-uterine contraceptive device 400
Diaphragms and caps 402
Female condom 403
Spermicides 404
Male condom 405
Fertility awareness methods (FAM) 407
Lactational amenorrhoea method (LAM) 408
Coitus interruptus or 'withdrawal' 408
Emergency contraception 409
Female sterilization 411
Male sterilization: vasectomy 413
Women living with HIV 414
Cautions and contraindications 416

Introduction

Despite the availability of wide variety of contraceptive methods, TOP rates remain high (UK data: 1 in 3 women have a TOP with a third requesting a repeat). Annually, about 190,000 TOPs are performed in England and Wales. At least 60% of these women report having used a contraceptive method at the time of conception, usually oral contraceptives or condoms, which require correct and consistent use. Table 34.1 compares failure rates for pills, condoms, and natural methods with typical and perfect use. At the first contraceptive consultation the HCP should:

* Consider the importance of efficacy and reversibility (is an unplanned pregnancy acceptable?).
* Find out if there is a particular interest in a contraceptive method?
* Take a comprehensive medical and sexual history. Dysmenorrhoea or heavy menstrual loss may indicate that a combined hormonal method, an injectable method, or a levonorgestrel intra-uterine system (IUS) would be ideal, offering therapeutic benefits.
* Dispel any contraceptive myths, e.g. the Pill makes you put on weight, injectables cause infertility, IUDs give you infections.
* Address the woman's worries and concerns, and explore why any previous contraceptive methods have been discontinued
* Discuss all options, focusing on long-acting and reliable contraceptive methods (LARCs).
* Explain how individual methods work, the advantages of each method, how to use the method, and any side effects that may occur and how they may be resolved.
* Provide accurate and up-to-date advice, including information on help lines and follow-up appointments.

Table 34.1 Summary table of contraceptive efficacy

Method	%♀ with unintended pregnancy in 1st year		%♀ continuing use at 1 year‡
	Typical use*	Perfect use†	
No method	85	85	–
Spermicides	28	18	42
Withdrawal	22	4	46
Fertility awareness methods	24	–	47
Diaphragm	12	6	57
Condom—female	21	5	41
Condom—male	18	2	43
Combined and progestogen-only pill	9	0.3	67
Evra® patch (transdermal combined hormone)	9	0.3	67
NuvaRing® (vaginal combined hormone)	9	0.3	67
Progestogen injectables	6	0.2	56
Intra-uterine T380A (copper T)	0.8	0.6	78
Intra-uterine (LNG-IUS) Mirena® system	0.2	0.2	80
Nexplanon®	0.05	0.05	84
Female sterilization	0.5	0.5	100
Male sterilization	0.15	0.1	100

*Among *typical* couples who initiate use of a method (not necessarily for the first time), the percentage who experience an accidental pregnancy during the first year if they do not stop use for any other reason.

†Among couples who initiate use of a method (not necessarily for the first time) and who use it *perfectly* (both consistently and correctly), the % who experience an accidental pregnancy during the first year if they do not stop use for any other reason.

‡Among couples attempting to avoid pregnancy, the % who continue to use a method for 1 year. Adapted from Trussell J (2011) Contraceptive failure in the United States. *Contraception* 83(5): 397–404, with permission from Elsevier.

Combined hormonal contraceptives (CHCs), including the combined pill, vaginal ring, and patch

CHCs are highly effective and quickly reversible, with failure rates of <1% per year when taken consistently and correctly (Table 34.1). ~3 million ♀ (16% of all in their reproductive years) in the UK take combined oral contraception (COC). >90% of sexually active ♀ have used the pill by the time they reach 30. COC is suitable from menarche to menopause, if no contraindicating risk factors or co-existing illnesses are identified.

Mechanism of action

- Inhibit ovulation.
- Alter cervical mucus, inhibiting spermatozoa penetration.
- Produce characteristic changes in the endometrium preventing implantation of the blastocyst.
- Modify sperm function/motility and cervico-uterine secretions.

Advantages of combined hormonal contraceptives

- Effective, reversible, convenient, non-intercourse related.
- Under the user's control.
- Regulates and ↓ menstrual loss, thereby improving iron-deficiency anaemia.
- Reduces dysmenorrhoea and relieves ovulation pain.
- May help premenstrual symptoms.
- May improve acne.
- Helps protect against ectopic pregnancies as it inhibits ovulation.
- Decreases incidence of benign breast disease.
- Long-term users are less likely to develop fibroids and functional ovarian cysts.
- Protects against PID and ↓ the risk of hospitalization for the disease.
- Reduces incidence of endometriosis, and a useful treatment and maintenance therapy for sufferers.
- Possible ↓ in the risk of developing rheumatoid arthritis and its associated symptoms.
- Reduces risk of ovarian cancer by 20% with every 5 years of use. ♀ who use this method for 15 years have half the risk of ovarian cancer compared with women who have never used this method.
- Reduces the risk of endometrial cancer by ~50%, with protection continuing for at least 20 years after the CHC is stopped.
- Reduced incidence of large bowel cancer by up to 40%.

Disadvantages of combined hormonal contraceptives

- Requires correct and consistent use to be effective (see Box 34.1 for instructions if taken incorrectly).
- Side effects may occur in the first few months, e.g. headaches, breast tenderness, breakthrough bleeding (although these tend to resolve quickly).

Box 34.1 Missed pill rules for COCs containing ethinylestradiol

- If missed one pill anywhere in the pack:
  - take forgotten pill, take next pill when due.
- If missed two pills (i.e. > 48 hours late) anywhere in the pack:
  - take forgotten last pill
  - take next pill when due
  - use a condom or abstain for 7 days
  - if pill-free interval in next 7 days do not stop pills, but start new packet straight away.
- If missed pills were in Week 1 of COC use and any unprotected sex has occurred in the 7 preceding days, then emergency contraception is required.

- Patches may cause a local skin reaction in about 10% of users with 2–3% discontinuing for this reason. 5–14% of ♀ using the vaginal ring complain of vaginitis.
- The vaginal ring can only be kept at room temperature for 4 months and requires a cold chain delivery system
- Potential drug interactions decrease the efficacy of these methods, e.g. use of liver-enzyme-inducing agents, St John's wort.
- No protection against STIs.
- May be associated with ↑ risk of breast cancer. The re-analysis data published in 1996 reported that current COC use ↑ the risk of developing breast cancer by 24%, but this fell back to background level 10 years or more after discontinuing the pill. However, five recently published studies have found no ↑ risk.
- After 5 years of use there may be an ↑ incidence of cervical intra-epithelial neoplasia and cancer of the cervix. COC appears to be a cofactor leading to persistence or repeated replication of oncogenic HPV. Regular cervical screening, as indicated by the NHS Cervical Screening Programme, should be advised.
- Possible small ↑ in the risk of myocardial infarction (MI) in non-smoking low-risk ♀. However, the risk may ↑ up to 20-fold in heavy smokers.
- Possible small ↑ (up to 2-fold) in the risk of ischaemic stroke in users, with about 3 ischaemic strokes occurring in 100,000 ♀ under 35 each year. Risk factors include hypertension, smoking, diabetes, and family history of stroke. No ↑ in the risk of haemorrhagic stroke in low-risk non-smoking ♀ with normal blood pressure.
- Increased risk of venous thromboembolism (VTE). Background risk of VTE in young ♀ is now thought to be about 2 per 10,000 ♀ each year. This risk increases to 5–7 per 10,000 women using CHC containing levonorgestrel, norethisterone, and norgestimate; 6–12 per 10,000 women using the vaginal ring or patch; and 9–12 per 10,000 women using CHC containing drospirenone, desogestrel, gestodene or cyproterone acetate. Increasing age, obesity, surgery, family history of VTE, and immobility ↑ the risk of developing a VTE.

Choice of CHC

Although all CHCs have the same mode of contraceptive action and similar efficacy they may have different side effects or benefits (e.g. less breakthrough bleeding or an improvement in acne). The first pill prescribed should be effective, suit the majority of ♀, have a proven safety record, and be inexpensive. A monophasic 30 mcg levonorgestrel pill (such as Microgynon® 30 or a branded generic pill) fulfils these criteria. 40% of ♀ may complain of side effects or perceived associated problems and request a change.

Combined hormonal contraceptive transdermal patch and vaginal ring

These LARC methods avoid daily pill taking, but have a similar efficacy as COC. Both give a regular monthly withdrawal bleed and are advantageous in ♀ who cannot remember to take a daily pill or who have gastrointestinal problems affecting pill absorption. The patch needs changing every 7 days with a patch-free week every 4th week. The vaginal ring is worn for 3 out of every 4 weeks. Minor and potentially serious, but rare, side effects are similar to those with COC.

Pill choice

- *First choice*: 30 mcg levonorgestrel, monophasic preparation (such as Microgynon30® or a branded generic pill).
- *To improve cycle control*: 30 mcg gestodene or 35 mcg norgestimate pill or vaginal ring once pathology, drug interaction, or poor compliance are excluded (e.g. Millinette 30/75®, Cilest®, NuvaRing®).
- *Oestrogen side effects*: include headaches, nausea, breast tenderness, or leg cramps. Reduce the dose of oestrogen to a pill containing 20 mcg ethinylestradiol (e.g. Millinette 20/75®, Loestrin20®, Gedarel 20/150®, Daylette®) or estradiol (Qlaira®, Zoely®), or change to a progestogen-only pill.
- *Progestogen side effects*: include mood change, bloating, and greasy skin. Change the progestogen in the pill. Cyproterone acetate and drospirenone in COCs are useful in ♀ with acne (e.g. Dianette®, Yasmin®, or branded generic).

Starting CHCs

See Table 34.2.

Table 34.2 Starting combined hormonal contraceptives

Circumstances	When to start	Extra precautions for 7 days?
Quick start	At any time, if it is reasonably certain not pregnant	Yes
Menstruating	Up to and including day 5	No
	After day 5	Yes
Amenorrhoeic	At any time, if it is reasonably certain not pregnant	Yes

Table 34.2 (Contd.)

Circumstances	When to start	Extra precautions for 7 days?
Post-abortion or miscarriage	Within 5 days	No
	After 5 days	Yes

Starting combined hormonal contraception post-partum

Circumstances	When to start	Extra precautions for 7 days?
Not breast-feeding	Start Day 21 post-partum (note it is not advised to start CHC until Day 21 in this group of women)	No
	From day 22 onwards (women with an additional risk factor for VTE should start CHC at 6 weeks)	Yes
Breastfeeding	From delivery until 6 weeks post-partum this method is not advised	N/A
	From 6 weeks post-partum CHC can be used safely in women with no contraindications	Yes
Switching from POP	Switch immediately from POP with a 3-hour window period	Yes
	Switch immediately from POP with 12-hour window period	No
Switching from implant	Switch any time before implant expires	No
Switching from injection	Any time before injection expires	No
Switching from IUS	Switch immediately post-removal (as long as no unprotected sex in previous 7 days)	Yes (or leave IUS *in situ* for a further 7 days and then remove)
Switching from IUD	Start up to and including day 5 of cycle. IUD can be removed at the same time	No
	After Day 5 of cycle start CHC on removal of IUD (as long as no unprotected sex in previous 7 days)	Yes (or leave IUD *in situ* for a further 7 days then remove)

Progestogen-only pill (POP)

Taken by 6% of ♀ in the UK. It is very effective when taken properly, but has typical failure rates of 9%.

Mechanism of action

- Ovulation may be suppressed in 50% of cycles by POPs containing levonorgestrel, or norethisterone, but in 97–99% by those containing desogestrel.
- All POPs alter the cervical mucus to reduce sperm penetration.
- POPs induce changes in the endometrium to prevent sperm survival and implantation of the blastocyst.
- Sperm motility and function is affected, preventing fertilization.

Cervical mucus effect peaks within 2–3 hours of oral ingestion and then slowly wanes. Desogestrel-containing POPs differ from more traditional POPs in that no extra contraceptive cover is required until 12 hours after a missed pill compared with 3 hours for other POPs.

POPs have frequently been restricted to ♀ who are breastfeeding or who have contraindications to taking synthetic oestrogen. However, users from all age groups may be interested in taking a POP, particularly as it is very safe and suitable for most women.

Advantages of progestogen-only pills

- Non-intercourse-related contraceptive.
- Simple and convenient to use.
- POPs are safe for ♀ who are breastfeeding.
- Ideal for ♀ who suffer from oestrogenic side effects when using CHCs, e.g. breast tenderness, headaches, fluid retention, or nausea.
- Suitable for ♀ over 35 years who smoke.
- Can be used in grossly obese ♀ with no dose adjustment required.
- Can be taken by ♀ with medical illnesses that contraindicate the use of synthetic oestrogen, e.g. those with hypertension, migraine with focal aura, or a previous personal history of VTE.
- No evidence of ↑ risk of cardiovascular disease, thromboembolism, or stroke.
- Minimal alteration in carbohydrate and lipid metabolism. Therefore, they are ideal for diabetics even with neuropathic or nephropathic complications.
- Can be used safely until the menopause and does not mask menopausal symptoms.

Disadvantages of progestogen-only pills

- POPs, excluding the desogestrel POP, are thought to be less effective than combined pills in practice as they are very reliant on regular pill taking (see Box 34.2 for advice on missed doses).
- May cause side effects, such as breast tenderness, mood changes, headaches, and acne.
- Can alter ovulation, thereby disrupting the menstrual bleeding pattern, with users reporting an ↑ in spotting, breakthrough bleeding, and amenorrhoea

- Functional ovarian cysts may develop in a small number of women; however, these tend to be transient and rarely require surgical intervention.
- Potential drug interactions decrease the efficacy of POP, e.g. use of liver-enzyme-inducing agents, St John's Wort.

Starting POPs

See Table 34.3.

Table 34.3 Starting regimens for progestogen-only pills

Circumstances	Start when?	Extra precautions for 48 hours
Quick start	Any time, if it is reasonably certain that ♀ is not pregnant	Yes
Menstruating	Up to and including day 5 of cycle	No
	After day 5 of the cycle	Yes
Amenorrhoeic	Any time, if it is reasonably certain that ♀ is not pregnant	Yes
Post-abortion or miscarriage	Within 5 days	No
	After 5 days	Yes
Starting progesterone-only pill post-partum		
Circumstances	When to start	Extra precautions for 7 days?
Breastfeeding or bottle-feeding	Upto and incl. 21 post-partum	No
	From day 22 onwards	Yes
Switching from CHC	Day 1–2 of hormone-free interval	No
	From day 2 onwards of hormone-free interval or during week 1 of CHC use	Yes
	During Week 2–3 of CHC use	No as long as CHC taken properly in the preceding 7 days
Switching from implant	Any time pre-expiry of implant	No
Switching from injectable contraception	Any time pre-expiry of injection	No
Switching from an IUS	Immediately post-removal (as long as no unprotected sex in previous 7 days)	Yes (or start POP then remove IUS after 48 hours)
Switching from an IUD	Start up to and including day 5 of cycle. IUD can be removed at the same time	No
	After Day 5 of cycle (as long as no unprotected sex in previous 7 days)	Yes (or start POP then remove IUD after 48 hours)

Box 34.2 Missed pill rules for POP

- If missed traditional POP by <3 hours or desogestrel POP by <12 hours: take forgotten pill and take next tablet when due.
- If missed traditional POP by >3 hours or desogestrel POP by >12 hours:
  - take last forgotten pill and next pill when due, and use condoms for 2 days.
  - Emergency contraception needed if any unprotected sex since the time of the missed pill.

Injectable contraception

Injectables are highly effective and have a safety record that spans 40 years. Intramuscular progestogen-only depot providing contraceptive cover for 2–3 months was one of the first long-acting hormonal preparations to be used. Progestogen-only injectables are used by ~3% of ♀ in the UK.

Three injectable contraceptive methods are available in the UK:

- Depo-Provera® (depot medroxyprogesterone acetate (DMPA-IM)) given every 13 weeks intra-muscularly normally into gluteus maximus.
- Noristerat® (norethisterone enantate (NET-EN) given every 8 weeks IM (used infrequently in the UK for short-term interim contraception).
- Sayana-Press® (DMPA-SC), given every 13 weeks subcutaneously into the anterior thigh or abdomen. This has been licensed for self-administration.

A significant number of ♀ fail to return for their second DMPA. Prolonged/ erratic bleeding is often cited as a reason for discontinuation. Pre-injection counselling, giving a realistic picture of potential side effects in the first few injection cycles, is important.

Mechanism of action

- DMPA and NET-EN inhibit ovulation by suppressing luteinizing hormone (LH) and, to a certain extent, FSH.
- Injectables alter the cervical mucus, inhibiting spermatozoa penetration.
- Injectables prevent implantation by inducing endometrial atrophy.
- Like other progestogens, injectables modify sperm function and motility.

Advantages of progestogen-only injectables

- Very effective, reversible, and discreet method of contraception with little dependence on the user.
- Non-intercourse-related contraceptive method.
- Very safe with no reported attributable deaths.
- Safe for breastfeeding mothers.
- Helpful for ♀ with premenstrual symptoms, ovulation pain, and painful heavy periods.
- Can be used in ♀ with sickle cell disease, with evidence suggesting a ↓ in crises
- Possesses most of the non-contraceptive benefits of CHCs, including protection against PID, extra-uterine pregnancies, endometriosis, functional ovarian cysts, and fibroid formation, ovarian cancer, and a 5-fold ↓ in the risk of endometrial cancer.
- Minimal metabolic effects occur, with recent research reporting no ↑ in the risk of acute myocardial infarction, VTE, or stroke.
- Safe to use in women taking liver enzyme-inducing drugs.

Disadvantages of progestogen-only injectables

- Irregular prolonged vaginal bleeding/amenorrhoea. ~1/3rd experience prolonged bleeding (>10 days) after receiving their first injection, but 50% are amenorrhoeic by 1 year.
- *IM or SC administration*: therefore, cannot be removed if side effects occur.
- Weight gain commonly reported, particularly in young women whose starting BMI is >30 km/m^2.
- Some may complain of progestogenic side effects, including mood changes, lassitude, loss of libido, bloating, and breast tenderness.
- Causes a short delay in the return to normal fertility with the mean time to ovulation being 5.3 months after the last injection.
- DMPA may adversely affect bone mineral density (BMD), but there are no good data suggesting that it causes osteoporosis or bone fracture. Present data suggest that BMD at the lumbar spine and femoral neck are ↓ in DMPA users compared with controls. BMD recovers to a similar level to never-users on discontinuation of DMPA (usually 3–5 years in adults and 18 months if <18 years).
- Committee on Safety of Medicines advice:
  - in adolescents, DMPA may be used as first-line contraception, but only after other methods have been discussed with the patient and considered to be unsuitable or unacceptable
  - in all ages, careful re-evaluation of the risks and benefits of treatment should be carried out in those who wish to continue use for >2 years
  - if significant lifestyle and/or medical risk factors for osteoporosis, other methods of contraception should be considered.
- There is no evidence that routinely giving 'add-back' oestrogen to DPMA users or additional investigations to check bone mineral density such as DEXA scans are warranted.
- ↑ low-density lipoprotein (LDL)-cholesterol and ↓ high-density lipoprotein (HDL)-cholesterol so needs to be used with caution in women who have multiple cardiovascular risk factors.
- Injection site reactions have been reported in 6% of women using Sayana-Press®
- Potential small increase in the risk of HIV acquisition, thus users of injectable contraception, as with any other method, should be advised about HIV preventative measures, such as male and female condoms.

Starting injectable contraceptives
See Table 34.4.

Table 34.4 Starting regimens for injectable contraceptives

Circumstances	When to start	Extra precautions for 7 days?
Quick start	At any time, if it is reasonably certain that ♀ is not pregnant	Yes
Menstruating	Up to and including day 5	No
	After day 5 of the cycle	Yes
Amenorrhoeic	Any time, if it is reasonably certain that ♀ is not pregnant	Yes
Post-abortion or miscarriage	Within 5 days	No
	After 5 days	Yes

Starting injectable contraception post-partum

Circumstances	When to start	Extra precautions for 7 days?
Breastfeeding or bottle-feeding	Upto and incl. 21 post-partum	No
	From day 22 onwards	Yes
Switching from CHC	Day 1–2 of hormone-free interval and week 2–3 of CHC use	No
		Yes
	From day 2 onwards of hormone-free interval and week 1 of CHC use	
Switching from POP	Switch anytime	Yes
Switching from implant	Anytime pre expiry	No
Switching from IUS	Immediately post-removal (providing no unprotected sex in previous 7 days)	Yes (or start injection then remove IUS after 7 days)
Switching from an IUD	Give the injection up to and including day 5 of cycle. IUD/IUS can be removed at the same time	No
	After Day 5 of the cycle start immediately post-removal (as long as no unprotected sex in previous 7 days)	Yes (or start injection then remove IUD after 7 days)

Contraceptive implant

A contraceptive implant offers an alternative way of delivering hormones providing long-acting low-dose reversible contraception. Norplant®, the levonorgestrel implant, was available in the UK from 1993 until 1999. It consists of 6 rods inserted subdermally ~8–10 cm above the elbow on the inner aspect of the non-dominant arm. It is licensed to provide contraception over a 5-year period. UK healthcare professionals may see ♀ from sub-Saharan Africa using this multi-rod contraceptive system or the two-rod system called Jadelle®.

Implanon®, containing a single rod of 68 mg etonogestrel (the active metabolite of desogestrel), was launched in the UK in 1999. It was replaced by Nexplanon® in 2010, which also contains 68 mg etonogestrel, but has a different preloaded applicator to decrease the risk of non-insertion, and contains barium, making it radiopaque so can be located on X-Ray and CT scan if need be.

It is used by 1% of ♀ in the UK and is licensed to provide contraception for 3 years. It is one of the most effective contraceptives with recent method failure rates quoted as 0.01 per 100 implants fitted.

Mechanism of action

- Etonogestrel inhibits ovulation by suppressing LH. However, up to 5% of users may ovulate in the third year.
- Implants also alter the cervical mucus, inhibiting sperm penetration and thereby preventing fertilization.
- Implants prevent implantation by inducing endometrial atrophy.
- Implants may modify sperm function and motility.

Advantages of contraceptive implants

- Long-lasting (3–5 years depending on the type of implant), effective, immediately reversible, and no effect on future fertility.
- Non-intercourse-related.
- Free from oestrogen side effects
- High user acceptability following pre-insertion counselling, with continuation rates between 67% and 78% at 12 months.
- Requires little medical attention, other than at insertion and removal.
- Can be used by those in whom synthetic oestrogen is contra-indicated.
- Safe for breast-feeding mothers.
- Nexplanon® does not adversely affect cardiovascular risk factors, thrombotic factors, CRP, cholesterol/HDL-cholesterol ratio, and nitrous oxide.
- Minimal effects on glucose metabolism and liver function.
- No adverse effect on systemic oestrogen levels or BMD.

Disadvantages of contraceptive implants

- Unpredictable and irregular bleeding patterns are common in Nexplanon® users with ~10% discontinuing because of prolonged and/or frequent bleeding with ~20% of 90-day reference cycles showing amenorrhoea, ~25% regular bleeding, ~30% infrequent bleeding, ~25% frequent and/or prolonged bleeding.
- Incidence of progestogen side effects with Nexplanon® similar to that with other progestogen-only methods. Side effects include headache, weight gain, acne, and mood changes.

- Insertion of implants requires a minor operative procedure under local anaesthetic by trained health professionals.
- Non-palpable implants have been reported in about 1 in 1000 insertions and are related to poor insertion technique. Very rarely, damage to the neurovascular bundle and intravascular migration has been reported. Referral to an 'expert' centre is advised for implant location using high frequency ultrasound scanning before removal. If the implant cannot be identified on imaging, a chest X-ray should be ordered and etonogestrel assays may be required.
- Some ♀ report mild discomfort and bruising following insertion or removal of the implants.
- Infection at the insertion or removal site, migration of the implants, and scarring are rare.
- Effectiveness may be reduced by concurrent usage of liver enzyme inducing drugs.

Contraceptive implants may not be a suitable method for some ♀ as discontinuation is not under their control.

Starting regimens for contraceptive implant
See Table 34.5.

Table 34.5 Starting regimens for contraceptive implants

Circumstances	When to start	Extra precautions for 7 days?
Quick start	At any time, if it is reasonably certain that ♀ is not pregnant	Yes
Menstruating	Up to and including day 5	No
	After day 5 of the cycle	Yes
Amenorrhoeic	Any time, if it is reasonably certain that ♀ is not pregnant	Yes
Post-abortion or miscarriage	Within 5 days	No
	After 5 days	Yes

Starting implant post-partum

Circumstances	When to start	Extra precautions for 7 days?
Breastfeeding or bottle-feeding	Upto and incl. 21 post-partum	No
	From day 22 onwards	Yes
Switching from CHC	Switching on Day 1–2 of the hormone-free interval or in week 2–3 of CHC use	No
	Switching from Day 2 of the hormone-free interval and in Week 1 of CHC use	Yes
Switching from POP	Switch anytime	No

(Continued)

Table 34.5 (*Contd.*)

Circumstances	When to start	Extra precautions for 7 days?
Switching from an injection	Switch any time before injection expires	No
Switching from IUS	Immediately post-removal (as long as no unprotected sex in previous 7 days)	Yes (or leave IUS in for another 7 days then remove)
Switching from IUD	Insert the implant up to and including day 5 of cycle. IUD can be removed at the same time	No
	After Day 5 of cycle switch immediately post-removal (as long as no unprotected sex in previous 7 days)	Yes (or leave IUD in for another 7 days then remove)

Levonorgestrel intra-uterine system

There are four different intrauterine systems available in the UK. Mirena®
has been available in the UK since May 1995 and used by ~2% of ♀. Mirena®
contains 52 mg levonorgestrel in a polydimethylsiloxane reservoir on the
vertical arm of a T-shaped plastic frame. Mirena® provides highly effective,
yet reversible contraception for 5 years. It is also licensed for the treatment
of heavy menstrual bleeding and as the progestogen component of HRT.

Jaydess® has been available in the UK since 2014. Jaydess® contains 13.5
mg levonorgestrel in a similar T-shaped frame to Mirena®. The Jaydess® inserter tube and device itself are slightly smaller than the Mirena® equivalent.
Jaydess® is licensed for 3 years and should be used for contraception only.

Levosert® has been available in the UK since 2015. Levosert® contains 52
mg levonorgestrel in a polyethylene T-shaped frame. The introducer differs
from Mirena® and Jaydess®, as the fitting requires a two-handed technique.
Levosert® is licensed to provide contraception and as a treatment for heavy
menstrual bleeding over a 4-year period.

Kyleena® has been available in the UK since 2018. Kyleena® contains 19.5
mg levonorgestrel in a similar T-shaped frame to Mirena®. It is licensed to
provide contraception for 5 years. The inserter tube and device are slightly
smaller than the Mirena® equivalent.

Mechanism of action

- Alters cervical mucus and utero-tubal fluid, inhibiting sperm migration.
- Prevents endometrial proliferation by causing atrophic changes over
  time. This precludes implantation.
- May affect sperm motility and function.
- May suppress ovulation in some in the first year, possibly by reducing the
  pre-ovulatory LH surge.

Advantages of IUS

- Long-acting (lasts 3–5 years, depending on the IUS) and independent of
  intercourse.
- Highly effective contraceptive (as effective as female sterilization) with
  an immediate return to fertility after removal. The ↑ in use of LARCs,
  such as the IUS has led to ↓ in requests for female sterilization in
  the UK.
- Reduces normal menstrual blood loss. After 3 years of use, 24%
  of women using Mirena® and 13% using Jaydess® have become
  amenorrhoeic. It is thought that Levosert® and Kyleena® have similar
  bleeding profiles to that of Mirena®.
- 90% after 12 months use have an ↑ in haemoglobin and serum ferritin.
  This has led to ↓ hysterectomies performed in the UK. They can be
  used in ♀ with coagulation disorders.
- Long-term use of Mirena® may prevent fibroid formation. Mirena®
  reduces heavy menstrual bleeding associated with fibroids and
  adenomyosis.

- Mirena® reduces the incidence of dysmenorrhoea.
- Mirena® may be a useful medical treatment for ♀ suffering from endometriosis-related problems with significant ↓ in severity and frequency of pain/menstrual symptoms. Good as maintenance therapy following conservative surgery for endometriosis.
- No evidence that serum oestradiol and BMD are affected.
- When used alongside oestrogen, Mirena® can be used in the treatment of premenstrual syndrome.
- May protect against the development of endometrial hyperplasia and cancer. Resolves endometrial hyperplasia without atypia in 92% of cases and endometrial hyperplasia with atypia in 67%. Not affected by concurrent use of liver enzyme-inducing drugs.

Disadvantages of IUS

- May cause irregular/prolonged bleeding in the first 3 months. Prolonged bleeding/spotting (>6 months following fitting) may occur in those with heavy menstrual bleeding, with or without fibroids. Pre-insertion counselling should include information on menstrual disturbance.
- May be expelled or displaced, particularly with intra-cavity fibroids or heavy menstrual loss.
- Fitting may be painful and seen as invasive by women.
- Small ↑ risk of PID within first 20 days after fitting, particularly in young ♀. Screen for STIs prior to fitting in those at risk.
- ~10% of women using Mirena® may develop functional ovarian cysts, but these tend to resolve over 6 months or so, and rarely require surgical intervention. Approximately 22% of women using Kyleena® in clinical trials have been found to have ovarian cysts, most of which are asymptomatic.
- Risk of uterine perforation when fitting IUS (< 2/1000 devices fitted). Risk rises to 6/1000 insertions in breastfeeding women.
- Some progestogenic symptoms in the first few months, i.e. breast tenderness, bloating, or acne. These usually settle.
- Overall incidence of ectopic pregnancy is lower than in the general population, but if IUS fails then it is thought that up to 50% of pregnancies may be ectopic. It can be used in ♀ with a past history of ectopic pregnancy.
- Cannot be used as an emergency form of contraception.

Starting regimens for intra-uterine systems

See Table 34.6.

Table 34.6 Starting regimens for intra-uterine systems

Circumstances	When to start	Extra precautions for 7 days?
Menstruating	Up to and including day 7 (avoiding insertion when menstrual flow is heavy, thereby reducing subsequent expulsion)	No
	After day 7 of the cycle, as long as it is reasonably certain that ♀ is not pregnant	Yes
Amenorrhoeic	Any time, if it is reasonably certain that ♀ is not pregnant	Yes
Post-abortion or miscarriage	Within 5 days	No (ensure no continuing pregnancy/retained products first)
	After 5 days	Yes (ensure no continuing pregnancy/retained products first)
	After surgical TOP	Insert at time of the surgical TOP

Starting intra-uterine system post-partum

Circumstances	When to start	Extra precautions for 7 days?
Breastfeeding or bottle-feeding	After day 28 (including following a Caesarean section)	Yes
Switching from CHC	Fit on Day 1 of hormone-free interval or during Week 2–3 of CHC use	No
	Fit from Day 2 of hormone-free interval and during Week 1 of CHC use	Yes (or fit IUS and continue CHC for another 7 days)
Switching from POP	Switch anytime	Yes
Switching from implant	Any time before implant expires	No
Switching from injection	Any time before injection expires	No
Switching from IUD	Switch methods immediately if Day 1–7 of cycle	No
	After day 7, advise no sexual intercourse for 7 days prior to switching the methods	Yes

Copper intra-uterine contraceptive device

IUDs are used by >110 million ♀ world-wide, with >50% of these users in China. Only 6% of ♀ in the UK use IUD, possibly because of concerns and myths attached to these methods. IUDs available in the UK are small copper-containing devices in varying shapes and sizes. Most have a central frame made of polyethylene impregnated with barium, making them radio-opaque. A frameless device called GyneFix® is also available. Most devices contain >300 mm^2 of copper, making them a highly effective, reversible, and inexpensive contraceptive option.

Mechanism of action

- Prevents fertilization as copper ions are toxic to sperm and ova (main mechanism).
- All IUDs ↑ the number of leucocytes in the endometrium, producing a typical 'sterile' inflammatory endometrial response, which helps prevent implantation. Copper enhances this reaction. The increased copper content of cervico-uterine mucus inhibits sperm penetration.
- An IUD is not an abortifacient.

Advantages of IUDs

- Long-term (up to 10 years), highly effective contraceptive with no delay in return to fertility following removal.
- Immediately effective.
- Non-intercourse related.
- No associated weight gain or hormonal side effects.
- Very effective as an emergency contraceptive. Can be fitted up to 5 days after unprotected sexual intercourse (UPSI) or 5 days after estimated time of ovulation, whichever is later.
- High acceptability and good continuation rates.
- Inexpensive and very cost-effective.
- Risk of ectopic pregnancy is low in devices with 300 mm^2 of copper. The incidence of ectopic pregnancy is 0.02 per 100 women-years, which is less than in those using no contraceptive method.

Disadvantages of IUDs

- May cause menstrual irregularities with intermenstrual bleeding and spotting more common in the first 6 months after insertion.
- Periods may become heavier, more prolonged, and painful, especially soon after insertion. ~10% of ♀ discontinue in the first year, citing menstrual bleeding and pain as the main reason.
- Users are more prone to bacterial vaginosis.
- ~1 in 20 IUDs are expelled; more likely within the first 3 months of fitting and similar for all types.
- Risk of PID associated with insertion, especially within the first 20 days. May be prevented by pre-insertion STI screening for those at risk.
- Rare complications, e.g. uterine perforation may occur in <2/1000 insertions (increased to 6/1000 insertions in breastfeeding ♀).

Starting regimens for IUDs

See Table 34.7.

Table 34.7 Starting regimens for intra-uterine devices

Circumstances	When to start	Extra precautions for 7 days?
Menstruating	At any time in the cycle if it is reasonably certain that the ♀ is not pregnant (avoiding insertion when menstrual flow is heavy, thereby ↑ subsequent expulsion)	No
Amenorrhoeic	Any time if it is reasonably certain that ♀ is not pregnant	No
Post-abortion or miscarriage	Immediately at the time of surgical TOP	No
	At any time following medical termination or miscarriage by an experienced clinician, as long as there is no concern that the pregnancy is not ongoing or that there are retained products of conception	No

Starting intra-uterine device post-partum

Circumstances	When to start	Extra precautions for 7 days?
Breastfeeding or bottle-feeding	After day 28 (including following a Caesarean section) if it is reasonably certain that ♀ is not pregnant	No
Switching from CHC	Switch immediately	No
Switching from POP	Switch immediately	No
Switching from implant	Any time before implant expires	No
Switching from injection	Any time before injection expires	No
Switching from IUS	Switch immediately – ensure the patient has not had unprotected sex in the 7 days prior to the change	No

Diaphragms and caps

These are often thought to be messy and difficult, and hence are used by <1% of ♀ in the UK. However, the ease of use and lack of interference with intercourse often surprises ♀. Must be used correctly and consistently, as typical failure rates in the first year can be high (12%). Should be fitted by a trained HCP who can advise about use of additional spermicide.

Mode of action

Physical and chemical barrier to sperm entering the upper female genital tract (when used with a spermicide). Diaphragms sit between the posterior fornix and the pubis to cover the cervix. Cervical caps fit directly over the cervix by suction and are ideal for ♀ with long cervices and ♀ with recurrent UTIs when using diaphragms.

Advantages of diaphragms and caps

- Effective with careful consistent use (6% failure rate with perfect use).
- Can be inserted anytime time before sex.
- No established health risks or systemic side effects.
- Silicone alternatives available for women with latex allergies.
- User controlled.

Disadvantages of diaphragms and caps

- High failure rates in practice (12% with typical use), therefore, requires careful use on all occasions.
- Must remain in place for 6 hours after the last episode of sexual intercourse, but should stay in for no longer than 48 hours
- May become dislodged during sex.
- May ↑ risk of cystitis or UTI.
- Potential risk of TSS if left *in situ* longer than the recommended time specified by the manufacturer.
- Should be used with a spermicide. More spermicide should be inserted into the vagina if the cap/diaphragm has been *in situ* for over 3 hours or before repeated sex occurs to ↑ efficacy.
- Spermicide is considered 'messy' by some users.
- Spermicide-induced vaginal irritation in some users.
- Needs to be fitted by a HCP.
- May need to be re-fitted after certain circumstances, for example weight changes of ±3 kg and having a baby.
- Can become damaged by oil-based lubricants.

Female condom

The female condom (Femidom®) was first marketed in the UK in 1992 but very few ♀ in the UK use this method. It can be bought in pharmacies and is acceptable to some ♀ who often alternate between using male and female barrier methods.

Mode of action

The female condom is a lubricated loose-fitting, polyurethane sheath with two flexible rings. The closed end with the loose ring is inserted into the vagina and the outer ring covers the vulva. It acts as a physical barrier between sperm and ovum.

Advantages of the female condom

- No known side effects.
- Acts as a contraceptive and may also protect against some STIs (inconsistent data).
- Theoretical benefit in helping to protect against HPV transmission and cancer of the cervix.
- Effective with careful use (5% failure rate with perfect use).
- Under direct control of the user.
- Can be inserted at any time before having sex.
- No additional spermicide required.
- Can be used with oil-based products.
- Polyurethane is stronger than latex and breakage is rare.
- No need for male erection before use.

Disadvantages of the female condom

- Has high failure rates in practice (typical failure rate 21%).
- Has a high slippage rate (about 6%).
- Requires thought before use and careful insertion to be effective.
- Can interrupt sex.
- Can be noisy and intrusive.

Spermicides

One of the oldest forms of contraception. Available in the UK as creams and pessaries. Many different substances have been used in the past, but preparations available in the UK contain nonoxynol-9.

Advantages of spermicides

- No serious side effects.
- Widely available in pharmacies and simple to use.
- Provide lubrication.
- Enhance efficacy of barrier methods.
- Useful during the peri-menopause (♀ >45 years with irregular cycles and some vasomotor symptoms).
- Can be used while breastfeeding (until menstruation returns and weaning begins).

Disadvantages of spermicides

- Must not be used as sole contraceptive in most circumstances (28% typical failure rate when used alone in fertile ♀).
- Can be messy and cause local irritation.
- Intercourse dependent.
- Waiting time of approximately 4 minutes after insertion of pessaries before they melt.
- Those available may damage the vaginal epithelium and have the potential to ↑ transmission of STIs.

Male condom

The condom or 'sheath' has been used to protect against transmission of STIs and prevent pregnancy over the centuries. It is still one of the most popular contraceptive methods and is used by 25% of British couples. They are readily available from a variety of outlets. Condoms must be used correctly and on all occasions when close sexual contact occurs to be effective. Typical failure rate is high (18%).

Male condoms come in different shapes, colours, sizes, and flavours. Most are made of latex, with the only contraindication being latex allergy. The majority of reactions are type IV hypersensitivity (mild genital inflammation), although rarely anaphylaxis can occur with type I hypersensitivity. Polyurethane, deproteinized latex, and polyisoprene condoms are available as alternatives. Condoms lubricated with a non-spermicidal agent are now advised since the addition of a spermicide may cause local genital irritation and thin the vaginal mucosa in ♀, leading to possible transmission of STIs. Additional spermicide does not improve the contraceptive efficacy of male condoms. Non-oil-based lubricants are recommended, especially for anal sex, to reduce the risk of breakage (3% breakage rate compared with 21.4% when lubricant is not used), but should not be applied directly to the penis under a condom as this may cause slippage.

Users should be advised to check their condoms for safety markings (CE markings or Kitemark) and expiry date.

Mode of action
- Acts as a physical barrier between sperm and ovum.

Advantages of the male condom
- No known serious side effects.
- Acts as a contraceptive and helps to provide protection against STIs and cervical neoplasia (Box 34.3).
- Effective with careful use (2% failure rate with perfect use).
- Latex-free condoms are available for those who have latex allergies.
- Under direct control of the user.

Disadvantages of the male condom
- High failure rates in practice.
- Transmission of STIs possible even with careful and consistent use.
- Oil-based lubricants and some vaginal preparations may affect latex condoms with ↑ risk of breakage. Aqueous-based lubricant should be used for anal sex to reduce the risk of breakage. 'Stronger' condoms result in similar breakage rates. Therefore, they are not recommended.
- Requires the penis to be erect before use.
- Has a high slippage rate if lubricant is placed in the condom.
- Can interrupt sex.

Box 34.3 **Male condoms and STI protection**

HIV infection

Effective condom use reduces HIV transmission by 85% (meta-analysis data ranges between 73% and 96%)

Data on other STIs is inconsistent and the degree of protection provided by male condoms is difficult to assess. However:

- *Gonorrhoea and chlamydia*: strong evidence that condoms reduce the risk of gonorrhoea and chlamydia in both men and women (review of 45 published studies).
- *Trichomoniasis*: conflicting data; however, TV is more likely to be found in inconsistent condoms users; therefore, correct and regular condom use is recommended.
- *Anogenital herpes*: conflicting data. Evidence of protection using male condom for HSV-2 sero-discordant couples or those with >4 sex partners, but no evidence for sex workers, their clients, and GUM male heterosexual attenders. Consistent and correct use of male condoms is recommended.
- *Syphilis*: limited data regarding the usefulness of condoms exists, although regular and correct condom use is recommended to protect against syphilis transmission.
- *Anogenital HPV*: risk of cervical and vulvo-vaginal HPV infection reduced with consistent condom use. Regression and clearance of flat penile warts and cervical intra-epithelial neoplasia has also been reported in association with condom use.
- *Hepatitis B virus*: reduced core antibody rates in female sex workers who consistently use condoms.

Using condoms with sex toys will also decrease the risk of STI acquisition.

Estimated minimum level of protection against infection provided by consistent condom use:

- HIV 85%.
- *C. trachomatis* 40%.
- *T. vaginalis* 60%.
- *N. gonorrhoeae* 49%.
- HSV infection in ♀ may be reduced but no evidence in ♂. Conflicting data on HPV infection but may ↓ incidence in ♂ and delay progression of CIN in ♀.

Fertility awareness methods (FAM)

FAM has replaced the terms 'rhythm method', 'natural family planning', or using the 'safe period'. FAM relies upon the detection of ovulation. It is effective if couples abstain from penetrative vaginal sex during the fertile period of the menstrual cycle or use a barrier method. Normally, a minimum of three menstrual cycles' information is needed for accurate prediction of the fertile phase. Efficacy is improved if several FAMs are used concurrently, such as menstrual records, basal body temperature, and cervical mucus indicators. The failure rate is 6% with perfect use of devices such as Persona®, which detect the fertile phase by measuring urinary oestriol-3-glucuronide and LH.

Fertility awareness is used by 2% of couples in the UK, but by many more worldwide to space their family.

Advantages of FAM

- Can be used to plan pregnancy, as well as prevent conception.
- If multiple methods are used together perfectly, the pregnancy rate may be as low as 4%.
- No known physical side effects.
- Non-intercourse-related method.
- No mechanical devices or hormones used.
- Acceptable to all cultures and religions.
- No follow-up is necessary once the user has learnt the method.

Disadvantages of FAM

- Relatively high failure rate in practice, if only one fertility awareness method is used (24%).
- Requires commitment of both partners.
- Needs to be taught by a trained practitioner in order to use successfully.
- Requires careful observation and record-keeping, which may take time to learn.
- Users must have high motivation, as long periods of abstinence from intercourse are required.
- No protection against STI transmission.

Lactational amenorrhoea method (LAM)

Breastfeeding is a natural way of spacing children, since suckling suppresses LH and FSH, resulting in amenorrhoea, and stimulates prolactin, leading to lactation. LAM is very effective, offering 98% protection against pregnancy under the following conditions:

- Fully or almost fully breast-feeding (feeding with no substitutes and at regular periods on demand, day and night).
- Baby is <6 months old.
- Menstruation has not returned.

Advantages of LAM

- Free of charge.
- Non-intercourse-related method.
- No mechanical devices or hormones used.
- Acceptable to all cultures and religions.
- Requires no prescription.
- Does not cause nausea or weight gain.
- Acceptable to many users and 'natural'.
- Failure rate low when the woman fulfils all the conditions of LAM.

Disadvantages of LAM

- Higher failure rate if the woman is supplementing with bottle feeding.
- No protection against STI transmission.

Coitus interruptus or 'withdrawal'

'Withdrawal' is the oldest method of birth control and is still one of the most popular natural contraceptive methods worldwide. In the UK 4% of couples use this method and it can be practiced by any couple at any time.

Advantages of coitus interruptus

- Free of charge.
- Requires no prescription.
- Does not cause nausea or weight gain.
- Acceptable to many users.

Disadvantages of coitus interruptus

- High failure rate (22% in practice).
- Intercourse is incomplete.
- May be unsatisfying for both partners.
- Partial ejaculation of semen can occur.
- No protection against STI transmission.

Emergency contraception

Emergency contraception (EC) involves methods that can be used in the event of UPSI to prevent pregnancy. These methods are not abortifacients as they do not disrupt implantation of the blastocyst.

Oral emergency contraception

Research began in the 1960s to develop post-coital contraception. A licensed preparation that became available in the UK in the early 1980s comprised two doses of 100 mcg ethinylestradiol and 500 mcg levonorgestrel to be taken within 72 hours of UPSI. We now know that progestogen-only emergency contraception containing 1500 mcg of levonorgestrel, taken in a single dose (Levonelle 1500® or branded generics) are more effective with fewer side effects.

Ulipristal acetate (EllaOne®), a selective progesterone receptor modulator, was launched in the UK in 2009. It has a similar mode of action to progestogen-only emergency contraception, but equally effective up to 5 days after UPSI.

Oral EC is now widely available with >50% being provided by a chemist or pharmacy, where it can be purchased or obtained 'free at the point of contact' through local patient group directions.

Levonorgestrel emergency contraception (LNG-EC)

LNG-EC works by delaying ovulation, rather than preventing implantation of the blastocyst, if taken before the start of the LH surge. No effect if taken after this time. Thought to prevent about 70% of pregnancies; may be more effective if taken as soon as possible after UPSI.

Providers should inform users of likely mode of action, to dispel some of the myths that oral EC 'causes abortions', contains 'dangerous hormones', and can affect future fertility.

A single dose of LNG-EC is licensed to be taken up to 72 hours after an episode of UPSI, and can be given multiples times in the same cycle if need be. ♀ taking liver-enzyme-inducing drugs, such as carbamazepine or St John's wort, should take two LNG-EC 1500 mcg tablets as a single dose. Additionally, women who weight more than 70 kg or have a BMI >26 kg/m² should take double-dose LNG-EC if they are unable to be fitted with an IUD or take ulipristal acetate emergency contraception (UPA-EC).

LNG-EC is available from GPs, nurses, community settings, and pharmacies. It has few side effects and no known teratogenicity. It can be prescribed in advance for those using barrier methods or 'perceived to be at risk'. It is the preferred oral EC option in women who are breast-feeding, wanting to 'quick-start' a hormonal method of contraception or require EC because of missed pills.

Ulipristal acetate EC

UPA-EC is a progesterone receptor modulator and works by stopping or delaying ovulation. It is effective throughout the fertile phase and at the start of the LH surge, but not once the LH surge has peaked. A single dose of UPA-EC can be taken up to 120 hours after UPSI and can be given more than once in the same cycle if needed. If taken within licensed indications, it will prevent 60–80% of pregnancies. UPA-EC is excreted in breastmilk, so if ♀ is breastfeeding, she must express and discard her breastmilk for the next 7 days. Not advisable to quick-start hormonal contraception for 5 days if UPA-EC has been taken, as its mode of action may be affected. Use of condoms or abstinence required during this time, until contraceptive method effective.

Also thought that hormonal contraception taken in the 7 days prior to taking UPA-EC will affect its action; therefore, LNG-EC or a copper IUD is the preferred choice.

UPA-EC is not recommended for use in women who are taking liver enzyme-inducing medication.

Copper IUD emergency contraception

Copper IUD (Cu-IUD) is the most effective method, preventing almost 100% of pregnancies if fitted within 120 hours of the first episode of UPSI any time in a menstrual cycle or after multiple episodes of UPSI, but no later than 5 days after the estimated time of ovulation. Cu-IUDs must be used, rather than the LNG- IUS.

Mode of action

Cu-IUDs ↓ viability of the ova, ↓ sperm numbers reaching the fallopian tubes; may prevent implantation by inducing endometrial changes.

A Cu-IUD should be offered to all ♀ requesting EC, as it is the most effective choice. However, oral EC should be prescribed if referral elsewhere is necessary or there is likely to be a delay in fitting a Cu-IUD. This will ensure that a method of EC has been provided if Cu-IUD insertion fails or the appointment is not kept.

Advantages of using Cu-IUDs for emergency contraception

- Suitable following multiple episodes of UPSI, but within 5 days after the estimated time of ovulation.
- Appropriate if vomiting follows oral EC.
- Ideal choice if requested as a long-term contraceptive method.
- Effective contraception for rest of menstrual cycle.
- Most effective method, especially if UPSI occurs close to the time of ovulation.

Disadvantages of using Cu-IUDs for emergency contraception

- Similar to Cu-IUDs used as a long-term contraceptive method.
- Possible pain at insertion, particularly if nulliparous.
- Some women perceive the fitting of an IUD to be 'invasive'.
- ↑ Risk of pelvic infection within the first 20 days. ▶ Screen for STIs prior to fitting. Some may consider antibiotic cover, while awaiting results in high-risk groups.
- Does not protect against STI transmission.

Female sterilization

Male and female sterilization is the main method of contraception for ~17% of couples in England and Wales. Female sterilization is normally performed as a day-case procedure. Regarded as permanent, as reversal, which requires surgery, may not be 100% successful.

Counsel use of effective contraception prior to surgery as up to 3% of ♀ may be pregnant at the time of sterilization. Sterilization should be postponed if there is any risk of pregnancy. Avoid routine sterilization immediately post-partum, post-abortion, or without considering other reversible options. Female sterilization has ↓ by >50% over the last 20 years, with the introduction of LARC.

Mode of action

Occlusion of fallopian tubes blocking the sperm and preventing fertilization. If done at laparoscopy or laparotomy, tubes are occluded by using clips, rings, or excising a part of the tube. If done hysteroscopically, micro-inserts placed into the tubes via the ostia. Hysteroscopic sterilization (Essure®) was discontinued in the UK in 2017.

Advantages of female sterilization

- Highly and immediately effective.
- High user satisfaction, removing fear of unplanned pregnancy.
- No 'hormonal' side effects.

Disadvantages of female sterilization

- Requires a general anaesthetic.
- Reversal requires a major surgical procedure and is not funded by the NHS.
- Other hormonal contraceptive methods are equally effective, and are reversible with additional non-contraceptive benefits.
- Has associated complications in 0.9–1.6 per 100 cases, with clips having the lowest complication rate of 0.47 per 100 cases (Box 34.4).

Box 34.4 Complications of female sterilization

Short term with laparoscopic sterilization
- *Anaesthetic complications*: overall mortality from anaesthetic complications is very low.
- *Operative complications*: occur in 0.5–1% of procedures.
- *Perforation of bowel, blood vessels, or bladder at the time of the procedure*: the need for laparotomy as a result of a serious complication is about 1.9 per 1000 procedures and risk of death is 1 in 12,000 laparoscopies.
- Wound infection.
- *Abdominal discomfort and shoulder tip pain*: from intra-peritoneal gas still remaining in the abdominal cavity. This slowly improves over 24–48 hours.

Long term
- *Late re-canalization of fallopian tubes*: Failure rates with Filshie clips are quoted as 2–3 per 1000 procedures. Occurs even up to 10 years after surgery with a cumulative ectopic pregnancy rate being as high as 31.9 per 1000 procedures, depending on the sterilization method used.
- *Complaints of heavy menstrual bleeding leading to hysterectomy*: Women often stop hormonal methods of contraception that have controlled their menstrual loss and pain. With advancing age, menstrual problems ↑ and this can lead to requests for treatment. There is a 17% cumulative probability of undergoing a hysterectomy when reviewed 14 years after female sterilization.
- *Regret*: not uncommon following sterilization, with 3–10% of couples reporting this. Regret is more common when the operation has been performed in those <30 years old and within a year of the birth of a child.

Male sterilization: vasectomy

In the UK ~11% of couples rely on male sterilization as their chosen method of contraception, with ~60% of all sterilization procedures performed on ♂. This ratio is different in other parts of the world, with ♀ ×10 more likely to be sterilized than their ♂ counterparts.

Mode of action

Male sterilization techniques in the UK aim to divide the vas deferens using ligation or coagulation, usually under local anaesthetic.

Advantages of vasectomy

- Very safe and effective with a failure rate of ~1/2000 in a lifetime after a negative 'clearance of sperm' test done at 12 weeks.
- Permanent method ameliorating concerns about future contraception or unplanned pregnancy.
- Minor surgical procedure, normally performed under local anaesthetic and taking 10–15 minutes.
- Can be done at a doctor's surgery or clinic.
- No evidence of ↑ risk of testicular/prostate cancer.
- No increased risk of coronary heart disease.

Disadvantages of vasectomy

- Reversal is not easy and is not funded by the NHS.
- Couples may regret this decision, especially if they are young (<30 years old).
- Not immediately effective, requiring a negative semen analysis before other methods can be abandoned.
- Surgical procedure with associated complications (Box 34.5).

Box 34.5 Complications of male sterilization

Short term

- *Local complications*: bruising and swelling with some discomfort or pain for a short time following the procedure. Scrotal haematoma formation occurs in 1–2% following vasectomy.
- *Wound infection*: in <2%. May require antibiotic treatment.
- *Failure to achieve azoospermia*: in ~0.5%. Further surgery may be required.

Long term

- *Sperm granulomata*: small tender lumps that form at the cut ends of the vas deferens, caused by leakage of sperm into the tissue from the cut ends, leading to local inflammation. Can be excised.
- *Chronic scrotal pain*: ~10% complain of chronic scrotal pain following vasectomy. May be made worse by sexual arousal or ejaculation. Local scar tissue formation and induration may be the cause. Further surgery to remove the epididymis and occluded vas may be indicated in some.

Women living with HIV

Why is the discussion of contraception important?

- The vast majority of ♀ infected with HIV are of reproductive age, with many relying solely on barrier methods and, therefore, at risk of an unplanned pregnancy.
- Effects of some antiretrovirals on the foetus may be severe (e.g. efavirenz, resulting in anencephaly in animal studies). Long-term effects are unknown, with concerns over haematological, metabolic and neurological abnormalities, and mitochondrial dysfunction.
- Drug interactions between hormonal contraceptives, some antiretrovirals and certain antibiotics. For up-to-date information, consult the online HIV drug interaction tracker: ℬ http://www.hiv-druginteractions.org (Box 34.6).
- Possible HIV transmission to the ♂ partner.

Male condom

Can be recommended for use by all HIV +ve ♀ and ♂, preferably in combination with another contraceptive method, if contraception is essential. If ♂ condom is unacceptable, consider ♀ condom.

Male/female sterilization

Both are safe in HIV infection, as operative risks are no greater than in those who are HIV –ve. However, if complications occur, they could be more serious in those with advanced HIV disease and other methods may be more acceptable. Caution should also be exercised in newly diagnosed patients who may be coming to terms with their condition and could change their views with regard to future pregnancies. A longer-term reversible method may be preferable.

Box 34.6 Interactions and hormonal contraception

Antibiotics

- Rifampicin and rifabutin: powerful enzyme inducers.
  - *CHC*—efficacy reduced therefore use not advised
  - *POP*—efficacy reduced, therefore, use not advised
  - *DMPA*—not affected
  - *IUS*—not affected
  - *Implant*—efficacy reduced, therefore, not recommended
  - *IUD*—not affected.
- *Broad-spectrum antibiotics*: not affected.

Antiretroviral drugs

- May ↑ or ↓ hormonal levels.
- All nucleoside reverse transcriptase inhibitors, including Combivir® and Truvada®, can be used safely.
- Efavirenz not compatible with oral methods, but DMPA is OK.
- Always check for antiretroviral drug interactions to identify potential drug interactions (ℬ www.hiv-druginteractions.org).

Combined hormonal contraceptives

There are no HIV-specific contraindications in those who are well and not on any treatment. Care must be taken to avoid any potential drug interactions.

Progestogen-only pills/subdermal implants

As with CHCs, there are no specific contraindications, but care needs to be taken to avoid drug interactions.

Depot medroxyprogesterone acetate (DMPA)

DMPA's efficacy is not affected by anti-retrovirals and the injection interval does not require altering from the standard 13 weeks. Some antiretrovirals may adversely affect bone mineral density, therefore, other progestogen-only contraceptive options may be preferred.

Intra-uterine contraceptives

- Cu-IUDs are highly effective and cost-effective.
- LNG-IUS are highly effective and can be used to treat menstrual problems, which are frequently seen in the Black African population.
- There are no drug interactions.
- IUD/IUS can be used without limitation in women whose CD4 count is >200 cells/mm^3.
- In women whose CD4 count is <200 cells/mm^3 IUD/IUS should be fitted with caution, although there is no issue with continuing to use the method if it is already *in situ*.
- Risks of complications and pelvic infection following IUD/IUS insertion are thought to be similar to those in HIV −ve ♀
- IUD/IUS use is not associated with ↑ risk of HIV transmission to a non-infected partner.

Cautions and contraindications

The UK Medical Eligibility Criteria for contraceptive use has adapted WHO guidance, and classifies the acceptability of each contraceptive method in different conditions into one of four categories.

UKMEC definition of category

- *Category 1*: a condition for which there is no restriction on the use of the contraceptive method.
- *Category 2*: a condition where the advantages of using the method generally outweigh the theoretical or proven risks.
- *Category 3*: a condition where the theoretical or proven risk generally outweighs the advantages of using the method. The provision of a method requires expert clinical judgement and/or referral to a specialist contraceptive provider, since use of the method is not usually recommended, unless other more appropriate methods are not available or not acceptable.
- *Category 4*: a condition that represents an unacceptable health risk if the contraceptive method is used.

UKMEC guidelines are summarized in Table 34.8.

Further information

UK Medical Eligibility Criteria for contraceptive use (UKMEC) 2016 Summary tables ℜ https://www.fsrh.org/standards-and-guidance/documents/ukmec-2016-summary-sheets/

Faculty of Sexual and Reproductive Health guidelines ℜ https://www.fsrh.org/standards-and-guidance/current-clinical- guidance/

Table 34.8 UK Medical eligibility criteria for contraceptive use guidelines (UKMEC) 2016*

UKMEC SUMMARY TABLE HORMONAL AND INTRAUTERINE CONTRACEPTION

Cu-IUD = Copper-bearing intrauterine device; LNG-IUS = Levonorgestrel-releasing intrauterine system;
IMP = Progestogen-only implant; DMPA = Progestogen-only injectable: depot medroxyprogesterone acetate;
POP = Progestogen-only pill; CHC = Combined hormonal contraception

CONDITION	Cu-IUD	LNG-IUS	IMP	DMPA	POP	CHC
			I = Initiation, C = Continuation			
PERSONAL CHARACTERISTICS AND REPRODUCTIVE HISTORY						
Pregnancy	NA	NA	NA	NA	NA	NA
Age	Menarche to <20=2, ≥20=1	Menarche to <20=2, ≥20=1	After menarche =1	Menarche to <18=2, 18-45=1, >45=2	After menarche =1	Menarche to <40=1, ≥40=2
Parity						
a) Nulliparous	1	1	1	1	1	1
b) Parous	1	1	1	1	1	1
Breastfeeding						
a) 0 to <6 weeks postpartum			1	2	1	4
b) ≥6 weeks to <6 months (primarily breastfeeding)	See below		1	1	1	2
c) ≥6 months postpartum			1	1	1	1
Postpartum (in non-breastfeeding women)						
a) 0 to <3 weeks						
(i) With other risk factors for VTE	See below		1	2	1	4
(ii) Without other risk factors			1	2	1	3
b) 3 to <6 weeks						
(i) With other risk factors for VTE			1	2	1	3
(ii) Without other risk factors	See below		1	1	1	2
c) ≥6 weeks			1	1	1	1

UKMEC	Definition of category
Category 1	A condition for which there is no restriction for the use of the method
Category 2	A condition where the advantages of using the method generally outweigh the theoretical or proven risks
Category 3	A condition where the theoretical or proven risks usually outweigh the advantages of using the method. The provision of a method requires expert clinical judgement and/or referral to a specialist contraceptive provider, since use of the method is not usually recommended unless other more appropriate methods are not available or not acceptable
Category 4	A condition which represents an unacceptable health risk if the method is used

(Continued)

Table 34.8 (*Contd.*)

UKMEC SUMMARY TABLE HORMONAL AND INTRAUTERINE CONTRACEPTION						
CONDITION	Cu-IUD	LNG-IUS	IMP	DMPA	POP	CHC
	I = Initiation, C = Continuation					
Postpartum (in breastfeeding or non-breastfeeding women, including post-caesarean section)						
a) 0 to <48 hours	1	1				
b) 48 hours to <4 weeks	3	3	See above			
c) ≥4 weeks	1	1				
d) Postpartum sepsis	4	4				
Post-abortion						
a) First trimester	1	1	1	1	1	1
b) Second trimester	2	2	1	1	1	1
c) Post-abortion sepsis	4	4	1	1	1	1
Past ectopic pregnancy	1	1	1	1	1	1
History of pelvic surgery	1	1	1	1	1	1
Smoking						
a) Age <35 years	1	1	1	1	1	2
b) Age ≥35 years						
(i) <15 cigarettes/day	1	1	1	1	1	3
(ii) ≥15 cigarettes/day	1	1	1	1	1	4
(iii) Stopped smoking <1 year	1	1	1	1	1	3
(iv) Stopped smoking ≥1 year	1	1	1	1	1	2
Obesity						
a) BMI ≥30–34 kg/m²	1	1	1	1	1	2
b) BMI ≥35 kg/m²	1	1	1	1	1	3

UKMEC	Definition of category
Category 1	A condition for which there is no restriction for the use of the method
Category 2	A condition where the advantages of using the method generally outweigh the theoretical or proven risks
Category 3	A condition where the theoretical or proven risks usually outweigh the advantages of using the method. The provision of a method requires expert clinical judgement and/or referral to a specialist contraceptive provider, since use of the method is not usually recommended unless other more appropriate methods are not available or not acceptable
Category 4	A condition which represents an unacceptable health risk if the method is used

Table 34.8 (Contd.)

UKMEC SUMMARY TABLE HORMONAL AND INTRAUTERINE CONTRACEPTION								
CONDITION	Cu-IUD	LNG-IUS		IMP		DMPA	POP	CHC
		I = Initiation, C = Continuation						
History of bariatric surgery								
a) With BMI <30 kg/m²	1	1		1		1	1	1
b) With BMI ≥30–34 kg/m²	1	1		1		1	1	2
c) With BMI ≥35 kg/m²	1	1		1		1	1	3
Organ transplant								
a) Complicated: graft failure (acute or chronic), rejection, cardiac allograft vasculopathy	I — 3 / C — 2	I — 3 / C — 2		2		2	2	3
b) Uncomplicated	2	2		2		2	2	2
CARDIOVASCULAR DISEASE (CVD)								
Multiple risk factors for CVD (such as smoking, diabetes, hypertension, obesity and dyslipidaemias)	1	2		2		3	2	3
Hypertension								
a) Adequately controlled hypertension	1	1		1		2	1	3
b) Consistently elevated BP levels (properly taken measurements)								
(i) Systolic >140–159 mmHg or diastolic >90–99 mmHg	1	1		1		1	1	3
(ii) Systolic ≥160 mmHg or diastolic ≥100 mmHg	1	1		1		2	1	4
c) Vascular disease	1	2		2		3	2	4
History of high BP during pregnancy	1	1		1		1	1	2
Current and history of ischaemic heart disease	1	I — 2 / C — 3		I — 2 / C — 3		3	I — 2 / C — 3	4
Stroke (history of cerebrovascular accident, including TIA)	1	I — 2 / C — 3		I — 2 / C — 3		3	I — 2 / C — 3	4
Known dyslipidaemias	1	2		2		2	2	2

UKMEC	Definition of category
Category 1	A condition for which there is no restriction for the use of the method
Category 2	A condition where the advantages of using the method generally outweigh the theoretical or proven risks
Category 3	A condition where the theoretical or proven risks usually outweigh the advantages of using the method. The provision of a method requires expert clinical judgement and/or referral to a specialist contraceptive provider, since use of the method is not usually recommended unless other more appropriate methods are not available or not acceptable
Category 4	A condition which represents an unacceptable health risk if the method is used

(Continued)

Table 34.8 (*Contd.*)

UKMEC SUMMARY TABLE HORMONAL AND INTRAUTERINE CONTRACEPTION						
CONDITION	Cu-IUD	LNG-IUS	IMP	DMPA	POP	CHC
	I = Initiation, C = Continuation					
Venous thromboembolism (VTE)						
a) History of VTE	1	2	2	2	2	4
b) Current VTE (on anticoagulants)	1	2	2	2	2	4
c) Family history of VTE						
(i) First-degree relative age <45 years	1	1	1	1	1	3
(ii) First-degree relative age ≥45 years	1	1	1	1	1	2
d) Major surgery						
(i) With prolonged immobilisation	1	2	2	2	2	4
(ii) Without prolonged immobilisation	1	1	1	1	1	2
e) Minor surgery without immobilisation	1	1	1	1	1	1
f) Immobility (unrelated to surgery) (e.g. wheelchair use, debilitating illness)	1	1	1	1	1	3
Superficial venous thrombosis						
a) Varicose veins	1	1	1	1	1	1
b) Superficial venous thrombosis	1	1	1	1	1	2
Known thrombogenic mutations (e.g. factor V Leiden, prothrombin mutation, protein S, protein C and antithrombin deficiencies)	1	2	2	2	2	4

UKMEC	Definition of category
Category 1	A condition for which there is no restriction for the use of the method
Category 2	A condition where the advantages of using the method generally outweigh the theoretical or proven risks
Category 3	A condition where the theoretical or proven risks usually outweigh the advantages of using the method. The provision of a method requires expert clinical judgement and/or referral to a specialist contraceptive provider, since use of the method is not usually recommended unless other more appropriate methods are not available or not acceptable
Category 4	A condition which represents an unacceptable health risk if the method is used

Table 34.8 (Contd.)

UKMEC SUMMARY TABLE HORMONAL AND INTRAUTERINE CONTRACEPTION									
CONDITION	Cu-IUD		LNG-IUS		IMP	DMPA	POP		CHC	
	I = Initiation, C = Continuation									
Valvular and congenital heart disease									
a) Uncomplicated	1		1		1	1	1		2	
b) Complicated (e.g. pulmonary hypertension, history of subacute bacterial endocarditis)	2		2		1	1	1		4	
Cardiomyopathy									
a) Normal cardiac function	1		1		1	1	1		2	
b) Impaired cardiac function	2		2		2	2	2		4	
Cardiac arrhythmias									
a) Atrial fibrillation	1		2		2	2	2		4	
b) Known long QT syndrome	I 3	C 1	I 3	C 1	1	2	1		2	
NEUROLOGICAL CONDITIONS									
Headaches									
a) Non-migrainous (mild or severe)	1		1		1	1	1		I 1	C 2
b) Migraine without aura, at any age	1		2		2	2	I 1	C 2	I 2	C 3
c) Migraine with aura, at any age	1		2		2	2	2		4	
d) History (≥5 years ago) of migraine with aura, any age	1		2		2	2	2		3	

UKMEC	Definition of category
Category 1	A condition for which there is no restriction for the use of the method
Category 2	A condition where the advantages of using the method generally outweigh the theoretical or proven risks
Category 3	A condition where the theoretical or proven risks usually outweigh the advantages of using the method. The provision of a method requires expert clinical judgement and/or referral to a specialist contraceptive provider, since use of the method is not usually recommended unless other more appropriate methods are not available or not acceptable
Category 4	A condition which represents an unacceptable health risk if the method is used

(Continued)

Table 34.8 (*Contd.*)

UKMEC SUMMARY TABLE HORMONAL AND INTRAUTERINE CONTRACEPTION						
CONDITION	Cu-IUD	LNG-IUS	IMP	DMPA	POP	CHC
	I = Initiation, C = Continuation					
Idiopathic intracranial hypertension (IIH)	1	1	1	1	1	2
Epilepsy	1	1	1	1	1	1
Taking anti-epileptic drugs	Certain anti-epileptic drugs have the potential to affect the bioavailability of steroid hormones in hormonal contraception. For up-to-date information on the potential drug interactions between hormonal contraception and anti-epileptic drugs, please refer to the online drug interaction checker available on the available on Stockley's Interaction Checker website (https://www.medicinescomplete.com/mc/alerts/current/drug-interactions.htm).					
DEPRESSIVE DISORDERS						
Depressive disorders	1	1	1	1	1	1
BREAST AND REPRODUCTIVE TRACT CONDITIONS						
Vaginal bleeding patterns						
a) Irregular pattern without heavy bleeding	1	1	2	2	2	1
b) Heavy or prolonged bleeding (includes regular and irregular patterns)	2	I: 1, C: 2	2	2	2	1
Unexplained vaginal bleeding (suspicious for serious condition) before evaluation	I: 4, C: 2	I: 4, C: 2	3	3	2	2
Endometriosis	2	1	1	1	1	1
Benign ovarian tumours (including cysts)	1	1	1	1	1	1
Severe dysmenorrhoea	2	1	1	1	1	1
Gestational trophoblastic disease (GTD)						
a) Undetectable hCG levels	1	1	1	1	1	1
b) Decreasing hCG levels	3	3	1	1	1	1
c) Persistently elevated hCG levels or malignant disease	4	4	1	1	1	1

UKMEC	Definition of category
Category 1	A condition for which there is no restriction for the use of the method
Category 2	A condition where the advantages of using the method generally outweigh the theoretical or proven risks
Category 3	A condition where the theoretical or proven risks usually outweigh the advantages of using the method. The provision of a method requires expert clinical judgement and/or referral to a specialist contraceptive provider, since use of the method is not usually recommended unless other more appropriate methods are not available or not acceptable
Category 4	A condition which represents an unacceptable health risk if the method is used

Table 34.8 (*Contd.*)

UKMEC SUMMARY TABLE HORMONAL AND INTRAUTERINE CONTRACEPTION								
CONDITION	Cu-IUD		LNG-IUS		IMP	DMPA	POP	CHC
	I = Initiation, C = Continuation							
Cervical ectropion	1		1		1	1	1	1
Cervical intraepithelial neoplasia (CIN)	1		2		1	2	1	2
Cervical cancer								
a) Awaiting treatment	**I** 4	**C** 2	**I** 4	**C** 2	2	2	1	2
b) Radical trachelectomy	3		3		2	2	1	2
Breast conditions								
a) Undiagnosed mass/breast symptoms	1		2		2	2	2	**I** 3 / **C** 2
b) Benign breast conditions	1		1		1	1	1	1
c) Family history of breast cancer	1		1		1	1	1	1
d) Carriers of known gene mutations associated with breast cancer (e.g. BRCA1/BRCA2)	1		2		2	2	2	3
e) Breast cancer								
(i) Current breast cancer	1		4		4	4	4	4
(ii) Past breast cancer	1		3		3	3	3	3
Endometrial cancer	**I** 4	**C** 2	**I** 4	**C** 2	1	1	1	1
Ovarian cancer	1		1		1	1	1	1

UKMEC	Definition of category
Category 1	A condition for which there is no restriction for the use of the method
Category 2	A condition where the advantages of using the method generally outweigh the theoretical or proven risks
Category 3	A condition where the theoretical or proven risks usually outweigh the advantages of using the method. The provision of a method requires expert clinical judgement and/or referral to a specialist contraceptive provider, since use of the method is not usually recommended unless other more appropriate methods are not available or not acceptable
Category 4	A condition which represents an unacceptable health risk if the method is used

(*Continued*)

Table 34.8 (*Contd.*)

UKMEC SUMMARY TABLE HORMONAL AND INTRAUTERINE CONTRACEPTION									
CONDITION	Cu-IUD		LNG-IUS		IMP	DMPA	POP	CHC
	I = Initiation, C = Continuation							
Uterine fibroids								
a) Without distortion of the uterine cavity	1		1		1	1	1	1
b) With distortion of the uterine cavity	3		3		1	1	1	1
Anatomical abnormalities								
a) Distorted uterine cavity	3		3					
b) Other abnormalities	2		2					
Pelvic inflammatory disease (PID)								
a) Past PID (assuming no current risk factor for STIs)	1		1		1	1	1	1
b) Current PID	**I** 4	**C** 2	**I** 4	**C** 2	1	1	1	1
Sexually transmitted infections (STIs)								
a) Chlamydial infection (current)	**I**	**C**	**I**	**C**				
(i) Symptomatic	4	2	4	2	1	1	1	1
(ii) Asymptomatic	3	2	3	2	1	1	1	1
b) Purulent cervicitis or gonorrhoea (current)	4	2	4	2	1	1	1	1
c) Other current STIs (excluding HIV & hepatitis)	2		2		1	1	1	1
d) Vaginitis (including Trichomonas vaginalis and bacterial vaginosis) (current)	2		2		1	1	1	1
e) Increased risk for STIs	2		2		1	1	1	1

UKMEC	Definition of category
Category 1	A condition for which there is no restriction for the use of the method
Category 2	A condition where the advantages of using the method generally outweigh the theoretical or proven risks
Category 3	A condition where the theoretical or proven risks usually outweigh the advantages of using the method. The provision of a method requires expert clinical judgement and/or referral to a specialist contraceptive provider, since use of the method is not usually recommended unless other more appropriate methods are not available or not acceptable
Category 4	A condition which represents an unacceptable health risk if the method is used

Table 34.8 (*Contd.*)

UKMEC SUMMARY TABLE HORMONAL AND INTRAUTERINE CONTRACEPTION							
CONDITION	Cu-IUD	LNG-IUS		IMP	DMPA	POP	CHC
		I = Initiation, C = Continuation					
HIV INFECTION							
HIV infection							
a) High risk of HIV infection	2	2		1	2	1	1
b) HIV infected							
(i) CD4 count ≥200 cells/mm³	2	2		1	1	1	1
(ii) CD4 count <200 cells/mm³	I 3	C 2	I 3 / C 2	1	1	1	1
c) Taking antiretroviral (ARV) drugs	Certain ARV drugs have the potential to affect the bioavailability of steroid hormones in hormonal contraception. For up-to-date information on the potential drug interactions between hormonal contraception and ARV drugs, please refer to the online HIV drugs interaction checker (www.hiv-druginteractions.org/interactions.aspx).						
OTHER INFECTIONS							
Tuberculosis							
a) Non-pelvic	1	1		1	1	1	1
b) Pelvic	I 4	C 3	I 4 / C 3	1	1	1	1
ENDOCRINE CONDITIONS							
Diabetes							
a) History of gestational disease	1	1		1	1	1	1
b) Non-vascular disease							
(i) Non-insulin dependent	1	2		2	2	2	2
(ii) Insulin dependent	1	2		2	2	2	2
c) Nephropathy/retinopathy/neuropathy	1	2		2	2	2	3
d) Other vascular disease	I	2		2	2	2	3

UKMEC	Definition of category
Category 1	A condition for which there is no restriction for the use of the method
Category 2	A condition where the advantages of using the method generally outweigh the theoretical or proven risks
Category 3	A condition where the theoretical or proven risks usually outweigh the advantages of using the method. The provision of a method requires expert clinical judgement and/or referral to a specialist contraceptive provider, since use of the method is not usually recommended unless other more appropriate methods are not available or not acceptable
Category 4	A condition which represents an unacceptable health risk if the method is used

(*Continued*)

Table 34.8 (*Contd.*)

UKMEC SUMMARY TABLE HORMONAL AND INTRAUTERINE CONTRACEPTION							
CONDITION	Cu-IUD	LNG-IUS	IMP	DMPA	POP	CHC	
	I = Initiation, C = Continuation						
Thyroid disorders							
a) Simple goitre	1	1	1	1	1	1	
b) Hyperthyroid	1	1	1	1	1	1	
c) Hypothyroid	1	1	1	1	1	1	
GASTROINTESTINAL CONDITIONS							
Gallbladder disease							
a) Symptomatic							
(i) Treated by cholecystectomy	1	2	2	2	2	2	
(ii) Medically treated	1	2	2	2	2	3	
(iii) Current	1	2	2	2	2	3	
b) Asymptomatic	1	2	2	2	2	2	
History of cholestasis							
a) Pregnancy related	1	1	1	1	1	2	
b) Past COC related	1	2	2	2	2	3	
Viral hepatitis							
a) Acute or flare	1	1	1	1	1	I	C
						3	2
b) Carrier	1	1	1	1	1	1	
c) Chronic	1	1	1	1	1	1	
Cirrhosis							
a) Mild (compensated without complications)	1	1	1	1	1	1	
b) Severe (decompensated)	1	3	3	3	3	4	

UKMEC	Definition of category
Category 1	A condition for which there is no restriction for the use of the method
Category 2	A condition where the advantages of using the method generally outweigh the theoretical or proven risks
Category 3	A condition where the theoretical or proven risks usually outweigh the advantages of using the method. The provision of a method requires expert clinical judgement and/or referral to a specialist contraceptive provider, since use of the method is not usually recommended unless other more appropriate methods are not available or not acceptable
Category 4	A condition which represents an unacceptable health risk if the method is used

Table 34.8 (*Contd.*)

UKMEC SUMMARY TABLE HORMONAL AND INTRAUTERINE CONTRACEPTION						
CONDITION	Cu-IUD	LNG-IUS	IMP	DMPA	POP	CHC
	I = Initiation, C = Continuation					
Liver tumours						
a) Benign						
(i) Focal nodular hyperplasia	1	2	2	2	2	2
(ii) Hepatocellular adenoma	1	3	3	3	3	4
b) Malignant (hepatocellular carcinoma)	1	3	3	3	3	4
Inflammatory bowel disease (including Crohn's disease and ulcerative colitis)	1	1	1	1	2	2
ANAEMIAS						
Thalassaemia	2	1	1	1	1	1
Sickle cell disease	2	1	1	1	1	2
Iron deficiency anaemia	2	1	1	1	1	1
RHEUMATIC DISEASES						
Rheumatoid arthritis	1	2	2	2	2	2
Systemic lupus erythematosus (SLE)						
a) No antiphospholipid antibodies	1	2	2	2	2	2
b) Positive antiphospholipid antibodies	1	2	2	2	2	4
Positive antiphospholipid antibodies	1	2	2	2	2	4
DRUG INTERACTIONS						
Taking medication	See section on drug interactions with hormonal contraception.					

UKMEC	Definition of category
Category 1	A condition for which there is no restriction for the use of the method
Category 2	A condition where the advantages of using the method generally outweigh the theoretical or proven risks
Category 3	A condition where the theoretical or proven risks usually outweigh the advantages of using the method. The provision of a method requires expert clinical judgement and/or referral to a specialist contraceptive provider, since use of the method is not usually recommended unless other more appropriate methods are not available or not acceptable
Category 4	A condition which represents an unacceptable health risk if the method is used

Psychological aspects and sexual problems

Psychological aspects associated with sexual health 430
Neuroses associated with sexual health 431
Sexual problems 432
Classification 433
Common female problems 434
Common male problems 436
Psychological problems in those with HIV infection 441

Psychological aspects associated with sexual health

Between 20 and 40% of new patients attending clinics for contraception or STI advice have high levels of anxiety. It is important to recognize and manage this during the consultation to help explore their presenting problem, as well as encourage further clinic attendances. The origins of this anxiety are multifactorial, but talking about sex and any associated problems can be embarrassing. Those worried about their sexuality or having contracted a potential STI, may feel stigma and shame. New diagnoses of HIV infection, anogenital herpes, or syphilis, together with discussions related to an unplanned pregnancy, generate the greatest anxiety.

The greatest psychological reaction usually arises from a diagnosis of HIV infection. It does not necessarily relate to the stage of the disease and may exhibit a 'bereavement'-type reaction—disbelief, denial, anxiety, and depression. There may also be suicidal tendencies. In addition, such feelings may be complicated by guilt, resentment, and stigmatization. Support is important, ensuring that information is given at and over a time best suited to the individual. Referral for specialist advice/counselling may also be required.

Certain procedures, e.g. colposcopy for abnormal cervical cytology, are associated with very high levels of anxiety. Stress and depression are common features of chronic conditions, e.g. HIV infection, provoked vestibulodynia, chronic pelvic/perineal pain, prostatitis, and persistent anogenital warts. Mental ill-health is also reported with conditions that persist or recur, such as anogenital herpes, genital warts, and vaginal candidiasis.

Asking open questions and giving patients sufficient time to express their concerns are important. Listening and empathizing are key communication skills to master. Remember that people disclosing sexual issues have chosen to talk to you, especially if you have asked 'do you have any sexual problems?' In a consultation, use your ears, eyes, and mouth, in that order.

Talking about sexual health concerns may help patients to reveal their innermost worries about their sexual performance. A careful discussion of the problem (with written information) may be all that is needed. Other may require appropriate signposting to other services, e.g. abortion clinics and psychosexual counselling.

Although therapeutic interventions, e.g. antiretroviral treatment for HIV, suppressive treatment for recurrent herpes, phosphodiesterase type 5 inhibitors (PDE5 inhibitors) for erectile dysfunction, may reduce psychological morbidity, patients may still find it difficult to disclose their diagnoses or condition to their sexual partners.

Neuroses associated with sexual health

Over-reaction and hypochondriasis

Examples include:

- Inappropriate reaction to the diagnosed condition.
- Undue vigorous penile squeezing to produce a urethral discharge.
- Obsessional attention to genital marks and irregularities.
- Repeated masturbation to confirm potency in those with erectile dysfunction.
- Repeated re-attendance for emergency contraception when an effective contraception method is used.
- Repeated attendance for PEPSE for low risk sexual exposure.

May be a symptom of some other underlying problem (e.g. rumours about a sexual partner). Manage by exploring the patient's anxieties and correcting misinformation.

Phobias

Excessive and inappropriate anxiety reactions, triggered by specific situations or objects, despite having an insight into the lack of reason or appropriateness.

Often triggered by stress and media publicity. Likely to be prompted by underlying guilt or a sexual concern, which should be addressed when formulating management strategies.

Factitious illness and Munchausen's syndrome

Attending sexual health clinics with an imagined HIV +ve test result. Presenting with symptoms and abdominal distention, suggesting pregnancy in pseudocyesis. Reasons and motivation are often unclear, but may be used to gain sympathy, hospital care, or social benefits. Psychiatric referral is often required.

Sexual problems

In the most recent NATSAL survey 42% of men and 51% of women reported having one or more sexual problems in the previous year. Over 70% never seek help and of those that decide to talk to a HCP, less than 50% will follow-up a referral to a psychosexual counsellor. HCPs interested in this work can train and become a member of the College of Sexual and Relationship Therapists (COSRT) or diplomate/member of the Institute of Psychosexual Medicine.

Different therapies are used to explore the sexual problem and the HCP will assess whether the sexual problem is psychological, physical, or a combination of the two. By discussing and using active listening techniques, the HCP will help patients gain a better understanding of their sexual problem and any potential underlying cause. The HCP may advise exercises or tasks for patients to undertake in their own time.

Patients can decide whether they would like to be seen individually and/or with their partner. The sessions last 30–50 minutes with most psychosexual counsellors working in community sexual health clinics undertaking short interventional work, seeing patients between 4 and 6 times.

Classification

- *Sexual desire disorders*:
  - hypoactive
  - sexual aversion
- Sexual arousal disorder
- Erectile dysfunction
- Premature ejaculation
- Orgasmic disorder
- *Sexual pain disorders*:
  - dyspareunia
  - vaginismus.

After organic problems have been identified and treated, the management of sexual problems requires motivation and cooperation of the patient, together with the support of their partner. Depending on the sexual issue, couple therapy may be indicated. Emotional issues that may underlie or complicate the presenting problem should be explored and addressed through counselling.

Simple, brief counselling can be undertaken by all HCPs with individuals or couples, and should include:
- basic information and correction of false ideas
- feeding back on transference and countertransference in the consultation
- using the genital examination as part of the therapy, e.g. addressing patient's concerns on the size of his penis or her labia
- making suggestions, e.g. positions during intercourse
- *providing permission and reassurances*: often linked with a new suggestion, e.g. the use of vibrators and other sex aids
- facilitating communication between partners, in particular to develop self-esteem, self-assertiveness, and self-protection.

This may lead to behavioural psychotherapy for individuals, couples, or sometimes groups. The framework consists of the following:
- setting behavioural tasks, i.e. 'homework'
- analysis of the patient's or couple's success, identifying obstacles, or difficulties
- provision of help, support, and advice to address the obstacles and problems
- review of the new situation with new tasks set or revised.

Common female problems

Low sexual desire/arousal and orgasmic dysfunction

Heterogeneous condition

Causal factors include:
- Partner conflict and disharmony.
- Ignorance.
- Psychological causes, e.g. anxiety, depression, body dysmorphism.
- *Physical causes*: local (e.g. provoked vestibulodynia, endometriosis, cystitis), systemic (e.g. diabetes mellitus, multiple sclerosis), drugs (e.g. antihypertensives, antidepressants), surgery affecting body image (e.g. hysterectomy, mastectomy).
- *Post-menopause*: low androgen levels after removal of both ovaries or in women in their 60s, vaginal atrophy.

Management
- *Defining and managing any underlying problems*: in post-menopausal women, local vaginal oestrogen and/or HRT, with androgenic activity may be beneficial (e.g. tibolone)
- *Testosterone gel* (Testim® or Testogel®): off-licensed use for female hypoactive sexual desire disorder, where both ovaries have been removed. Contents of one tube or sachet (50 mg/5 g) to be applied over a 10-day period, therefore 3 tubes/sachets a month. Women should receive concomitant HRT. Adverse effects include hirsutism and acne.
- *Sensate focus*: a 3-stage programme in which the couple progresses stepwise from non-genital pleasuring through genital pleasuring to non-demanding coitus under the control of the woman.
- *Insufficient data on drugs*: flibanserin licensed in the US provides a modest improvement in sexual satisfaction for pre-menopausal women. Phosphodiesterase-5 inhibitors appear to be disappointing.

Dyspareunia

Genital pain just before, during, or after sexual intercourse. Worsened by vaginismus (involuntary bulbocavernosus muscle spasm) and exacerbated by psychological factors, especially anxiety and partner disharmony.

Vulvo-vaginal problems

- *Congenital*: e.g. vaginal septum.
- *Physiological*: inadequate lubrication (e.g. oestrogen deficiency, breast feeding).
- *Traumatic*: e.g. episiotomy, radiation therapy.
- *Inflammatory*:
  - *infective*—e.g. candidiasis, trichomoniasis
  - *ulcerative*—e.g. genital herpes, syphilis, aphthosis, Behçet's disease
  - *dermatological*—e.g. irritant dermatitis, lichen sclerosis or planus
  - *degenerative*—atrophic vaginitis
  - provoked vestibulodynia.
- *Neoplastic*: e.g. squamous cell carcinoma.
- *Bartholin gland*: abscess, cyst.

Uterine/pelvic problems

Retroverted uterus, pelvic congestion, cervicitis, endometritis, PID, pelvic adhesions, endometriosis, fibroids, adnexal pathology (e.g. ovarian cysts, tumours).

Anal/intestinal problems

Anal fissure/fistula, irritable bowel syndrome, inflammatory bowel disease.

Urinary problems

Urethritis, urethral caruncle, cystitis, painful bladder syndrome.

Vaginismus

A learned response, often 2° to dyspareunia (e.g. from provoked vestibulodynia, atrophic vaginitis, trauma), leading to recurrent or persistent involuntary contraction of the musculature of the outer third of the vagina, interfering with coitus, and causing distress. Other causes/factors include fear of pregnancy, loss of control, association of intercourse with violence, previous sexual abuse, relationship difficulties, and religious/cultural taboos. Tampons are usually avoided and sanitary towels are used for menstruation. Involuntary perineal spasms may occur while preparing for/conducting a pelvic examination, which is often evaded.

Management

Management is in stages—problem-orientated therapy with behavioural and desensitization exercises:
- Exclude or manage physical causes and psychological factors. Discuss and explore any misconceptions related to sexual functioning, with the partner's involvement if agreeable.
- Encourage the woman to become comfortable touching her genitalia and inserting a finger into the vagina.
- Encourage her to firmly massage the vulval vestibule and posterior fourchette.
- Proceed to more fingers and/or the use of lubricated, graded vaginal dilators.
- *Advise Kegel's exercise*: perineal contraction [against inserted finger(s) or dilators] followed by relaxation (as when passing urine), to help muscle control.
- *Suggest partner involvement*: gentle introduction of a finger into the vagina, slowly escalating to more fingers or dilators.
- When comfortable, proceed to penetrative sexual intercourse with the woman adopting a position (e.g. superior) to maintain control.

Common male problems

Erectile dysfunction (ED)

See Table 35.1.
Common, affecting 8% of men in their 40s, increasing to 40% in their 60s reporting ED: 60% organic, 15% psychogenic, 25% mixed.

Main causes

- *Lifestyle factors*: obesity, smoking, alcohol, recreational drugs (e.g. amphetamines, barbiturates, cocaine, marijuana, heroin).
- *Trauma and iatrogenic*: e.g. prolonged bicycle riding, prostatic/pelvic surgery, pelvic fracture, and local radiation treatment.
- *Drugs*: e.g. antidepressants [most with bupropion, mirtazapine have the least effects], antipsychotics (many), antihypertensives (most), androgen inhibitors (e.g. finasteride for benign prostatic hypertrophy with alpha blockers having a lower risk of ED)].
- *Vascular*: responsible for nearly 50% of cases in those aged >50 years, e.g. ischaemic heart disease (IHD), hypertension, peripheral vascular disease. Coexisting IHD (up to 40%) manifests a mean of 38 months after ED (penile arteries 1–2 mm, coronary 3–4 mm).
- *Endocrine*: diabetes mellitus (>50% over 55 years have ED), neurogenic and vascular factors; hyper/hypothyroidism; hypogonadism, both physiological and pathological; hyperprolactinaemia.
- *Neurological*: multiple sclerosis; Parkinson's disease.
- *Psychogenic (depression, anxiety)*: increase in sympathetic tone. Performance anxiety may become self-perpetuating.

Basic assessment

- *History*: for risk factors; libido (presence of morning erections, use of pornography, masturbation issues), shaving (need and frequency).
- *Examination*: genital abnormalities, including hypogonadism, facial/body hair, neurological (S2–S4 dermatomes), BP/peripheral pulses.
- *Investigations*: exclude diabetes (urinalysis/blood glucose); consider serum testosterone, prolactin + other endocrine tests (thyroid, pituitary function), lipid profile, etc. Ultrasonography and angiography rarely required.

First-line management

- Psychosexual therapy (alone or in combination).
- *PDE 5 inhibitors*:
  - *Sildenafil*—recommended dose 50 mg (range 25–100 mg) 1 hour before intercourse. Advise 1 dose in 24 hours (100 mg maximum). 29% fall in plasma concentration if taken with food. Half-life, 4–5 hours.
  - *Vardenafil*—recommended dose 10 mg (range 2.5–20 mg) 25–60 minutes before intercourse. Advise 1 dose in 24 hours (20 mg maximum). 20% fall in plasma concentration with food. Half-life, 4.8–6 hours.
  - *Tadalafil*—recommended dose 10 mg (range 10–20 mg) 30 minutes–12 hours before intercourse. Maximum dose over 24 hours, 20 mg. No decline in plasma concentration with food. Half-life, 17.5–21 hours. Can be taken daily when anticipated sexual activity is at least twice weekly – dose 5 mg a day. Adjust dose according to response.

Table 35.1 International index of erectile function-5 (IIEF-5) scoring system

Over the past 6 months	Score				
	1	2	3	4	5
Confidence in getting and keeping an erection	Very low	Low	Moderate	High	Very high
Erections on sexual stimulation hard enough for penetration	Never/ almost never	<50% of the time	750% of the time	>50% of the time	Always/ almost always
Maintaining erection after penetration	Never/ almost never	<50% of the time	750% of the time	>50% of the time	Always/ almost always
Maintaining erection to completion of intercourse	Extremely difficult	Very difficult	Difficult	Slightly difficult	Not difficult
Satisfactory intercourse	Never/ almost never	<50% of the time	750% of the time	>50% of the time	Always/ almost always

IIEF-5: severe (5–7); moderate (8–11); mild to moderate (12–16); mild (17–21); and no ED (22–25).

Reprinted from Rosen, Cappelleri, Smith et al. (2000) Development and evaluation of an abridged, 5-item version of the International Index of Erectile Function (IIEF-5) as a diagnostic tool for erectile dysfunction. *International Journal of Impotence Research* 11(6): 319–26, with permission from Springer Nature.

- *Avanafil*—recommended dose 100 mg (range 50–200 mg) 15–30 minutes before intercourse. Advise 1 dose in 24 hours (200 mg maximum). 39% lower in plasma concentration following a fatty meal. Half-life, 6-17 hours.
- Success rates (erection suitable for intercourse) of PDE 5 inhibitors up to 75%, but high placebo rates (22–38%).
- Contraindicated in patients taking nitrates (both therapeutic and recreational), and those with hypotension, unstable angina, recent cerebrovascular accident, or myocardial infarction.
- Avoid alpha-blockers for 4 hours after taking sildenafil, use minimum dose for avanafil, lowest dose and 6 hours after vardenafil

Alternative management methods
- *Synthetic prostaglandin E₁ agent* (e.g. alprostadil) available as:
  - *Intra-urethral pellets*—usual starting dose 250 mcg up to 1 mg. Maximum 2 doses a day/7 doses a week.
  - *Urethral cream*—3 mg per 1 g in applicator applied to tip of penis 5–30 minutes before sexual activity. Maximum 1 dose in 24 hours not more than 2–3 times per week.

- *Intra-cavernosal injection*—usual dose range 5–20 mcg. Not more than 2–3 times per week with at least 24 hours between injections. Reduce dose if erection lasts more than 2 hours
- Up to 90% response rate with alprostadil injection and 40–60% with pellets/cream.
- *Testosterone (IM or transdermal)*: should only be considered when ED is related to hypogonadism, otherwise no evidence of benefit.
- *Pelvic floor exercises with biofeedback* (including perineal muscle electrical stimulation): only if ED related to venous leakage or occlusion (success rate ~50%).
- *Mechanical aids*:
  - *vacuum devices*—suck venous blood into the penis, causing erection maintained by a firm constricting band. Lacks spontaneity, may cause bruising, and produces a venous (cold/blue) erection
  - *implants*—e.g. inflatable devices, malleable rods inserted surgically into the penis. 90–95% produce erections suitable for intercourse with satisfaction rates of 80–90%.

Premature ejaculation

Most common sexual dysfunction in men under 40 years, reported in about 30%. Difficult to define as dependent on sexual partner and may indicate delayed partner orgasm, but generally indicative of ejaculation with minimal penile stimulation resulting in reduced sexual satisfaction. Generally considered to be a psychological problem; rarely reported with chronic prostatitis.

- *Primary*—patient has always ejaculated prematurely. Often considered to be a conditioned response from teenage masturbatory practices, but may reflect sexual performance anxiety, deep sexual concerns from childhood traumatic experiences, including sexual assault and/or familial conflict. Current research also suggests genetic susceptibility and decreased central serotonin (5-hydroxy tryptamine - 5-HT) mediated neurotransmission.
- *Secondary*—previous ejaculatory control. Probably largely related to performance anxiety.

Management

If associated with ED, treat ED first. Encourage communication between the couple to discuss anxieties and issues.

- Distraction techniques (concentrating on something not linked to sex, such as thinking of countries of the World beginning with A).
- Taking a deep breath just before ejaculation. This can delay ejaculation and reduce the stimulation.
- Concentrate on foreplay to provide greater partner satisfaction.
- *Stop/start*: manual stimulation (initially) by partner or patient until ejaculation is imminent. Then cease for 30 seconds before resuming. The sequence is repeated until ejaculation is required.
- *Squeeze technique*: similar approach but firm pressure is applied across the penis at the frenulum, aborting imminent ejaculation. Over time these methods progress to vulval contact and then vaginal penetration, stopping for 30 seconds, or withdrawing and squeezing as ejaculation approaches. Success rate 65–90% with active participation of partner.

- *Ejaculation 1–2 hours before coitus*: results in longer latent period for coital ejaculation, especially if the partner is superior. Older men may have problems attaining a further erection.
- *Reduce sensation*:
  - local anaesthetic gel/ointment, e.g. lidocaine (provided that there is no allergy)
  - use of condoms containing local anaesthetic gel or thicker condoms.
- *Drug treatment (licensed)*: dapoxetine initially 30 mg 1–3 hours before sex. Maximum dose 60 mg/day or 30 mg if taking certain drugs, including clarithromycin, erythromycin, fluconazole. Increase in intravaginal ejaculatory latency time from 0.9 minutes to 1.9, 3.1, and 3.6 minutes, respectively, for placebo, dapoxetine 30 mg and dapoxetine 60 mg.
- *Drug treatment (not licensed)*: selective serotonin re-uptake inhibitors (SSRIs) and clomipramine delay ejaculation by their effect on central 5-HT receptors. SSRIs take at least 3 weeks to produce the effect, but clomipramine is effective after a single dose. Regimens shown to be effective:
  - *daily*—clomipramine 10–40 mg or SSRI (paroxetine 20–40 mg, sertraline 50–100 mg, or fluoxetine 20 mg).
  - *'On-demand'*—clomipramine 10–50 mg 5–6 hours before coitus.
- Pelvic floor (Kegel) exercises to improve ejaculatory control.

Retarded ejaculation

Difficulty, delay, or absence of orgasm following sufficient sexual stimulation, which causes personal distress.

Aetiology

- *Physiological*: decreased sensitivity, inadequate stimulation.
- *Congenital*: Wolffian and Mullerian duct malformations.
- Benign prostatic hypertrophy, prostatic carcinoma.
- *Increasing age*: neuronal degeneration, decreased sensitivity associated with falling levels of testosterone.
- *Pelvic surgery*: e.g. prostatectomy (transurethral/radical), bladder neck surgery, proctocolectomy.
- *Neurological*: e.g. multiple sclerosis, spinal cord damage.
- *Endocrine*: diabetes mellitus (neuropathy), hypogonadism.
- *Drugs*: e.g. alcohol, most anti-depressants and drugs for treating obsessive–compulsive disorders, alpha- and beta-blockers, anticholinergic agents.
- *Psychological*: e.g. fear of being seen, pregnancy, infection, from strict, religious background.

Management

Treat underlying cause, when relevant. If associated ED, this should be managed first. If drug-related, consider altering medication or adding pharmacological adjuvants, such as amantadine (100–400 mg 2 days before sex or 75–100 mg 2–3 times daily), bupropion (75–150 mg as needed or 75 mg 2–3 times a day), buspirone (15–60 mg as needed or 5–15 mg bd), cyproheptadine (4–12 mg as needed).

- *Psychological approach*: more common in those with controlling personalities, which may be inward focused. Issues with showing emotions and letting go.
- Reduce masturbation as the penis may have become conditioned to a firmer stimulus of 'hands', rather than 'vagina'.
- Explore and resolve any underlying anxieties or relationship issues.
- Establish extragenital ejaculation, with suitable stimulation (mechanical, such as a vibrator or visual as required), gradually introducing vaginal contact and insertion into the programme.
- *Male superior position*: facilitates ejaculation.

Dyspareunia

Genital

- *Congenital/post-traumatic*: e.g. phimosis, tight frenulum.
- *Inflammatory*: urethritis, genital herpes, syphilis, candidiasis, dermatological (e.g. lichen sclerosis), aphthosis, Behçet's disease.
- Peyronie's disease.
- Iatrogenic (e.g. intracorporeal and transurethral alprostadil; rarely priapism following PDE-5 inhibitor use).
- *Testicular lesions*: e.g. epididymitis, torsion.
- *Neoplastic*: e.g. SCC.

Ejaculatory pain

- *Seminal vesicle disorders*: calculi, cystic malformations, metastatic cancer.
- *Other pelvic causes*: chronic prostatitis, benign prostatic hypertrophy and prostatic carcinoma, urethral stricture, pelvic arteriovenous malformation, hernia repair.
- *Drugs*: antidepressants, neuroleptics.
- Mercury poisoning.
- *Psychogenic*: e.g. fear of being seen.

Anal

Anal dyspareunia during receptive anal intercourse may be due to psychogenic factors or intestinal tract diseases, including anal fissures, inflammatory disease, and irritable bowel disease.

Examination and investigations

Examine genitals to detect dermatological conditions, curvature of the penis/Peyronie's plaques, phimosis, short frenulum, prostate tenderness. Investigations may include STI screen, urinary microscopy, cystoscopy, ultrasonography of lower abdomen, etc.

Treatment

Treat underlying condition. Alpha-blockers or topiramate may be helpful in some with painful ejaculation and pain after hernia operations. Surgery may be an option in those with large Peyronie plaques, severe phimosis and pudendal nerve entrapment. Where no physical cause found, refer for psychotherapy.

Psychological problems in those with HIV infection

Psychological problems are common amongst people living with HIV, and risk of HIV acquisition is higher amongst people with mental illness. Stigma, isolation, guilt, shame, disgust (self-stigma), pre-existing mental illness, post-traumatic stress, substance use, living with a chronic medical condition, neuropsychiatric side effects of antiretrovirals, all contribute.

Mental health and substance misuse not only impact upon quality of life, but can lead to disengagement with clinical care and non-adherence to ART.

Psychological screening should be a routine part of assessment and follow-up appointments.

Online forums, apps, one-to-one support, and peer support groups can help, as well as psychological therapies. Many HIV services will have access to dedicated clinical psychologists. Third sector and charitable organizations offer support in many areas. Signpost and/or refer as necessary.

Other issues that may arise include:

- *Bereavement reaction with new HIV-positive result*: extreme anxiety and phobia generated by HIV diagnosis and prospect of life-long ART. Psychological therapy and peer support may help
- *HIV infection may be associated with reduced testosterone levels and its cause is multifactorial, leading to reduced libido and ED*: ART, together with testosterone supplementation may help symptoms of androgen deficiency (reduced muscle mass, decreased strength, fatigue, depression, difficulty concentrating, decreased libido).
- *Sexual dysfunction is common amongst both men and women living with HIV and contributes to reduced quality of life*: physiological causes should be excluded by appropriate examination, medication review, and investigations. As the HIV cohort ages co-morbidities, poly-pharmacy contributes, as well as psychological factors.
- *Recreational and 'chemsex' drugs* used by some HIV-infected MSM may increase unsafe sex and contribute to poor therapeutic adherence.
- *Cognitive disorders* (memory, language, problems solving, attention) are frequently reported in people living with HIV despite effective ART. Establishing causation can be challenging, with interplay of mental health, substance use, medication side effects and effects of HIV itself. Screening for cognitive impairment is recommended with referral for further neuropsychological assessment if problems detected.

HIV: prevention

Introduction *444*
Post-exposure prophylaxis *445*
Pre-exposure prophylaxis *447*

Introduction

HIV prevention is multifaceted and requires input from a range of disciplines.

Public health campaigns, and education in schools and high risk groups to increase awareness, condom use, and safe sex. Education and support around chemsex and binge drinking may also reduce high-risk sexual behaviour. Reducing STIs and improving genital health also has some role to play in reducing HIV transmission. Circumcision has also been associated with reduced risk of HIV acquisition.

Amongst some groups of MSM, sexual practices to reduce transmission are sometimes used, such as 'sero-sorting', where those with HIV infection choose partners who also have HIV infection and vice versa. 'Sero-positioning' is where the HIV −ve partner will choose a sexual position associated with lower risk of transmission. The effectiveness of these strategies is unproven, so cannot be recommended.

The '90 90 90' WHO target for HIV, aims to have 90% diagnosed, 90% on treatment, and 90% undetectable by 2020. In the UK, 12% of people with HIV remain undiagnosed. Undiagnosed HIV infection accounts for disproportionate onward transmissions. Campaigns such as HIV testing week, and universal testing in medical admission units and GP surgeries in areas where prevalence in greater than 2/1000, availability of POCT in voluntary sector centres, postal HIV testing kits, as well as raising awareness of HIV indicator diseases, where a HIV test should be considered, will all help reduce undiagnosed HIV.

Guidelines recommend ART for all diagnosed with HIV, regardless of CD4 count, but those who have not started treatment should be offered treatment in the context of a discordant relationship, frequent partner changes or casual partners. This is referred to as TasP (treatment as prevention ➔ Chapter 55, 'HIV: management', pp. 621–51). With effective ART, consistently undetectable viral load, and the absence of genital ulcer disease or concurrent STI, the risk of onward transmission is negligible.

Universal antenatal HIV testing has been part of routine practice since 2000 and for mothers diagnosed with HIV, medical, obstetric, and postnatal infant management (➔ Chapter 56, 'HIV: pregnancy', pp. 653–8) transmission of HIV from mother to infant has reduced significantly to <1% in the UK.

PEP following an HIV risk has been available for several years, but more recently, PrEP has been shown to be effective for certain high-risk individuals. Both should be considered as part of the HIV prevention tool kit.

Post-exposure prophylaxis

PEP and post-exposure prophylaxis after sexual exposure (PEPSE) are the administration of antiretroviral agents after a risk exposure to HIV in order to prevent HIV acquisition. Studies suggest antiretrovirals (ARVs) given <48–72 hours after exposure, reduce dissemination and replication.

Indications for PEP(SE)

Where the risk of acquisition is >1/1000, PEP should be offered and where the risk is between 1/1000 and 1/10,000 PEP should be considered. Transmission varies according to type of exposure, infectivity of the source and host characteristics. PEP is not recommended where the HIV +ve source has viral load (VL) <20 for >6 months on effective therapy (J℅ www.bhiva.org/PEPSE-guidelines.aspx).

Risk of transmission = Risk or source having HIV × exposure risk

Insertive anal sex × UK MSM = 1/90 × 5.9/100 = 5.9/9000 = 1/1525

Factors that increase risk of transmission
- ↑ VL of source.
- *Breaches to mucosal barrier*: ulceration/trauma/infection.
- STI in source or host.
- Ejaculation.
- Non-circumcision.

Estimated HIV prevalence in UK (2014)
- *MSM*:
  - UK overall 5.9%
  - London 12.5%
  - Brighton 13.7%
  - Manchester 8.6%
  - Elsewhere 3.8%.
- *Heterosexuals*:
  - Black African ethnicity ♂ 4.1%, ♀ 7.1%
  - non-Black African ethnicity ♀ and ♂ 0.06%.
- Injecting drug user ♀ and ♂ ≤1.1%.

Estimated risk of exposure type with known HIV viraemic source
- *Receptive anal intercourse 1/90*: with1/65 or without 1/170 ejaculation.
- *Insertive anal intercourse 1/666*: with 1/909 or without 1/161 circumcision.
- Receptive vaginal intercourse 1/1000.
- Insertive vaginal intercourse 1/1219.
- Giving or receiving fellatio <1/10,000.
- Semen splash in eye <1/10,000.
- Blood transfusion 1/1.
- Needlestick injury 1/333.
- Needle/equipment sharing 1/149.
- Human bite <1/10,000.

Situations where PEPSE is recommended
- Unprotected receptive anal sex, where source has VL>200.
- Unprotected insertive anal sex, where source has VL>200.
- Unprotected receptive vaginal sex, where source has VL>200.
- Unprotected receptive anal sex, where source is from high-risk group/country.
- Where risk of transmission is 1/1000–1/10,000 with additional factors that increase transmission, e.g. sexual assault (traumatic sex).

Post-exposure prophylaxis prescribing and management

- *Try to determine HIV status of source*: if occupational exposure, wash wound and gently encourage bleeding. Another HCW should gain consent from source for blood-borne virus screening.
- If known HIV +ve source, try to establish VL.
- Baseline investigations should include HBV sAg, HCV, HIV, U&E, LFT, urinalysis, and if sexual exposure also syphilis, STI screen and pregnancy test.
- Patient should see a HIV specialist at earliest opportunity.
- Consider if PrEP appropriate following completion of PEPSE.

Recommended PEP regimen
- Tenofovir/emtricitabine od + raltegravir 400 mg bd.
- Started <72 hours after (most recent) exposure.
- Continued for 28 days.
- If further exposure within 2 days of completion, continue PEP for 48 hours after last exposure risk.

Top tip

The decision for PEP should be based on risk of HIV acquisition and not to treat anxiety. Referral to health psychology or a HA may be beneficial for anxiety related to HIV transmission.

Pre-exposure prophylaxis

Estimated UK incidence of HIV has not fallen over the past decade. Undiagnosed prevalence remains high at 12%, with the undiagnosed population thought to account for the majority of new transmissions. PrEP is one of many strategies to reduce new HIV transmissions. It has been shown to be cost-effective in certain high-risk individuals.

Indications for PrEP

People at ↑ risk of HIV acquisition who may benefit from PrEP
- MSM, transmen, and transwomen having condomless anal sex.
- Sexual partners of people with detectable HIV viraemia or within 6 months of viral suppression.
- Heterosexual reporting condomless sex with HIV +ve person(s), with ongoing risk.
- Person who has had PEPSE, bacterial STI, or Hep C in past year.
- People may also present already taking PrEP bought online.

PrEP regimes

For MSM, two regimens have been shown to be effective:
- *Event-based TDF/emtricitabine (FTC)*: 2 tablets 2–24 hours before sex + 1 tablet od for next 48 hours. Most appropriate if having unprotected anal intercourse (UPAI) <1 weekly
- *Oral daily TDF/FTC*: most appropriate if UPAI >1 weekly, or unable to predict UPAI, or if HBV co-infected.

For heterosexuals, trans men and trans women 1 tablet daily TDF or TDF/FTC.

For anal sex, PrEP is effective after 2–24 hours if initiated with double-dose TDF/FTC; should be continued until 48 hours after last risk.

For vaginal sex PrEP is effective after 7 days of daily PrEP and should be continued for 7 days after the last risk.

Where to obtain PrEP

Availability varies in the different countries of the UK:
- *Scotland and Wales*: available in NHS sexual health clinics.
- *England*: available in some centres as part of PrEP impact trial.
- Also available to buy online.

For further information and where to obtain PrEP go to:
  ℘ www.aidsmap.com
  ℘ www.iwantprepnow.co.uk
  ℘ www.prepster.info

PrEP consultation

History
- Reason for seeking PrEP.
- Timing and type of condomless sex.
- Previous STI/HIV screen, last HIV test.
- Previous medical history (renal/bone disease/Hep B).
- Drug history (prescribed/recreational).
- If already sourced PrEP online check source, consider therapeutic drug monitoring (TDM).

PrEP discussion
- Importance of adherence to PrEP.
- Risk of HIV infection and resistance with poor adherence.
- 3-monthly STI/HIV screen (annual if stable heterosexual couple).
- Potential side effects, including renal impairment and reduced bone mineral density.
- Risk reduction, including condoms and chemsex support.
- Symptoms of HIV seroconversion illness.

Baseline investigations
- 4th-generation HIV test +/−POCT HIV.
- STI, hepatitis B and C screen.
- Urinalysis and serum creatinine.

Offer
- PEPSE if appropriate.
- Information on where to obtain PrEP.
- If POCT −ve can start PrEP same day.
- 3-monthly follow-up or sooner if within window for STI/HIV screen.

Follow-up consultation
- Check and support adherence to PrEP.
- STI/HIV/hepatitis C screen 3-monthly (6–12-monthly if stable heterosexual couple).
- Serum creatinine + eGFR annually, if eGFR >90 and age <40, at least 6-monthly, if eGFR 60–90, age >40 or other risk factors. If eGFR <60, careful risk assessment and renal advice recommended.

Further information

British HIV Association guidelines: ℘ http://www.bhiva.org/guidelines.aspx

HIV: introduction and epidemiology

History 450
Origin of HIV 451
The viruses and their epidemiology 451
Biological implications of HIV types and subtypes 452
Prevalence 453
Risk factors and transmission routes 454

History

In June 1981, the USA Centers for Disease Control and Prevention reported a number of unusual infections and rare cancers in previously healthy young MSM. They all shared severe damage to the immune system and the acronym Acquired Immune Deficiency Syndrome (AIDS) was used for the first time in 1982. Previous research on animal viruses provided the basis for a USA group to publish their work in 1980 on the identification of a human T-cell leukaemia virus (later known as HTLV-1) as the first pathogenic human retrovirus. In 1981, the same group discovered HTLV-2 in a different T-cell type. HIV-1 was isolated in 1981 by a French group and, independently, by a USA group, and they published their research in the *Lancet*, April 1984, and *Science*, May 1984, respectively. The new virus isolates were collectively designated HTLV-3, a term no longer in use as the virus is officially called human immunodeficiency virus (HIV). HIV-2 was discovered in 1986.

HIV belongs to the genus lentivirus, a member of retroviruses family. Unlike other RNA viruses, retroviruses replicate their genome through a double-stranded viral DNA intermediate in the host nucleus.

Significant dates and events

- Zidovudine was approved by the USA Food and Drug Administration (FDA), as the first antiretroviral drug in March 1987.
- In 1988, 1 December was designated by WHO and supported by the UN as World AIDS Day.
- June 1995, the FDA approved the first protease inhibitor. (Saquinavir) ushering in a new era of highly active antiretroviral therapy (ART).
- June 1996, Nevirapine was the first non-nucleoside reverse transcriptase inhibitor (NNRTI) to be approved.
- The 11th International Conference on AIDS (Vancouver, July 1996) marked the first data to show evidence of (triple therapy) ART effectiveness and was quickly incorporated into clinical practice.
- October 2007, the FDA approved the first integrase inhibitor (Raltegravir).
- 2012, the FDA approved Truvada® for PrEP.
- In 2014, UNAIDS set the '90-90-90' targets, aiming to diagnose 90% of all HIV positive people, provide ART for 90% of those diagnosed, and achieve undetectable HIV RNA for 90% of those on treatment by 2020.
- *Treatment as prevention (TasP)*: there is enough evidence that patients on effective ART with an undetectable viral load cannot transmit HIV to others. Treatment as a tool for prevention is endorsed by many organizations.
- 'Undetectable equals untransmittable' (U=U) is a Consensus Statement produced by the Prevention Access Campaign. Backed by many organizations including the BHIVA and UNAIDS.

Origin of HIV

The reasons for the sudden emergence and the epidemic spread of HIV are still subjects of debate. Old World monkeys are infected with >40 different lentiviruses, simian immunodeficiency viruses (SIVs). They are largely non-pathogenic in their natural hosts. SIVmac causes immune deficiency in captive macaques (an Asian primate) and it is not a natural pathogen. Chimpanzees, sooty mangabey monkeys, and gorillas are natural hosts of SIVcpz, SIVsmm, and SIVgor, respectively; all of them are potential sources of human infection. Phylogenetically, HIV-1 is closely related to SIVcpz and HIV-2 to HIVsmm and SIVmac. Based on biological properties, and on phylogenetic and statistical analysis, transmission of these simian viruses to humans must have occurred through cutaneous or mucous membrane exposure of infected ape-blood and/or body fluids. Such exposure occurs most commonly in the context of bush meat hunting in central West Africa. Large scale vaccination campaigns at the beginning of the 20th century, together with rapid expansion of cities, disruption of the social structure, and increase rates of STIs, including genital ulcer disease, may have facilitated the dissemination and the adaptation of both HIV-1 and HIV-2.

The viruses and their epidemiology

HIV-1 is divided into 4 groups (M, N, O, and P) that were thought to have resulted from independent transmission events. Group M (major) was discovered first and is responsible for the pandemic. Molecular testing has dated the onset of group M and N (non-major) to the beginning of the 20th century. Groups O (outlier) and P are more recent. Genetic testing of infected blood and tissue samples collected from residents of Kinshasa (Democratic Republic of Congo) in 1959 and 1960, respectively, revealed that HIV had already diversified into different groups. Group M is further classified into 9 subtypes (A–D, F–H, J, and K), as well as >70 circulating recombinant forms (CRFs). A&D originated in central Africa, but established epidemics in eastern Africa. C was introduced to, and predominates in southern Africa, then spread to India and other Asian countries. Subtype B (accounts for the majority of HIV-1 in Europe and the Americas) arose from a single African strain that spread to Haiti in the 1960s then onwards to the USA and other western countries. CRF01 dominates in Southeast Asia.

HIV-1 is worldwide, whereas HIV-2 is restricted to West Africa (and countries with socio-economic links). HIV-2 is further divided into 8 groups (A–H), each represents an independent host transfer.

Biological implications of HIV types and subtypes

- HIV-2 is less aggressive and patients have lower viral loads. This leads to lower transmission rates and near complete absence of mother-to-child HIV transmission. Most infected patients do not progress to AIDS, but those who do show clinical disease indistinguishable from HIV-1.
- *Mode of transmission of HIV-1 subtypes:*
  - subtype B is mainly found in MSM
  - subtypes E (CRF01_AE) and C are more commonly seen in heterosexuals. They replicate more easily than subtype B in Langerhans' cells (normally found in the vagina, cervix, and prepuce, but not in the rectum)
- *Infectivity*: subtype E (CRF01_AE) is transmitted more easily than subtype B.
- The different geographical distribution may be a result of biological differences between types and subtypes.
- Group D has been associated with greater pathogenicity and increased incidence of cognitive impairment.
- HIV-2 is intrinsically resistant NNRTIs.
- Unclear whether a vaccine would provide subtype cross-protection.
- Diagnostic and screening tests must reliably detect all known types, subtypes, and CRFs.

Prevalence

Worldwide

See Table 37.1.

76.1 million people have become infected with HIV since the start of the epidemic, and 35.0 million people have died from AIDS-related illnesses since the start of the epidemic. UNAIDS estimated that by the end of 2016 there were 36.7 million people living with HIV (PLWH). In 2016, 1.8 million adults and children were newly infected, 64% of them are in sub-Saharan Africa. Due to availability of effective therapy and other strategies, the number of PLWH is likely to ↑ and new infections are likely to continue declining.

UK (2016 data)

- By the end of 2016, there were 89,400 PLWH in England, 11.6% of them were undiagnosed.
- 71% of males living with HIV were MSM.
- Due to changes in immigration patterns, there has been a continued decline in new HIV diagnoses among Black African heterosexual men and women in the past 10 years.
- New diagnoses were rising until 2015, followed by 18% decline in 2016.
- In 2016, new HIV diagnoses among MSM fell for the first time since the start of the epidemic.
- Late diagnosis remains a challenge. In 2016, 42% of diagnoses happened at a late stage of infection (CD4 count <350 cells/μL).
- In 2016, 96% of those diagnosed are accessing treatment and 94% are virally suppressed.
- One in three of PLWH accessing care are aged 50 years or older, and 5% are 65 or older.

Table 37.1 UNAIDS 2016 figures

Region	Number (in millions)
Asia and the Pacific	5.1
Eastern and Southern Africa	19.4
Eastern Europe and Central Asia	1.6
Latin America	1.8
Caribbean	0.31
Middle East and North Africa	0.23
Western and central Africa	6.1
Western and central Europe and North America	2.1

Risk factors and transmission routes

HIV is exclusively transmitted through body fluids. Routes of transmission include:

- *Sexual intercourse between women and men, men and men, and rarely women and women*: sex between men and men is the major route of transmission in the USA, Western Europe, and Australia, elsewhere it is typically heterosexually spread.
- Sharing contaminated needles, syringes, and other equipment among drug users.
- *Transfusion of blood and blood products*: now very rare in countries where blood is screened for HIV. Transmission may occur in developing world through the re-use of contaminated surgical equipment and needles.
- *Vertically from an infected mother to baby*: antepartum, intrapartum, and post-partum (breastfeeding)
- *Occupational*: to HCW. In the UK there is only one documented case of a HCW transmitting HIV to patients.

Risk factors

Table 37.2 HIV transmission risk following a single exposure to HIV infection*

Sexual intercourse	
Anal: receptive	0.1–3%
Anal: insertive	0.06%
Vaginal: receptive	0.1–0.2%
Vaginal: insertive	0.03–0.09%
Oral (fellatio): receptive	Up to 0.04%
Oral: cunnilingus and insertive fellatio	No data, but estimated to be at least half receptive rate
Other	
Sharing injecting equipment	0.7%
Single unit of blood	90–100%
Occupational	
Needlestick injury	0.3%
Mucous membrane contact	0.1%

*Influenced by plasma and genital VLs, breaks in mucosal surfaces, e.g. trauma, genital ulcer disease.

Frequently asked questions

What is HIV?

HIV is a virus that damages the body's immune system. HIV destroys a type of WBC called the CD4 cell. This cell spearheads/leads the body's defence against infection. When a person's CD4 count becomes low, he/she is more susceptible to certain infections.

What is AIDS?

AIDS is the final stage of HIV infection. When the CD4 cells drop to a very low level (usually <200 cells/µL), the ability to resist certain infections is seriously impaired. Certain opportunistic conditions (AIDS-defining illnesses) can develop, e.g. *Pneumocystis jiroveci* (*carinii*) pneumonia (PCP), KS.

How is HIV transmitted?

- Having unprotected sex with an infected person.
- Sharing a needle/equipment to take drugs.
- Receiving a blood transfusion from an infected person (unlikely in the UK, where blood has been tested for HIV since 1985).
- Transmission from a positive mother to her baby during pregnancy or delivery, and by breastfeeding.

Can it be passed on by kissing?

There is no evidence of transmission by kissing, and viral levels in saliva are very low. Body fluids which contain high levels of HIV correlating with infection are blood, seminal fluid, vaginal/menstrual fluid, and breastmilk.

Can it be passed on by oral sex?

Yes, especially with receptive fellatio.

Does HIV have symptoms?

Some people have flu-like symptoms 4–8 weeks after infection. They usually settle within 1–2 weeks. A person can have HIV for many years before developing symptoms (and may never do so).

Does a negative HIV antibody test mean I have not contracted HIV?

This depends on when your last risk activity was. An antibody test can be negative in the first few weeks after transmission. A further negative test at 3 months should confirm that transmission has not occurred.

Delay between infection and a positive HIV antibody test

Although most infected people test positive within 2–6 weeks, it can take up to 3 months for enough antibodies to be produced to give a positive HIV antibody test. During this time the person is often very infectious with a high VL.

Pathogenesis of HIV

HIV structure 458
Genetic organization of HIV 459
HIV replicative cycle 460
HIV and its receptors 462
Factors influencing HIV disease progression 463

HIV structure

Icosahedral with the following components (see Fig. 38.1):

- *Envelope*: a lipid bilayer formed from host cell lipids and viral proteins. Nine to ten spikes (gp160) are embedded in the envelope, involved in binding and membrane fusion. These spikes are composed of 2 loosely attached viral surface glycoprotein, gp120, and transmembrane glycoprotein, gp41.
- *Matrix*: encapsulated by the envelope, made up of viral protein p17.
- *Core*: Conical and comprises:
  - *RNA dimer*—two identical copies of single-stranded RNA, each containing ≈9500 nucleotides. Tightly bound to p7 nucleocapsid proteins and late assembly protein p6.
  - *Capsid protein p24* encapsulates the ribonucleoprotein core, which contains three enzymes; reverse transcriptase (p51), integrase (p32), and protease (p11).

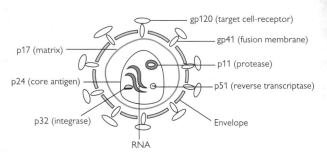

Fig. 38.1 HIV structure: gp and p refer to glycoprotein and protein, respectively, and the numerical values (×10³) indicate molecular weight

Genetic organization of HIV

- Genetic information is stored as RNA.
- Gene maps for HIV1 and HIV2 are similar, except that HIV2 has vpx instead of vpu.
- Both sides of the HIV provirus are flanked by a repeated sequence, known as the long-terminal repeat (LTR).
- HIV genes and their major functions are outlined in Table 38.1.

Table 38.1 HIV genes and their major functions

Major structural proteins	Gag	Encodes for capsid, matrix, and nucleocapsid
	Pol	Encodes for viral enzymes
	Env	Encodes for envelope glycoproteins
Regulatory proteins	Tat	Regulates HIV transcription
	Rev	Stimulates HIV proteins production and suppresses expression of HIV regulatory genes
Accessory proteins	vpu	Helps the assembly and budding of new virus particles and enhances the degradation of CD4 proteins.
	vpr	Accelerates HIV proteins production, nuclear localization of PIC and slows host cell growth cycle.
	vif	Promotes infectivity by interfering with cellular defences.
	nef	↓ Regulates cell surface expression of CD4 and stimulates HIV infectivity

HIV replicative cycle

Replication occurs in the following sequence: binding → fusion and entry → reverse transcription → integration → proviral transcription and translation → assembly and budding → maturation.

Binding/attachment

Glycoprotein120 binds to the extracellular component of the CD4 receptor (expressed in helper T-cells, macrophages, monocytes, microglial, dendritic, and Langerhans' cells). This results in conformational change facilitating 2° interaction with a second receptor (a chemokine co-receptor) CCR5 or CXCR4.

Fusion

The distal tips of gp41 are inserted in to the cellular membrane followed by conformational changes folding in half to form coiled loops. This process pulls the viral and cellular membranes together, and fusing them with subsequent uncoating of the viral capsid, and the release of the HIV RNA dimer and proteins into the host cell cytoplasm.

Reverse transcription

In this process, viral ssRNA is transcribed by the viral reverse transcriptase (RT) into double-stranded DNA (dsDNA). HIV uses cellular tRNA^{Lys3} as a primer. The primer hybridizes to a specific site (primer binding site, PBS) of the virus RNA genome to initiate reverse transcription. Transcription takes place in 5' → 3' direction to form a minus-strand complementary DNA (cDNA). The RNA:DNA hybrid is then degraded by RNase H domain of reverse transcriptase. DNA:tRNA is transferred to the 3'-end of the template to complete synthesis of the first strand DNA. The rest of viral ssRNA is degraded by RNase H, except for a purine-rich sequence (named polypurine tract, ppt), which subsequently serves as a primer for initiation of the second strand ssDNA synthesis. RT then elongates the ppt primer from the 3'-end of the template. tRNA is then degraded by RNase. PBS from the second strand hybridizes with the complementary PBS of the first strand. Extension of both strands produces a complete viral dsDNA.

Reverse transcription yields a pre-integration complex (PIC), composed of linear dsDNA, cellular host proteins, transcriptase, nucleocapsid, matrix, vpr, and integrase. PIC enters the nucleus through the nuclear pore complex.

Due to its poor proofreading ability, reverse transcriptase has a high error rate when transcribing RNA into DNA. This allows mutations to accumulate, which in turn, have a role in the development of drug resistance and escape from immune surveillance.

Integration

Integrase binds to the end of each LTR of the HIV double-stranded cDNA. The final outcome, after a series of reactions, is a 'cut-and-paste' clipping of the host DNA and joining the proviral genome to the clipped ends.

Proviral transcription and translation

Proviral genome remained latent until CD4 cell is activated. Certain cellular transcription factors (NF-kB is the most important) must be present for active virus production, which are then up-regulated when T-cells get activated. Early in the transcription process, short completely spliced mRNAs that codes for Tat and Rev are produced. As transcription rate increases, larger incompletely spliced mRNAs are produced. These code for Env, vif, vpr, and vpu. Late in the process, full length transcripts are produced, which act as virion genomic RNA. Spliced mRNAs are exported from the nucleus and translated in the endoplasmic reticulum into structural proteins Gag and Env, and others into the regulatory proteins Tat and Rev. Gag proteins bind to copies of the virus RNA genome to package them into new virus particles.

Virion assembly and budding

Assembly occurs at the plasma membrane. Gag (and Gag-Pro-Pol) polyprotein mediates the essential events in virion assembly, including binding the plasma membrane, making the protein–protein interactions necessary to create spherical particles, concentrating the viral Env protein, and packaging the genomic RNA. Conformational change(s) within Gag couples membrane binding, virion assembly, and RNA packaging. Although Gag itself can bind membranes and assemble into spherical particles, the budding event that releases the virion from the plasma membrane is mediated by host machinery

Maturation

Viral maturation begins concomitant with (or immediately following) budding and is driven by viral protease cleavage of the Gag and Gag-Pro-Pol polyproteins at 10 different sites, ultimately producing the fully processed MA, CA, NC, p6, PR, RT, and IN proteins. Over the course of maturation, these processed proteins rearrange to create the mature infectious virion.

Mature virions are released ready to infect new cells and begin the replication cycle once again. This process is very active, 10^8 –10^{10} viral particles produced each day.

HIV and its receptors

- The primary cellular receptor for HIV entry is CD4. Expression of CD4 on a target cell is necessary, but not sufficient for HIV entry.
- CD4 antigen is the principal receptor, mainly expressed on the surface of helper T lymphocytes. It is also expressed, but to a lesser degree in CD4 dendritic cells including Langerhans' cells and CD4 monocytes, macrophages, and microglial cells.
- *Co-receptors*: several described, act as co-factors that allow HIV entry when co-expressed with CD4 on a cell surface. CCR5 and CXCR4 are the most important, and they act in concert with CD4 to facilitate HIV and cell membrane fusion. CCR5, which is expressed on macrophages and on some T cells. M-tropic HIV isolates appear to use some T cells. CXCR4 is expressed on T cells, but not usually on macrophages. Other chemokine co-receptors, e.g. CCR3, expressed on eosinophils and microglia, is used by some strains of HIV for infection of the microglia resulting CNS pathology.

Factors influencing HIV disease progression

Host factors

- *Age*: ↑ age is associated with ↑ progression.
- *Co-infection*: may affect immune system resulting in ↑ progression (e.g. tuberculosis and hepatitis C). CMV associated with ↑ progression in haemophiliacs.
- *Gender*: ♀ appear to have higher VLs at any CD4 level and may progress more rapidly.
- *Psychosocial factors*: depression, impaired intellectual functioning, drug use, social deprivation may be associated with ↑ progression.
- *Genetic susceptibility*:
  - 4–15% of Caucasians have a deletion in *CCR5* gene resulting in a mutant co-receptor (CCR5Δ32). The effect is a truncated co-receptor not expressed at the cell surface. People of Northern European descent have the higher frequency of these deletions. Homozygous individuals (1–2% of the Caucasian population) are almost resistant to HIV infection and heterozygotes are slow progressors. Other alleles of *CCR5* genes were described in Africans and Asians, and have different effects on co-receptor expression.
  - CCR2 (a minor co-receptor) deletion (CCR-V641) is widespread in all ethnic groups and results in slower progression to AIDS
  - certain HLA types associated with ↑ or ↓ progression
  - *possession or lack of certain genes*—e.g. low copy number of CCL3L1 associated with ↑ susceptibility.
- *Nutrition*: poor premorbid state associated with ↑ progression.
- *Pharmacological variability*: individual drug metabolism and elimination modify response to therapy.

Viral factors

Changes in the phenotype and the genotype of the virus enable it to 'escape' control by the immune system. In late HIV infection switching from CCR5 to CXCR4 tropism leads to infection of both active and resting immune cells resulting in ↑ disease progression. Mutations may alter viral 'fitness' influencing pathogenicity. Gene mutation involving nef is associated with ↓ progression and some drug-resistant mutations (e.g. M184V, which induces lamivudine resistance) may ↓ viral fitness.

Drug susceptibility depends largely on HIV genotypic and phenotypic characteristics with genotype mutations rendering some drugs ineffective. Other factors, such as efflux pumps, may also be involved.

Staging, classification, and natural history of HIV disease

Clinical staging 466
Natural history of untreated HIV infection 468

Clinical staging

Early in the epidemic, before HIV was discovered, diagnosis of AIDS was largely based on finding *Pneumocystis jirovecii* pneumonia or Kaposi's sarcoma. Revised WHO Clinical Staging of HIV/AIDS for Adults and Adolescents is also based on clinical progression and is used in third world countries and as a research tool (Tables 39.1 and 39.2). The Centers for Disease Control and Prevention devised a classification system, revised in 1993, based on clinical features, AIDS-defining illnesses and CD4 counts, see Table 39.3. The CD4 count is a useful predictor for the development of opportunistic infections (OIs) and malignancies, but it should be recognized that this may be influenced by other factors such as inter-current infection.

Table 39.1 Revised WHO clinical staging of HIV/AIDS for adults and adolescents

Stage	Characteristics
Primary HIV infection	• Asymptomatic HIV infection • Acute retroviral syndrome
Clinical stage 1	• Asymptomatic • Persistent generalized lymphadenopathy

Clinical stage 2	• Weight loss (>10% body weight)
	• Recurrent respiratory tract infections
	  • sinusitis
	  • bronchitis
	  • otitis media
	• Angular cheilitis
	• Recurrent oral ulceration
	• Herpes zoster
	• Papular pruritic eruptions
	• Seborrhoiec dermatitis
	• Onychomycosis

Clinical stage 3	• Unexplained chronic diarrhoea >1 month • Severe weight loss (>10% body weight) • Oral hairy leukoplakia • Severe bacterial infection, e.g. empyema, osteomyelitis, pneumonia, meningitis • Unexplained anaemia (<80 g/l), neutropaenia (<500/μl), thrombocytopaenia (<50000/μl) for >1 month • Fever intermittent or chronic >1 month • Oral candidiasis • Pulmonary TB (in last 2 years) • Acute necrotizing gingivitis, stomatitis, or periodontitis

Data sourced from World Health Organization WHO (2007) Case definitions of HIV for surveillance and revised clinical staging and immunological classification of HIV-related disease in adults and children. Geneva, World Health Organization. ℬ www.who.int/hiv/pub/guidelines/HIVstaging150307.pdf

The revised WHO clinical staging of HIV/AIDS for adults and adolescents

See Table 39.1 for the clinical staging of HIV, and Table 39.2 for AIDS-defining conditions.

Table 39.2 Clinical Stage 4 (AIDS defining conditions)

Conditions where presumptive diagnosis may be made based on clinical symptoms/signs	Conditions where diagnostic tests are required
• HIV wasting syndrome	• Invasive cervical cancer
• Oesophageal candidiasis	• Visceral leishmaniasis
• KS	• Isosporiasis
• Extrapulmonary cryptococcosis	• *Mycobacterium avium* complex
• Invasive cervical cancer	• *Mycobacterium* tuberculosis
• Pneumonia (recurrent severe)	• Any disseminated mycosis, e.g. coccidioidomycosis, histoplasmosis
• Pneumocystis pneumonia	• Cerebral toxoplasmosis
• HIV encephalopathy	• Pneumonia (recurrent severe)
• Herpes simplex:	• Progressive multifocal leucoencephalopathy
• chronic (>1 month)	• Salmonella (septicaemia, recurrent)
• oesophageal	• Cryptosporidiosis
	• CMV
	• Lymphoma (cerebral or B cell non-Hodgkins)

Data sourced from World Health Organization WHO (2007) Case definitions of HIV for surveillance and revised clinical staging and immunological classification of HIV-related disease in adults and children. Geneva, World Health Organization. ℘ www.who.int/hiv/pub/guidelines/HIVstaging150307.pdf

Table 39.3 Revised classification of HIV disease (CDC January 1993)

Categories CD4 (cells/µL)	A	B*	C
	Asymptomatic, acute HIV, or PGL	Symptomatic conditions, not A or C	AIDS-indicator conditions
≥500 cells/µL	A1	B1	C1
200–499 cells/µL	A2	B2	C2
<200 cells/µL	A3	B3	C3

PGL, persistent generalized lymphadenopathy.

*Category B symptomatic conditions are defined as symptomatic conditions occurring in an HIV-infected adolescent or adult that meet at least one of the following criteria:

• They are attributed to HIV infection or indicate a defect in cell-mediated immunity.

• They are considered to have a clinical course or management that is complicated by HIV infection.

Data sourced from National Center for Infection Diseases Division of HIV/AIDS (1993) Revised Classification System for HIV Infection and Expanded Surveillance Case Definition for AIDS Among Adolescents and Adults. *MMWR Recomm Rep.* 41(RR-17): 1–19.

Natural history of untreated HIV infection

Characterized by progressive loss of immune function allowing the development of some virulent bacterial infections, certain opportunistic infections, and malignancies that define AIDS (Fig. 39.1). Progression rate varies depending on interactions between host, viral, and environmental factors. The average time between HIV acquisition and AIDS is 10 years if untreated.

The course of the disease can be divided into five continuous stages: seroconverion followed by early, middle, advanced, and late stages. There is significant individual variation between patients in the same clinical stage.

- *HIV infection*: disseminates widely in the body at seroconversion, usually with a very high VL and a rapid CD4 cell ↓, which is spontaneously, but not fully reversible.
- *Early stage*: CD4 count >500 cells/μL, viraemia ↓ (rarely becoming undetectable). Usually asymptomatic apart from generalized lymphadenopathy and certain skin disorders (e.g. seborrhoeic dermatitis, aphthous ulcers, eosinophilic dermatitis, and psoriasis).
- *Middle stage*: CD4 count 200–500 cells/μL, mostly asymptomatic/mildly symptomatic. Skin disorders of early stage may worsen. Recurrent HSV, varicella zoster (VZV), diarrhoea, weight loss, and intermittent fever may develop. Lung infections caused by community-acquired organisms, such as *Streptococcus pneumoniae, Haemophilus influenzae*, and *Mycobacterium tuberculosis* become more common.
- *Advanced stage*: CD4 count 50–200 cells/μL. ↑ VL with classical manifestations of AIDS, especially PCP, KS, lymphomas, and *Mycobacterium avium* complex (MAC) infection.
- *Late stage*: CD4 count <50 cells/μL. Very high levels of viraemia. Further development of conditions associated with severe immune deficiency, e.g. CMV retinitis, disseminated MAC. Neurological manifestations ↑ due to brain lymphoma, multifocal leukoencephalopathy, and dementia. HIV wasting disease is commonly seen at this stage.

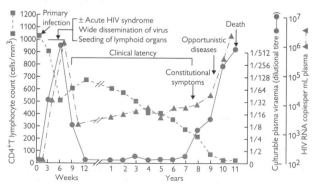

Fig. 39.1 Schematic representation of progression of HIV infection with time. Reproduced with permission of Professor Giuseppe Pantaleo, Centre Hospitalier Universitaire Vaudois.

HIV: diagnosis and assessment

Introduction 470
HIV testing and risk assessment 471
Post-test counselling 476
Assessment of newly diagnosed patients 477

Introduction

The Joint United Nations program on HIV/AIDS (UNAIDS) aim to eliminate the HIV epidemic by 2030 and has set a target towards this goal of 90% cases of HIV aware of their diagnosis, 90% of those diagnosed being on treatment, and 90% of those on treatment achieved viral suppression. When this target is achieved 73% of people living with HIV will have suppressed VL. The UK has achieved the second and third target, but 12% of people with HIV remain undiagnosed. Globally, the target is a long way off, with significant variation between countries.

People living with undiagnosed HIV infection are more likely to be diagnosed late with increased mortality and morbidity, and an estimated 50% of transmissions are from people unaware of their infection. Thus, reducing the undiagnosed HIV population reduces late diagnoses and onward transmission rates.

People with CD4 count is <350 at the time of diagnosis are considered to be diagnosed late and have been living with their infection for at least 3 years. They have ×10 ↑ mortality in the first year after diagnosis compared with people with CD4 >350 at the time of diagnosis. Many late diagnoses have had contact with health professionals in the years preceding diagnosis, with missed opportunities for testing.

By increasing testing in healthcare, voluntary sector, and other settings, we have increased the proportion of people who are aware of their diagnosis from 2/3 to 87%, and reduced late diagnoses from >50% to 39% over the past decade. Further improvements are required to eliminate the epidemic and improve patient outcomes.

HIV testing and risk assessment

Normalizing HIV testing amongst HCPs and the general population is necessary in order to improve testing rates. It has been shown that universal screening in certain populations, health settings, and risk groups where the rate of infection exceeds 0.05% is cost effective. Benefits of opt out testing include increased uptake, early diagnosis, normalization of testing, and reduced onward transmission, including mother to child transmission (MTCT). Universal antenatal HIV opt-out screening has been in place in the UK since 2000 and reduced MTCT to <0.5%.

Who to test

HIV testing is recommended in the following situations:
- If HIV or PHI comes into the diagnosis (Box 40.1).
- Anyone diagnosed with an STI.
- All MSM and female partners of MSM.
- Anyone with history of intravenous drug users (IVDUs) or sexual partner of IVDU.
- Sexual partner of person known to have HIV infection.
- Anyone with risk factors for HIV acquisition (Table 40.1).
- Anyone from high prevalence area (➲ Chapter 37, 'HIV: introduction and epidemiology', pp. 449–54).
- Anyone with sexual partner from high prevalence area.
- In areas where prevalence of HIV ≥2/1000 all ♀ + ♂:
  - registering with GP
  - general medical admission.
- Where universal screening is recommended (Box 40.2).

How to test

Pre-test discussion should not be a barrier to testing and, in most settings, can be kept to a minimum. In many sexual health services, it is routine to carry out a risk assessment prior to screening (Table 37.2). Essential component to obtain verbal consent to perform an HIV test. All trained HCWs should be able to obtain consent and perform HIV testing. HIV testing should be normalized and thought of in the same way as ordering a chest X-ray or blood glucose.

> **Top tip: How to ask for consent to perform an HIV test**
>
> *If there is a low/moderate risk of HIV*
> 'It is routine practice for us to offer an HIV test, are you happy to go ahead with that?'
>   'I would like to do some routine tests that include (e.g. glucose, blood count, etc.), and an HIV test. Is that OK?'
>
> *If there is a high risk of HIV*
> 'We recommend testing for HIV in anyone with this condition. If HIV is an underlying cause effective treatment is available and it is much better to for us to know the diagnosis so we can treat you'.

Box 40.1 Clinical indicator conditions (↑ prevalence of HIV)

- *Reticulo-endothelial abnormalities*:
  - impaired immunity
  - unexplained lymphadenopathy
  - blood dyscrasia.
- *Infections*:
  - TB*or atypical mycobacterial infection
  - *Pneumocystis jiroveci* pneumonia*
  - cerebral toxoplasmosis*
  - oral or oesophageal candidiasis
  - recurrent or multi-dermatomal herpes zoster
  - CMV retinitis*
  - aseptic meningitis
  - transverse myelitis
  - peripheral neuropathy.
- *Malignancies*:
  - lymphoma (Hodgkins, non-Hodgkins*, cerebral*)
  - cervical cancer* and CIN ≥2
  - lung cancer
  - head and neck cancer
  - anal cancer.
- *Dermatological conditions*:
  - seborrhoeic dermatitis
  - recalcitrant psoriasis.
- *General*:
  - oral hairy leukoplakia*
  - unexplained weight loss
  - unexplained diarrhoea
  - night sweats
  - pyrexia of unknown origin
  - symptoms of seroconversion illness (➔ Chapter 41 pp. 479–84).

*AIDS defining conditions.

Giving results

In outpatient settings, arrangements for obtaining the results should be discussed. Many services will provide results by text message within 7–10 days; however, if someone is high risk or anxious POCT or 24-48hour testing with results given face-to-face may be appropriate.

With in-patients the results should be given by the person/team who requested the test. (➔ Chapter 40, 'Post-test counselling', p. 476).

Patients declining testing

People who decline HIV testing are at higher risk of HIV. Many decline testing because of stigma, out-of-date understanding of HIV, and implications of testing. It is important to address:

- *Why they are declining the test*:
  - needle phobia
  - afraid of result
  - known people who have died from AIDS
  - stigma.

Box 40.2 Universal HIV screening in the UK

Opt out testing is offered to everyone accessing the following:
- Antenatal services.
- Termination of pregnancy services.
- Drug dependency programmes.
- Sexual health services.
- Services for people with HBV, HCV, lymphoma, and TB.
- Blood donation.
- Organ donation or recipient.
- Dialysis.
- At GP registration/acute hospital admission in areas where prevalence >2/1000.

Table 40.1 HIV pre-test check list

Risk factors	Y/N	Further information
If risk <72 hours ago ➲ Chapter 36, 'Post-exposure prophylaxis', pp. 445–6		
Previous HIV test		When
Blood product recipient (abroad or pre-1992 in UK)		When and where
Injecting drug use		When
Medical/surgical treatment abroad		When and where
Tattoo abroad/non-professional		When
Lived in ↑ prevalence area		Which country
Sex with person from ↑ prevalence area		Which country, when
MSM or sex with MSM		When, type of sex*
Sex with person with HIV		Viral load, type of sex*
Commercial sex worker (CSW) or sex with CSW		When
Non-consensual sex		When, who
Information provided		
Benefits of testing/early diagnosis		
Window period (8 weeks from risk)		
Receiving results		
Consent given (verbal)		If not, why not?
Repeat test required		When

* ➲ Chapter 36, 'Estimated risk of exposure type with known viraemic source' p. 445.

- *Dispel myths and misconceptions*:
  - negative test has no effect on insurance and now possible to get insurance with a positive test
  - finger prick or buccal swab POCT available
  - treatment free in UK.
- *Advise of benefits of testing*:
  - benefits of early diagnosis/worse outcome with late diagnosis
  - good prognosis with treatment
  - reduced anxiety if negative result.
- Give others opportunities to test.

Repeat testing

Repeat testing may be required and should be offered if:
- *Ongoing risk factors*: repeat 3–12-monthly depending on risk.
- *Initial test was within window period*: repeat 8 weeks from risk.
- *Previous testing declined*: repeat at any point.

Window period is the time from acquisition of infection to when the test will detect it and is 8 weeks with fourth generation HIV tests.
- recommended that MSM have STI/HIV testing annually, or more often depending on risk or presence of symptoms
- injecting drug users should be offered testing annually
- women who have refused antenatal screening should be re-offered throughout pregnancy and at time of delivery.

Where to test

Asymptomatic individuals can request routine HIV testing:
- GP practice
- sexual health service (express clinics often available)
- voluntary sector services
- home testing/sampling may be available.

Types of tests available

See Table 40.2.

Laboratory tests

Recommended first-line assays should be 4th-generation tests. These detect p24 antigen (Ag) and HIV 1+2 antibodies (Abs), with low false positive rate <0.2%. p24 Ag can be detected from 10 to 14 days after acquisition of

Table 40.2 HIV test types

Test	Time to result	Obtaining result
Serum laboratory test	1–14 days	Text/call/in clinic
Confirmatory test	24–48 hours	Face-to-face
Clinic POCT (buccal or capillary sample)	1–20 minutes	Face-to-face
Home sampling	5–7 days	Text/email/call
Home testing	15–20 minutes	Self

the infection, but HIV Abs take 4–12 weeks to appear. If suspected primary HIV infection (PHI) or 2–4 weeks after high risk exposure HIV RNA testing (plasma sample) can be requested.

Confirmatory testing
Three independent assays should be performed on initial positive samples, either in-house or sent to referral laboratory. Before a new diagnosis of HIV can be made a separate sample should also be tested.

Point of care tests
Near patient tests use either buccal swab or finger prick capillary blood sample. Fourth-generation tests are available with good −ve predictive value, but +ve predictive values are lower, i.e. a −ve result is likely to be a true result, but there is a higher rate of false +ves. All +ves, therefore, require a serum sample for confirmation.

Home sampling and home testing
Home sampling tests include a kit to provide capillary blood spot that is sent away for testing. Home testing kits (available in the UK since 2015) provide the POCT with instructions and a helpline contact number. The test is performed and interpreted by the individual.

Post-test counselling

Giving a positive result

This should ideally be given face-to-face by the clinician who requested the test. If given by a non-specialist, initial points to cover include:

- assess psychological stage and offer psychology
- need for confirmatory testing
- referral to HIV specialist for further management.

Giving a negative result

Tailor to reason for testing. It is an opportunity to provide education on HIV transmission and risk reduction. Recommended discussion points:

- repeat testing if still within window period or ongoing risk
- give safe sex advice
- post-exposure prophylaxis
- pre-exposure prophylaxis.

Counselling someone newly diagnosed with HIV

This may be done over more than one session.

- address anxieties/mental state, refer to psychology if needed
- information on natural history HIV
- efficacy of treatment/good prognosis
- few restrictions on lifestyle, travel, employment
- information on reducing onward transmission
- condoms/PEPSE/family planning
- disclosure to sexual partners/legal implications
- onward management tailored to patients needs
- follow up, further investigations, and treatment
- details of support services
- health advisor referral/contact tracing.

Assessment of newly diagnosed patients

The baseline assessment is to ascertain their general state of mental and physical health including symptoms of OI, stage of HIV infection, assess urgency for treatment, and identify any issues that require additional support.

History

General

- Current symptoms
- Thorough Systematic enquiry
- Psychological and neurocognitive screen
- Past medical history including tuberculosis/OI
- Medications, remedies, supplements, allergies
- Vaccination history

Sexual and reproductive health

- Partner notification and HIV status
- Previous STI
- Reproductive history
- HIV status of children
- Contraception
- Risk of pregnancy
- Cervical cytology

Social history and lifestyle

- Lifetime travel history
- Substance misuse/IVDU, chemsex, alcohol, smoking
- Safeguarding, vulnerability, intimate partner violence

Examination

General examination

- Weight, height, BMI waist circumference, blood pressure
- Cardiovascular, respiratory, abdominal, neurological

Specific examination

- Skin – rashes, Kaposi's sarcoma, molluscum, warts
- Eyes – slit lamp fundoscopy if CD4 <50 to look for CMV retinitis
- Oral – candidiasis, oral hairy leukoplakia, dental health
- Lymph nodes – position, size, texture, symmetry, tenderness
- Anogenital examination – discharge, ulcers, warts, masses

Investigations

Routine tests

- Full blood count, urea, electrolytes, eGFR, liver function, bone profile,
- Urinalysis - if protein + on dipstick add urine protein/creatinine ratio
- Cervical cytology – ♀ age 25-64 if not performed in past 12 months

HIV specific tests
- Confirmation of HIV-1 or 2
- Recent infection testing algorithm – assesses if infection is recent
- HIV viral load – informs likely rate of progression
- CD4 count – predicts risk of opportunistic infection
- HIV viral resistance – informs choice of ART
- HLA-B*57:01 if abacavir therapy considered

Infection/immunity
- STI screen- Chlamydia, gonorrhoea, syphilis - all
- Hepatitis A, B, C – all
- Measles, Varicella – according to vaccination history
- Rubella – all ♀ according to vaccination history
- Interferon gamma release assay (IGRA) if TB risk and low CD4
- Tropical screen if relevant travel and persistent eosinophilia
  - Stool for ova, cysts and parasites
  - Filaria and schistosomiasis serology

Risk assessment
- Lipid profile, HbA1c/glucose – all >40 years
- Cardiovascular risk (QRISK2) – all >40 years
- Fragility fracture risk (FRAX) – all >50, risk factors, postmenopausal

Prophylaxis against infection

Prophylaxis requirement is determined by CD4 count and exposure history, and is recommended in the following situations (➔ Chapter 55, 'Prophylaxis against infections', pp. 650–1):
- *Pneumocystis jiroveci* - if CD4 <200
- Toxoplasma – if CD4 <100
- Tuberculosis – travel history or contact of TB
- Varicella – if IgG negative and <72 of significant exposure
- *Mycobacterium avium* complex – if CD4 <50

Vaccinations

➔ Chapter 55, 'Vaccinations', p. 638.

It is recommended that all patients with HIV are offered the following vaccinations. If CD4 <200 risk of infection should be weighed against improved immunogenicity once CD4 count improves with ART.
- hepatitis B – if non-immune
- hepatitis A – if non-immune
- seasonal influenza – annual
- pneumococcal PCV 13 – once.

HIV: primary infection

Introduction *480*
Immune responses *481*
Acute seroconversion illness *482*
Diagnosis *484*
Management of primary HIV infection *484*

Introduction

PHI is usually defined as the first 6 months after infection with HIV. It is the period of time from the onset of infection until immune system establishes a balance with viral replication. Characterized by rapidly increasing viraemia with transient immune suppression. Seroconversion occurs during this time, usually within 12 weeks of infections; this may be symptomatic or asymptomatic. Acute seroconversion illness is the symptomatic development of HIV-specific antibodies.

Immune responses

Cellular response

HIV-specific cellular responses, particularly cytotoxic CD8 cells, influence the natural history of HIV infection. It develops earlier and is more important than humoral immunity in containing HIV infection.

In 1° infection active viral replication is followed by very high plasma viraemia, as HIV disseminates throughout the body, particularly to the lymphoid system. HIV integrates into the genome of infected cells, which are generally activated and killed by the immune system. In the first few days of infection, both CD4 and CD8 cells are suppressed, resulting in lymphopenia approaching levels seen in advanced disease. This is followed by relative lymphocytosis, predominantly CD8 cells, which declines when acute seroconversion is complete. The CD4 count, although increasing, does not return to baseline values with consequent reversal of the CD4/CD8 ratio to <1. In acute HIV infection, rapid depletion of CD4 cells in the gut lymphoid tissue is also seen, which persists despite immune reconstitution with ART.

HIV viraemia ↓ with HIV-specific immune responses, gradually stabilizing within 6–12 months to reach a 'viral set-point'. Higher set-points indicate ↑ risk of disease progression.

Some infected CD4 cells revert to a resting state, and the integrated latent pro-virus they contain remains undetected by the immune system and unaffected by ART. However, they can reactivate again to produce infectious virus, presenting a barrier to eradication. Other reservoir sites include infected macrophages, astrocytes, and dendritic cells in gut, genital tract, lymph nodes, and the central nervous system.

Humoral response

Antibody response is usually detectable within 10–21 days of the onset of symptoms, but may take up to 3 months from infection. Antibodies to gp160 and p24 develop first, followed by anti-gp120 and anti-gp41. Anti-p24 diminishes with time and may disappear in advanced disease. Anti-gp120 and anti-gp41 persist for life. Poor prognosis if inadequate HIV antibody response. Neutralizing antibodies are usually detected 1–8 weeks after resolution of the viraemic peak. Non-neutralizing antibodies to envelope and p24 antigens develop earlier, coinciding with seroconversion.

Acute seroconversion illness

Seroconversion, the development of HIV specific antibodies, usually occurs within 12 weeks of infection; this may be symptomatic (acute seroconversion illness) or asymptomatic.

Prevalence

Difficult to determine because of the wide spectrum of clinical presentations, which may be mild and non-specific (Table 41.1). This explains the wide range of reported prevalence of 30–93% in those recently infected. Clinician awareness and high index of suspicion ↑ diagnostic rate. It is unclear what determines the severity of symptoms. The inoculum size, HIV strain virulence, and patient's immune status may be factors. Almost all reports of acute seroconversion illness are in adults with HIV-1.

Clinical features

Symptoms usually begin 2–6 weeks after infection, typically lasting 5–10 days and rarely >14 days. Subjective symptoms, such as fatigue may continue for several weeks or even months, but eventually almost all patients enter an asymptomatic phase that may last for years. Within 2–4 weeks of infection very high levels of free HIV and p24 antigen can be detected in the peripheral blood. Symptoms coincide with peak levels of plasma viraemia.

Common clinical features of acute seroconversion include fever followed by lymphadenopathy, pharyngitis, and maculopapular skin rash (face, neck, and trunk > limbs). Other less common clinical features include:

- Mucosal ulceration of genitals, mouth, and oesophagus.
- Pustules, urticaria, erythema multiforme, and alopecia.
- Thrombocytic purpura.
- *Infectious mononucleosis (EBV)-like illness*:
  - oral ulceration (highly suggestive of acute seroconversion)
  - no prominent tonsillar involvement (unlike EBV).
- *Evidence of immune deficiency*:
  - oral and oesophageal candidiasis
  - *Pneumocystis jiroveci* (carinii) pneumonia.
- *Neurological manifestation*: aseptic meningitis, peripheral neuropathy, brachial neuritis, Bell's palsy, myelopathy, encephalitis, Guillain–Barré syndrome, mononeuritis, transverse myelitis, and radiculopathy.

Severe and prolonged illness, especially with neurological manifestations, is associated with a poorer prognosis. Resolution of symptoms coincides with ↓ viraemia and the development of a CD8 cell-specific immune response with the later emergence of HIV-specific antibodies (usually within 4–6 weeks of infection, but may be up to 3 months).

Table 41.1 Acute seroconversion illness; frequency of clinical features

Fever 80–97%	Lymphadenopathy 40–77%
Pharyngitis 44–73%	Skin rashes 51–70%
Myalgia or arthralgia 49–70%	Thrombocytopenia 45–51%
Leucopenia 35–40%	Diarrhoea 32–33%
Headache 30–70%	↑ Serum transaminases 21–23%
Nausea and vomiting 20–60%	Hepatosplenomegaly 14–17%
Weight loss 13–32%	Oral candidiasis 10–12%
Encephalopathy 8%	Neuropathy 8%

Diagnosis

PHI usually presents before the development of antibodies and there-fore is diagnosed by p24 antigen or HIV RNA tests. Fourth-generation HIV tests detect p24 antigen, and are usually positive by 4 weeks following infection but can be falsely negative in the early stages. HIV VL is usually extremely high in the early stages, often >10^6copies/mL.

Atypical lymphocytes are commonly seen in the peripheral blood with levels up to 30%. Anaemia, thrombocytopenia, abnormal liver function tests, or ↑ inflammatory markers may also be found (Box 41.1 for differential diagnoses).

> **Box 41.1 Differential diagnosis of acute seroconversion illness**
> - EBV (infectious mononucleosis)
> - CMV infection.
> - Toxoplasmosis.
> - Viral hepatitis.
> - Secondary syphilis.
> - Rubella.
> - Primary HSV infection.
> - Drug reaction.
> - Meningitis.
> - Streptococcal pharyngitis.

Management of primary HIV infection

PHI is the time of highest infectivity in HIV infection. The plasma HIV VL strongly predicts the progression rate. PHI may be diagnosed through routine screening with recent negative test, low avidity, or when the patient presents with symptoms.

Early initiation of ART has advantages, such ↓ viral reservoir (number of infected cells), preserved HIV-specific immune responses, and has been shown to improve patient outcomes. Benefits of treatment should be weighed against drug toxicity/side effects, adherence, and readiness of patient for life-long therapy. Patients with neurological symptoms, AIDS defining illness, CD4 <350 should be strongly encouraged to start ART.

Benefits of diagnosing PHI
- Improved prognosis with early detection and treatment.
- Minimizing late HIV diagnosis (CD4 <350) which carries increased mortality and morbidity.
- Reduced onward transmission: safer sex counselling.
- Treatment to ↓ viraemia and, therefore, ↓ transmission (➔ Chapter 55, 'HIV: management', pp. 621–51)
- Early identification of partners at risk, for testing and risk reduction counselling.

HIV: gastrointestinal disorders

Introduction *486*
Oral diseases *487*
Oesophageal diseases *493*
Enteric diseases *495*
Anal diseases *501*
Pancreatic diseases *503*
Hepatic and biliary tract diseases *504*

Introduction

The gut contains the largest and the most complex lymphoid tissue of the body [gut-associated lymphoid tissue (GALT)]. The GALT contains 70–80% of the total body lymphocytes. More than 60% of CD4 cells are depleted in the first 2–4 weeks after HIV infection and are not replenished, even after immune reconstitution with ART seen in the peripheral blood in the majority of treated patients. HIV directly infects the gut mucosal cells and interaction between gp120 and certain mucosal proteins results in efficient cell-to-cell spread of HIV. Alteration in gut permeability and microbial translocation are thought to play a role in immune activation and disease progression. Similar to peripheral blood mononuclear cells, there is evidence of HIV persistence in GALT in aviraemic-treated patients. This may imply cross-infection between these 2 cellular compartments and may have a role in HIV persistence (reservoirs), despite long-term viral suppression.

In the pre-ART era opportunistic mucosal infections were a common feature of disease progression. With treatment, it is evident that patients do not demonstrate any short-term effects from the profound loss of CD4 cells of the gut.

Oral diseases

Very common; oral lesions may alert professionals to HIV as the underlying cause. Detailed oral examination should be part of the assessment of all newly diagnosed HIV +ve individuals. Various lesions of ulcerative, raised, white, or pigmented appearance may be encountered (Boxes 42.1 and 42.2). Advice from a dentist and oral or maxillofacial surgeon should be obtained when necessary.

Viral infections

Herpes simplex virus

HSV infection is very common, with seropositivity rates approaching 80% in homosexual men living with HIV. Oral HSV, like herpes infection elsewhere, is characterized by latency (in the trigeminal ganglia). The majority are caused by HSV-1:

- 1° *episodes*: can occur at any age, but most common in children and young adults. May be asymptomatic to severe gingivo-stomatitis. Vesicles, typically itchy, appear on the lips, tongue, gums, buccal mucosa, or gingiva and hard palate. Unlike herpes zoster 1° HSV infection is not associated with viraemia. Lesions are initially vesicular, followed by ulcers, crusting then healing. It may take up to 3 weeks for 1° HSV lesions to heal. The duration is longer in the severely immunocompromised.
- *Recurrent HSV*: tends to localize to the vermilion border of the lips. Some patients experience pain or tingling sensation before the appearance of the lesions. It may take 7–10 days for oral HSV lesions to heal. Recurrent HSV infection may be more common in patients with symptomatic HIV disease, and severely immunocompromised patients tend to have more frequent and more severe attacks.
- *Complications*:
  - Ocular keratitis occurs with the same frequency as in HIV −ve individuals.
  - HSV oesophagitis usually with severe odynophagia occurs more frequently in patients with late HIV disease, but not necessarily associated with concomitant oral herpes.
  - HSV meningitis is more likely to follow 1° genital herpes, but can occur in acute oral herpes.
- *Management*: labial herpes may be treated with topical acyclovir 4–6 times a day (systemic treatment; see Chapter 42, 'Anal disease', pp. 501–2).

Box 42.1 Differential diagnosis of white lesions in the oral cavity

- Candidiasis.
- OHL.
- Frictional keratosis.
- Tobacco-induced leukoplakia.
- Lichen planus.
- White sponge naevus.
- Geographical tongue.
- Primary syphilis and syphilitic mucous patches.
- SCC.

Cytomegalovirus

Seroprevalence rates rise with age. >90% prevalence rates have been found in homosexual men living with HIV.

CMV oral ulcers

- mucosal, intra-oral, typically solitary, deep, necrotic with a red margin and a white halo; difficult to differentiate from those of other aetiology
- arise when the CD4 count is <50 cells/µL
- usually occur as part of disseminated CMV disease and attempts must be made to exclude other organs involvement, e.g. the retina
- diagnosis is established by the biopsy finding of typical owl's eye inclusions; CMV PCR on tissue sample may help

Management: For systemic management see Chapter 44, 'Treatment', (pp. 518–19).

Varicella zoster virus

Reactivation of VZV causes herpes zoster (HZ)/shingles in the immuno-compromised host, including HIV infection at any stage. Rarely presents as a 1° infection in those without previous exposure to the virus. People with HIV infection are 15 times more likely to have HZ than age-matched controls. Oral HZ is latent in the trigeminal ganglion. Mandibular branch involvement presents with lesions on the lower lip and lateral border of the tongue, and maxillary branch involvement presents with lesions on the hard palate. Oral vesicles last for a few hours followed by painful ulcers, while the concomitant skin lesions may last for 2–4 weeks.

For diagnosis and management, see Chapter 47, 'Varicella zoster virus infection', pp. 553–4.

Oral hairy leukoplakia (OHL)

White adherent vertically corrugated lesion, only found in the mouth, most commonly the lateral aspect of the tongue, and can be on one side only (Plate 26). The affected area may fluctuate in size.

Caused by EBV. Usually asymptomatic, but a few patients may complain of pain, and altered sensation and taste. Reported in all risk groups but more frequent in adults, men and smokers. It is not pathognomonic and occurs in other immunocompromised individuals, such as bone marrow and renal transplant recipients. Incidence and persistence increase with advancing HIV disease and declining CD4 counts. Its occurrence is associated with faster progression towards AIDS even after adjustment for CD4 count. It is not premalignant and does not need specific treatment, but re-gresses with improved immune function associated with ART.

Human papilloma virus

Incidence dropped dramatically with the advent of ART. HPV type 44, 32, 7, 13, and 18 are the most commonly identified causes of oral warts in PLWH. Mutant strains are frequently identified. Oral warts are more common than in the general population, but there is no association with the stage of infection. HPV-16 has been associated with oral SCC in HIV-infected men. Although mostly localized to the oral cavity, laryngeal warts may occur, and may be solitary or multiple, pedunculated, or sessile with small papilliferous or cauliflower-like projections.

Management
Surgical excision, laser, or cryotherapy.

Bacterial diseases

Periodontal disease
The ↑ incidence of gum and periodontal disease in PLWH makes dental hygiene particularly important. Periodontal disease should be managed in consultation with the dentist, and/or the maxillofacial or dental surgeon. Mild gingivitis and dental abscesses are common at all stages of HIV infection. Linear gingival erythema (LGE), necrotizing ulcerative periodontitis (NUP) and necrotizing stomatitis (NS) occur more frequently in HIV infection. They are characterized by rapid onset, increased severity, and poor response to conventional treatment.

- *LGE*: patients present with spontaneous painless gum bleeding. Examination reveals an oedematous erythematous band parallel to the free gingival margin, which may be a precursor of NUP. Commonly isolated organisms include *Bacteroides gingivalis, Fusobacterium nucleatum*, and *Actinobacilli*. Response to treatment is poor, but attention to oral hygiene and chlorhexidine mouthwashes are helpful. Systemic metronidazole may be required.
- *Necrotizing periodontal diseases (NPD)*: acute-onset severe rapidly progressive disease, usually seen in patients with advanced HIV. Includes NUG and NS. Appears to be related to diminished resistance to bacterial infection and only differ in the severity of tissue involvement, with NUP extending into periodontal attachment resulting in more destruction. Patients complain of spontaneous bleeding, foul mouth smell and deep jaw pain. Severe gum pain precedes the appearance of signs, which include soft tissue necrosis with destruction of periodontal ligament and bone. NUP may resemble intra-oral lymphoma. Management includes oral hygiene, chlorhexidine mouthwashes and oral antibiotics e.g. metronidazole and amoxicillin together with gentle debridement.

Tuberculosis
The most common oral manifestation is irregular ulceration of the tongue or palate. Culture has low sensitivity detection rates (2–17%) so PCR should be considered.

Fungal diseases

Oral and pharyngeal candidiasis
Probably the most common opportunistic infection (OI) in HIV. >90% would have oropharyngeal candidiasis at some stage. Commonly caused by *Candida albicans*, but other species, such as *Candida glabrata* and *Candida tropicalis* are implicated. Although oropharyngeal candidiasis may occur at acute seroconversion, it is more frequent as the CD4 count ↓.

Clinical features
- *Pseudomembranous candidiasis*: the pseudomembranous appearance results from overgrowth of candidal hyphae, mixed with desquamated epithelium and inflammatory cells. Appears as white plaques at any site

of the mouth or pharynx, and leaves an erythematous raw bleeding mucosa on scraping. Patient may complain of soreness and altered taste (Plate 25).

- *Erythematous candidiasis*: appears as flat, red patches of varying morphology that can be difficult to recognize and, therefore, diagnosis may be delayed. Most common sites are palate and dorsal surface of the tongue. Usually asymptomatic, but soreness and burning sensation may be reported, especially after eating salty or spicy food.
- *Angular cheilitis*: may appear solely or in conjunction with other forms of oropharyngeal candidiasis, resulting in redness, ulcers, and fissuring of one or both corners of the mouth.
- *Hyperplastic candidiasis*: the rarest form of candidiasis in PLWH. Chronic, white, and nodular, and cannot be wiped off.

Diagnosis

Can be made on the clinical appearance. Candidal hyphae can be demonstrated on Gram or periodic acid Schiff staining of smears from lesions. Culture may be used, particularly in recalcitrant infection, to identify the candidal type, which may guide treatment. Sensitivities may be difficult to interpret. It does not help in making the diagnosis, as candida is a commensal of the oropharynx.

Management

- *Systemic antifungal (standard mode of therapy)*:
  - *fluconazole*—50–100 mg od for 7–14 days
  - *itraconazole solution*—100–200 mg od for 7–14 days.
- *Topical antifungal (consider in mild cases)*:
  - *nystatin (as oral suspension)*—100,000 units qds for 7 days and continue for 48 hours after lesions resolution
  - *miconazole oral gel*—2.5 mL after food qds, continue for at least 7 days after lesions resolution.

Topical treatment must be retained in the mouth in contact with lesions for sufficient time.

Prognosis

Relapses are common and may be the result of poor compliance, rather than resistance to antifungals. Consider prophylactic therapy (fluconazole 50 mg daily) when recurrences are common, but risk of resistance.

Neoplasia

Kaposi's sarcoma

See Chapter 54, 'Kaposi's sarcoma', pp. 611–13.

Oral KS was among the first recognized features in the early AIDS epidemic. More common in MSM. Usually presents as a blue, purple, or red lesion that may be flat, papular, nodular, or rarely a large tumour (Plate 27). Large nodular lesions may ulcerate and be secondarily infected. Occasionally, the adjacent mucosa is yellow stained (due to haemosiderin). Commonest site is the hard palate, but may be seen on the gingiva, tongue, soft palate, and buccal mucosa. Local pain may be a feature in secondarily infected, ulcerative lesions. Mucosal lesions may indicate more extensive visceral involvement requiring good systemic enquiry and radiological investigation with chest X-ray and possibly computerized tomography (CT) scanning.

Management:
See Chapter 54,'Kaposi's sarcoma', pp. 611–13.
- immune reconstitution accomplished by art may result in KS resolution, improves survival, and response to therapy
- small lesions respond to local therapy, e.g. surgical excision (may bleed excessively), laser excision, and intralesional chemotherapy
- larger lesions may be treated with radiation therapy, which may be complicated by mucositis.

Oral lymphoma
EBV is implicated in the majority of cases. The vast majority are B-cell non-Hodgkin's lymphomas. Oral lymphoma may precede the development of lymphomas at other sites. Presents as a rapidly growing tumour at any site in the mouth (Plate 28). May be diffuse or discrete nodules, or may present as ulcers of variable morphology. May mimic periodontal disease. Diagnosis by tissue biopsy.

Management
Once the diagnosis is established, lymphoma must be staged by appropriate imaging. Systemic chemotherapy and local radiation are the main stay of therapy in collaboration with the maxillofacial surgeons to minimize oral side-effects.

Idiopathic aphthous ulcers
Recurrent oral ulceration resembling aphthous ulcers is a common phenomenon in PLWH, usually well circumscribed, superficial, and varying in size:
- *Herpetiform*: painful clusters of 1–2 mm ulcers, usually in the mouth and soft palate.
- *Minor*—usually solitary, 0.5–1.0 cm in diameter, causing minimal symptoms.
- *Major*—2–4 cm in size and necrotic. Usually found on the tonsils and tongue base, and rarely the pharynx and nasopharynx. Typically, very painful, persisting for several weeks.

Management
- *Local analgesics*: lidocaine hydrochloride 5% ointment or 10% solution as a spray; apply thinly to the ulcer using a cotton bud.
- *Topical steroids*: e.g. hydrocortisone muco-adhesive buccal tablets as 1 qds (allow to dissolve slowly in mouth in contact with ulcer).
- Systemic steroids may be used if associated with oesophageal ulcers 40–60 mg daily for 7–10 days. Infective aetiology must be excluded.
- *Thalidomide* (50–200 mg/day) produces an excellent response in resistant cases. Prescribing thalidomide needs compliance with certain requirements, especially the avoidance of pregnancy.

Salivary gland disease
Salivary glands may become infiltrated with lymphocytes, predominantly CD8 cells, leading to enlargement especially the parotids.

Xerostomia may be caused by drugs such as didanosine (DDI), antihistamines, and antidepressants, but also as a manifestation of HIV infection, where the precise aetiology is unclear. Salivary amylase levels may be raised in drug-related cases.

Management
- Salivary stimulants, such as sugarless sweets and chewing gum for symptomatic relief.
- Artificial saliva as necessary.
- Careful dental hygiene.

Parotid gland enlargement

- *Diffuse infiltrating lymphocytosis syndrome (DILS)*: due to CD8 expansion, may also involve the cervical lymph nodes and lungs. Presents with dry mouth and parotid glands enlargement.
- *Benign lympho-epithelial cysts*: usually painless and soft, may be single or multiple, and may enlarge gradually to involve the superficial lobes of both glands.

Imaging techniques and fine needle aspiration help to confirm diagnosis. Parotidectomy rarely needed other than for cosmetic reasons.

Box 42.2 Differential diagnosis of oral–pharyngeal ulcers

- *Viral*:
  - HSV
  - CMV
  - HZV.
- *Bacterial*:
  - necrotizing ulcerative periodontitis
  - necrotizing ulcerative gingivitis
  - *Mycobacterium tuberculosis*
  - *Mycobacterium avium* complex
  - *Treponema pallidum*.
- *Fungal*: histoplasmosis.
- *Malignancies*:
  - lymphoma
  - KS
- *Other causes*: aphthous ulcers.
- Behçets disease.

Oesophageal diseases

Dysphagia +/− odynophagia are the main symptoms. However, symptoms and signs are not discriminative enough to establish an underlying aetiology (Box 42.3). Assessment of the nutritional status and hydration is essential in managing such patients.

Dysphagia investigations

- Endoscopy and biopsy required to establish a definitive diagnosis.
- Double-contrast barium swallow may differentiate between infection and neoplasm, but rarely diagnostic.
- More than one pathology may co-exist and, therefore, multiple biopsies (>6) from different sites are advisable.
- Generally, culture of oesophageal specimens is not helpful as does not differentiate between colonization and actual tissue invasion, but may be useful in identifying viral and mycobacterial pathogens.

Candidal oesophagitis

Most common cause of oesophagitis in HIV infection. Patient with oral candidiasis and odynophagia can be treated empirically for oesophageal candidiasis, and investigated if it fails to respond. Usually occurs when CD4 count <200 cells/μL and rarely asymptomatic. Endoscopic appearance classically diffuse raised plaques that can be removed from the mucosa by the endoscope. Brushing or biopsy of plaques shows candida hyphae, spores, and diffuse inflammatory infiltrates.

Management

- fluconazole 100–200mg daily for 7–14 days.
- itraconazole 200 mg daily in 1-2 divided doses (the suspension formulation of itraconazole has a better bioavailability than the capsular form). This is especially useful in fluconazole-resistant candidiasis (rare and seen in those with very low CD4 count who have had repeated courses of fluconazole).
- liposomal amphotericin B (e.g. Amphocil®, AmbiSome®)
- voriconazole, in refractory cases and in fluconazole-resistance.

Box 42.3 Causes of oesophagitis

Infections
- *Candida* spp.
- CMV.
- HSV.
- *Mycobacterium avium* complex.

Malignancies
- KS.
- Lymphoma.

Idiopathic oesophageal ulceration (non-HIV-related)
- Reflux oesophagitis.
- Pill-induced oesophagitis, e.g. zidovudine.

CMV oesophagitis

CMV causes large distal oesophageal ulcers. Biopsy required to con-firm, and exclude other or concomitant causes of oesophagitis.

Management

CMV disease is treated with ganciclovir or foscarnet until clinical improve-ment. Patients may be given maintenance oral valganciclovir to prevent CMV retinitis (see Chapter 44, 'CMV retinitis', pp. 518–19).

Enteric diseases

Diarrhoea is an extremely common symptom in HIV infection. Can be debilitating, and require extensive and invasive investigation. In patients with CD4 >200 cells/μL, usually caused by virulent organisms and managed as in the immunocompetent. When CD4 <200 cells/μL, it is usually more severe, more likely caused by OIs, more difficult to diagnose and is less responsive to treatment. Large bowel diarrhoea is typically of small volume, may be blood-stained, and associated with lower abdominal pain and tenesmus. Small bowel diarrhoea is characteristically of large volume, offensive, and of pale colour. Diarrhoea is chronic if persists >1 month. Although infection with campylobacter and other enteric pathogens occur (see Chapter 20, 'Proctocolitis and enteric sexually acquired infections', pp. 259–66), particularly important organisms are cryptosporidium, microsporidium, cystoisospora, and salmonella.

Cryptosporidiosis

Cryptosporidium spp. are protozoan parasites that primarily cause enteric illness in humans and animals. They have worldwide distribution and lack host specificity. The two species that infect humans most frequently are *Cryptosporidium hominis* and *Cryptosporidium parvum*. They are 4–6 μm intracellular protozoa and have a complete life cycle (with a sexual and an asexual stage) in the intestinal mucosa of a single host. The oocyst can survive in the environment for >3 months. Given its small size, it may bypass water filtration systems. It has an outer shell making it resistant to standard home and hospital disinfectants. It is highly infectious; the infectious dose for *C. hominis* 10–83 oocysts. Infection is self-limiting and is usually asymptomatic in the immunocompetent host, but can cause debilitating symptoms in patients with advanced HIV disease. Human disease is usually limited to the jejunum, but may involve all the GI and respiratory epithelium in the immunocompromised.

The incidence of cryptosporidiosis in PLWH has declined dramatically since the introduction of ART.

Important factors in transmission

- *Zoonotic infection*: e.g. rural communities. Contact with infected lambs and calves.
- Outbreaks have been linked to drinking or swimming in contaminated water.
- Travellers to countries with poor sanitation systems.
- Human-to-human transmission, which may include sexual contact.
- Oocysts may be excreted for 2 weeks after recovery.

Clinical features

- *PLWH with preserved immune function*: similar to HIV –ve immunocompetent. Acute, self-limiting profuse, watery diarrhoea with weight loss, abdominal pain, anorexia, and fatigue. Symptoms resolve within 2–3 weeks.
- *In advanced HIV disease*: persistent watery diarrhoea of variable frequency and volume (1–15 L/day). Commonly associated with nausea, abdominal cramps, malabsorption, weight loss, and electrolyte disturbances. Sclerosing cholangitis, interstitial lung disease, chronic sinusitis, and otitis media are rare features.

Diagnosis
The parasite can be easily missed on routine stool analysis, inform lab that diagnosis is considered. Special staining techniques such as auramine-phenol (fluorescent stain) are required. Intestinal mucosal biopsies may identify the organism.

Management
Attention to fluid and nutrition is important. No proven effective agent, although paromomycin, azithromycin, and other antibiotics are used with variable degrees of success.
• Best response is by improving the immune function with ART.
• *Antidiarrhoeal agents*:
  • loperamide
  • opiates
  • diphenoxylate
  • octreotide (somatostatin analogue)—effective in secretory diarrhoea.

Prevention
• Raising awareness of modes of transmission.
• *If CD4 <50 cells/μL*: boil water for minimum 10 minutes.
• Use of fine filters to the mains water supplies.

Microsporidiosis

Microsporidia are small (1–5 μm) obligate intracellular fungi of which several hundred species were identified, but only a few cause human disease. They develop in enterocytes and are excreted in faeces. Transmitted by the ingestion of contaminated food or water, and possibly through contact with infected animals. Incidence in PLWH ↓ dramatically with the introduction of ART. The commonest microsporidia that cause disease in patients with advanced HIV infection are:
• *Encephalitazoon intestinalis*: accounts for the majority of microsporidial diarrhoea. It is associated with cholangitis, dermatitis, disseminated infection, superficial keratoconjunctivitis, and weight loss.
• *Enterocytozoon bieneusi*: accounts for most of remainder of microsporidial diarrhoea. It is associated with malabsorption, pulmonary disease, and cholangitis.

Diagnosis
Identification of the organism in the stools with modified trichrome stain and immunofluorescent stains such as calcofluor stain. Molecular identification using species-specific PCR assays are also available. Various staining methods are used to visualize the organism in tissue biopsies. Transmission electron microscopy of intestinal biopsies considered as gold standard if available.

Management
• Immune reconstitution with ART as the most effective treatment.
• Albendazole 400mg twice daily for 4 weeks produces best results for Encephalitazoon infection.
• Some relief of symptoms has been described with metronidazole,
• Co-trimoxazole, erythromycin and octreotide but all fail to eradicate the organism.

Cystoisosporiasis (formerly known as isosporiasis)

Cystoisospora belli (formerly known as *Isospora belli*) is a common cause of epidemic diarrhoea in tropical countries and travellers. Infection occurs by ingestion of the mature (fully sporulated) oocysts contaminating food and water. Infection is usually confined to the small intestine, but may cause acalculous cholecystitis and may disseminate in patients with advanced HIV disease.

Clinical features
- Crampy abdominal pain, watery diarrhoea, and weight loss similar to cryptosporidiosis.
- Steatorrhoea (involvement of the pancreatic and biliary tracts).
- Eosinophilia.
- Rarely involves the spleen, liver, and abdominal lymph nodes.

Diagnosis
Oocysts (25–30 × 10–19 µm) are visualized in the stools by using special stains such as modified Ziehl–Neelson or in duodenal aspirate or biopsy.

Management
- Co-trimoxazole 960 mg 2–4 times a day for 2–4 weeks gives good results.
- 2° prophylaxis recommended as relapses are common, e.g. co-trimoxazole as for PCP.
- ART results in significant improvement of symptoms.

Salmonellosis

Salmonellae are Gram –ve non-spore-forming rods belonging to the Enterobacteriaceae family. Non-typhoidal salmonella infections occur with ↑ frequency in PLWH, particularly with *Salmonella typhimurium*. Major sources are poultry and eggs. Salmonella multiplies in the intestinal epithelium and, if not contained, it invades the mesenteric lymph nodes and disseminates. Cellular immune responses are important defence mechanisms.

Clinical features
In HIV infection, salmonella tends to cause more systemic symptoms. A common feature is severe gastroenteritis and fever. Localized extraintestinal focal infection may occur. Bacteraemia is common in patients with advanced HIV disease, may be recurrent and may not be accompanied by gastrointestinal symptoms.

Diagnosis
- isolation of the organism is necessary for a definitive diagnosis
- salmonella may be isolated in the blood before stools become +ve
- diagnosis should be considered in all PLWH with fever +/– diarrhoea, and blood and stool cultures taken.

Management
Salmonella requires prompt treatment in PLWH because of severity, high relapse rates, and higher risk of dissemination:
- fluid and electrolyte replacement
- oral ciprofloxacin 750 mg bd (the drug of choice)
- ceftriaxone 1–2 g daily
- amoxicillin, but bacterial resistance is ↑.

Prevention
- Avoid eating undercooked food with particular care during travel.
- Long-term suppressive antibiotic therapy may be required if recurrent episodes. It may be possible to stop such therapy if there is significant immune reconstitution with ART. Ciprofloxacin is the drug of choice though co-trimoxazole has some effect.
- AIDS patients have ↑ rates of carriage, which has implications in those working in the food industry.

Shigellosis

Shigellae are Gram −ve bacteria that can colonize and invade the intestinal cells, causing disease ranging from mild gastroenteritis to severe acute watery diarrhoea, which may have blood or mucus. The genus Shigella belongs to the family Enterobacteriacae and consists of four species; *Shigella dysenteriae, S. flexneri, S. boydii,* and *S. sonnei.* Historically, in the UK, most cases of shigellosis were associated with travel. Recently, there is a sustained outbreak of *S. flexneri* amongst MSM. Sexual practices such as rimming (oro-anal contact), sharing of sex toys, and multiple partners play a role. These practices are often linked to parties and chemsex (the use of certain substances that lead to disinhibition and engagement in high risk sexual practices).

Diagnosis
By stools culture or PCR

Management
Attention to hygiene and fluid intake needed. Usually self-limiting and does not require antibiotics. Antibiotic treatment, if needed, better guided by sensitivity testing, as *Shigella* often resistant to multiple antibiotics. Ciprofloxacin can be commenced pending lab results.

HIV enteropathy

An idiopathic form of diarrhoea that can occur during the acute phase of HIV infection through advanced disease. Histologically, villous blunting, crypt hyperplasia, inflammatory infiltrates of the lamina propria, immune activation, impaired mucosal repair and regeneration. Absorption and secretory functions are also affected. The pathogenic mechanism/s remains unclear, but may involve effects of HIV itself on the GI tract and the GALT. Viral proteins secreted or shed from infected cells may have toxic effects on cells of the GI tract. HIV can affect the local humoral immunity and gut motility as a result of autonomic dysfunction. This leads to rapid cell turnover and functional immaturity of intestinal epithelium, resulting in lower enzyme production, which leads to impaired absorption. Evidence of malabsorption, such as abnormal D-xylose test, low vitamin B12 levels, and impaired triolein breath tests are described in patients with advanced HIV. These abnormalities may occur in the absence of intestinal disease. HIV enteropathy is a diagnosis of exclusion (Fig 42.1). It improves with ART, but it may also occur in patients receiving ART.

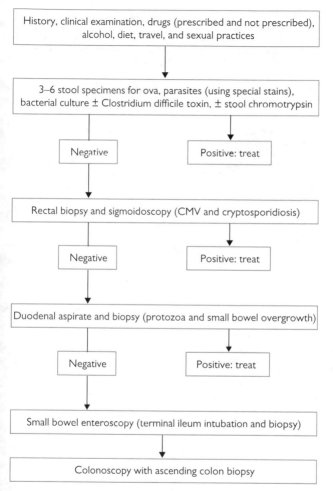

Fig 42.1 Evaluation of chronic diarrhoea in PLWH

Management

Every attempt should be made to find an underling cause, especially infection (Box 42.4). Address factors contributing to diarrhoea, such as alcoholism and drugs. Principles of therapy are attention to nutrition and symptomatic control of diarrhoea. Improves with ART.

Box 42.4 Common causes of diarrhoea in HIV

Infections
- Bacterial:
  - Salmonella, Shigella, Campylobacter, E. coli, C. difficile
  - CD4 < 50 cells/μl — MAC.
- Parasitic:
  - Giardia, Cryptosporidium, Microsporidum, Cystoisospora & Entamoeba
  - CD4 < 50 cells/μl—Cryptosporidium, Microsporidium.
- Viral:
  - Enteroviruses
  - HIV enteropathy
  - CD4 < 50 cells/μl— CMV, HSV.

Other causes
- Drugs: most anti-retroviral drugs.
- Chronic pancreatitis.
- Lymphoma.
- Bowel cancer.

Anal diseases

Anal complaints and anal lesions are frequent presentations in those with HIV infection, especially MSM. Anal pain, pruritus, discharge, and bleeding should be assessed by enquiring about sexual practices, followed by anal and rectal examination by proctoscopy. Gonorrhoea, chlamydia, syphilis, and anogenital warts are common and must be excluded.

Anal HSV infection

Although hsv2 causes the majority of infection, hsv1 is ↑. Patients with advanced hiv disease tend to have more recurrences and prolonged episodes that are less likely to resolve spontaneously.

Typical painful vesicles and ulcers occur in the anal and peri-anal region. Severe disease may result in diffuse peri-anal ulceration. The distal rectum may be involved, resulting in anal discharge, painful defaecation, rectal bleeding, and tenesmus. Fever and painful inguinal adenopathy occur more commonly in primary attacks.

Diagnosis:

See Chapter 22, 'Anogenital herpes', pp. 277–89.

Management

Prompt treatment with specific antiviral drugs reduces the duration of symptoms and viral shedding. Chronic episodes (>4 weeks) occur more frequently in patients with advanced HIV disease. Acyclovir-resistant hsv has been reported in association with hiv infection. Valaciclovir and famciclovir have better bioavailability.

Recommended initial treatment in the immunocompromised:
- aciclovir 400 mg 5 times a day for 10 days
- famciclovir 500 mg bd for 10 days (cost may limit use)
- valaciclovir 1000 mg bd for 10 days.

Suppressive treatment (interrupted and reviewed every 6–12 months):
- aciclovir 200 mg qds (or 400 mg bd)
- valaciclovir 500 mg bd
- famciclovir 500 mg bd (cost may limit use).

Human papilloma virus infection

Anal warts common in PLWH, especially MSM. HPV6 and 11 are the most frequent types, but others including 16, 18, 31, and 33 have been detected. Patients with advanced HIV may have exuberant plaques in the peri-anal region, as well as flexural areas. Extensive anal and peri-anal warts may present with rectal bleeding and constipation.

Management

➜ Chapter 23, 'Anogenital warts', pp. 291–304.

No treatment ensures HPV eradication and is similar to the HIV −ve, although persistence and recurrences are more common, but may improve with immune reconstitution produced by ART.

Prevention

In the UK, an HPV vaccination scheme is offered to MSM up to and including the age of 45 years using the quadrivalent vaccine (HPV types 6, 11, 16 and 18).

Anal intraepithelial neoplasia (AIN)

The epithelium of the transitional zone between the anus and colonic mucosa is susceptible to intra-epithelial neoplasia and invasive cancer, similar to those seen in the female cervix. AIN1–3 precedes the development of anal cancer, similar to cervical cancer. HPV (type 16 and 18) infection, receptive anal intercourse, and HIV infection are co-factors for the development of these changes. The incidence of AIN and anal carcinoma, especially in MSM, is ↑ as life expectancy rises with availability of ART, which does not appear to be protective.

Anal carcinoma may be prevented by the early detection and treatment of AIN3. Anal cytology can be used to detect dyskaryosis, although this is not routine clinical practice. In the absence of anal cytology annual digital rectal examination is recommended to detect early lesions.

Low grade AIN lesions can be treated conservatively by regular monitoring and high grade lesions (AIN3) by ablative surgical techniques.

Pancreatic diseases

Pancreatic involvement in HIV infection is common, but is usually asymptomatic. Drugs, alcohol, and OIs are the usual causes. Pancreatic disease tends to occur in conjunction with hepatic and hepatobiliary disease. Presentation may be with acute or chronic pancreatitis. Elevation of serum amylase or lipase may predate symptoms development.

Acute pancreatitis

Patients usually severely ill, in shock, with acute abdominal pain, nausea, and vomiting. Causes include:

- *OIs*:
  - *CMV*—most common infective cause
  - cryptococcus and toxoplasmosis
  - cryptosporidiosis
  - hsv.
- *Malignancies*:
  - non-Hodgkin's lymphoma
  - ks (less common).
- Drugs such as didanosine, co-trimoxazole, and pentamidine.
- Very high levels of triglycerides associated with protease inhibitors.

The serum amylase is elevated and CT scan demonstrates an oedematous, enlarged pancreas with surrounding fluid. Admission to a high dependency unit for cardiovascular and electrolyte support is usually required.

Chronic pancreatitis

Typically presents with pancreatic exocrine deficiency. Chronic diarrhoea and malabsorption are the usual presenting features. As with HIV –ve patients, the discontinuation of any offending drugs and alcohol may result in symptomatic improvement. HIV related cholangiopathy is a recognized underlying cause.

Diagnosis

Chronic abdominal pain (especially if history of acute pancreatitis) is suggestive of chronic pancreatitis. This may be accompanied by pancreatic insufficiency symptoms, e.g. steatorrhoea, weight loss, and other evidence of malabsorption. Screen by measuring faecal elastase, or chromotrypsin and triolein breath tests (serum amylase and lipase are usually normal). The best diagnostic test is endoscopic retrograde cholangiopancreatography (ERCP). Magnetic resonance cholangiopancreatography and endoscopic ultrasonography can be helpful.

Management

- pain control
- pancreatic enzyme supplement.

Hepatic and biliary tract diseases

HIV itself has been found in Kupffer cells, hepatic macrophages, and hepatocytes. Prior to ART, the most common causes of liver dysfunction were OIs (including CMV and mycobacterium infections) and AIDS-related neoplasms, such as lymphoma and KS. In the ART era the spectrum of liver disease has shifted to concomitant infection with chronic HCV and HBV, medication-related hepatotoxicity, alcohol abuse, and non-alcoholic fatty liver disease. In ART era, liver disease is the most common non-AIDS-related cause of death among PLWH, accounting for 14–18% of all deaths. In some series, ~ half of deaths among hospitalized PLWH in the ART era have been attributed to liver disease.

Hepatic disease

>80% of those with HIV infection are estimated to have abnormal LFTs at some time during the course of their life. This does not necessarily indicate the presence of liver disease. Important causes of abnormal LFTs and liver disease are (Box 42.5):

- *Viral co-infections*: HCV, HBV, HDV, CMV, EBV.
- *Drugs*:
  - *Antiretrovirals*—all may cause raised ALT, more common in hepatitis co-infection. Abnormal LFTs were seen in 14–20% of patients starting ART. The overall frequency of grade 3/4 ALT elevation occurs in 1–18% patients starting any ART. Atazanavir causes clinically insignificant raised bilirubin due to uridine-glucuronosyltransferase inhibition.
  - Many of the drugs used in prophylaxis and treatment of OI lead to liver toxicity.
  - Nucleotide reverse transcriptase inhibitors (NRTIs) particularly DDI and zidovudine (AZT) may cause mitochondrial toxicity, leading to hepatic steatosis.
- Alcohol.
- Bacterial, fungal, and protozoal infections, and neoplasms occur much less frequently. The pattern of LFTs and the clinical stage of HIV infection may help to narrow the diagnostic options.

Box 42.5 Main causes of liver disease in HIV patients

- *Viral*:
  - HBV
  - HCV
  - CMV.
- Alcohol.
- *Drugs*:
  - recreational
  - therapeutic, e.g. antiretroviral and antituberculous
- *Other infections*:
  - mycobacteriosis.
- *Malignancies*:
  - lymphoma
  - KS.

- IRIS, a paradoxical worsening of pre-existing infection due to rapid immune restoration in the setting of successful HIV RNA suppression
- 'Chemsex' is an emerging phenomenon, where substances such as mephedrone, crystal meth, and gamma hydroxybutyrate (GHB)/ gamma-butyrolactone (GB) are used in parties where participants are disinhibited and are engaged in high-risk condomless sex with multiple partners. In these parties, drugs are commonly injected (slamming), resulting in increase in blood-borne virus infections, including hepatitis B, hepatitis C, and HIV, and ↑ rates of STIs.

Liver damage may lead to:
- Hepatic steatosis is common in HIV, due to NRTI-induced mitochondrial toxicity, or part of metabolic syndrome associated with protease inhibitor (PI), and HCV co-infection. May lead to steatohepatitis and cirrhosis.
- Cirrhosis is a common cause of morbidity and mortality. Generally associated with viral hepatitis, but 10% may be related to drugs.
- Nodular regenerative hyperplasia is a cause of portal hypertension and variceal bleed in the absence of fibrosis and may be caused by HIV +/−anti-retrovirals, e.g. DDI

History
Prior infection with viral hepatitis, alcohol intake, prescribed and recreational drug use, anti-retroviral history, and recent travel.

Examination
Fever, hypotension, signs of chronic liver disease, and nutritional status (obesity and malnutrition).

Abnormal LFTs
Mixed hepatic and obstructive liver enzyme abnormalities are common, but rarely diagnostic in isolation.
- Predominant ↑ of serum transaminases usually indicate hepatitis, but lacks sensitivity and specificity. A new hepatitis viral infection or reactivation of hepatitis B and/or C infection with immune reconstitution should be excluded. Consider drug hepatotoxicity and investigate for other infections.
- Predominant ↑ of serum alkaline phosphatase usually indicates biliary obstruction. Initial assessment is by ultrasound scan, or CT of the liver and abdomen. Lesions identified can be targeted by image-guided biopsy. ERCP must be considered if imaging techniques reveal intrahepatic and/or extrahepatic duct dilatation.

Biliary tract disease

Presents with right upper quadrant abdominal pain, weight loss. Investigations to exclude common biliary conditions, such as cholelithiasis should proceed before attributing to HIV infection.

hiv-associated cholangiopathy
Similar to sclerosing cholangitis, presenting with right upper abdominal pain associated with nausea, vomiting, fever, and marked elevation of serum alkaline phosphatase. Ultrasound shows dilated intra- and/or extrahepatic bile ducts. ERCP provides further structural delineation. Some cases are associated with cryptosporidial and CMV infections.

Acalculous cholecystitis

Presents with similar symptoms to HIV-associated cholangiopathy. Ultrasound of the abdomen normally shows thickened dilated gall bladder, but may be normal. Can be complicated by recurrent cholangitis. Associated with CMV, *Cryptosporidium parvum*, microsporidia, and MAC infection, but no cause in >50%.

Diagnosis by ultrasound or technetium scintigraphy.

Treatment is cholecystectomy.

HIV: hepatitis virus co-infection

Introduction *508*
HIV–hepatitis B virus co-infection *509*
HIV–hepatitis C virus co-infection *511*

Introduction

Liver-related mortality among PLWH has ↑. Hepatitis B (and D), hepatitis C, and HIV can all be transmitted variably via blood and sexual contact, and consequently, co-infection is common.

Assessment of co-infection requires a multidisciplinary approach with attention to ongoing drug and alcohol use, psychiatric illness, progressive liver disease, and degree of HIV immune suppression. Alcohol should be strongly discouraged. PWID should be supported to enter a maintenance programme.

Vaccination against hepatitis A and/or B should be offered to PLWH who have not previously exposed or vaccinated.

HIV–hepatitis B virus co-infection

Epidemiology

The worldwide rate of HBV in PLWH is between 5 and 20%, equating to around 2.7 million people. For HBV in high endemic areas of sub-Saharan Africa, eastern Europe, south and southeast Asia co-infection rates are highest. In the UK, HBV/HIV co-infection is 5–8% and more common in haemophiliacs, PWID, and those from high prevalence areas. Co-infection rates vary regionally within the UK.

Natural history and clinical features

Co-infection is usually associated with a higher HBV viraemia and a more rapid progression to cirrhosis and ↑ risk of hepatocellular carcinoma (HCC). HBV does not appear to influence the natural history of HIV. There is ↑ risk of hepatotoxicity in relation to antiretroviral therapy. HBV reactivation can occur in those who appear to have cleared their HBV infection with transient HB surface antigenaemia more frequently seen when CD4 counts are ↓. In addition, the natural clearance of HBe antigen is ↓, but spontaneous recovery from chronic HBV infection may occur in those whose CD4 count ↑.

Co-infection with hepatitis D (HDV) leads to more rapid progress of liver disease and should be considered if evidence of more significant liver disease in those with ↑ ALT despite low HBV VL.

Diagnosis and investigations

- As for HBV and HIV (➲ Chapter 25, 'Diagnosis', p. 314; Chapter 40, 'HIV: Diagnosis and assessment', pp. 469–78). However, if ALT is raised persistently, HBV DNA should be measured to exclude occult HBV disease.
- It is important to repeat HBV serology regularly in immuno-naive patients with HIV infection.
- All HBsAg +ve PWLH should be screened for hepatitis D.
- Alpha-foetoprotein (AFP) and liver ultrasound should be performed in all at diagnosis and 6-monthly if cirrhotic. Furthermore, 6-monthly screening should be considered in those with severe fibrosis, family history of HCC, and if HBV VL high and ALT abnormal.
- If ALT raised, screen for other causes of liver disease.
- *Aminotransferase platelet ratio index (APRI) score*: a product of ALT, AST, and platelets predicts cirrhosis if >2 and non-cirrhosis if <1.
- Fibroscan® ≥13.1 KPa is suggestive of cirrhosis.
- Liver biopsy may be considered, particularly if other cause of liver disease considered or there is concern regarding more severe disease, despite the above.
- Test for resistance.

Management

See Box 43.1.

In chronic HBV–HIV co-infection, the aim of HBV treatment is to suppress viral replication. Only rarely is it curative (loss of surface antigen).

Box 43.1 HIV–HBV co-infection management
- *Initial investigations*: CD4, LFT, FBC, AFP, clotting, albumin, hepatitis B viral load, HDV Ab, US liver.
- *Stage liver fibrosis*: APRI Score, Fibroscan®, possibly liver biopsy.
- *Consider treatment in all patients*: ART with HBV activity.

Treatment regime
- Co-infected patients requiring ART should be treated with a regime containing tenofovir disoproxil fumarate (TDF) or tenofovir alafenamide (TAF) and emtricitabine AF or lamivudine. Lamivudine or emtricitabine should not be used without adequate second agent. If ART regimens containing lamivudine with TDF or TAF achieve good HBV response, but need to be changed, TDF or TAF should be maintained in the new ART combination. If TAF or TDF cannot be given entacavir can be used with effective ART, adefovir may need to be added if known HBV resistance.
- PLWH who have co-infection should be assessed for liver transplantation if decompensated cirrhosis or HCC develops.
- Co-infection with HDV is very difficult to treat.

HIV–hepatitis C virus co-infection

Epidemiology
Worldwide HCV is found among 2–15% of PLWH (2.75 million people), 90% of those co-infected are PWID. In the UK, HCV co-infection is found in 10–12% of PLWH, it is found more commonly in patients from high endemic areas, PWID and MSM. HCV transmission is seen in MSM particularly if anal sex, chemsex, co-existing STI, or low CD4 count.

Heterosexual HCV transmission is infrequent, but may be more likely with anal sex or with co-existing STIs.

Natural history and clinical features
Co-infection with HCV accelerates the progression of HIV and results in a poorer CD4 increase with ART.

HCV/HIV co-infected patients have a faster progression to cirrhosis if untreated (median time decreases from 32 to 23 years with ~50% cirrhotic at 30 years post-HCV infection) with death from ESLD more common. Vertical transmission of HCV ↑ from 1-5% to 14–17% if co-infected.

Otherwise clinical features as for mono-infection (➜ Chapter 25, 'Clinical features', p. 318).

Diagnosis and investigations
- As for HCV and HIV (➜ Chapter 25, 'Diagnosis and investigations', pp. 318–19; ➜ Chapter 40, 'HIV diagnosis and assessment', pp. 469–78), including HCV genotype testing. HCV Ab should be checked at diagnosis and yearly if MSM, PWID, or others at risk. HIV patients may have occult HCV (3.2% HCV PCR +ve, HCV Ab –ve; ↑ with low CD4) and HCV VL should be measured if ALT persistently raised and HCV Ab –ve.
- APRI score or Fibroscan® should be considered, there may be overestimation of fibrosis in co-infection if standard cut-off of 12 kPa used for cirrhosis.
- Patients with cirrhosis should be monitored with AFP and 6-monthly ultrasound liver for HCC.

Management
See Box 43.2.

Treatment should be considered in all patients. Directly acting antiviral drugs (DAA) acting against HCV are highly effective with no difference in effectiveness due to HIV co-infection (➜ Chapter 25, 'Hepatitis C virus (HCV) infection', pp. 318–21).

Box 43.2 HIV–HCV co-infection management
- *Baseline tests*: LFTs, clotting, albumin, *HCV* genotype, HCV RNA, CD4.
- *Liver fibrosis assessment*: APRI score and if available Fibroscan® or fibrosis biomarkers.
- *ART + DAA +/– ribavirin*: consider drug interactions/toxicity.
- During treatment measure HCV RNA at 4 and 12.
- *Duration of treatment*: dependent on genotype and treatment.

Pre-treatment

Consider the following:

- Check HBV, *HCV* genotype, HCV VL, consider resistance testing if previous HCV treatment, not normally needed.
- ART should be started in patients with HCV co-infection. Potential interactions should be considered (see Box 43.3).
- Those with CD4>500 cells/μL with low HIV VL can be considered for DAA for HCV prior to ART, if no significant delay.
- Didanosine and zidovudine should be avoided in combination with ribavirin (increased side effects).

Treatment regime

- Treatment for HIV/HCV co-infection does not differ significantly from mono-infection (see Chapter 22, 'Management', pp. 319–21).
- Check HCV VL at 4 weeks, end of treatment, 3 months and 6 months post treatment.
- As above consider interactions.

Box 43.3 HCV drug interactions with HIV medications

- *Sofosbuvir*: no significant interaction.
- *Daclatasvir*: decrease dose to 30 mg when used with atazanavir (ATV)/r or EVG/c, increase dose to 90 mg with efavirenz (Elvitegravir, EFV)
- *Elbasvir/Grazoprevir*: cannot be co-administered with PIs, EVG/c, or NNRTI. Integrase no significant interaction.
- *Paritaprevir/r/ombitasvir/dasabuvir*: cannot be co-administered with regimes containing cobicistat, NNRTI (rilpivirine may ↑ QT can be used with significant caution), Maraviroc may need to be ↓. Unboosted ATV or DRV (Darunavir, dose 800 mg od) may be used.
- *Paritaprevir/r/ombitasvir*: as above; in addition DRV or ATV should not be co-administered.
- *Sofosbuvir/Ledipasvir*: need to carefully monitor renal function if TDF used in regime.
- *Sofosbuvir/Velpatasvir*: should not be administered with NNRTI other than rilpivirine. Need to carefully monitor renal function if TDF used in regime.

HIV: disorders of the eye

Introduction *514*
Ocular surface and adnexa of the eye (eyebrow,
    conjunctiva, eyelids, and lacrimal apparatus) *515*
Anterior segment of the eye (cornea, anterior
    chamber and iris) *517*
Posterior segment of the eye *518*
Neuro-ophthalmic manifestations *521*

Introduction

Before ART, up to 70% of PLWH developed some form of ocular involvement as a result of OIs, HIV-associated tumours, or direct infection by HIV. Ocular manifestations ↑ in frequency as the CD4 count ↓. Patients with CD4 count <200 cells/μL should be closely examined for signs of ocular disease which may be asymptomatic in the early stages. Close cooperation with ophthalmology is essential to ensure timely therapeutic interventions to ↓ risk of visual impairment and blindness. ART ↓ the incidence of ocular complications by 26-50% and altered the natural history of many OIs.

Ophthalmic manifestations of HIV infection can be classified as:

- *Ocular surface and adnexa of the eye:*
  - sicca syndrome
  - conjunctival microvasculopathy
  - Herpes zoster ophthalmicus
  - KS
  - *Molluscum contagiosum*
  - Conjunctival SCC.
- *Anterior segment of the eye:*
  - superficial candidal keratitis
  - anterior uveitis
  - immune-recovery uveitis.
- *Posterior segment of the eye:*
  - retinal microvasculopathy
  - CMV retinitis
  - acute retinal necrosis
  - progressive outer retinal necrosis
  - toxoplasmosis retinochoroiditis
  - Candida endophthalmitis.
- Neuro-ophthalmic manifestation.

Ocular surface and adnexa of the eye (eyebrow, conjunctiva, eyelids, and lacrimal apparatus)

Sicca syndrome

Dry eye is frequent among PLWH. Results from HIV-mediated inflammation and damage to the lacrimal glands. Patients complain of burning uncomfortable red eyes.

Treatment is with artificial tears and lubricating ointments.

Conjunctival microvasculopathy

Occurs in 70–80% of PLWH. Exact aetiology not known, but may be related to ↑ viscosity and immune complex deposits. Conjunctival changes are found near the limbus and can only be detected by slit-lamp examination. Features include segmental vascular dilation and narrowing, microaneurysms and appearance of comma-shaped vascular fragments.

Herpes zoster ophthalmicus

Results from reactivation of a latent infection by VZV in the dorsal root of the trigeminal root ganglion. It is recognized by characteristic vesicular eruptions, which is often preceded by pain. Usually involves the upper lid, does not cross the midline, and may be associated with blepharitis, conjunctivitis, keratitis, uveitis, and necrotizing retinitis, which may occur at same time or soon afterwards. Complications and post-herpetic neuralgia ↑ in the immunosuppressed.

Early retinal lesions similar to CMV, but rapidly progressive, deep, and multifocal with ↑ risk of retinal detachment, which may lead to blindness in days without prompt treatment.

Diagnosis

Characteristic rash and its distribution are usually sufficient to establish the diagnosis. Serological tests and PCR rarely needed.

Treatment

IV aciclovir is the treatment of choice along with aciclovir eye drops if corneal involvement. Valaciclovir can be used after initial improvement or mild disease with good CD4 count. Other problems, such as anterior uveitis are treated with topical steroids and mydriatics.

Kaposi's sarcoma

KS is a vascular neoplasm, which is almost exclusively seen in patients with AIDS. Up to 20% of patients with skin KS have eyelid and conjunctival lesions. Lesions appear as violaceous non-tender nodules on the eyelid or conjunctiva, although conjunctival lesions may resemble traumatic haemorrhages.

Treatment

Options include surgical removal, cryotherapy, α-interferon and intralesional chemotherapy. Systemic chemotherapy may be needed if extensive disease (see Chapter 54, 'Kaposi's sarcoma,' pp. 611–13). Radiation is effective, but may be complicated by loss of eyelashes and conjunctivitis.

Molluscum contagiosum

Discrete, rounded, pearly white umbilicated lesions of the eyelids can be a presenting ocular feature of HIV disease. The eyelid is involved in 5% of HIV. Lesions can be extensive and disfiguring with severe immune deficiency.

Treatment

Options include incision and curettage, cryotherapy, and trichloroacetic acid. However, spontaneous regression may occur with ART.

Conjunctival squamous cell carcinoma

May be due to an interaction between HIV, sunlight, and HPV infection. Tumour appears as a pink, gelatinous growth, usually in the interpalpebral area and may extend onto the cornea. An engorged blood vessel feeding the tumour is seen.

Treatment

Options are local excision, and local excision and cryotherapy.

Anterior segment of the eye (cornea, anterior chamber, and iris)

Infectious keratitis

- *Viral*: HSV and VZV are the most common infections, may recur and may be resistant to treatment. VZV keratitis is associated with herpes zoster ophthalmicus.
- *Bacterial*: rare in HIV, but severe.
- *Fungal*: Candida albicans and Candida parapsilosis are the commonest fungal infections in HIV, albeit rare, and normally seen in advanced HIV. Symptoms include eye pain, photophobia, and discharge and foreign-body sensation. Slit-lamp examination reveals corneal stromal infiltrate with a feathery border. Associated small focal lesions around the 1° corneal infiltrate are often present, along with conjunctival injection, anterior chamber reaction, and hypopyon. Diagnosis can be established by identifying fungal elements in corneal scrapings and fungal culture. Responds well to topical antifungals.

Iridocyclitis

Causes:
- *Infections*:
  - mild with CMV, HSV, and VZV
  - severe with ocular toxoplasmosis, tuberculosis, syphilis, bacterial, and fungal retinitis.
- Retinitis and retinochoroiditis sequelae.
- Drugs (rifabutin).
- Part of generalized autoimmune and endogenous uveitis (e.g. Reiter syndrome).

Anterior uveitis

Can be a direct manifestation of HIV infection, autoimmune or drug-induced (rifabutin), secondary to direct toxic effect upon the non-pigmented epithelium of the ciliary body and infections e.g. VZV, HSV, CMV, *Toxoplasma gondii*, and *Toxoplasma syphilis*.

Immune-recovery uveitis

A syndrome where PLWH with prior CMV retinitis experience an increase in intra-ocular inflammation following ART. Mainly involves anterior uveal tract and vitreous, and is commonly associated with a marked disturbance of visual function due to macular oedema and epi-retinal membrane formation. The marked cellular infiltration of the vitreous (in the absence of an active retinal or chorioretinal lesion) is the hallmark of this phenomenon. Responds well to systemic steroids.

Posterior segment of the eye

Retinal microvasculopathy

Asymptomatic and occurs in >50% of PLWH. Seen as transient cotton wool spots (light-coloured retinal deposits 2° to infarcts of the nerve fibre layer), intra-retinal haemorrhages and micro-aneurysms. Often occurs simultaneously in the conjunctiva. Aetiology not known, but thought 2° to HIV infection of retinal vascular cells.

Treatment is based on delaying the progression of the disease associated with HIV

CMV retinitis

CMV retinitis results from reactivation of infection acquired in childhood or early adult life. The most common eye OI in the pre ART era occurring in 30–40% of patients with CD4 count <50 cells/μL. Bilateral in 30–50% and optic nerve papillitis in 5%. Serious visual complications can be avoided by detecting early features with regular dilated fundal examination for at risk patients (CD4 <100 cells/μL).

Clinical features

Symptoms depend on site and extent of retinal involvement. Peripheral retinal lesions are asymptomatic. Earliest and most common symptoms are floaters (representing foci of inflammatory cells in the vitreous, attempting to contain the infection). Other symptoms include flashing lights, blurring/loss of central vision and scotomata. Initial focus of retinal inflammation expands peripherally, inducing retinal necrosis.

Early active lesions appear as multiple granular white dots with occasional haemorrhages. With further progress, areas of retinitis enlarge by following the vascular arcades, resulting in an arcuate or triangular zone of infection. Areas of active infection may also be linear, following the retinal vessels or nerve-fibre layer into the periphery. Early CMV lesions may be confused with cotton-wool spots (due to HIV vasculopathy), which may co-exist. Serial drawings or retinal photographs are helpful in differentiation. Continuing activity of the necrotic process results in atrophic features with thinning of the retina resulting in visualization of the underlying choroid. Other features of CMV retinitis include vascular attenuation, vessel occlusion, vitritis, and anterior uveitis (Plate 31). May be complicated by retinal detachment and cataract.

Occasionally, it may be difficult to establish the cause of retinitis.

Diagnosis

Usually clinical, all patients presenting with CD4 <100 cells/μL should have slit lamp examination. Confirmed by obtaining a vitreous sample for CMV PCR. A rising CMV VL, detected by PCR, is associated with ↑ eye and other organ disease.

Treatment

ART improves response to treatment, prognosis, and ↓ relapse rates.

IV ganciclovir, given as an induction course for 2–3 weeks (5 mg/kg body weight 12-hourly) followed by maintenance therapy (5 mg/kg body weight 7 days a week or 6 mg/kg body weight 5 days a week). Side-effects include rigors and neutropenia that may require discontinuation of treatment or the use of granulocyte colony stimulating factor. Oral valganciclovir 900 mg bd for 3 weeks followed by 900 mg od produces blood levels comparable with IV ganciclovir. Main side-effects are bone marrow suppression and GI upset.

Intravitreal ganciclovir implants are very effective, but need to be replaced after 6–9 months; does not give protection to the other eye or protect against systemic disease.

IV foscarnet, given as an induction course for 2–3 weeks (60 mg/kg body weight 8-hourly) followed by maintenance therapy (90–120 mg/kg body weight od). Given when ganciclovir is not tolerated due to its toxicity. Side-effects include nephrotoxicity, convulsions, meatal ulceration, and electrolyte disturbance. Has ↑ infusion time and requires an infusion pump.

IV cidofovir plus oral probenecid is effective in ganciclovir-resistant CMV, but is highly nephrotoxic and myelosuppressive.

Prognosis
Response to therapy achieved in 80–90%. Without immune reconstitution, the median time to relapse is 50–120 days using standard anti-CMV treatment. Maintenance therapy can be stopped once immune reconstitution is achieved.

Acute retinal necrosis (ARN)
ARN is usually due to VZV infection, and less commonly HSV or CMV. Can occur at any stage of HIV infection. Presents with eye pain associated with scotomata progressing rapidly to visual loss. The other eye is involved in one-third. Fundal examination shows prominent anterior chamber reaction, marked vitritis, occlusive retinal and choroidal vasculitis, and full-thickness retinal necrosis. It can lead to retinal detachment in 75% of cases and blindness in 64% of cases within 2–3 months. May be complicated by proliferative retinopathy and retinal detachment. The diagnosis is mainly clinical and is confirmed by PCR assays on vitreous samples.

Treatment
IV aciclovir or oral valaciclovir or famciclovir combined with laser treatment to prevent retinal detachment.

Progressive Outer Retinal Necrosis (PORN)
PORN is severe viral retinitis without vitritis or retinal vasculitis. The main cause is VZV. HSV, CMV and Epstein–Barr virus are also implicated. It is usually seen in patients with severe immune deficiency, an average CD4 count of 20 cells/uL. Typical features are multifocal retinal opacities starting at the peripheral retina, involving the posterior pole in 30% of cases, rapidly coalescent and progressing to complete retinal necrosis. The main symptom is rapid loss of vision. The retina typically shows a white lesion with no haemorrhages or exudates. Diagnosis with vitreal biopsy and viral PCR.

Treatment
IV aciclovir can be associated with progression. IV ganciclovir can be associated with significant toxicity. Intra-vitreal ganciclovir and foscarnet may be superior.

Prognosis

Very poor and retinal detachment is common. Resolution may leave a white plaque with the appearance of 'cracked mud'.

Toxoplasma retinochoroiditis

Accounts for only 1–2% of retinitis in PLWH, 30–50% of them have concurrent CNS involvement. Unlike the immunocompetent patients, PLWH often have bilateral and multifocal disease associated with anterior uveitis, and later on vitritis, and no pigmented scars adjacent to the areas of retinal necrosis. Toxoplasmosis in immunocompromised patients is not self-limiting.

Diagnosis

Fundal examination reveals characteristic extensive fluffy areas of retinal whitening with accompanying vitritis, but unlike CMV infection retinal haemorrhaging is less likely. Toxoplasma serological tests are unreliable to make a diagnosis, but the absence of toxoplasma IgG antibodies makes it less likely.

Treatment

Pyrimethamine plus sulfadiazine or clindamycin plus folinic acid. Equally good response may be obtained with atovaquone. Long-term maintenance treatment with clindamycin and pyrimethamine usually required.

Candidal endophthalmitis

Posterior segment infection is seen in advanced HIV disease. More common in PWID and may be associated with infected lines in the seriously sick. In the initial stages, floaters are the main symptom. With progression, whitish 'puff-balls' and vitreous strands develop. Later, similar infiltrates appear in the choroid and retina, and may extend into the overlying vitreous. Majority of patients have systemic candidiasis.

Diagnosis

Blood cultures, and vitreous aspiration and diagnostic vitrectomy for fungal culture and histological examination.

Treatment

Depends on severity of ocular involvement and presence of systemic disease. Original foci should be looked for and removed (e.g. central line). Systemic antifungals, e.g. liposomal amphotericin, voriconazole, and fluconazole.

Neuro-ophthalmic manifestations

Occur in 10%. Most common features include papilloedema, cranial nerve palsies, ophthalmoplegia, and visual field defects. Caused by lymphoma and any CNS infection, most frequently cryptococcal meningitis, neurosyphilis, and toxoplasmosis. HIV encephalopathy and progressive multi-focal leukoencephalopathy may have similar complications.

Investigate by magnetic resonance imaging, lumbar puncture (CSF-cell count, cytology, culture, and serology).

Neuro-ophthalmic manifestations

HIV: respiratory disorders

Introduction *524*
Bacterial pneumonia *527*
Pneumocystis pneumonia *528*
Tuberculosis *531*
Immune reconstitution syndrome *534*
Opportunist mycobacterial infections *534*
Other fungal infections *535*
Other conditions *537*

Introduction

Respiratory tract involvement is very common in HIV infection. Reported incidence ranged from >90% early in the epidemic to 70% in the ART era. Symptoms represent a wide disease spectrum (Box 45.1) that include conditions not directly related to HIV. Bacterial infections, e.g. sinusitis, bronchitis, otitis, and pneumonia are among the most common infectious complications, occurring with increased frequency at all CD4 counts.

Box 45.1 Spectrum of respiratory illnesses in HIV +ve patients

- *Bacteria*:
  - *Streptococcus pneumoniae*
  - *Haemophilus influenzae*
  - Gram –ve bacilli (*Pseudomonas aeruginosa, Klebsiella pneumoniae*)
  - *Staphylococcus aureus*
  - *Mycobacterium tuberculosis*
  - Atypical mycobacteria (*Mycobacterium kansasii*, MAC)
  - *Rhodococcus equi*
  - Nocardia.
- *Fungi*:
  - PCP
  - *Cryptococcus neoformans*
  - *Histoplasma capsulatum*
  - *Aspergillus* spp.
  - *Candida* spp.
  - *Coccidioides immitis*
- *Viruses*:
  - CMV
  - HSV.
- *Parasites*:
  - *Strongyloides stercoralis*
  - *Toxoplasma gondii*
- *Neoplasia*:
  - KS
  - non-Hodgkin's lymphoma
  - bronchogenic carcinoma.
- *Other respiratory illnesses*:
  - upper respiratory tract infection (sinusitis, pharyngitis)
  - Lymphocytic interstitial pneumonitis
  - non-specific interstitial pneumonitis
  - acute bronchitis
  - obstructive lung disease (asthma, chronic bronchitis)
  - bronchiectasis
  - emphysema
  - pulmonary vascular disease
  - illicit-drug-induced lung disease
  - medication-induced lung disease
  - primary pulmonary hypertension
  - *Bronchiolitis obliterans* organizing pneumonia.

In HIV infection

- HIV itself, without pulmonary OI, leads to ↓ lung function.
- ↑ Frequency of respiratory diseases with falling CD4 count and ↑ duration of HIV infection.
- The CD4 count is a good indicator of risk of developing a specific OI:
  - *any CD4 count*—upper respiratory tract infections, bacterial pneumonias, obstructive airway disease, TB, and bronchogenic carcinoma are more common than in the general population, and their rates increase with declining CD4 count
  - *<500 cells/μL*: recurrent bacterial pneumonia
  - *<200 cells/μL*: ↑ incidence bacterial pneumonia associated with bacteraemia, *M. tuberculosis*, which is often extrapulmonary or disseminated, PCP and *Cryptococcus neoformans* pneumonia
  - *<100 cells/μL*: ↑ *Staphylococcus aureus*, *Pseudomonas aeruginosa*, pulmonary KS, and *Toxoplasma gondii*
  - *<50 cells/μL*: MAC, respiratory infections by endemic (e.g. *Histoplasma capsulatum, Coccidioides immitis*), and non-endemic fungi (e.g. *Aspergillus* spp.) and certain viruses (most commonly CMV). These infections are often associated with extrapulmonary or disseminated disease that dominates the clinical presentation.
- Risks of OI ↑ by other factors, e.g. cigarette smoking (further damages lung defences).
- Significant ↓ in the burden of HIV-associated respiratory disease in the ART era.

Pathology
Varies with:
- *Age*: e.g. lymphocytic interstitial pneumonitis (LIP) occurs predominantly in children.
- *Exposure (travel to or residence in endemic areas for specific pathogens)*: e.g. histoplasmosis.
- Level of immune function.
- *Specific immune defects*: e.g. failure to produce antibodies against pneumococcal capsular antigen (independent of CD4 count).
- Altered/atypical clinical presentations not uncommon in the immuno-compromised
- Altered results of investigations e.g. ↓ rate of sputum smear positivity in pulmonary TB.

Considerable overlap of symptoms and signs, and dual infections may occur. It is rare for a particular constellation of symptoms, clinical findings, and radiological abnormalities, to be definitively diagnostic and a full investigation is usually required. However, radiological appearances may suggest different groups of conditions (See Table 45.1). As deterioration can sometimes be rapid it is important that 'best guess' therapy is initiated, while awaiting the result of microbiology.

Table 45.1 Chest X-ray appearances

Interstitial	PCP, LIP (usually in children), rarely CMV
Lobar	Bacterial infection
Nodular	KS, septic emboli, fungal infection, non-Hodgkin's lymphoma
Miliary	TB
Pneumatocele	PCP, staphylococcal pneumonia
Pleural effusion	KS, TB, lymphoma (including primary effusion lymphoma)
Mediastinal and /or hilar lymphadenopathy	Mycobacteriosis, lymphoma, fungal infection

Bacterial pneumonia

Has a higher incidence than in HIV −ve people. In the pre-ART era, bacterial pneumonia was the most frequent pulmonary complication occurring in up to 42% in autopsy studies. Since the introduction of ART, the incidence of bacterial pneumonia continued to decline. An episode of bacterial pneumonia is associated with subsequent ↑ morbidity and mortality.

Aetiology

As in the general population, *S. pneumoniae* and *H. influenzae* are the most frequently identified causes of community-acquired bacterial pneumonia. *S. aureus* and *P. aeruginosa* are more frequent than in the HIV −ve population. There are higher bacteraemia rates in pneumococcal infection and there may be ↑ incidence of penicillin-resistant isolates. IV drug use further ↑ the risk of bacterial pneumonia. Atypical bacterial pathogens, such as *Legionella pneumophila* and *Mycoplasma pneumoniae* are infrequent causes of community-acquired bacterial pneumonia in HIV +ve individuals. Less common causes include *Rhodococcus equi*, which produces a cavitary pneumonia of insidious onset.

Clinical and diagnostic features

Most bacterial pneumonias present acutely with symptoms and radiological patterns similar to those seen in HIV −ve patients. *S. pneumoniae* or *H. influenza* typically present with consolidation. However, the radiological presentation may be indistinguishable from other OIs. *H. influenzae* can present with diffuse opacities, mimicking PCP. With progression of immunodeficiency pneumonias due to *S. aureus* and *P. aeruginosa* become more important and may produce cavitation.

Management

In a patient presenting with a clinical diagnosis of bacterial pneumonia, assess and correct hypoxia, volume depletion, and hypotension, gauge severity by presence of confusion, ↑ blood urea, ↑ respiratory rate, ↓ BP, older age group and co-morbidities. Obtain sputum and blood cultures. Consider urine testing for legionella antigen and pneumococcal antigen. Check inflammatory markers and WCC, although white cell response may be ↓ in HIV-induced marrow suppression. If severe (use CURB65 >2 or severe sepsis) commence IV antibiotic therapy with either cefuroxime 1.5 g tid plus a macrolide (e.g. clarithromycin 500 mg bd), or amoxicillin 1 g tid plus a macrolide. Consider modification to these combinations if there are features suggesting *S. aureus*, *P. aeruginosa*, or atypical organisms, such as *R. equi*. If recurrent and evidence of ↓ antibody production consider IVIg therapy or prophylactic antibiotics. For outpatient and less severe pneumonia oral amoxicillin and a macrolide may suffice.

Pneumocystis pneumonia

Caused by *Pneumocystis jirovecii*, a ubiquitous fungus. *Pneumocystis carinii* now refers to the pneumocystis that infects rats and *P. jirovecii* refers to the distinct species that infects humans. The abbreviation PCP is still in use to designate pneumocystis pneumonia. PCP results from new acquisition or from reactivation of latent infection acquired earlier in life. It was an AIDS defining illness in 70–80% of patients before the widespread use of PCP prophylaxis and ART. ~90% of cases occurred in patients with CD4 counts <200 cells/μL.

Clinical features

Usually presents sub-acutely with symptoms ↑ over weeks with night sweats, systemic symptoms and weight loss, dry cough, progressive dyspnoea, initially on exertion and eventually at rest, occasionally with spontaneous pneumothorax. Abnormalities on respiratory examination often minimal or absent, and significant ↓ of pulmonary function may occur despite minimal chest X-ray changes.

Diagnosis

Empirical treatment may need to be started if unable to get definitive diagnosis through induced sputum or bronchoalveolar lavage (BAL)

Oximetry

If history suspicious but normal resting oxygen saturations, exercise oximetry showing ↓ in oxygen saturation by 5% or to <90% highly suggestive of PCP.

Radiology

* High resolution CT shows ground glass appearance of interstitial pathology.
* Chest X-ray may be normal in early and mild disease, but in severe cases, the typical pattern is bi-basal perihilar interstitial infiltrates (Plate 29). Less commonly unilateral infiltrates and pneumatoceles, and rarely pneumothorax and pleural effusion.
* Atypical upper lobe involvement may be seen in patients on nebulized pentamidine prophylaxis. They may also develop extrapulmonary involvement of various organs, including eyes, spleen, and skin (due to lack of systemic effect).

Respiratory secretions/lung tissue

Specific diagnosis requires demonstration of *P. jirovecii* cysts in respiratory secretions or lung tissue. Patients with borderline lung function may require sputum induction and bronchoscopy. Sputum/respiratory specimen is stained with immunofluorescence or histochemistry. PCR has a sensitivity of 97–98% and a specificity of 68–96%. PCR cannot differentiate between active infection and colonization:

* Induced sputum by 3% saline using an ultrasonic nebulizer. Most laboratories perform:
  * fibre optic BAL-sensitivity 90–95%
  * open lung biopsy sensitivity or transbronchial biopsy with histology of fixed tissue-sensitivity 95–100%. Not routinely performed as pneumothorax is common in PCP.

Management

Prior to initiating investigations in those presenting with a history suggestive of PCP, it is essential to assess pulmonary impairment and the need for oxygen supplements by pulse oximetry and arterial blood gases.

If there is pulmonary impairment, delays in initiating PCP therapy should be kept to a minimum. ART should not be deferred beyond 1 week after acute PCP treatment, as there is an ↑ risk of death if delayed.

Gold standard antibiotic therapy is co-trimoxazole 120 mg/kg in 4 divided doses daily for 3 days, if stable/improving reduce to 90 mg/kg/day for further 18 days. Haematology, LFTs, and the skin (rash seen in 1%) must be monitored carefully for evidence of toxicity or developing hypersensitivity. Folinic acid supplements may be considered if there is evidence of impaired marrow function. For non-responders or hypersensitive patients alternative regimens include clindamycin (600mg tid) plus primaquine (30 mg/day), dapsone (100 mg/day) plus trimethoprim (5 mg/kg every 6–8 hours), atovaquone (750 mg bd) and IV pentamidine (4 mg/kg).

In patients with arterial oxygen pressures <9.3 kPa or O_2 saturations <92% steroid therapy is recommended, as it ↓ risk of respiratory failure and mortality. Conventional regimen is prednisolone, or equivalent, 40 mg bd for 5 days, 40 mg od for 5 days followed by 20 mg daily for 5–10 days. There is no significant ↑ in risk of other OIs, except *Candida* spp. and local HSV.

Patients with severe PCP may progress to respiratory failure requiring ventilatory support with constant positive airways pressure (CPAP), or intubation and ventilation. Pneumothorax may require chest drain insertion. Adverse prognostic indicators include ↑ serum lactic dehydrogenase (LDH) levels, need for high ventilatory pressures and prolonged intensive therapy unit stay.

PCP prophylaxis

Primary prophylaxis

PCP is almost completely preventable by primary prophylaxis.

Indications
- CD4 counts <200 cells/mm³
- CD4 cell percentage <14%
- oral candidiasis
- presentation with an AIDS-defining illness.

Secondary prophylaxis

Prophylaxis with the same regimen should be continued after successful treatment of PCP.

Drugs for PCP prophylaxis
- Co-trimoxazole [480 mg OD or 960 mg on alternate days (3 times a week)] is the drug of choice. Cutaneous hypersensitivity reactions are common, but 80% of HIV +ve patients can be desensitized by the use of gradually ↑ doses.
- Dapsone (100 mg od) need to add pyrimethamine to protect against toxoplasmosis,
- Atovaquone (750 mg bd)
- Pentamidine isetionate (by inhalation of nebulized solution, 300 mg every 4 weeks). Does not protect against toxoplasmosis

Withdrawal of PCP prophylaxis
- 1° PCP prophylaxis can be discontinued when the CD4 count has been >200 cells/μL for at least 3–6 months (rate of OIs do not ↓ until after 2 months of ART).
- Careful consideration is needed before stopping prophylaxis in patients who have had PCP or other AIDS defining illness, perhaps deferring interruption until complete viral suppression and sustained CD4 count ↑ for 6 months.

Tuberculosis

TB is the leading cause of morbidity and mortality among people living with HIV (PLWH) worldwide. Globally PLWH are 26 times more likely to develop active TB disease than the general population. Sub-Saharan Africa bears the highest TB/HIV burden and over 50% of TB patients are co-infected with HIV. In the UK, the annual incidence of TB ↓ since 2012. In 2016, the rate of TB is ×15 higher in the non-UK born population.

The most common route of infection is inhalation of droplets containing *Mycobacterium* tubercles. The immune response limits the multiplication of tubercle bacilli, but viable ones may persist for years (latent TB infection). Active TB disease develops soon after exposure to (primary disease) or after reactivation of latent infection. The risk of reactivation is much higher with untreated HIV compared with the general population. TB can occur at any CD4 count, although the risk increases with ↓ CD4 counts.

ART results in significant ↓ in the incidence of TB. However, even with the beneficial effects of ART, the risk and incidence of TB disease among PLWH remains higher than in the general population.

Patients diagnosed or suspected with TB should be risk-assessed and tested for HIV. PLWH presenting with a pulmonary illness should have TB excluded. Proven or suspected TB should be notified to public health authorities and contact tracing initiated.

Clinical features

Classic presentation of pulmonary TB is night sweats/fever, cough, pleuritic chest pain, haemoptysis, and weight loss. Less typical presentations occur as CD4 count ↓. Lobar distribution of pulmonary infection may be atypical and mimic community-acquired pneumonia. Disseminated and extrapulmonary disease are more common with ↓ CD4 count. Although most cases are caused by reactivation of latent infection, 1° infection with rapid progression to active TB can occur when CD4 count <100 cells/μL. TB has an additional immunosuppressive effect in HIV infection.

Diagnosis

- Microscopy for acid fast bacilli (AFB) on respiratory samples (expectorated sputum, induced sputum, or BAL), followed by molecular testing in conjunction with culture and drug sensitivity testing. Examination of at least 3 sputum samples is the standard practice. Careful control of infection precautions are required to avoid nosocomial transmission of TB during such procedures. Smear positivity ↓ if advanced immunodeficiency.
- *TB pleural effusion*: obtain cultures on pulmonary samples even in the absence of obvious parenchymal involvement, as the yield of sputum culture in induced samples approaches 55%. Diagnosis is established by detection of *M. tuberculosis* in pleural fluid or pleural biopsy by finding caseating granulomas, together with AFB.
- *Radiology*: in patients with preserved immune function typical upper lobe cavitary changes occur. In those with ↓ CD4 counts appearances may be more extensive mimicking other infections.

- If extra-pulmonary findings (e.g. lymphadenopathy, bone marrow abnormalities) tissue histology and cultures may be diagnostic.
- *Latent TB*: interferon-gamma release assay (IGRA) is recommended for all PLWH at high risk of TB (those with recent exposure and those from high and medium TB-incidence countries) regardless of their CD4 count and ART.
- *Diagnosis of multi-drug resistant TB*: molecular techniques (rifampicin resistance gene probe), in addition to phenotypic drug susceptibilities should be performed to achieve rapid detection of drug/s resistant strains.

Management

Drug therapy of TB-co-infected PLWH is complex due ↑ drug toxicities, drug–drug interactions, and paradoxical reactions. If TB is strongly suspected, empirical therapy, after appropriate cultures taken, with 4 drugs should be initiated immediately. Even if cultures are negative, a full course may be required if there is clinical response. Treatment of active TB may lead to ↑ in CD4 counts.

For fully sensitive organisms, a 6-month course of TB therapy is sufficient for respiratory and most extrapulmonary TB. Initial phase with quadruple therapy of isoniazid (300 mg daily), rifampicin (600 mg daily), pyrazinamide (1.5–2 g daily), and ethambutol (15 mg/kg/day) with monitoring precautions until mycobacterial drug sensitivities are known. Intensive phase of 2 months with quadruple therapy should be followed by 4 months continuation phase of rifampicin and isoniazid, if fully sensitive. If MDRTB suspected seek expert advice on initial regimen and further management

Monitor for visual symptoms and LFTs regularly.

▶ Check visual acuity prior to starting ethambutol.

▶ There are very important drug–drug interactions between anti-TB and ART drugs because of their varying enzyme inducing and enzyme inhibiting effects (➲ Chapter 55, 'Antiretroviral drug–drug interactions', p. 643).

▶ *Choice and timing of ART initiation*
- If not on therapy, ART should be started as soon as practical and within 8 weeks of TB diagnosis.
- *If CD4 count ≤ 100 cells/μL*: start ART as soon as practical and within 2 weeks.
- Efavirenz, raltegravir or dolutegravir may be used with tenofovir/ emtricitabine or abacavir/lamivudine.
- Rifabutin (150 mg od or 350 mg ×3/week) instead of rifampicin, where ART regimen includes a ritonavir-boosted protease inhibitor.
- Do not use fixed-dose combinations containing tenofovir alafenamide (TAF) when co-administered with rifampicin or rifabutin.
- Avoid nevirapine in ART-naïve individuals, when TB regimen includes rifampicin.

▶ If already established on ART with fully suppressed VL:
- ART should not be interrupted.
- Start rifampicin-based TB regimen if ART consists of efavirenz, nevirapine, dolutegravir, or raltegravir, plus two NRTIs.
- Rifabutin instead of rifampicin where established ART necessitate use of ritonavir.

Where there is no suspicion of resistant organism the patient would be regarded as no longer an infection risk after 2 weeks of therapy.

Management of latent TB

IGRA is recommended for all PLWH. If +ve, consider treatment of latent infection in individuals at high risk of TB (those with recent exposure, and those from high and medium TB-incidence countries) and no evidence of active tuberculosis (asymptomatic, normal CXR) regardless of their CD4 count and ART.

• Isoniazid od for 6–9 months, or isoniazid and rifampicin for 3 months

Immune reconstitution syndrome

See Chapter 55, 'Immune reconstitution', p. 642.

Characterized by the worsening of existing or the development of new symptoms, signs, or radiological abnormalities after the initiation of ART. These are not explained by another disease or TB treatment failure. IRIS is, therefore, a diagnosis of exclusion. It is thought to result from unmasking of an occult OI, not clinically apparent before ART. It is more common with low CD4 count, after a prompt ↑ of CD4 count and rapid ↓ of HIV VL. It is usually short-lived, but may last for several months. May require steroids or interruption of ART until TB is better controlled.

Opportunist mycobacterial infections

MAC consists of *M. avium*, *M. intracellulare*, and *M. chimaera*, and are ubiquitous in the environment. MAC is the most common cause of non-tuberculous mycobacterial infection in patients with AIDS, typically when the CD4 counts <50 cells/μL. The incidence is 20–40% in the absence of effective ART. The incidence among PLWH has fallen dramatically with ART.

Characteristically produce generalized bacteraemic disease, often in patients with wasting syndrome. MAC infection in the ART era is almost always localized and related to IRIS. During immune reconstitution as a result of ART, previously subclinical infection in the lungs may become apparent as an inflammatory response leading to pulmonary inflammation and X-ray changes.

Other fungal infections

Pulmonary cryptococcosis

The incidence of cryptococcosis has declined substantially with ART. Most new infections are recognized in newly diagnosed HIV with CD4 counts typically <100 cells/µL. Pulmonary disease is less frequent than meningitis, although the lung is the most likely portal of entry. Pulmonary involvement can be asymptomatic, but precedes the onset of disseminated disease in the majority of patients.

Symptoms
Cough (productive and unproductive), fever, malaise, shortness of breath, and pleuritic chest pain.

Diagnosis
- Chest X-ray may be normal, or show focal or diffuse infiltrates that mimic PCP, solitary nodules, consolidation, hilar and mediastinal lymphadenopathy, and pleural effusions.
- High resolution CT scan must be performed if pulmonary involvement is suspected. May show diffuse, small lesions similar to TB or infiltrates similar to bronchopneumonia. Cavitation and bronchiectasis may also be present.
- Organism are more likely isolated from BAL, rather than sputum.
- Cryptococcal antigen can be detected in blood, BAL, or pleural fluid and biopsy specimens.

Management
Early treatment of pulmonary lesions can prevent disseminated disease. Treatment consists of liposomal amphotericin B, combined with flucytosine as induction therapy, followed by fluconazole or itraconazole (see Chapter 16, 'HIV: neurological disorders', p. 544).

Pulmonary aspergillosis

Aspergillus spp. colonize the lungs of individuals with underlying lung pathology. Invasive aspergillosis occurs when lung parenchymal infection disseminates to other organs. This can occur in PLWH, but is rare in the absence of other risk factors, such as neutropenia, transplantation, or steroid use.

Symptoms include fever, dyspnoea, cough, chest pain, and haemoptysis. 20% have unilateral or bilateral diffuse or nodular infiltrates.

Diagnosis
- *Chest X-ray*:
  - ≈30% have thick-walled upper lobe cavities.
  - ≈20% have unilateral or bilateral diffuse or nodular infiltrates.
- CT chest may show 'Halo' sign.
- *Microbiology*:
  - Sputum, BAL, blood, bone marrow, and/or tissue biopsies should be examined by microscopy and cultured for fungi. Only 10–30% have positive findings on sputum culture. BAL has a higher yield.
  - Culture is required as can be difficult to distinguish aspergillus from other fungal species by microscopy alone.
  - Serum PCR and/or galactomannan ELISA may be helpful, but need careful interpretation

Management
- *Liposomal amphotericin*: test dose 1 mg (give over 10 minutes) then 3–5 mg/kg od.
- Voriconazole 6 mg/kg bd 24 hours, as a loading dose, followed by 4 mg/kg 7 days. 200 mg bd (often used as first line). Isavuconazole or posaconazole may be alternatives.
- Caspofungin 70 mg stat then 50 mg/day

In patients with severe neutropenia granulocyte macrophage colony stimulating factor may have an adjunctive role. Interactions must be reviewed (see Chapter 55, 'Antiretroviral drug–drug interactions', p. 643).

Other conditions

Cytomegalovirus pneumonitis

Patients with PCP often have CMV isolated from bronchial washings or lung biopsy. In most cases, this represents viral replication without pneumonitis and the patient responds to PCP therapy alone. Active pneumonitis occurs much less frequently than in patients taking immuno-suppressive therapy after transplant. Hypoxia is usual.

Diagnosis
- Chest X-ray shows diffuse interstitial infiltrates.
- CMV PCR is not specific and often +ve, representing high levels in blood, rather than lung disease; definitive diagnosis is through histology and identification of CMV in lung tissue.

Management
Patients with interstitial pneumonia and positive CMV identification in lung tissue should be treated with anti-CMV therapy using ganciclovir or foscarnet (see Chapter 46, 'Distal symmetric polyneuropathy', p. 548).

Mediastinal and hilar lymphadenopathy

Patients with HIV-related persistent generalized lymphadenopathy have sub-diaphragmatic lymphadenopathy, but do not have significant hilar or mediastinal node enlargement. Hilar or mediastinal adenopathy implies significant pathology. The differential diagnosis includes:
- lymphoma
- KS
- TB
- fungal disease.

May be seen in active PCP, but other radiological abnormalities usually co exist. A careful search for peripheral lymphadenopathy, skin lesions, and other abnormalities that could be subjected to histological and microbiological examinations should be sought. If necessary, mediastinoscopy and biopsy can be performed.

Pulmonary vascular disease

1° Pulmonary hypertension can occur as a consequence of HIV infection (0.5% in PLWH vs 0.0015% if HIV –ve). IV drug users may develop pulmonary small vessel obstruction due to injection of particulate material or may suffer recurrent pulmonary emboli.

Intense fatigue, breathlessness, and faintness on exertion are features of severe pulmonary hypertension. Clinical features include accentuated pulmonary component of the second heart sound, third heart sound, left lower parasternal heave, pan-systolic murmur indicative of tricuspid valve regurgitation, jugular venous distension, hepatojugular reflux, ascites, and peripheral oedema. Should be considered in unexplained shortness of breath

Diagnosis
- *ECG*: RV strain, RBBB, right axis deviation.
- Echocardiography.
- Ultrasonography of the deep veins of the leg.
- Pulmonary angiography.
- Right heart catheterization is the gold standard diagnostic test.

Management
- ART may improve mortality and morbidity.
- Specific drug therapy in collaboration with specialist (anticoagulants, calcium channel blockers, endothelin receptor antagonists and phosphodiesterase type-5 inhibitors).

HIV: neurological disorders

Introduction *540*
Cerebral disorders *542*
Meningitis *544*
Autonomic neuropathy *545*
Spinal cord disease *546*
Peripheral nerve disease *547*
Miscellaneous *549*

Introduction

HIV enters the central nervous system (CNS) soon after 1° infection, either carried by infected mononuclear cells or by cell-free transfer across the blood–brain barrier. Infected monocytes then differentiate into macrophages, and produce virions that can infect astrocytes and microglia (brain macrophages). Neurons are not infected, but they are lost and become dysfunctional in HIV brain disease.

Neurological disease is common and may be the presenting clinical syndrome in 30% of HIV infections occurring at any stage, but most often presents following seroconversion or with severe immunodeficiency. Neurological features have been reported in 40–70% of patients with AIDS, 90% at post-mortem examination (Box 46.1). Abnormal CSF findings including ↑ lymphocytes, protein, immunoglobulin, and oligoclonal bands may be found in patients with no neurological symptoms or signs. The presence or absence of neurological disease is independent of CSF viral load.

Mechanisms of CNS injury and the spectrum of neurological disease vary with the stage of HIV infection and the degree of immune deficiency.

- At *seroconversion*: viraemia and inflammation resulting from the initial immunological response to HIV infection predominate, inducing aseptic meningitis, meningoencephalitis, ataxic neuropathy, Guillain–Barré syndrome, acute myelopathy, multiple-sclerosis-like syndrome, acute brachial neuritis, Bell's palsy, and acute meningoradiculitis. Patients presenting with these syndromes should be offered HIV screening.
- *In chronic HIV infection*: asymptomatic neurocognitive impairment can be found in 5–20% of patients (60% in those with AIDS diagnosis). This tends to improve with ART.
- As *HIV progresses*: altered CNS cytokine production and direct neurotoxic effects of HIV components (e.g. gp120) are pathogenic.
- *With immunodeficiency*: OIs/tumours and complications of treatment predominate.

ART has changed the epidemiology of the neurological manifestations of HIV resulting in ↓ CNS OIs, ↓ incidence of HIV dementia complex, and improved prognosis for some infections that were previously difficult to treat, such as progressive multifocal leukoencephalopathy (PML). However, there has been ↑ of drug-induced CNS and peripheral nerve disease.

Box 46.1 HIV-related neurological and neuromuscular disease may present with a number of symptom complexes

Headaches

May be an important symptom of neuropathology, such as 1° or opportunist meningitis, intracerebral opportunist pathologies, or the side-effects of drugs, such as zidovudine or co-trimoxazole. Non-HIV-related problems, such as migraine or psychogenic headache may occur.

Altered peripheral sensation

May occur with or without motor abnormalities and is a significant symptom in peripheral neuropathy 2° to HIV, drugs or OI.

Leg weakness

May result from muscular weakness due to myopathic processes, but intrinsic or extrinsic spinal cord disease should be considered and sensory levels searched for.

Seizures

↑ Risk. First seizure may be a first presentation of HIV, 5–9% lifetime risk. Most commonly 2° to OI in AIDS:
- OIs such as toxoplasmosis, cryptococcosis, and PML.
- CNS lymphomas.
- Cerebrovascular disease.
- Metabolic encephalopathy.

Focal neurological signs and symptoms

Particularly with cerebral toxoplasmosis, 1° cerebral lymphoma, and PML.

Cerebral disorders

HIV associated neuro-cognitive disorder

HIV-associated neurocognitive disorders (HAND) vary from relatively asymptomatic deficits, through minor cognitive impairment to HIV-associated dementia (HAD). Prior to ART dementia was a common cause of morbidity and mortality, seen in up to 50% of patients before death. Generally seen with ↓ CD4 count. Pathogenesis may include altered cytokine levels, free radicals, and the neurotoxic effects of gp120. Histological abnormalities include perivascular infiltrates, microglial nodules, multinuclear giant cells, and pruning of dendritic processes in the white matter (leading to significant gliosis) and subcortical gray matter with relative sparing of the cortex.

Presentation

HAND presents with variable severity of poor concentration, decreased executive functioning, impaired short-term memory, and slowed thought and reaction times. HAD is associated with clumsiness, gait disturbance may follow, with corticospinal tract abnormalities. Psychiatric illness and personality change may also be presenting features. Depression, effects of substance abuse, cerebrovascular disease, and neurosyphilis should be excluded.

Diagnosis

Blood and CSF serological tests for syphilis should be carried out and vitamin B_{12} deficiency excluded. Other conditions, such as CNS infections (TB, toxoplasmosis, CMV encephalitis), PML, lymphoma, and toxic metabolic states (e.g. alcoholism, adverse medication effects, drug interaction, recreational drug use) should be excluded as dictated by the clinical presentation.

MRI (more sensitive) or CT brain scan reveal cerebral atrophy with abnormality of the periventricular white matter. Neuropsychological examination reveals ↓ executive thought processes and ↓ short-term memory. CSF should be examined to exclude other pathologies and OIs. Electroencephalogram (EEG) may reveal non-specific sencephalopathic changes.

Management

ART, consider including zidovudine (proven efficacy) or other drugs that cross the blood–brain barrier, can produce marked improvement in intellectual function and return to independent living. The patient may require psychological and social support, including help to take medication.

Viral encephalitis

VZV is a rare cause of meningo-encephalitis, is seen when CD4 count <50 cells/μL. Due to direct CNS infection, rather than reactivation of dormant virus, as is the case with shingles. The pathological process is large- and small-vessel vaculopathy leading to ischaemic and demyelinating lesions. 33–50% of patients do not have the typical rash. CT or MRI may show necrotizing encephalitis and help differentiate from toxoplasmosis and PML, but changes are not specific. CSF should be examined by PCR (highly sensitive and specific). Treatment with aciclovir 10 mg/kg 8-hourly should be given for at least 14 days, followed by prophylaxis until CD4 >100 cells/mm³.

CMV encephalitis occurs when CD4 <50 cells/mm³ and may be suspected when there is evidence of CMV disease in other organs, or blood and CSF

PCR is positive and patient presents with drowsiness, cognitive dysfunction, and seizures. CMV directly toxic to neurons. Treatment as for CMV retinitis.

HSV is an uncommon cause, but diagnosis should be considered in patients with meningo-encephalitis, aseptic meningitis, myelitis, or polyradiculitis. DNA detection in the CSF is very useful, with high sensitivity and specificity.

Progressive multifocal leukoencephalopathy

Unlike other OIs, the prevalence of PML has not significantly ↓ with ART. It is a demyelinating disease caused by reactivation of John Cunningham virus (JCV), occurs in 4–8% of patients with advanced HIV infection. Fulminant disease with dementia and coma can occur, but the usual picture is of sub-acute or chronic progressive disease with focal deficits. These include personality change, aphasia, hemiparesis, dizziness, gait disturbance, visual field defects, and seizures.

MRI scan usually reveals single or multiple lesions (non-enhancing, hyperintense on T2-weighting) without mass effect in the white matter, particularly in the parieto-occipital region (Plate 30). CSF JCV PCR is +ve in ~60% of cases and ↑ JCV VL associated with poorer prognosis.

Prognosis is poor, especially without ART. ART leads to significant improvement in 10%, but 33% die within 2 years. Some individuals, especially those with very low CD4 counts, can develop IRIS with worsening of PML or new-onset PML after the initiation of ART. Treatment trials with cidofovir, interferon alfa α, and topotecan were unsuccessful. Case reports of improvement with mefloquine and/or mirtazapine.

Cerebral toxoplasmosis (*Toxoplasma gondii*)

The most common cause of mass lesions in HIV prior to the introduction of PCP prophylaxis, which has ↓ incidence. Results from reactivation of a previously acquired infection when CD4 declines (<200 cells/mm³). Often contracted from contaminated soil or direct contact with cats.

Presentation
Typically includes confusion, headache, personality change, hemiparesis, focal sensory disturbances, seizures, and fever.

Diagnosis
MRI or CT scanning reveal ring-enhancing lesions with oedema, usually multiple, particularly in the cortex at gray–white matter interface and thalamus. The differential diagnosis, particularly if lesions are single, includes primary cerebral lymphoma, cryptococcoma, and tuberculomas. CSF changes are non-specific. Positive serum toxoplasma IgG in 90%. CSF PCR is helpful if +ve (sensitivity 50%, specificity 100%).

Management
Standard therapy for cerebral toxoplasmosis is sulfadiazine 1–2 g qds and pyrimethamine 200 mg loading dose followed by 50–100 mg/day with folinic acid to reduce bone marrow toxicity. Clindamycin 600 mg IV/PO qds if allergic to sulfonamide. Neuro-imaging should be repeated after 2 weeks followed by brain biopsy to exclude other pathologies if no improvement. 2° prophylaxis (pyrimethamine 50 mg od and sulfadiazine 2–3g/day in 2–4 divided doses or clindamycin 300 mg tds), should be given until immune reconstitution with ART (CD4 >200 cells/µL for >6 months). 1° prophylaxis as for PCP.

Meningitis

Cryptococcal meningitis

Cryptococcus neoformans (an encapsulated yeast, common in environment, found in bird droppings)—most common fungal pathogen in the CNS. Usually when CD4 <100 cells/mm^3.

Presentation

Usually as subacute meningitis (may initially be surprisingly mild) with headache and fever. Evidence of meningism occurs in only 30%. A high index of suspicion must be maintained to avoid delays in diagnosis. Other presentations include acute confusional state and cranial nerve palsies.

Diagnosis

CSF pressures can be markedly raised, normally raised protein, low glucose and pleocytosis; but pleocytosis may be absent, and protein and glucose levels normal. The organism may be visualized by India ink staining. Mainstay of diagnosis is detection of CSF and serum cryptococcal antigen, which is highly sensitive. Neuro-imaging is usually normal, but cryptococcomas can occur, usually in the basal ganglia.

Management

Daily lumbar punctures (LPs) may be required until CSF pressures normalize. If CSF pressure does not ↓ with LPs, a lumbar drain may be used. Antifungal therapy with IV liposomal amphotericin B 4mg/kg/day IV in combination with flucytosine 100mg/kg/day for 2 weeks followed by fluconazole 400 mg daily. Renal function should be monitored. Ongoing suppressive therapy with fluconazole (superior to itraconazole) is required to minimize significant relapse rates. Continue until immune reconstitution is achieved with ART.

Commence ART 2 weeks after initiation of antifungals.

Aseptic meningitis

Most commonly presents at seroconversion, but may be recurrent or become chronic. Usually presents with headache. Cranial nerve palsies and altered mental state can occur. Lumbar puncture, following neuro-imaging, when focal deficits are present, needed to exclude other pathologies. Mildly ↑ CSF lymphocyte counts and protein level with normal glucose are typical findings.

Autonomic neuropathy

Evidence of autonomic dysfunction can be found at various stages of HIV infection. Measurement of pulse rate variation in response to standing, deep breathing, Valsalva manoeuvre, and cold exposure reveal autonomic dysfunction in ~15% (probably underdiagnosed). Frequency related to the level of immune function, but unlike sensory neuropathy, not the use of non-nucleoside reverse transcriptase inhibitors.

Symptomatic autonomic neuropathy occurs in advanced immunodeficiency, and may result in severe postural hypotension and syncope. Cardiac denervation may lead to serious cardiac dysrhythmias.

Those developing postural dizziness or syncope should have postural blood pressure recordings, tests of autonomic function, and assessment of sodium intake. Adrenal insufficiency should be excluded by carrying out a short Synacthen® test.

Therapy with mineralocorticoid (fludrocortisone 50–200 mcg daily), sodium supplements, compression stockings, and α-adrenergic agents, such as midodrine, may reduce postural blood pressure falls and alleviate symptoms. There may be improvement in autonomic function with ART.

Spinal cord disease

Vacuolar myelopathy

Post-mortem studies have shown vacuolar myelopathy in up to 30% of cases, but clinically far less common. Pathological mechanisms are probably the same as in HIV dementia complex. Often associated with dementia, but may be isolated when the clinical picture mimics that of vitamin B$_{12}$ deficiency spinal cord disease.

Presentation

Typically, with subacute progressive motor and sensory deficits with paraesthesiae, but brisk tendon reflexes—commonly lower limb. Uncharacteristic findings may occur if there is concomitant peripheral neuropathy or other cause.

Diagnosis

Investigations should include measurement of vitamin B$_{12}$ level and radiological imaging to exclude structural lesions. Areas of ↑ T2 signal may occasionally be seen on MRI scan. CSF may be normal or show only non-specific abnormalities, such as low-level pleocytosis or mildly ↑ protein levels.

Management

Spasticity may require anti-spasmodic therapy, such as baclofen 10–30 mg tid, and dysesthesia may require amitriptyline or gabapentin. Physiotherapy and occupational therapy input. Improvements in function may occur with ART.

HTLV1-associated myelopathy

In patients from areas of significant risk for HTLV1 infection, such as Japan, the Caribbean, and parts of Central and Latin America, subacute myelopathy may result from HTLV1 infection and anti-HTLV1 antibodies should be assayed. HTLV1 viral load can be performed from serum or CSF.

Acute myelopathy

Acute spinal cord disease may occasionally occur as a seroconversion event. Other important causes are spinal cord compression from lymphomatous metastases, tuberculous or bacterial abscesses, and acute infections with VZV.

Presentation

Typically, rapidly developing neurological deficit, such as leg weakness and sphincter disturbance, with evidence of a sensory level.

Diagnosis

Emergency investigation required with spinal MRI or CT. In the absence of compression CSF and/or biopsy of compressive lesion, patient should be examined for evidence of infectious and neoplastic causes, including HIV, VZV, and CMV viral PCR and cytology.

Management

Supportive with specific treatment directed at the identified cause.

Peripheral nerve disease

Neuritis

Herpes zoster (shingles)

May occur at any stage of HIV infection with a typical distribution and course. Atypical multi-dermatomal involvement, viraemic dissemination of lesions, and recurrences more common as CD4 counts ↓.

Presentation

Frequently prodromal pain of dermatomal distribution followed by an erythematous maculopapular eruption, evolving into vesicles, which then pustulate and crust. Bullous haemorrhagic and necrotic lesions may occur. Lesions will be at various stages at any one time. With low CD4 dissemination of lesions possible. Pain during the acute phase can be severe and disabling; post-herpetic neuralgia may follow.

Diagnosis

Clinical picture is usually characteristic. VZV can be detected by viral swab of burst vesicle by PCR.

Management

Pain often does not respond well to conventional analgesics and adjuvants. Amitriptyline 25–150 mg/day or gabapentin up to 2.4 g/day in divided doses may be required. In disseminated or eyesight-threatening ophthalmic shingles, consider IV aciclovir 10 mg/kg 8-hourly as early as possible (most effective within 24 hours, but useful even if given later in immunocompromised) and switch to valaciclovir 1 g tid when lesions cease to progress for a total course of at least 7 days or until all lesions have dried and crusted. Oral valaciclovir may be used in dermatomal shingles, most effective if started within 72 hours, in immunosuppressed often required to prevent deterioration/dissemination.

Ophthalmology review if ophthalmic branch of trigeminal nerve affected (forehead and to tip of nose), aciclovir eye drops may be used if cornea involved.

Mononeuritis multiplex

Usually occurs in patients with advanced HIV disease. Typical presentation is with subacute onset of multifocal or asymmetric sensory deficits, including Bell's palsy. Nerve conduction studies show demyelination and axonal loss. May be associated with CMV infection in advanced immunodeficiency. Differential diagnosis includes nerve compression in severe wasting syndrome, neoplastic infiltration, and neurotropic viral infections (e.g. VZV). Consider treatment with ganciclovir if circumstantial evidence of CMV infection (e.g. positive blood PCR).

Neuropathy

Drug toxicity

The toxicity of therapeutic drugs, notably didanosine, zalcitabine, and stavudine (20% effected after 6 months), is responsible for ↑ proportion of peripheral neuropathy.

Distal symmetric polyneuropathy

Occurs in 35% of patients with advanced HIV disease. 15% of those with asymptomatic HIV infection have abnormal nerve conduction studies. Typical symptoms are tingling, numbness, and burning pain, beginning in the toes or plantar surfaces, often ascending over time. Involvement of hands is rare. Examination shows ↓ ankle reflex, vibration sense, appreciation of temperature, and fine touch. Unexpectedly brisk reflexes should raise the question of additional spinal cord or brain disease. Differential diagnosis includes effects of alcohol, drug toxicity, and vitamin deficiency. Treatment is directed towards controlling neuropathic pain with drugs, such as amitriptyline 25–150 mg daily or gabapentin (300 mg 8-hourly, maximum of 2.4 g daily) or pregabalin (75 mg bd to max of 300 mg daily).

Inflammatory demyelinating neuropathy (Guillain–Barré syndrome)

May occur with seroconversion or during late stages of HIV infection. Manifestations as in non-HIV status with progressive symmetric weakness in the limbs and loss of tendon jerks, but CSF pleocytosis may occur. Treatment is immunoglobulin 400 mg/kg/day for 5 days or plasmapheresis up to six exchanges over 2 weeks. Patients with the chronic form may need monthly cycles of treatment until stabilization.

Progressive lumbosacral polyradiculopathy

Caused by CMV infection in patients with CD4 counts <50 cells/mm³. Rarely caused by tuberculosis. There may be evidence of CMV disease elsewhere. Bilateral leg weakness progresses over several weeks, sometimes to flaccid paraplegia. Sphincter disturbance is common and sensory loss combined with painful dysaesthesia is usual. Sensory symptoms differentiate this from myopathy, and sphincter disturbance with sparing of the upper limbs distinguishes it from other forms of neuropathy. Cord compression (2° to lymphoma, toxoplasma, TB, etc.) should be excluded by MRI of spine, MRI is non-specific, but may show thickening of nerve roots or enhancement of cauda equina. CSF usually pleocytosis—40–50% neutrophils, ↑ protein, and normal glucose. CSF PCR for CMV is +ve and the patient should be treated with ganciclovir or foscarnet.

Miscellaneous

Cerebrovascular disease

Strokes and transient ischaemic attacks are reported in 0.5–8% of HIV-infected patients. Prevention should include attention to vascular risk factors, such as smoking, hypertension, and hyperlipidaemia. Cocaine use and alcoholic binges may lead to thrombotic strokes. Embolic strokes may result from cardiac or carotid artery disease. Cardiogenic emboli may result from infective or non-infective endocarditis, following myocardial infarction or from dysrhythmias.

Cerebral vasculitis, particularly due to VZV or syphilis, may cause cerebral thrombosis. The hyper-coagulable state that may occur with HIV may contribute.

Haemorrhage may complicate VZV cerebral vasculitis and thrombocytopenia, rarely due to metastatic KS.

Neurosyphilis

Can affect most parts of the nervous system (see Chapter 7, 'Neurosyphilis', p. 122).

Neoplastic disease

KS, although the most common systemic neoplasm in HIV infection, rarely involves the nervous system.

The CNS may be invaded by non-Hodgkin's lymphoma, leading to malignant meningitis and compressive symptoms requiring intrathecal cytotoxic therapy and radiotherapy.

1° cerebral lymphoma occurs in patients with advanced immunodeficiency and presents with confusion, lethargy, personality change, focal neurological deficits, seizures, ataxia, and aphasia. On MRI or CT scanning, lesions are ring-enhancing, and about 50% are associated with cerebral oedema and mass effect. The finding of a single lesion favours the diagnosis of lymphoma over cerebral toxoplasmosis. +ve EBV PCR is suggestive, but not diagnostic of 1° cerebral lymphoma. Treatment for toxoplasma empirically may be considered with brain biopsy if no clinical response after 2 weeks. Cerebral radiotherapy may improve survival. Prognosis very poor with 3 months median survival.

HIV: dermatological disorders

Introduction *552*
Infections *553*
Inflammatory conditions *558*
Pruritic follicular and papular eruptions *559*
Neoplasia *560*
Drug reactions *562*

Introduction

Skin conditions are extremely common and may occur at any stage of HIV infection. Appearance of certain skin conditions should alert physicians to possibility of undiagnosed HIV infection. Pre-existing skin conditions may worsen after its acquisition. Immunodeficiency is associated with atypical presentations, severe manifestations, and a poor response to treatment. In general, improved immunity with ART resolves or improves them.

Culture and biopsy are important in diagnosis. Particularly in patients with significant immunosuppression specimens should be sent for histology, and separately for fungal, bacterial, and TB culture. Where indicated, viral PCR may be needed.

Infections

Viral infections

Acute seroconversion (acute retroviral syndrome)

Skin rash occurs in up to 70% cases. It is often part of an infectious mononucleosis-like illness. Typically, symmetrical and non-itchy, extending over the trunk and upper limbs, and macular or maculopapular in appearance, although it can be vesicular, pustular, or urticarial. May be associated with oro-pharyngeal and genital ulceration. Resolves spontaneously within 1–2 weeks.

Herpes simplex virus

1° and recurrent HSV present with genital and orofacial clusters of vesicles that ulcerate, crust, and heal within 2–3 weeks during the early stages of HIV infection. With advanced disease, ulcers become atypical or chronic and may coalesce to form large painful crusted lesions commonly seen peri-anally, but may involve the peri-oral and rarely the peri-ungual region. Though dissemination is rare, lesions may be auto-inoculated to distant sites. HSV infection rarely presents with necrotizing folliculitis (difficult to diagnose without biopsy).

A swab sent for HSV/PCR testing of skin lesions is very sensitive and specific. Biopsy and histological examination may be necessary for atyp-ical presentations, demonstrating multinucleated giant epithelial cells, and immunohistochemistry can stain for HSV.

Treatment

➔ Chapter 22, 'Management: treatment', pp. 284–5.

Varicella zoster virus infection

Those with no previous exposure to VZV develop chickenpox, which may be severe and associated with visceral involvement.

Most adults have been infected by VZV and so present with shingles. Vesicular eruption is normally preceded by tingling and a burning sensa-tion. In the immunocompromised affects multiple dermatomes, commonly the thoracic and the trigeminal nerves. In advanced HIV, disease tends to have painful bullous haemorrhagic necrotic lesions that may persist for sev-eral weeks and heal with severe scarring. Recurrences and dissemination ↑. Disseminated disease is characterized by dermatomal and non-dermatomal eruptions. Rarely, VZV presents with chronic widespread ulcers or hyperkeratotic lesions.

Clinical diagnosis is usually accurate in typical dermatomal involvement, but skin biopsy is required for atypical, chronic ulcerative, and hyper-keratotic lesions.

Prompt treatment with high-dose aciclovir ↓ risk of dissemination and shortens its course. Clinical presentation and degree of immune deficiency determine mode and length of therapy, which is usually continued until le-sions start to crust.

- IV aciclovir (10 mg/kg body weight tid) for disseminated infection, CD4 count <200 cells/µL, or with involvement of the ophthalmic division of the trigeminal nerve. May be replaced with oral valaciclovir once lesions start to crust.

- Famciclovir (500 mg tid, usually for 10 days) and valaciclovir (1 g tid, usually for 7 days) have better bio-availability than aciclovir.
- Oral aciclovir (800 mg five times daily) may be given to those with limited disease and preserved immune function.

Skin care with bathing with water and mild soap is helpful. Analgesics for pain control.

Molluscum contagiosum

Caused by a *molluscum contagiosum* virus and when widespread is a marker of advanced HIV disease. Lesion is typically a flesh-coloured, 2–3 mm domed, umbilicated papule, with a faint whitish core. Those with relatively preserved immune function may have mollusca in the groin, which may be chronic. With advanced HIV disease, lesions may reach 1 cm in size and may be widespread, involving the face, trunk, eyelids, and rarely the mucous membranes (conjunctivae and lips). Mollusca are commonly seen in the beard area (related to trauma of shaving) where they are difficult to treat.

Treatment comprises cryotherapy or curettage, and is given for cosmetic reasons; no cure is available.

Human papilloma virus infection (warts)

Widespread, resistant, and recurrent warts, which may have atypical appearances, are seen more frequently in those immunosuppressed. Facial involvement, otherwise rare, is well recognized in HIV infection.

Principles of therapy are as for those not infected by HIV. Ablative treatment is used depending on morphology, location, and number.

Bacterial infections

Staphylococcal skin infection

Staphylococcus aureus nasal carriage is common, explaining ↑ rates of infection with this organism. *S. aureus* skin infection are often associated with a golden yellow crusting and presents as:

- *folliculitis*: commonly in the hirsute areas, e.g. groin, axilla, face, and trunk; infection may involve deeper tissues, forming abscesses
- *hidradenitis-like plaques*: many adjacent follicles infected, forming large discoloured lesions several centimetres deep
- *bullous impetigo*: commonly seen on the groin and axillae as superficial vesicles or ulcers with yellow crusts
- *ecthyma*: an eroded or ulcerated lesion with an adherent crust covering an abscess
- *scalded skin syndrome*: part of systemic *S. aureus* infection.

Swab should be taken for culture to rule out MRSA. Superficial infection responds to standard anti-staphylococcal antibiotics (e.g. flucloxacillin 500 mg qds for 7–10 days).

Deep infection may require abscess drainage and prolonged courses of combined antibiotics, based on bacterial sensitivities. Washing the area with antiseptics helps by removing crusts and ↓ bacterial concentration.

Bacillary angiomatosis

Caused by *Bartonella henselae* (transmitted by flea and scratch from infected animals) and *Bartonella quintana* (transmitted by body louse), small

Gram −ve aerobic fastidious bacilli. In addition, *B. henselae* causes cat scratch fever and *B. quintana* causes trench fever. Angiogenic lesions are most often recognized in cutaneous or SC tissues and can be difficult to differentiate from KS. *B. henselae* causes lesions in lymph nodes, liver (peliosis hepatitis), and spleen. *B. quintana* has a predilection for subcutaneous deep soft tissues and bones.

Clinical presentation
- *Bacilliary angioma*: friable, easy bleeding hyperpigmented papules, nodules, or plaques, but in the early stages may be purplish to bright red in colour, up to several centimetres in diameter. Lesions solitary or multiple, and widespread on the skin. Need to be differentiated from KS and pyogenic granuloma.
- *Bacteraemia*: presenting as pyrexia of unknown origin.
- *Organ involvement*: e.g. liver, spleen, brain, and lymph nodes.

Diagnosis
- Abnormal vascular proliferation and a mixed inflammatory infiltrate on histological examination of tissues.
- *Special stains*: e.g. Warthin–Starry, Steiner and Steiner, required.
- Electron microscopy.
- PCR of tissue and blood samples.

Serological tests are not reliable in HIV infection.

Treatment
Prolonged course of antibiotics, e.g. erythromycin 500 mg qds, doxycycline 100 mg bd, or azithromycin 0.5–1.0 g daily, until lesions heal.

Mycobacterial infection
1° Mycobacterial skin infection is rare. Skin may be involved in up to 10% of disseminated *Mycobacterium avium* complex infection, typically when the CD4 count is <50 cells/µL. Most frequent presentations are chronic sinuses overlying an infected lymph node (scrofuloderma) and chronic skin ulcer. Rare presentations include violaceous nodules, necrotic papules, plaques, panniculitis, and erythema nodosum.

Mycobacterial infection should be considered in any chronic non-healing skin ulcer. Diagnose by demonstration of acid-fast bacilli in smears and by culture for TB. Caseating granuloma is usually absent.

Treatment
➔ Chapter 45, 'Tuberculosis', pp. 531–3; Chapter 48, '*Mycobacterium avium* complex', p. 569.

Fungal infections
Cutaneous candidiasis
Skin infection with *Candida* spp. occurs in different forms, including *Tinea unguium* (leuconychia, nail ridging, flaking, onycholysis, and atrophy), acute paronychia (tender fluctuation of the nailbed), chronic paronychia, and intertrigo (an erosive painful erythematous rash on flexures associated with satellite pustules). Acute candidal paronychia must be differentiated from that caused by HSV infection using appropriate tests.

- *Tinea unguium* requires prolonged systemic antifungals (e.g. itraconazole).
- Acute paronychia and intertrigo respond well to topical antifungals (e.g. miconazole).

Dermatophytosis

Very common in HIV infection. May be atypical and extensive, and may mimic inflammatory skin conditions, such as seborrhoeic dermatitis or psoriasis.

- *Tinea pedis*: usually presents with interdigital maceration and scaling of the soles, rarely with hyperkeratosis of the soles. Usually, associated with *Tinea unguium*. Caused by *Trichophyton rubrum*. 2° bacterial infection common and may result in cellulitis.
- *Onychomycosis*: results in subungual hyperkeratosis and toenail atrophy.
- *Tinea cruris*: symmetrical, erythematous scaling rash with central clearance on the groin, sometimes extending to buttocks and thighs. May resemble seborrhoeic dermatitis because of absence of central clearance.
- *Tinea corporis*: annular scaling plaques with central clearance.
- *Tinea capitis*: localized scaling discoid patch or generalized scaling resembling seborrhoeic dermatitis.
- *Tinea faciale*: differentiated from seborrhoeic dermatitis by asymmetrical distribution and well-demarcated edge.

Apart from tinea pedis, which can be treated with topical antifungals, other forms need systemic antifungals, such as terbinafine (250 mg daily for several weeks) or a triazole (e.g. fluconazole 50 mg daily).

Cryptococcosis

Skin involvement occurs in up to 20% of systemic cryptococcal infection. Most common skin manifestation is a nodule or papule with central umbilication resembling *Molluscum contagiosum*, usually on the face. Plaques and tender SC lesions are rare. Diagnosed by skin biopsy with fungal culture and histology.

Treatment

Patient should be evaluated for systemic and neurological cryptococcal infection, and managed accordingly (➔ Chapter 46, 'Management', p. 544).

Penicilliosis

Endemic to southeast Asia. Caused by *Penicillium marneffei*. Presents with fever, skin lesions, anaemia, lymphadenopathy, and hepatosplenomegaly. Skin lesions resemble haemorrhagic *Molluscum contagiosum*. Diagnosed by fungal culture of blood, bone marrow, and skin scrapings. Responds well to liposomal amphotericin followed by itraconazole, but relapses are common and long-term prophylaxis with itraconazole recommended.

Histoplasmosis

Cutaneous histoplasmosis has been reported in up to 10% of patients with systemic infection, which usually occurs in endemic areas (central/eastern USA, some parts of southeast Asia, and Africa). Diagnosis by biopsy and fungal culture of papules, nodules, or ulcers. Treat with liposomal amphotericin or high-dose itraconazole followed by itraconazole maintenance.

Scabies

In advanced HIV disease crusted (Norwegian) scabies may occur, characterized by widespread scaly erythematous lesions on the face and scalp, together with hyperkeratotic lesions on the hands and feet, giving the characteristic 'breadcrumb' appearance. Appearances can be very atypical and may require biopsy to diagnose. Highly infectious because of heavy infestation.

Treatment

Patients with crusted scabies must be barrier nursed and, in addition to topical treatment (permethrin 5% or malathion 0.5%), may be given ivermectin (200 mcg/kg as a single dose). Topical steroids may be needed for eczematous nodules.

Inflammatory conditions

Seborrhoeic dermatitis

Occurs in up to 85% and may be a first indicator of HIV infection. Severity and recurrences ↑ with ↓ CD4 count. Related to infection with *Pityrosporum* spp., ↑ sebum production, and a genetic predisposition.

Presents as an itchy erythematous rash with a yellow greasy scale, but in severe cases, plaques and hyperkeratotic lesions occur. Usually affects paranasal area, but may involve eyebrows, post-auricular areas, and scalp. May also affect intertriginous areas and chest. Severe cases may resemble psoriasis. Facial lesions must be differentiated from lupus erythematosus and rosacea.

Treatment
* Topical antifungals and steroids, e.g. miconazole and hydrocortisone.
* *Scalp lesions*: tar-containing shampoos, selenium sulfide, salicylic acid, and ketoconazole.
* Severe disease responds well to systemic triazoles, such as itraconazole.

Psoriasis

A chronic disease, characterized by erythematous plaques or papules covered by silvery adherent scales. May appear for the first time or pre-existing disease may become worse with HIV infection. Several forms of psoriasis may co-exist.
* Chronic plaque psoriasis classically involves elbows, knees, and scalp, and may be associated with nail dystrophy.
* Flexural psoriasis affects axillae, groin, and intergluteal cleft; more common in advanced HIV disease.
* Guttate psoriasis presents with widespread raindrop-size lesions.

Treatment
* Treatment of HIV may improve.
* Mild to moderate disease can be treated with a regular emollient plus moderately potent topical steroid, calcitriol, tar-containing ointments, or dithranol.
* Severe disease can be treated with systemic agents, e.g. methotrexate (especially in the presence of psoriatic arthritis), acitretin, and ciclosporin. Biological agents may also be considered. Closer monitoring of VL may be required.

Beware of effects of these drugs (apart from acitretin) on immune system.

Eczema

Seen in up to 30% of cases. Severity and frequency ↑ as CD4 count ↓. Xerosis (dry skin) is a common complaint and may be associated with an itchy papular scaly rash on the arms and legs. Skin may be damaged as a result of excessive scratching, resulting in excoriation, lichenification, eczematous changes, and discoloration. May be colonized with *S. aureus*.

Treatment
Treatment includes topical steroids and emollients.

Pruritic follicular and papular eruptions

Pruritus is a common occurrence. Follicular, papular, or nodular lesions may be altered by excoriation and lichenification.

Eosinophilic pustular folliculitis

Chronic, intensely itchy, follicular rash affecting face, upper trunk, and extensor surfaces of the arms. Usually seen when CD4 count <200 cells/μL. Sterile papular, papulopustular, or urticarial papules, centred around hair follicles found. May be ↑ IgE with eosinophilia.

Treatment

Responds best to phototherapy. Emollients for eczematous lesions. Antihistamines not usually helpful. ART may improve.

HIV-associated pruritus

Diagnosis of exclusion of other causes of pruritus. Clinical features 2° to scratching—excoriation, linear lesions, lichenified eczematous changes, and post-inflammatory pigmentation.

Treatment

Regular emollients, topical steroids for eczematous changes, and anti-histamines.

Malassezia furfur folliculitis

Yeast overgrowth producing folliculitis through production of fatty acids and scale formation blocking follicular ostea. Presents with chronic or relapsing pruritic follicular-centred papules on the scalp, flexures, upper trunk, and face.

Treatment

Oral itraconazole (preferred option) 200 mg daily for 7 days. If patient has AIDS, maintenance (200 mg od) or intermittent 'pulse' therapy should be considered. Other options are oral fluconazole and 2% ketoconazole cream. Scalp relapses are best treated with intermittent ketoconazole shampoo.

Neoplasia

Kaposi's sarcoma

➔ Chapter 54, 'Kaposi's sarcoma', pp. 611–13.

Incidence ↓ since the introduction of ART. HHV-8 identified in 1994 as the causative agent. Although the skin is usual site, KS may develop in visceral organs.

Typically, KS lesions appear on the nose and hard palate, but may arise anywhere on the skin. Disease usually has an insidious course with new lesions appearing as existing ones enlarge. Rapidly aggressive disease may occur, but is rare. Initially, starts as a painless non-pruritic pink or red macule, or a papule that gradually darkens to resemble a bruise. May be surrounded by a yellow halo due to extravasated red cells (Plate 32). May be dark and difficult to recognize in black people (see Plates 34 and 35). KS lesions vary in size from a few millimetres to several centimetres (Plates 33 and 35). Extensive plaques with scaling can develop on the legs and may break down, producing local pain and oedema. Lesions on the soles may be particularly troublesome as they interfere with walking. Facial and genital KS is cosmetically unsightly. With treatment, the lesion becomes flat and the colour fades, but some pigmentation persists, even in the absence of residual tumour.

Non-pitting oedema is commonly associated with KS, especially affecting the lower limbs. May be due to skin lymphatic involvement or 2° to vasoactive substances produced by KS. Degree of oedema occasionally disproportionate to size of KS lesions (i.e. feature of the disease itself, rather than 2° to lymph node enlargement/lymphatic obstruction).

Diagnosis

Typical skin KS lesions are diagnosed clinically, but biopsy provides an absolute diagnosis in atypical lesions. Patients with significant mucosal involvement, fever, symptoms, or signs suggestive of other organ involvement should be evaluated by CT to look for visceral involvement or other HHV8 associated conditions. Patients with severe oedema may require CT to exclude localized obstruction or accompanying pathology.

Treatment

➔ Chapter 54, 'Kaposi's sarcoma', pp. 611–13.

Treatment for skin KS is for cosmetic reasons and to alleviate symptoms.

Lymphomas

➔ Chapter 54, 'Non-Hodgkin's lymphoma', pp. 614–16.

Extranodal cutaneous involvement occurs in up to 8% of those with B-cell non-Hodgkin's lymphoma. Presents with an enlarging violaceous nodule or plaque, which may ulcerate.

Cutaneous T-cell lymphoma presents as a scaly patch or plaque with erythema, hypo- or hyperpigmentation, and atrophy. It may be mis-diagnosed as chronic eczema.

The skin may be involved when lymphoma (usually B-cell) involves an underlying lymph node.

Treatment

⊃ Chapter 54, 'Non-Hodgkin's lymphoma', pp. 614–16.

The principles of management of non-Hodgkin's lymphoma are the same as for lymphoma elsewhere and chemotherapy is usually given.

Drug reactions

Cutaneous drug reactions ↑, as does the development of hypersensitivity reactions to previously tolerated drugs. Mild drug eruptions do not always necessitate the cessation of the causative drug, especially if it is the most effective agent and is given for a short time (e.g. co-trimoxazole for *Pneumocystis jiroveci* pneumonia). Desensitization may be possible for essential drugs. Cross-sensitivities may occur, e.g. between dapsone and co-trimoxazole.

Hypersensitivity reactions are common with certain antiretroviral drugs, such as nevirapine and abacavir, which may cause a fatal reaction. Special attention (with counselling) to patients on these treatments is important to ensure early recognition and prompt action.

- Morbilliform (erythematous maculopapular) drug eruption is common and may be associated with systemic symptoms. Most frequent causative drugs are amoxicillin and sulfonamides. Progresses in a caudocephalic direction, resolving within 3–5 days, but occasionally persisting for weeks after its withdrawal. Many viral infections cause a similar rash.
- Erythroderma occurs when a morbilliform rash becomes confluent and involves the whole body. May result in hypothermia and shock.
- Erythema multiforme, SJS, and toxic epidermal necrolysis ↑ in HIV infection. Offending drug must be stopped. If severe patients best managed in high-dependency units, where attention to electrolyte and fluid balance and skin care are of paramount importance.
- Nail and oral pigmentation 2° to zidovudine.
- Penile ulceration due to foscarnet.

HIV: pyrexia
of unknown origin

Introduction *564*
HIV-related aetiology (data from Europe and USA) *565*
Diagnosis *566*
Management *568*
Mycobacterium avium complex *569*
Visceral leishmaniasis *570*

Introduction

Pyrexia of unknown origin (PUO) was defined by R. G. Petersdorf and P. B. Beeson (*Medicine* **40**, 1–30, 1961) as a temperature of >38.3°C on multiple occasions over a period of >3 weeks with failure to reach a diagnosis after 1 week of investigation.

HIV-related diseases are an important cause of prolonged fever and must be considered in patients with PUO. In patients with known HIV infection PUO may arise during follow-up. D. T. Durack and A. C. Street (*Curr Clin Top Infect Dis* **11**, 35–51, 1991) produced a definition of HIV-associated PUO, including temperatures >38.3°C on multiple occasions over a period of >4 weeks for outpatients or 3 days for inpatients, with negative microbiological results after at least 2 days incubation.

PUO occurs predominantly in the late stages of infection with CD4 counts <100 cells/μL and is less common in patients on effective ART. In the general population, infections account for only 33% of PUO. However, infectious diseases are the predominant cause in PLWH, accounting for 80–90% with neoplasia (lymphoma commonest) and drug reactions accounting for most of the others.

A cause can be found in 80%. In those with undetermined diagnoses fever may settle spontaneously. In the general population a single pathology is almost universal, but two or more simultaneous pathologies may be found in about 20% of HIV-related cases. Even if patients are taking standard prophylaxis against agents, such as *Pneumocystis jiroveci* or MAC, these cannot be excluded without appropriate investigation.

There are important geographical differences, e.g. tuberculosis and leishmaniasis are much more common in Europe than in the USA. It is also important to consider non-HIV-related causes and other infections, whose presentation may be modified by immunodeficiency. Strenuous diagnostic efforts are important in PUO as it may enable the diagnosis and treatment of infections before the onset of specific organ dysfunction (e.g. a PCP). A careful history, including sexual, lifetime history of travel, immunization, consumption and source of dairy products, family history, animal contact, and drugs (prescribed and non-prescribed) is mandatory.

HIV-related aetiology (data from Europe and USA)

- *Mycobacterial infection*:
  - *Mycobacterium tuberculosis*—7% (USA) to 37% (Europe). CD4 count may be normal
  - *MAC*—12–31% (CD4 count <100 cells/μL).
  - *Others (e.g. M. kansasii, M. genavense)*—1–5%.
- *PCP*—5–13% (CD4 count <200 cells/μL).
- *Viral*:
  - *CMV*—5–9% (CD4 count <50 cells/μL)
  - *HIV itself, HSV, VZV, parvovirus B19, adenovirus, HBV, and HCV*—2–7%.
- *Bacterial*: 5–7%.
- *Fungal (cryptococcosis, candidaemia, disseminated histoplasmosis, aspergillosis, Penicillium marneffei)*: 2–8% (CD4 count <200 cells/μL).
- *Parasitic*:
  - *Leishmaniasis*—0% (USA) to 12% (Europe)
  - *Toxoplasmosis*—1–3%
  - *Others (isosporiasis, cryptosporidiosis)*—<1%.
- *Neoplasia*:
  - *Lymphoma*—5–10% (CD4 count may be normal)
  - *KS*—isolated reports.
- *Drugs*: <1%.
- Other unusual causes include Reiter's syndrome, non-specific hepatitis, Castleman's disease, and angiofollicular hyperplasia.

Diagnosis

Careful history-taking, including length of symptoms, systemic enquiry, sexual, lifetime history of travel, immunization, consumption and source of dairy products, family history, occupational history, personality change, animal contact, contact with ticks and insect bites, past medical history, and drugs (prescribed and non-prescribed) is mandatory.

Examination especially for lymphadenopathy, abdominal (hepatosplenomegaly), skin rash, full cardiology (looking for murmurs, splinter haemorrhages) respiratory (listening for crackles, effusions), neurological (full neurological examination essential, and should include tests of memory and collateral for change in personality), and retinal abnormalities (through dilated pupils). Examination should be repeated over time.

All patients should have first level (non-invasive) investigation proceeding to second level (invasive) if diagnosis is not established.

First level includes
- FBC/differential WCC, LFTs, CRP, ESR, ferritin, urinalysis, CD4 count, and HIV VL.
- Pulse oximetry.
- Chest X-ray.
- Repeated cultures of blood, sputum, urine, and faeces as indicated for bacteria, mycobacteria (requires specific mycobacteria culture bottles), and fungi. STI screen.
- Blood film examination.
- Serum cryptococcal antigen (if CD4<200 cells/µl).
- Serology for syphilis and other specific serologies indicated by travel or exposure history.
- Echocardiography if murmur.

Further investigation is dictated by level of immunosuppression, results of 1st level investigation, and clinical examination/history.

2nd level as indicated
Include:
- abdominal and thoracic CT
- CT head and /or MRI brain
- exercise oximetry
- bronchoscopy with broncho-alveolar lavage
- fluorodeoxyglucose positron emission tomography (PET) is helpful to guide biopsy and highlight areas of abnormality not picked up on routine imaging.
- Biopsy (histology and microbiology—*must include fungal and mycobacterial culture*): bone marrow (useful if significant immunosuppression, anaemia, or cytopaenia), liver (particularly if enlarged or raised alkaline phosphatase—mycobacterial infection), lymph node (including mediastinoscopic or endoscopic ultrasound), skin rash, intestinal (if loose stool), oesophageal mucosa (if dysphagia/odynophagia).
- Lumbar puncture.
- CMV PCR (CD4 <200 cells/µl), EBV PCR (may be raised in lymphoma).

Causes of PUO unrelated to HIV must not be forgotten (Box 48.1) and may require other investigations, e.g. auto-antibody screen and isotope-labelled white cell scan.

Box 48.1 Non-HIV-related causes of PUO

Infection

Bacterial
- *Site-specific*: abscesses, urinary tract infection, prostatitis, pelvic inflammatory disease, endocarditis, hepatobiliary infection, osteomyelitis.
- *General*: syphilis, relapsing fever, Lyme disease, gonorrhoea, lymphogranuloma venereum, psittacosis, salmonellosis, Q-fever.

Viral
CMV, EBV, hepatitis viruses.

Fungi (usually only if immunosuppressed):
Candidiasis.

Parasites
Malaria, toxoplasmosis.

Connective tissue/autoimmune diseases
Rheumatoid arthritis, Still's disease, systemic lupus erythematosus.

Vasculitis
Giant cell arteritis, polymyalgia rheumatica, polyarteritis nodosa.

Granulomatous diseases
Sarcoidosis, regional enteritis, granulomatous hepatitis.

Neoplasia
Lymphomas, Hodgkin's disease, leukaemias, solid tumours (especially renal cell carcinoma), malignant histiocytosis.

Inherited diseases
Familial Mediterranean fever.

Drugs
Antibiotic reactions.

Endocrine
- Hyperthyroidism.

Factitious

Consider serology depending on history, country of origin/travel, and examination for: CMV, EBV, toxoplasma, parvovirus, coxiella, mycoplasma, *Chlamydia pneumoniae*, syphilis, bartonella, brucella, rickettsia, leptospirosis, borrelia, histoplasma, coccidioidomycosis, and cryptococcus.

Consider serum PCR for CMV (rising or high CMV PCR correlates with development of end-organ disease, but not diagnostic), parvovirus (particularly if anaemic), EBV (may be positive in lymphoma), and HHV-8 (associated with KS and Castleman's disease).

Consider drugs, including antiretrovirals and antituberculous medication. These should be considered, particularly in the setting of eosinophilia or significant liver injury following initiation of therapy.

Consider IRIS particularly in patients with a diagnosis of TB/MAC/other deep-seated infection who have had response to treatment (CD4 ↑, HIV VL decrease >1 log), and no new infection found or adverse drug reaction.

Management

Management depends on the underlying cause. Cases where no underlying additional pathology is found may respond to ART, if not already treated. As in any fever, general measures, such as good hydration, antipyretics, and reassurance, are important. In patients with late-stage HIV disease and limited treatment options, palliation with steroids may be necessary. MAC infections and, less commonly, leishmaniasis often present with unexplained pyrexia without focal organ involvement. IRIS may require steroids if severe systemic symptoms or danger of focal damage, e.g. neurological.

Other causes of HIV-related PUO, which may present with clinical features specific to their infection site are described elsewhere in this book.

Mycobacterium avium complex

Ubiquitous and frequently isolated from soil, food, and water. Infection usually affects those with CD4 counts <100 cells/μL (median 10 cells/μL). Any organ can be affected; most commonly lymph nodes, spleen, GI tract, lungs, and bone marrow, but often patients develop disseminated infection without prior localization.

Clinical features

Most common is pyrexia (in ~9%) with night sweats, fatigue, diarrhoea/abdominal pain/nausea and vomiting/weight loss, lymph-adenopathy, and hepato-splenomegaly.

Investigations and diagnosis

- *FBC*: anaemia (common and often severe).
- *LFTs*: ↑ alkaline phosphatase (common).
- Blood cultures (>95% sensitivity for disseminated MAC).
- Culture of material from bone marrow, lymph nodes, and liver.
- Staining of material from bone marrow, lymph nodes (Plate 6), and liver for mycobacteria (marrow provides rapid diagnosis in ~3%).
- X-rays may show internal lymphadenopathy with a typical abscess pattern on CT.

Management

Three or four drug regimens are recommended as multi-resistance is usual, macrolide use associated with better outcome.

A macrolide (clarithromycin 500 mg bd or azithromycin 500 mg daily) plus ethambutol 15 mg/kg daily +/− rifamycin (rifabutin 300 mg/day or rifampicin 450–600 mg/day), particularly if severe disease or a quinolone (e.g. moxifloxacin 400 mg daily) or if unable to use any one first-line drug. Data to advise on the duration of treatment are lacking, but it should be a minimum of 12 months or until virological and clinical response and CD4 >100 cells/μL for at least 3 months. ART should also be commenced, taking into account potential drug interactions. Steroids may be required to ameliorate severe fever.

1° prophylaxis is now rarely required because of the effectiveness of ART, but may be considered for those with a CD4 count <50 cells/μL. Azithromycin recommended (1250 mg weekly). Combination with rifabutin does not increase survival and leads to drug interactions, and is not recommended. Prophylaxis can be stopped once CD4 is >50 cells/L for >3–6 months on ART.

Visceral leishmaniasis

Caused by *Leishmania* spp., protozoa transmitted by sandflies from rodents, small carnivores, dogs, foxes, and humans. Typically, presents with fever, malaise, weight loss, hepatosplenomegaly, and lymphadenopathy. Pancytopenia may occur.

Consider if PUO, hepatosplenomegaly, or bone marrow dysfunction. Diagnosed by identifying organism in tissue by microscopy (Leishman–Donovan bodies in macrophages), culture, or PCR. Fine-needle aspiration of spleen is most sensitive (about 98%), but bone marrow aspiration is safer with 54–86% sensitivity. Serology (immunofluorescent antibody test and direct agglutination test) is insensitive unless high protozoal load.

Treat with sodium stibogluconate 20 mg/kg/day IV/IM for 28 days or liposomal amphotericin B. 2° prophylaxis with amphotericin or sodium stibogluconate every 2–4 weeks is essential to prevent recurrence (occurs in 60–90% without prophylaxis). Daily itraconazole may be effective prophylaxis.

HIV: endocrine and metabolic disorders

Introduction *572*
Endocrine disturbances *573*
Metabolic disorders *576*
HIV-associated wasting syndrome *580*

Introduction

A wide range of endocrinopathies and metabolic disturbances occur at all stages of HIV disease. In patients with advanced disease in the pre-ART era, endocrine disturbances were often a result of a direct effect of HIV itself, and/or infiltration by neoplasms and OIs. However, commonly, endocrine abnormalities are due to functional disturbances, or 2° to drugs and inter-current severe illnesses.

HIV infection is a persistent inflammatory state, even in those taking ART with fully suppressed blood virus. The persistent inflammation is multifactorial, in part due to immune dysregulation, coagulopathy, and occult viral replication. Elevated inflammatory factors (e.g. tumour necrosis factor-α) may alter the hypothalamus-pituitary-adrenal/thyroid/gonadal axes, which directly affect hormonal secretion at the cellular level.

In ART era, coupled with the survival benefit, there is ↑ prevalence of metabolic disorders, such as insulin resistance, dyslipidaemia, abnormal body fat distribution, and abnormal bone metabolism.

Endocrine disturbances

Pituitary function

Pituitary gland involvement was seen in 30% of autopsies carried out in AIDS patients. Panhypopituitarism is rare, but selective failure, e.g. gonadotrophins is more common. Like other endocrine glands, the pituitary may be affected by OIs, infarction, haemorrhage, and neoplasms. Growth hormone deficiency (may contribute to insulin resistance), galactorrhoea, unexplained hyponatremia, syndrome of inappropriate antidiuretic hormone secretion (SIADH), and central diabetes insipidus have all been described. Drugs and pathophysiological mechanisms are proposed reasons for these abnormalities.

Thyroid disease

Thyroid glands infiltration with malignancies and OIs seen in autopsies is not usually associated with abnormal thyroid function tests (TFTs). TFTs are often abnormal in HIV patients, but the prevalence of overt thyroid disorder is not higher than in the general population. CD4 count correlates inversely with thyroid-binding globulin (TBG). These changes may be a response to the stress of advanced disease state or comorbidities. Occasionally, the biochemical picture does not fully fit with sick euthyroid disease. Progression of HIV disease exhibits ↓ T3, ↑ TBG and ↓ reverse triiodothyronine (rT3) levels over time. Observations showed increased prevalence of overt and subclinical 1° hypothyroidism with absent antithyroid antibodies.

Thyroid dysfunction has also been described as a component of IRIS. Some of these patients have autoimmune thyroid disorder, Graves' disease been the commonest.

In subclinical hypothyroidism with mildly elevated thyroid-stimulating hormone (TSH), the TSH level should be rechecked in 1–3 months. Levothyroxine may be considered with persistently elevated levels of TSH >10 mU/L. Routine screening of TFTs is not recommended in asymptomatic patients.

Gonadal function

Dysfunction occurs in both sexes, especially in the late stages of HIV disease and in those with weight loss. Sex hormone-binding globulin levels are increased in 30–50%. Free testosterone levels are more reliable in the assessment of hypogonadism. The aetiology of gonadal dysfunction is often multifactorial. Severe systemic illness, OIs, malnutrition, weight loss, recreational drug use, chronic alcoholism, and increased levels of cytokines may be contributory. HIV-related gonadal failure results in loss of muscle mass, fatigue, sexual dysfunction, and decreased quality of life. Unlike HIV −ve men there is no increase in fat mass.

Testicular function

Male gonadal dysfunction is common. Two-thirds of male patients with advanced HIV disease complain of loss of libido. Erectile dysfunction is reported in up to 60% of HIV +ve male patients, which has no correlation with hypogonadism. HIV +ve men are prone to an early 'andropause' marked by dysregulation of hypothalamic–pituitary axis. Biochemical hypogonadism was reported in up to 50% of male AIDS patients. This dropped to around 20% in those receiving ART. Testicular dysfunction is mostly 2° to low gonadotropin levels due to inflammation, infection, undernutrition, and the effects of several drugs on gonadotropin production. Increased prolactin levels and gynecomastia have been reported. Gynecomastia has been seen in a small percentage of male patients with hepatitis C and lipodystrophy.

Free testosterone assay is recommended to diagnose hypogonadism.

Testicular function is affected by drugs such as:
- *opiates*—associated with hypogonadotropic hypogonadism.
- *ketoconazole*—causing oligospermia and gynaecomastia.
- *megestrol acetate*—inhibiting gonadotropin secretion.

Testosterone replacement ↑ lean body mass, body weight, and well-being.

Ovarian function

Ovarian dysfunction among female AIDS patients is less common. Amenorrhoea, irregular periods, and oligomenorrhoea occur with increasing frequency with HIV disease progression. Early menopause has been seen in up to 8% of HIV +ve female patients. Up to 67% of females with AIDS wasting syndrome have low levels of free testosterone. The mechanism of this is not known.

Adrenal function

The adrenal gland is the most commonly affected endocrine gland leading to glucocorticoid, and less commonly, aldosterone deficiency. Hypothalamic–pituitary–adrenal axis abnormalities in HIV are usually due to medications, destruction of the adrenals, or the anterior pituitary by OIs and malignancies, autoimmune adrenalitis, and abnormal cytokine levels. The adrenals may be directly infected by HIV. CMV adrenal gland involvement (found in 40–85% of autopsies) may lead to acute adrenal insufficiency.

In AIDS patients, subtle impairment of adrenal function is manifested as fatigue, hyponatremia, or rarely with clinical symptoms of adrenal insufficiency. Biochemical abnormalities of adrenal insufficiency are relatively common in hospitalized patients.

Increased cortisol levels may be seen in HIV-infected patients; mostly, a stress response to the disease burden. Cushing's syndrome has been reported, from concomitant use of PI and steroids (e.g. inhaled high dose steroids). Rarely, glucocorticoid resistance at receptor level has been shown in advanced disease. Such patients have increased cortisol and ACTH level with Addisonian symptoms. If suspected, risk factors (OIs, drugs) for adrenal insufficiency should be sought. Although chronic steroid replacement at supraphysiologic doses is not advocated in AIDS to prevent further immunosuppression, HIV is not a contraindication to pharmacologic steroid therapy.

Features of adrenocortical disturbances found in HIV infection:
- ↑ levels of dehydroepiandrosterone with ↑ cortisol.
- ↓ basal adrenal androgen levels.
- ↓ adrenal responses to adrenocorticotrophic hormone (ACTH).

Drugs may also compromise adrenal function:
- megestrol acetate (used as an appetite stimulant) ↓ plasma cortisol level and may lead to acute adrenal crisis if stopped abruptly after prolonged use
- Azoles results in ↓ cortisol and testosterone levels
- rifampicin enhances hepatic cortisol metabolism and causes adrenal insufficiency in patients with Addison's disease who are on replacement therapy or in those with limited adrenal function.

Patients with fatigue, loss of weight, postural hypotension, hyponatraemia, and hyperkalaemia should be assessed with a short synacthen test. Primary adrenal insufficiency can be identified by measuring ACTH simultaneously with serum cortisol.

Aldosterone deficiency may occur (often with glucocorticoid deficiency) leading to persistent hyponatraemia, hyperkalaemia, and metabolic acidosis requiring replacement therapy.

Management
Patients with glucocorticoid insufficiency should receive replacement therapy with hydrocortisone 30 mg/day in divided doses.

Patients with aldosterone deficiency should receive fludrocortisone 50–300 µg/day.

Pancreatic function
Both exocrine and endocrine functions can be affected in HIV. The pancreas is a target for OIs and malignancies (lymphoma, KS), but clinically significant endocrine dysfunction is rare. Major clinical manifestations are pancreatitis and hypoglycaemia. Pancreatitis is commonly seen as a drug effect (pentamidine, trimethoprim and didanosine). Elevated amylase levels may be due to macroamylasaemia or salivary gland disease. Hypoglycaemia can result from islet cell inflammation and insulin release by pentamidine with subsequent chronic hyperglycaemia. Megestrol acetate is associated with new-onset diabetes mellitus

Pancreatic endocrine function
Insulin resistance occurs more frequently especially in those treated with PIs and those with wasting syndrome. Diabetes is more likely to occur in those with other predisposing factors e.g. family history. Pentamidine is toxic to pancreatic β cells inducing hypoglycaemia in 15–28% (2–3 times more common than in HIV –ve patients). Substantial destruction of β cells may later lead to diabetes mellitus. Management of diabetes follows the same principles as for HIV –ve individuals.

Pancreatic exocrine function
Reduced exocrine pancreatic function is common in HIV infection and may be asymptomatic. Severe chronic pancreatic insufficiency results in severe diarrhoea and can be caused by HIV drugs, e.g. didanosine. Feacal elastase may be low. May require pancreatic enzyme supplements.

Metabolic disorders

Lipodystrophy syndrome

HIV lipodystrophy syndrome is characterized by abnormal body fat distribution and metabolic derangements. These features are often seen in combination, but may occur in isolation. While there is some resemblance to Cushing's syndrome, HIV lipodystrophy lacks myopathy, bruising, and facial plethora, and has normal cortisol level with its normal diurnal variation and adequate suppressibility to dexamethasone. May arise spontaneously, but much more commonly associated with the use of ART, especially if containing PIs. The frequency and severity depend on gender, genetic factors and ethnicity, age, duration of HIV infection, length, and type of antiretroviral drugs.

Cardiovascular risk ↑, especially in patients on ART

Lipodystrophy

Found in ≈4% of those with untreated HIV infection. Rate for those taking ART is difficult to determine because of inconsistent diagnostic criteria, but ranges from 20% to 75% (median development time, 18 months). Magnitude varies with individual PIs. Prevalence also related to duration of NRTI use, especially thymidine analogues such as zidovudine. More common in whites and almost twice as common in ♀.

Lipohypertrophy (especially associated with PIs)
- *Dorsocervical fat pad*: buffalo hump.
- Increased neck circumference (by 5–10 cm).
- Breast hypertrophy (♀ and ♂).
- *Central truncal adiposity*: pot belly due to ↑ intraperitoneal fat.
- Lipomas occur in ≈10% of these patients.

Lipoatrophy (especially associated with NRTIs, particularly stavudine)
- *Loss of SC fat from cheeks*: emaciated appearance, can be disfiguring, may identify patients as having HIV infection, and may affect quality of life and compliance to drugs
- Loss of SC fat from arms, shoulders, thighs, and buttocks.

Dyslipidaemia

HIV infection may cause abnormalities in lipid metabolism, which include:
- ↑ serum triglyceride
- ↑ total cholesterol, but HDL may be elevated in early stages and decrease with advanced disease.
- ↓ LDL
- predominance of small, dense LDL particles.

It is reported in up to 80% of those taking ART and especially if PI-based. Typical abnormalities include:
- hypercholesterolaemia, mostly very-LDL, but also intermediate density lipoproteins. HDL unchanged or ↑
- hypertriglyceridaemia.

More frequent and severe with ritonavir and lopinavir–ritonavir, followed by amprenavir and nelfinavir with indinavir and saquinavir having the fewest effects. Atazanavir and darunavir appear to have little effect.

NRTIs are implicated less, although stavudine is more likely to be associated with ↑ in cholesterol and triglycerides unlike lamivudine, emtricitabine, tenofovir and abacavir, which appear to have minimal or no effect on lipid metabolism.

NNRTIs can cause alterations in the lipid profiles, but to a lesser extent than PIs. Nevirapine produces marginally smaller changes than efavirenz and improvements in lipid levels when switching from PIs. Rilpivirine has a better effect on lipids than efavifenz.

Integrase inhibitors have very favourable lipid profile.

Hyperglycaemia

New-onset diabetes mellitus, diabetic ketoacidosis, and exacerbations of pre-existing diabetes mellitus have all been reported with ↑ rates of other risk factors, e.g. family history, pregnancy. Diabetes is directly associated with HIV infection, reported in 3.3% and increased to 5.9% with concomitant HCV infection. Impaired glucose tolerance and insulin resistance precede weight loss. Insulin resistance, rather than insulin deficiency, is usually implicated in the pathogenesis of diabetes in HIV-infected patients. Autoimmune diabetes has been reported in some HIV-infected patients after immune restoration during ART. Concurrent use of opiates may alter beta-cell function, while heroin addiction is associated with insulin resistance. HIV-associated insulin resistance and glucose dysregulation may lead to atherosclerosis and coronary heart disease. Stronger link is observed with most PIs. Darunavir and atazanavir are the least associated.

Assessment

Patients on ART should have body weight, lipids, and blood sugar measured at regular intervals. Clinical examination and self-reporting of body shape changes help detect early signs. Photographs may aid in the early recognition of facial lipoatrophy. Additional cardiovascular risks, such as life style, smoking, hypertension, family history and age should also be assessed and managed as in the HIV –ve individuals.

Management

- General advice:
  - nutrition—assessment, dietetic advice and possible benefit from dietary supplements (fibre, omega-3 fatty acids)
  - exercise—↑ physical activity and exercise to build muscles, improve abdominal shape, and combat peripheral wasting.
- Start ART before CD4 <200 cells/µL or development of AIDS.
- Take care with choice of initial regimen if possible:
  - avoid PIs and NRTI combinations with highest risk
  - use lamivudine, emtricitabine, tenofovir instead of zidovudine.
- Switch to drugs with low or no association. Benefit of switching is inconsistent, morphological changes being more resistant.
- Fibrates and statins: used according to lipid profile.
  - Hypercholesterolaemia managed with low-fat diet and statins.
  - Hypertriglyceridaemia responds best to low-fat diet, fibrates, and statins.
  - Most PIs inhibit the metabolism of most statins and can significantly increase serum statin levels, thus increasing the risk of toxicity, including myopathy and rhabdomyolysis. Pravastatin is the preferred statin as it is least likely to interact with PIs. Fluvastatin is an

alternative. Atorvastatin must be used with caution. Simvastatin and lovastatin should be avoided. NNRTIs are enzyme inducers and higher levels of statins may be required.
• Fibrates (gemfibrozil, bezafibrate, fenofibrate) are usually used in combination with statins as more effective than fibrate monotherapy. Seek advice from lipidologist before starting.
  ↑ risk of rhabdomyolysis and hepatotoxicity.
• *Other drugs*:
  • metformin (avoid if lipoatrophy) for insulin resistance, dyslipidaemia and fat accumulation
  • glitazones for insulin resistance with weight loss.
• *Invasive methods for lipodystrophy*:
  • plastic surgery, e.g. liposuction and breast reduction
  • polylactic acid (New-Fill®) injections for lipoatrophy.

Electrolytes and water imbalance

Sodium and water

Hyponatraemia is a common finding in advanced HIV disease. It is reported in up to 20% of HIV +ve outpatients and up to 60% of hospitalized patients, when mostly due to GI loss associated with hypovolaemia. Respiratory and CNS infections, or certain drugs, e.g. antidepressants, may cause the SIADH. This is characterized by hyponatraemia, inappropriately ↑ urinary osmolality/Na for the degree of serum hypo-osmolality and normal blood volume in the context of normal adrenal and thyroid functions. Severe hyponatraemia causes confusion, seizures, and coma. Decreased water clearance from HIV-related nephropathy may exacerbate hyponatraemia. Manage SIADH by removing/treating the underlying cause, fluid restriction.

Hyporeninaemic hypoaldosteronism should be considered when hyponatraemia is associated with hyperkalaemia, providing normally functioning kidneys and adrenals. Hyporeninaemic hypoaldosteronism can rarely be caused by drugs like miconazole and pentamidine (pentamidine tubulopathy).

Hypernatremia may be seen in foscarnet-induced nephrogenic diabetes insipidus.

Potassium

High dose co-trimoxazole may result in hyperkalaemia especially if pre-existing renal impairment. Pentamidine-associated tubular nephropathy, HIV-nephropathy, and 1° adrenal insufficiency are other causes of hyperkalaemia. Trimethoprim (similar structure to amiloride) reported the commonest cause of hyperkalaemia, occurring in nearly 20–50% AIDS patients. Trimethoprim inhibits tubular potassium excretion.

Calcium and phosphate

Serum calcium concentration decreases progressively with stage of HIV disease. Around half of the patients with hypocalcaemia have vitamin D deficiency, but without compensatory increase in parathyroid hormone (PTH). The reason for this is not known

Causes of hypocalcaemia include:
• HIV enteropathy.
• *Vitamin D deficiency*:
  • malabsorption (AIDS enteropathy)
  • decreased hydroxylation (PI-induced).

- Fanconi syndrome with hypophosphatemia (tenofovir).
- Severe intercurrent illnesses.
- *Drugs*:
  - foscarnet binds calcium resulting in decreased ionized calcium
  - ketoconazole inhibits 1,25-dihydroxycholecalciferol synthesis
  - pentamidine causes renal loss of magnesium with 2° hypocalcaemia.

Hypercalcaemia is rarely reported in AIDS, granuloma (tuberculosis, lymphoma), enhanced local osteoclastic resorption of bone (disseminated CMV), or activation of PTH-related protein (HTLV1).

Hypophosphataemia is very common in HIV +ve patients, occurs in 10% of patients not taking ART and in 20–31% of those on ART. Main causes are malnutrition, GI losses, osteomalacia, hyperparathyroidism, alcoholism, and intercurrent illness. Tenofovir causes hypophosphataemia by its effect on tubular function.

Bone mineral dysfunction

Osteopenia, osteoporosis, and fractures are more common in HIV +ve individuals compared with the general population, especially with ↑ age in the ART era. Tenofovir is associated with osteopenia.

Risk factors for low bone mineral density (BMD)

- HIV itself
- older age
- white ethnicity
- hypogonadism
- post-menopausal status
- low body mass
- smoking
- high alcohol intake
- glucocorticoid use.

Evaluation and management

- Fracture risk assessment (using FRAX score) at the time of diagnosis in all patients over 50 (>40 years if major risk factors), post-menopausal women, or in the presence of other risk factors. Stratify according to score:
  - *<10%*—reassure and repeat after 3 years
  - *10–20%*—consider dual energy X-ray absorptiometry (DEXA) scan to refine risk estimate; if >10% fracture risk, provide lifestyle advice and optimize risk factors including vitamin D deficiency correction
  - *>20%*—optimize risk factors, review ART (tenofovir) and lifestyle factors, and refer for osteoporosis treatment.
- Vitamin D/parathyroid hormone levels if increased fracture risk.

HIV-associated wasting syndrome

An AIDS-defining illness, defined by Centers for Disease Control (CDC) as involuntary loss of >10% of body weight, plus >30 days of either diarrhoea or weakness, and fever in the absence of illnesses other than HIV. It is becoming less common with the wide availability of ART. Independently associated with an increased risk of OIs, disease progression, and death. Mainly loss of lean body mass and, to a lesser extent, loss of fat.

Additional factors that exacerbate wasting include
- Depression.
- Nutritional factors, e.g. anorexia, dysphagia, poor nutrient absorption.
- OIs.
- Metabolism, e.g. ↑ resting metabolic rate, ↑ protein turnover ↑ production of cytokines, hypertriglyceridemia, and hypogonadism.

Assessment
- Weight and BMI at regular intervals help with early recognition and monitoring.
- Specialist nutritional review.
- Testosterone measurement.
- Techniques such as DEXA scan and MRI provide more accurate measurement of body composition.

Management
- Treatment of contributing factors.
- ART
- Improving food intake by dietary supplements, enteral, and parenteral feeding.
- *Pharmacologic agents*:
  - Testosterone may be considered to reverse muscle loss, but beware of the adverse effects of long-term administration.
  - Megestrol an appetite stimulant (side effects—hypogonadism, adrenal insufficiency, deep venous thrombosis, and avascular necrosis).
  - Growth hormone administration may increase lean body mass, but is expensive and benefit may be lost after discontinuation.
  - Thalidomide results in significant weight gain, but has strict prescribing guidelines and has potential serious side effects.
  - Anabolic hormones, e.g. oxymetholone, side-effects include liver toxicity. Nandrolone is effective in increasing lean body mass in both men and women, but long-term side effects are not known.

HIV: renal disorders

Introduction 582
HIV-associated nephropathy (HIVAN) 583
Immune-mediated renal disease 584
Thrombotic microangiopathy 585
Interstitial nephritis 585
Acute renal failure and HIV seroconversion 585
Drugs and renal disease 586
Other diseases (less commonly reported) 588
End-stage renal disease 588

Introduction

Kidney disease was relatively common before the ART era. Proteinuria may be found in up to 30%. Necropsy studies in the USA have shown renal pathological abnormalities in 3–7%. In the ART era 1° renal diseases, diabetes, hypertension, vascular disease, and drug toxicity (including antiretrovirals) are more common than HIV-associated nephropathy.

Initial presentation may be as acute renal failure, especially in advanced HIV disease, 2° to the following:
- Dehydration and electrolyte disturbances (e.g. following vomiting and diarrhoea).
- *Acute tubular necrosis due to:*
  - sepsis
  - hypotension
  - drug nephrotoxicity (e.g. tenofovir, adefovir, aminoglycosides, pentamidine, aciclovir, cidofovir, foscarnet, amphotericin B)
  - rhabdomyolysis can occur with use of statins in combination with PI.
- *Obstruction (2° to nephrolithiasis and crystalluria):*
  - *Nephrolithiasis*—indinavir, rarely atazanavir.
  - *sulfadiazine and aciclovir*—can cause crystalluria especially in high dosage and with dehydration.

HIV-related infection (e.g. TB) can involve the kidney.

The general management of renal failure should follow the same principles as for HIV −ve patients, i.e. fluid replacement, dietary restriction, renal replacement therapy, erythropoietin, vitamin D analogues, reducing dose of drugs, etc.

Assessment of HIV +ve patients for renal disease

Address all risk factors such as smoking, hypertension, dyslipidaemia, hyperuricaemia, metabolic syndrome, vascular disease. The following should be measured routinely:
- Dipstick for protein in urine and, if +ve, quantify with 24-hour urine protein or urine spot sample for urine PCR (uPCR). 24-hour urine collection may not be reliable.
- Serum creatinine should be complimented by an estimated glomerular filtration rate (eGFR) using MDRD or Cockcroft–Gault equations. If uPCR >45 or eGFR <60, renal ultrasound and consider referral to nephrology (definitely if uPCR>100 mg/mmol); otherwise minimum annual measurements.
- Patients at high risk for development of renal dysfunction, i.e. HIV VL >4000 copies/mL, CD4 <200 cells/μL, black race, diabetes, HCV co-infection, or HBV, may need to have renal function monitored more frequently.

HIV-associated nephropathy (HIVAN)

First described in 1984. Early studies from USA demonstrated that it accounted for >50% of HIV-related renal disease. Renal glomerular and tubular epithelial cells have been shown to be infected by HIV, although the mechanisms of viral-induced injury are unclear.

Predominantly found in black ♂ of African origin and, currently, the third most common cause of end-stage renal disease (ESRD) in 20–64-year-old African Americans. Low incidence amongst follow-up patients (0.25/1000 patient-years) and higher (1%) in newly diagnosed black people. 10:1 M:F ratio.

Clinical features

Presents with nephrotic syndrome—proteinuria (>3.5 g/day), hypo-albuminaemia, oedema, and hyperlipidaemia. Typically, no hypertension. Leads to progressive renal insufficiency, which is modified with ART.

Diagnosis

- CD4 count usually <200 cells/μL.
- Urinalysis shows leucocytes, hyaline casts, and oval fat bodies, but no cellular casts.
- Renal ultrasound typically shows normal or enlarged renal size with ↑ echogenicity.
- Markedly impaired renal function.
- Renal biopsy may be required if diagnosis in doubt (e.g. patient with other risk factors for renal disease or not responding to ART). Definitive diagnosis is made by renal biopsy showing focal segmental glomerulosclerosis, collapse of glomerular tuft associated with tubular ectasia, and tubulo-interstitial nephritis.

Management

- ART, with dose adjustment when GFR<50 mL/min, avoid nephrotoxic ART e.g. tenofovir, PI. Leads to >20% ↑ in creatinine clearance. ↓ need for renal replacement therapy.
- Prednisolone if not improving (improves renal function by ↓ HIV-initiated inflammatory process).
- Angiotensin-converting enzyme inhibitors, if initiated prior to severe renal insufficiency may offer long-term renal survival benefits. Angiotensin receptor blockers are alternatives.
- Dialysis if needed.
- Transplant should not be withheld if clinically warranted.

Immune-mediated renal disease

Less common than HIVAN, but reported as the main cause of HIV-related renal disease in non-black races. Found in 10–80% of autopsy and biopsy studies in HIV +ve patients from different European and Asian countries. Most common form is membranoproliferative glomerulo-nephritis. Membranous nephropathy, post-infectious glomerulonephritis, fibrillary glomerulonephritis, and IgA nephropathy (majority Caucasians and Hispanics) are other described forms of immune-mediated renal disease.

HBV and HCV both more common in injecting IV drug users, are important co-infections and may individually cause renal disease.

HCV-associated cryoglobulinaemic glomerulonephritis is found in both HIV- and non-HIV-infected patients, but is more aggressive in the former. Typical presentation includes purpura, arthralgias, and peripheral neuropathy, Raynaud's phenomena in addition to renal insufficiency.

HBV, syphilis, and malignancy may all cause membranous nephropathy, and are all found more frequently in those with HIV infection.

Clinical features

Slowly progressive and mild compared with HIVAN. Typical early features are asymptomatic proteinuria and microscopic haematuria, with mild renal insufficiency.

Diagnosis

- Serum cryoglobulin measurement (blood collected must not be allowed to cool, generally kept warm in sand).
- Complement level ↓.
- Detection of other infection(s), e.g. syphilis, HBV, and HCV.
- Renal biopsy if required: membranoproliferative glomerulonephritis.

Management

- Treat any co-infection or malignancy.
- ART.

Thrombotic microangiopathy

Appears to be the most common microvascular injury associated with HIV. May be associated with malignancy (lymphoma), other infections (herpes, CMV), or drugs (valaciclovir, circumstantial). Thrombotic thrombocytopenic purpura and haemolytic uraemic syndrome occur, characterized by micro-angiopathic haemolytic anaemia with renal insufficiency, thrombocytopenia, fever, and neurological changes. Mean age at presentation 35 years with 80% males. Poor prognosis in HIV, with mortality of 66–100%. Investigations may show fragmented red cells on blood film, thrombocytopaenia, anaemia, ↑ bilirubin, ↑ LDH, renal dysfunction. Massive proteinuria is uncommon (unlike immune-mediated disease and HIVAN). ART and plasmapheresis are the mainstay of therapy. Steroids may be helpful. Splenectomy may be helpful in refractory cases.

Interstitial nephritis

Not uncommon and may be associated with other renal pathology, such as HIVAN. Equal prevalence in black and Caucasian people. May present with proteinuria, renal failure, or nephrotic syndrome. Acute interstitial nephritis related to allergic drug reactions presents with acute renal failure, skin rash, and eosinophilia. NSAIDs are a common cause.

Acute renal failure and HIV seroconversion

Acute renal failure and nephrotic syndrome may be presenting features of acute HIV seroconversion. Renal biopsy typically shows acute tubular necrosis and mesangio-proliferative glomerulonephritis, with tubuloreticular inclusions.

Drugs and renal disease

- The overall incidence of severe renal dysfunction in patients taking anti-retrovirals is <1%.
- *Indinavir*: ~4% develop nephrolithiasis, prevented by ample fluid intake (>2 L/day). Nephrolithiasis reported with other PIs (e.g. atazanavir, 0.97% prevalence, high risk of recurrence).
- *Ritonavir*: interstitial nephritis.
- *Tenofovir*: far more common with TDF than TAF—renal tubular dysfunction with hypophosphataemia, normoglycaemic glycosuria, and proteinuria (late phenomenon). Fanconi's syndrome may develop. Phosphate should be monitored monthly, then 3-monthly after 1 year.
- Dose adjustment is not necessary for PI and NNRTI, but most NRTI require dose adjustment (see Table 50.1) with renal dysfunction and creatinine clearance <60 mL/min. Need to split fixed-dose combinations.

Table 50.1 NRTI dose adjustments

Antiretroviral		Dose adjustment	
Protease inhibitors, NNRTI, integrase inhibitors, abacavir, and enfuviritide		No dose adjustment (fixed dose combinations need to be split)	
	Normal dose	eGFR	Dose
Emtricitabine	200mg od	30–49	200mg 48-hourly
		15–29	200mg 72-hourly
		<15 or HD*	200mg 96-hourly
Lamivudine	300mg od	30–49	150mg 24-hourly
		15–29	×1 150 mg then 100 mg 24-hourly
		5–14	×1 150 mg then 50 mg 24-hourly
		<5 or HD	×1 50 mg then 25 mg 24-hourly
Tenofovir disoproxil fumarate	300mg od	30–49	300mg 48-hourly
		10–29	300mg twice weekly (72–96-hourly)
		<10	No recommendation
		HD	300mg every 7 days
Tenofovir alafenamide/ emtricitabine (Descovy®)	od	<30	Not recommended
Tenofovir disoproxil fumarate/ emtricitabine (Truvada®)	od	30–49	1tablet every 48 hours
		<30	Not recommended
Maraviroc	Differs depending on combination	<30 without CYP3A inducer/ inhibitor	300mg bd
		<30 with CYP3A inducer/ inhibitor	Not recommended

*HD, haemodialysis.

Other diseases (less commonly reported)

- Minimal change disease.
- Amyloidosis.
- Renal malignancy.

End-stage renal disease

Dialysis should be considered (haemodialysis is currently the preferred method). May only be required on a temporary basis until ART is introduced. Cadaver renal transplantation has been performed with no evidence of ↑ rate of opportunistic infections or rejection.

HIV: cardiovascular disorders

Introduction *590*
Pericardial effusion *590*
Myocarditis *590*
Dilated cardiomyopathy *591*
Endocarditis *591*
Pulmonary hypertension *592*
Venous thrombosis *592*
Cardiac neoplasia *592*
Vascular disease *593*
Drug-associated disorders *593*

Introduction

Reports of the prevalence of cardiac involvement in patients with AIDS vary from 28% to 73%, with the first case of myocardial KS, found at autopsy in 1983.

Since the introduction of ART, a sharp ↓ in mortality and morbidity has been observed. New risk factors for coronary heart disease such as increased insulin resistance, dyslipidaemia, and lipodystrophy syndrome, which can be associated with ART, may accelerate underlying arteriosclerosis in HIV-infected patients.

Pericardial effusion

Prior to the introduction of ART, the frequency of this complication was estimated to be 5–46%, and fibrinous pericarditis has been identified at autopsy in 9–62% of deceased AIDS patients. It is often small with no haemodynamic consequences, although if large, it may cause tamponade. It is associated with low CD4 count and reported causes include bacteria, *Mycobacterium* spp., *Cryptococcus neoformans*, CMV, tumours (lymphoma, KS). Clinically similar to non-HIV-infected patients, and although usually seen in advanced HIV infection, rarely causes death.

Pericardial aspiration, +/– biopsy may be needed, particularly if no other source of infection found, often culture negative. Should be sent for bacterial, fungal, and TB culture. Histology should be done and special staining for viruses, fungal, and TB carried out.

Treatment is of the underlying cause.

Myocarditis

Prior to ART autopsy, evidence was found in 40–52% of those with AIDS, with a specific cause found in <20% (the most common being *Toxoplasma gondii, Mycobacterium tuberculosis, Histoplasma* and *Cryptococcus neoformans*). HIV alone can cause myocarditis, HIV or its proteins have been found in the myocardium of patients with or without cardiac disease.

Presents with chest pain and symptoms of cardiac dysfunction. May have abnormal ECG (T-wave inversion common or saddle-shaped ST elevation if associated with pericarditis) in the absence of ischaemic heart disease.

Myocardial biopsy may be indicated, especially if CD4 ↓, severe dysfunction, and no other cause evident.

Dilated cardiomyopathy

Prevalence in patients with AIDS is 10–30% by echocardiographic and autopsy studies. Associated with advanced disease. Several studies have supported a direct role for HIV as the cause of cardiac injury, but the mechanism remains unclear. Other viruses, such as group B coxsackie virus, CMV, or EBV have been implicated (found in >80% of heart histology specimens). Consider drugs and alcohol. The patient will present with shortness of breath, persistent tachycardia, and signs of heart failure. Echocardiogram is of use in diagnosis. Myocardial biopsy may be indicated to identify a cause, but associated with mortality. The overall prognosis is poor.

Endocarditis

Non-bacterial thrombotic endocarditis

Friable fibrinous clumps of platelets and red blood cells adherent to cardiac valves (usually tricuspid in HIV infection) without an inflammatory reaction. Occurs in 3–5% of those with AIDS, usually aged >50 years. Associated with malignancy, hypercoagulable states, and chronic wasting disease. Emboli may occur in up to 42%, normally involving lungs, but if on left side, valves may involve the brain, spleen, kidneys, and coronary arteries. They are usually asymptomatic, but rarely may be fatal.

Infective endocarditis

Occurs most commonly in PWIDs, usually affecting the tricuspid valve. The main causative organisms are *Staphylococcus aureus* (75%) and *Streptococcus viridans* (20%). *Candida*, and *Aspergillus* spp. may rarely cause endocarditis.

Usually presents with fever, sweats, weight loss, peripheral signs of endocarditis (splinter haemorrhages, Osler nodes, Janeway lesions, and Roth's spots), and co-existing pneumonia (often necrotic with abscess formation), mycotic aneurysms and/or meningitis. A murmur is normally heard. Transthoracic echocardiogram is important, if negative may need to do transoesophageal echocardiogram to confirm diagnosis. ↑ Mortality in advanced HIV.

Treatment is with IV antibiotics, sensitive *S. aureus* 4–6 weeks IV flucloxacillin, *S. viridans* 2–4 weeks amoxicillin.

Pulmonary hypertension

→ Chapter 45, 'Pulmonary vascular disease', pp. 537–8.

HIV is an independent risk factor for the development of pulmonary hypertension. The true incidence is not known, but reported incidence in symptomatic patients is 0.3–0.5%, × 50 that in the general population. The precise pathogenesis is unknown. The stage of HIV infection is unrelated to the development and progression of pulmonary hypertension and it may pre-date the diagnosis of HIV disease. Found most commonly in young ♂.

Progressive dyspnoea followed by ankle oedema are the usual presenting features. Diagnosed after excluding other causes, e.g. thrombo-embolism, talc granuloma (particularly in PWIDs). Echocardiogram may show right ventricular dilatation and right heart vascular studies may be required to confirm the diagnosis. The response to pulmonary vasodilator agents, and anticoagulation therapy is variable. The prognosis is poor compared with 1° pulmonary hypertension. Inconsistent reports of improvement with ART.

Venous thrombosis

↑ Risk of venous thromboembolic disease leading to deep venous thrombosis and consequently pulmonary embolism. Related to changes in coagulation (see Chapter 53, 'Coagulation disorders', p. 606).

Cardiac neoplasia

Kaposi's sarcoma

In autopsy studies, mostly MSM incidence of cardiac KS prior to ART was 12–28% (usually part of disseminated involvement). Typical cardiac sites are the visceral layer of serous pericardium or sub-epicardial fat (especially beside a major coronary artery). Clinical features are often negligible. May cause pericardial effusion, which can produce cardiac tamponade requiring emergency paracentesis. If suspected, diagnosis can be confirmed by biopsy through a pericardial window, which also provides decompression.

Non-Hodgkin's lymphoma

Usually part of disseminated neoplasia, rather than primary cardiac lymphoma (very rare). Typically high grade, with spread often early in those with AIDS. Any heart chamber may be involved, but right atrium is the most common. Usually, no specific symptoms, but may present with progressive congestive heart failure, pericardial effusion, cardiac arrhythmia, or cardiac tamponade. Nodular or polypoid lymphomas may appear, predominantly involving the pericardium with variable myocardial infiltration. Their removal may alleviate mechanical obstruction. Prognosis is poor, although clinical remission has been observed with ART and combination chemotherapy.

Cardiovascular disease

May be directly caused by HIV with infected monocytes and macrophages, producing atheroma by adhesion or angiitis. There is also evidence of inflammation and T-cell changes leading to increased risk of atherosclerosis, elite controllers of HIV have higher rate of coronary artery plaques than HIV −ve. PLWH on average are more likely to have risk factors for cardiovascular disease, including smoking, hypertension, and dyslipidaemia. Co-infection with HCV increases risk of cardiovascular disease.

Overall the risk of MI is ×2 among HIV +ve vs HIV −ve population. This risk is increased in those with CD4 <200 cells/μl and may not be significantly increased in those with well-preserved CD4 counts. The risk of stroke is also increased.

ART, especially containing PIs, except atazanavir, may cause hyperlipidaemia leading to atherosclerosis and thrombosis. Hyperlipidaemia is found to a lesser extent with the nucleoside/nucleotide reverse transcriptase inhibitors (especially stavudine) and the non-nucleoside reverse transcriptase inhibitors. Insulin resistance (associated with PIs) is an independent risk factor for MI and death. Although abacavir was implicated in early cohort studies large meta-analysis are less supportive of this. Overall, ART leads to reduced risk of MI and benefits outweigh risk associated with higher lipid levels. ART treatment interruption appears to ↑ risk probably through inflammatory mechanisms.

Other cardiovascular risk factors are important to consider, especially cigarette smoking as higher rates have been reported in MSM with HIV infection. Advice on low-fat diets, regular exercise, BP control, lipid-lowering drugs, and smoking cessation are important in patient care (see Chapter 49, 'Metabolic disorders', pp. 576–9).

Drug-associated disorders

Cardiomyopathy may be caused by zidovudine (also myocarditis), doxorubicin, amphotericin B, and foscarnet, dysrhythmias by ganciclovir and interferon alfa α, and conduction defects by co-trimoxazole, pentamidine, and pyrimethamine.

Chapter 52

HIV: musculoskeletal disorders

Introduction 596
Pathogenesis of autoimmunity in HIV 596
Inflammatory arthropathies 597
Infections 599
Osteopenia and osteoporosis 600
Neoplasia 600
Muscle disease 601
Rheumatic disease in ART era 601

Introduction

Before the use of ART, diseases characterized by CD8 expansion dominated, e.g. reactive arthritis, painful articular syndrome, DILS, and psoriatic arthritis. With ART, new phenomena emerged, such as osteoporosis, immune reconstitution inflammatory syndrome, sarcoidosis, and metabolic abnormalities.

Musculoskeletal problems are commonly reported in PLWH, up to 65% in some sub-Saharan Africa cohorts. However, studies show that they are likely to be influenced by HIV risk factors:

- People who inject drugs (PWIDs) and haemophiliacs are more susceptible to septic arthritis and osteomyelitis.
- MSM are more likely to develop SARA.

Joint symptoms may also be a feature of other conditions found more commonly in those with HIV infection, e.g. haemophilia (with haemarthrosis), syphilis, gonorrhoea, HBV and HCV, and chlamydial infections. They may also be due to the side effects of drugs used to treat HIV and related conditions.

Autoantibodies are commonly produced (although in low titres), except when CD4 counts are very low and may re-appear with immune reconstitution following ART. When CD4 count is >500 cells/µL following treatment, autoimmune diseases may occur. Diseases reported very rarely include systemic lupus erythematosus, vasculitis, polymyositis, Raynaud's phenomenon, Behçet's disease, 1° biliary cirrhosis, and Graves' disease. Immune complex vasculitis is associated with counts of 200–499 cells/µL and spondyloarthropathy with counts <200 cells/µL.

Pathogenesis of autoimmunity in HIV

Rheumatic diseases encountered in HIV correlate with the degree of immune suppression. T-regulatory cells expressing CD4 are specifically depleted in HIV infection. They are responsible for the maintenance of self-tolerance and help protect against the development of autoimmunity. The death of T-cells may release proteins that prompt formation of autoreactive CD8+ cells. Cytokine production is important in HIV pathogenesis, and possibly contributes to the development of autoimmune complications. During 1° HIV infection, tumour necrosis factor, IL-6, Il-12, and interferon-γ can be detected. These cytokines are associated with chronic inflammation. Molecular mimicry similar to other virus-triggered/mediated autoimmune diseases may also occur.

Inflammatory arthropathies

Arthralgia

Most common joint manifestation occurring in up to 45% of cases. Pathology is unclear but may involve cytokines or transient bone ischaemia. Can occur at any stage of HIV disease and may be the first manifestation. Usually mild to moderate in intensity.

In up to 10% of those with advanced HIV infection, a painful transient articular syndrome, characterized by an acute onset of severe pain in up to four joints, has been described. Knee most commonly affected, with shoulder and elbow also involved. Symptoms may mimic acute septic arthritis, but no effusion, synovitis, or ↑ in joint fluid white cells. Radiology normal or may show peri-articular osteopenia. Treat with standard analgesics/NSAIDs, although opioids may be required.

Diffuse idiopathic lymphocytic syndrome

Similar to Sjögren's syndrome and found at any stage of HIV infection, caused by CD8+ T-cell oligoclonal expansion. Presents with salivary gland enlargement (parotid swelling may be massive), xerostomia, xerophthalmia, peripheral neuropathy, myositis, and arthralgia. Occasional pulmonary infiltrates can mimic pneumocystis. The incidence of DILS has ↓ since the introduction of ART. Treat with artificial saliva and tears in addition to ART.

Acute symmetrical polyarthritis

Presentation similar to rheumatoid arthritis (RA), with involvement of small joints of the hand leading to ulnar deviation of the digits and swan-neck deformities. May be differentiated from RA by acute onset and negative rheumatoid factor. Radiological appearances similar to RA with peri-articular osteopenia, joint-space narrowing, and marginal erosions.

Patients with RA may go into remission when they become infected with HIV, but some progress to destructive disease, despite having low CD4 counts. IRIS has been associated with new-onset RA. Respond to standard disease-modifying anti-rheumatic drugs (DMARDs). Gold treatment may be required. Immunosuppression may be relatively contraindicated.

HIV-associated arthritis

Asymmetrical oligoarticular arthritis. Possibly caused by effects of local infection (HIV detected in joint fluid). More common in ♂. Typically, presents with sudden onset of severe pain, mainly affecting knees and ankles. Self-limiting, usually lasting from a few weeks to 6 months. Synovial fluid commonly contains up to 2500 white blood cells/μL, negative autoimmune screen. Radiology may show osteopenia, but no erosions. A chronic mononuclear cell infiltrate is found on synovial biopsy. Treat with NSAIDs or intra-articular corticosteroid injections for symptomatic relief.

Hypertrophic osteoarthropathy

May appear as a complication of PCP. Affects bones, joints, and soft tissues. Presents with severe pain in the lower limbs, arthralgia, non-pitting oedema, and finger clubbing. Skin over affected areas (ankle, knees, and elbows) is shiny, warm, and oedematous. Extensive periosteal reaction and sub-periosteal proliferative changes in the long bones of the legs are found on radiology, with bone scans showing ↑ uptake along the cortical surfaces. Usually responds to treatment of underlying PCP.

Reactive arthritis

Probably no more frequent in those with HIV infection, but tends to be more severe. Lower limb peripheral arthritis predominates. Synovial fluid is inflammatory (a few thousand polymorphonuclear leucocytes per ml) and sterile with a glucose level at least 66% of the serum level. Treat initially with NSAIDs (as in HIV –ve patients). Other drugs may be required, e.g. gold, methotrexate (with caution as immunosuppressive), and other disease-modifying agents. ART is likely to be beneficial.

Psoriatic arthritis

More common (×20–40) and severe than in HIV –ve individuals. Usually polyarticular and asymmetrical. Extra-articular manifestations occur in >50%. Usually insidious, with the appearance of bone erosions within weeks or months. Radiological findings include peri-articular erosions, asymmetric destruction of distal interphalangeal joints. Joint and tendon involvement in HIV-associated psoriatic arthritis tends to be less responsive to NSAIDs (still first line therapy). Methotrexate and azathioprine are effective, but require careful monitoring because of myelosuppression. Sulfasalazine may be helpful, but skin rash occurs in 30%. Low-dose systemic corticosteroids are ineffective. Retinoids, phototherapy, etanercept, adalimumab, and infliximab reported to improve the skin and joints in some.

Osteonecrosis (avascular necrosis)

Result of direct damage to the vascular supply, leading to death of subchondral bone. Additional risks are prior use of corticosteroids, testosterone, or anabolic steroids, hyperlipidaemia, hypercoagulability, sickle cell disease, alcohol abuse, and smoking. No link to ART found. Most common site is femoral head followed by humeral head, with bilateral involvement in 40%. May be asymptomatic or cause severe disabling deep pain. Plain X-rays may be normal; MRI is recommended. In early stages rest may be adequate, but in advanced disease joint replacement or other surgery may be required.

Infections

Septic arthritis

Usually, mono-articular, with the hip being most frequently affected, although in PWIDs there may be sternoclavicular joint involvement. *Staphylococcus aureus* followed by *Streptococcus pneumoniae* are the most common causative organisms. If CD4 count <100 cells/µL multiple joint involvement and associated skin infection may occur with opportunistic infections (e.g. MAC, cryptococcosis, sporotrichosis). Diagnosed by Gram stain and culture of synovial fluid. Blood cultures may be positive before synovial cultures. Treat with appropriate antibiotics (usually IV flucloxacillin or cephalosporin) and monitor inflammatory markers.

Osteomyelitis

- *Septic osteomyelitis*: may follow direct extension or haematogenous spread from an infected joint. Suspect if septic arthritis fails to respond despite adequate treatment.
- *Tuberculous osteomyelitis*: develops from the haematogenous spread of an acute or reactivated infection. The spine, especially the thoracic and lumbar regions, is most commonly affected, starting in the vertebral body, and spreading to the adjacent disc spaces. Vertebral wedging leads to gibbus formation. In addition to antibiotics, surgical intervention with irrigation and debridement may be required.

Bacillary angiomatosis due to *Bartonella henselae* may cause osteomyelitis. Occurs in the immunosuppressed and is characterized by vascular proliferation involving the nervous system (aseptic meningitis, intracerebral mass lesions), liver (peliosis hepatitis), lymph nodes (adenitis), and bone.

Osteopenia and osteoporosis

HIV infection is associated with ↓ BMD determined by measurement of X-ray absorption, e.g. DEXA scan. A DEXA scan T-score (number of SDs from the mean value in young, healthy individuals) is diagnostic. Scores between −1 and −2.5 indicate osteopenia (pre-symptomatic) and −2.5 or less indicates osteoporosis.

Osteopenia is found in up to 65% of those with HIV infection and osteoporosis in up to 25%. Duration of infection is significantly associated. Other factors are HIV wasting, low BMI, malnutrition, immobilization, hypogonadism, menopause, steroids, alcohol excess, and smoking. ART, especially with protease inhibitors, has been suggested as a contributor, but evidence is conflicting. Tenofovir leads to ↓ BMD; hypophosphataemia may be a contributing factor.

Occur mainly in the vertebrae, lower arms, and hips. Osteoporosis is often asymptomatic, but may cause pain (low back, neck, hip), loss of height, kyphosis, and fractures.

Estimate fracture risk with online FRAX score. Consider DEXA if postmenopausal, men ≥50 years, 40–50 years history of fracture, and chronic steroid use with high FRAX high fracture risk (age dependent) 10-year fracture risk.

Bone metabolism should be assessed (serum calcium, phosphate, and alkaline phosphatase, vitamin D level).

Management should include advice on diet and exercise, and avoidance of alcohol/nicotine. Osteopenia can be managed with vitamin D (400–800 IU daily) if vit D deficient and calcium supplements (calcium-rich diet or calcium tablets 1.2 g/day). Osteoporosis should be treated with bisphosphonates (with additional vitamin D and calcium supplementation), repeat DEXA at 2 years and reassess need for bisphosphonates at 3-5yrs.

Neoplasia

Non-Hodgkin's lymphoma

Bone involvement occurs in 20–30%. May present as a pathological fracture, especially of the lower limbs. Radiology shows an area of osteolysis with cortical destruction. A periosteal reaction and soft tissue mass may also be present. Findings similar to bacterial osteomyelitis, therefore, biopsy recommended. Treated with chemotherapy, radiation, and possibly surgical debridement.

Kaposi's sarcoma

Rarely reported and usually associated with widespread dissemination. Frequently asymptomatic, otherwise bone pain, with radiology either normal or demonstrating lesions usually lytic, occasionally sclerotic. Diagnosis by biopsy. Radiotherapy may alleviate bone pain.

Muscle disease

Myopathy is uncommon and a polymyositis syndrome occurs very rarely. The most important cause of myopathy is prolonged zidovudine therapy, associated with ↑ creatinine kinase level in 16% and symptomatic weakness in 6%. Treatment involves discontinuation of the drug and NSAIDs, but some patients may require prednisolone (starting with 60–80 mg daily, reducing over several months) to restore muscle strength.

Myopathy may occur with previous D4T/DDI treatment and may be progressive over lifetime. It is probably caused by mitochondrial dysfunction because of the inhibition of mitochondrial DNA γ-polymerase by NRTI (AZT, D4T or DDI). Muscle weakness and wasting is proximal, with preserved reflexes and sensory function. Electromyographical evidence of myopathy is found in >90%. Ragged red fibres (due to the accumulation of abnormal mitochondria) may be seen on muscle biopsy.

Rheumatic disease in ART era

A new spectrum of disorders has appeared, e.g. osteonecrosis, rhabdomyolysis, and IRIS. The frequency of reactive arthritis and psoriatic arthritis ↓ in ART era.

Rhabdomyolysis is more frequently a complication of anti-lipid drugs, e.g. when PIs are combined with statins.

Adhesive capsulitis, Dupuytren contractures, tenosynovitis, and temporomandibular joint dysfunction have been reported as a consequence of indinavir treatment.

Hypergammaglobulinaemia, positive rheumatoid factor, antinuclear antibodies, cryoglobulinaemia (consider HCV or HBV co-infection), and anticardiolipin antibodies (low titres), all previously more common, are less frequent with ART.

Immune reconstitution inflammatory syndrome

Unexpected exacerbation of inflammatory disease and atypical clinical features that resemble the symptoms of autoimmune disease can arise as part of IRIS. Autoimmune diseases such as Graves autoimmune thyroiditis, pulmonary sarcoidosis, systemic lupus erythematosus, RA, and polymyositis may occur. Most cases arise *de novo*, but >20% are flares of pre-existing diseases (often mild) that were in remission due to immunosuppression 2° to HIV. IRIS most often a reaction to underlying undiagnosed infections e.g. MAC.

ART should be continued with IRIS as most symptoms will resolve. However, if the inflammatory process involves certain areas, e.g. CNS where damage is likely to occur, steroids should be considered, ART may need to be held.

HIV: reticulo-endothelial disorders

Haematological disorders 604
Persistent generalized lymphadenopathy 607

Haematological disorders

Haematological abnormalities may be direct effect of HIV itself or 2° to concurrent infection, malignancy, or therapeutic agents. Common findings are ↓ haemopoiesis, altered coagulation, and immune-mediated cytopenias with ↓ bone marrow cellularity and dysplasia.

Anaemia

Most common form of cytopenia and an independent prognostic factor; 8% of all PLWH and 50–75% of patients with AIDS. Usually due to ↓ erythropoiesis, but other mechanisms (e.g. infection, drug toxicity, malignancy, dietary deficiencies, alcohol abuse, blood loss) may contribute. Chronic anaemia causes fatigue, exertional dyspnoea, and a hyperdynamic state that, if severe, may lead to angina, congestive cardiac failure, and confusion.

Diagnosis and evaluation

Examine and test for iron, vitamin B_{12}, and folate deficiencies, haemolysis, and blood loss according to red cell indices. Eliminate possible causes by excluding infection and malignancy, and reviewing drug therapy. Bone marrow examination may be required, particularly if pancytopaenia and common causes excluded.

- *HIV-related*: normocytic normochromic anaemia ↑ in frequency and severity as HIV progresses. May be a direct effect of HIV on bone marrow progenitor cells, ↓ erythropoietin production, and ↑ cytokines (inhibit haemopoiesis). Improves or normalizes with ART provided that drug effects do not supervene.
- *Drug toxicity*:
  - *Macrocytosis and normal haemoglobin*—typical with AZT.
  - *Macrocytic anaemia*—caused by AZT. AZT exerts broader myelosuppressive effects, more frequent in patients receiving higher doses (in ≈1% receiving 500 mg/day) and those with advanced disease. Improves following discontinuation. Anaemia may require blood transfusion following discontinuation of AZT.
  - *Normocytic normochromic anaemia*—associated with normal or ↓ reticulocyte count, 2° to bone marrow suppression. Causes include anaemia of chronic infection and drugs (e.g. ganciclovir, co-trimoxazole, amphotericin, and interferons).
  - Haemolytic *anaemia*—features are macrocytosis, ↓ haptoglobin, and ↑ lactic dehydrogenase, indirect bilirubin, and ↑ reticulocyte count. Common causes include drugs, e.g. dapsone (with methaemoglobinaemia), ribavirin, and primaquine. Glucose 6 phosphate dehydrogenase (G6PD) deficiency predisposes to dapsone and primaquine haemolysis. Autoimmune haemolytic anaemia (AIHA) with positive Coombs' test also occurs.
  - *Bone marrow infiltration (usually causes pancytopenia)*:
  - *OI*—most commonly MAC (also TB and CMV).
  - *Tumours*—lymphoma and rarely KS.

- Parvovirus B19 infects erythroid precursors. In immune deficiency, persistent infection may result in severe chronic normocytic normochromic anaemia. Diagnosed by detecting B19 parvovirus antibodies and PCR for B19 in serum and/or bone marrow. Responds well to high-dose IV immunoglobulins (0.4 g/kg/day), which contain parvovirus antibodies, but may require repeated blood transfusions.

Thrombocytopenia

Occurs in around 6–9%. HIV-related immune thrombocytopenia is a frequent early finding, tending to deteriorate as HIV progresses. Commonly an isolated haematological abnormality. Results from clearance of immunoglobulin-coated platelets by reticulo-endothelial system. with ↑ levels of antiplatelet immunoglobulin. May be result of drug toxicity, immune and non- immune destruction, or defective platelet production.

Diagnosis and evaluation
Exclude underlying causes, e.g. drug toxicity, liver disease, alcoholism, and lymphoma. Further investigation not usually necessary, presence of normal or ↑ megakaryocytes on bone marrow examination is sufficient to diagnose HIV-induced thrombocytopenia.

Treatment
- Mild and *asymptomatic*: ART, switch/discontinue implicated drugs.
- *Symptomatic or before surgical procedures*: IV immunoglobulins, steroids, and ART.
- *Substantial bleeding*: packed red cells and platelet transfusion.

Thrombotic thrombocytopenic purpura

Rare, of unknown aetiology, usually seen in early stages of HIV infection. Characterized by hyaline microvascular deposits on biopsy. Clinical features include fever, renal impairment, neurological deficit, and microangiopathic haemolytic anaemia. Mortality rate 65% without treatment. There may be response to plasmapheresis, steroids, ART, and antiplatelets (e.g. aspirin).

Neutropenia

HIV directly implicated, especially in advanced stages. More commonly due to drug toxicity, associated infection, and bone marrow infiltration. Risk of bacterial infection ↑ significantly when absolute neutrophil count <500 cells/µL. Drugs causing neutropenia include AZT, ganciclovir, co-trimoxazole, pentamidine, interferon alfa α, and chemotherapeutic agents.

Diagnosis and evaluation
Careful review of medication. Withdraw offending drug(s) if absolute neutrophil count <500 cells/µL. If cause uncertain, consider bone marrow examination.

Treatment
- *ART*: variable response.
- *Granulocyte colony stimulating factor*:
  - HIV-induced
  - drug-induced (if implicated drug cannot be reduced or stopped).

Coagulation disorders

↑ Risk of thrombotic disease associated with low CD4 counts, OIs, neo-plasms, and HIV-associated autoimmune disorders.

- *High inflammatory state*: ↑ D-dimer and cytokines are found in advanced disease.
- Lupus anticoagulant may be detected with thrombo-embolic disease.
- ↓ Levels of active protein S frequently found, not associated with immune suppression.
- Contributing prothrombotic factors include ↓ plasminogen activator inhibitor level, abnormal platelet aggregation, and ↑ von Willebrand factor.
- ART does not fully reverse pro-coagulant effect of HIV.

Persistent generalized lymphadenopathy

Generalized lymphadenopathy involving two extra-inguinal sites persisting for more than 3 months. Of no prognostic significance, but other causes of generalized lymphadenopathy should be excluded (see box). Occurs in up to 70% of patients within 1 year of seroconversion, but may co-exist with other manifestations of HIV infection. Lymph nodes usually symmetrical, >1 cm in size, rubbery, and non-tender. May be accompanied by hepatosplenomegaly. Biopsy for histology and culture should be done in those with systemic symptoms of fever, weight loss or if inflammatory markers are raised or large lymph nodes that increase in size overtime. Mediastinal lymphadenopathy usually has other causes and should be investigated.

Important diagnoses to consider in HIV-associated lymphadenopathy
- Persistent generalized lymphadenopathy.
- Bacterial infections (including mycobacteria).
- 2° syphilis.
- Lymphoma.
- Histoplasmosis.
- Multicentric Castleman's disease.

HIV: malignancies

Introduction 610
Kaposi's sarcoma 611
Non-Hodgkin's lymphoma 614
Multicentric Castleman's disease 617
Hodgkin's disease 617
Invasive cervical carcinoma 617
Anal carcinoma 618
Leiomyosarcoma 618
Lung cancer 618
Hepatocellular carcinoma 619

Introduction

The overall incidence of many malignancies ↑ in patients with HIV. The incidence increases as the CD4 count falls below 500 cells/μL. Certain malignancies occur more frequently in HIV infection, especially when immunosuppressed, and are often associated with other viral co-infection.

The following are designated as AIDS-defining illnesses:

- KS
- high-grade B-cell non-Hodgkin lymphoma (NHL) and primary cerebral lymphoma (PCL)
- Invasive cervical carcinoma (ICC).

Other associated malignant conditions include SCC (anogenital, conjunctival, labial, and glossal), multicentric Castleman's disease, testicular tumours (seminomas), melanomas, Hodgkin's disease, multiple myeloma, leiomyosarcoma in children, liver cancer, and lung cancer. Some data suggest no ↑ risk of other cancers, e.g. colon and breast cancer.

The following viral infections contribute to the induction of malignant disease HIV-infected patients.

- *HHV-8*: KS and 1° effusion lymphomas. Found in 100% of multicentric Castleman's disease.
- *HPV*: anogenital and occasionally oral carcinomas.
- *EBV*: NHL.
- *HBV and HCV*: hepatocellular carcinoma.

Other factors, such as sexual practices and cigarette smoking, may play a part.

Overall risk of malignancy is doubled in a HIV-infected population. Natural history of malignancy may be altered in HIV infection with advanced rapidly progressive disease more likely. Treatment may be made difficult because of ↑ sensitivity to side effects of chemotherapy if immunosuppressed, drug interactions, and ↓ bone marrow reserve. ART has had a dramatic effect on the incidence of some tumours, particularly cerebral lymphoma; however, lifetime risk of some cancers, such as liver and anal cancer remains ↑ despite ART.

ART: PI-r therapy often avoided when chemotherapy considered as significant interactions, NNRTI or INSTI with backbone preferred.

All patients should be treated in large centres with good liaison between HIV physician, oncology, haematology, palliative care, specialist pharmacists, and nurse.

Kaposi's sarcoma

Initially described in 1872 by Moritz Kaposi and rare before HIV epidemic. There are four different types:

- *Classic*: usually elderly ♂ from eastern Mediterranean/Europe. Causes multiple skin lesions of lower limbs.
- *Endemic*: equatorial Africa. More virulent than classic, often affecting lower limbs.
- *Acquired*: people on immunosuppressant therapy. Resolves when drugs stopped.
- *Epidemic*: associated with HIV infection. Variable, but generally more aggressive than other types.

Caused by HHV-8 (found in >90% of KS lesions) spread sexually, by mother-to-child contact and organ transplant. In MSM, new HHV-8 infection is associated with an HIV +ve partner. No evidence to support transmission by semen (HHV-8 rarely detected) and conflicting data on the role of rimming.

Epidemic KS

Most common malignancy associated with HIV infection. Before ART, it was the AIDS-defining disease in 15–20% of MSM (found in up to 50% of patients with AIDS by mid-1980s). The incidence of KS has ↓ after ART introduction, still ×500 more likely in HIV +ve vs HIV −ve population. Predominantly found in MSM and rare among IDU, haemophiliacs and ♀ (where more aggressive and usually associated with HIV acquisition from bisexual ♂). KS found more commonly in those with advanced disease, but may occur with preserved CD4 count. Prevalence of KS in different HIV populations reflects the background seroprevalence for HHV-8.

Clinical features

Skin lesions

May occur on any part of the body, but facial involvement common (margin of nostrils, tip of the nose, and eyelids; Plate 34). Typical pigmented macules, papules, plaques, and nodules ranging in size from several millimetres to many centimetres. Colour varies from pink to deep purple with a yellow or green halo (extravasated erythrocyte pigments) characteristically surrounding them (plates 32–35). Colourless SC nodules may also be found. In dark-skinned people the lesions are dark brown or black (plate 34, 35). Ulceration of nodules may lead to bleeding or infection. Large painful plaques may appear, especially on thighs and soles of feet. Pain suggests more progressive disease.

 Biopsy should be taken to confirm diagnosis.

Oral lesions

Found in around 33% of those with epidemic KS, usually affecting hard palate (also gingiva, tongue, uvula, tonsils, pharynx, and trachea). Often asymptomatic. Usually appear as focal or diffuse red/purple plaques, which may become nodular and ulcerate. May indicate more extensive mucosal involvement.

Others

- Visceral disease occurs in 14%.
- *GI tract*: unless symptomatic their presence does not influence prognosis. May occur without skin lesions, and may cause GI bleeding or obstruction.
- *Respiratory*: may involve lung parenchyma, bronchial tree, and pleura, leading to large blood-stained pleural effusions. Usual symptoms dyspnoea, haemoptysis, cough, and wheezing. Radiology often shows ill-defined nodules or areas of infiltration. Biopsy generally not recommended due to risk of bleeding.
- *Lymph nodes*: modest lymphadenopathy common. Rarely massive lymphadenopathy (possibly without KS elsewhere) necessitating diagnostic biopsy. Extensive lymphadenopathy may suggest co-existing Castleman's disease.
- *Lymphoedema*: non-pitting, most commonly affecting feet and legs, and may be complicated by ulceration and infection. May result from direct KS dermal lymphatic involvement.
- Hepatic, splenic, cardiac, pericardial, bone marrow involvement all rarely reported, usually at autopsy.

Social/emotional implications

Lesions often obvious and disfiguring, acting as a constant reminder, and leading to isolation, anxiety, and depression.

Diagnosis and assessment

- Biopsy should be taken to confirm diagnosis of cutaneous KS can be graded histologically into patch, plaque, or nodular. Lymph node biopsy should be considered for large lymph nodes.
- If extensive mucocutaneous disease, systemic symptoms or specific symptoms as above. Appropriate investigations include—CT scan, endoscopy, bronchoscopy.
- *HHV-8 VL tests*: higher levels are associated with poorer prognosis and may indicate other HHV8-associated diseases. HHV8 VL ↓ when KS treated with chemotherapy and ART.

Pre-ART poorer prognosis associated with severe oedema and/or ulceration, extensive mucosal lesions, visceral disease, CD4 <150 cells/μl, Karnovsky performance <70, or other HIV-related illness. Prognostic score developed in ART era-score 10 for KS; if first AIDS-defining illness −3, for each complete CD4 of 100 cells/mm^3 −1, for age ≥50 years +3, for other AIDS/poor performance status +2.

Management

ART often significantly improves KS (in up to 80%) without further intervention. ART should be offered to all patients. Additional treatment options depend on prognostic score/extent of KS These therapeutic interventions have been shown to improve survival and prolong time to KS treatment failure.

No interventional treatment: ART alone

Consider if only skin lesions and/or mild KS-associated lymphadenopathy and no additional problems. Disfiguring lesions can be cosmetically camouflaged.

Local therapy

- *Cryotherapy*: small flat lesions on thin skin (e.g. face, genitals). Repeat treatment usually required. May leave hypopigmented scar.
- *Radiotherapy*: for lesions that are painful, causing lymphatic obstruction, oropharyngeal, or ophthalmic. Side effects include local erythema, hair loss, mucositis, and pigmented scarring. Reported response rate is 74–91%. Regrowth common if no ART.
- *9-cis-retinoic acid (alitretinoin) 0.1% gel*: not licensed in Europe.
- *Intra-lesional vinblastine, vincristine, or interferon alfa α*: limited mucocutaneous disease. Painful injections causing inflammatory response before lesions shrink or disappear leaving a scar. Repeat injections required and relapse within 6 months is common.
- Excision for small lesions.

Chemotherapy

Chemotherapy strongly consider if patients have prognostic score >12, consider in clinically advanced KS, particularly with prognostic score >5. All patients should be treated with ART. Prophylaxis against PCP should be provided during chemotherapy because of risk of immunosuppression.

Liposomal chemotherapy

Liposomal doxorubicin and liposomal daunorubicin now standard of care for KS where treatment indicated. Liposomal daunorubicin (40 mg/m^2 every 2 weeks) or pegylated liposomal doxorubicin (20 mg/m^2 every 3 weeks). Preferentially absorbed by vascular KS lesions, producing targeted chemotherapy with ↓ side effects. Main side effects are bone marrow suppression (occurs in 50%), neutropenia can be treated with G-CSF, alopecia, and vomiting.

Paclitaxel

Second-line chemotherapy at a dose of 100 mg/m^2 every 14 days plus ART. More toxicity seen, including bone marrow suppression, myalgia, alopecia, and allergic reactions.

Interferon alfa α

Rarely used in the era of ART. May have a place in those with residual/progressive KS after chemotherapy. Main side-effects are flu-like symptoms, depression, and neutropenia.

Non-Hodgkin's lymphoma

NHL is the second most common HIV-associated malignancy ×12 more likely than non-HIV +ve. First cases were reported in MSM in 1982. Prior to ART, it accounted for 2–3% of AIDS-defining illnesses, with haemophiliacs and those with other clotting disorders having the highest incidence. The incidence of AIDS-related NHL has decreased since the introduction of ART, although the percentage as first AIDS-defining illness has increased.

Most NHLs are clinically aggressive monoclonal B-cell lymphomas, especially diffuse large B-cell lymphomas (DLBCL) and Burkitt's or Burkitt-like lymphomas (BLs). More common in ♂ and Caucasians. EBV episome is found in 40–50% overall, ranging from 100% of PCL to 20% of DLBCL. Other much less frequent subtypes of HIV-related lymphomas include PCL, 1° effusion lymphomas (αHHV8) and plasmablastic lymphomas.

Systemic lymphoma

Wide range of CD4 count at presentation, including normal levels, but median is 100 cells/µL. Typically, presents with lymphadenopathy, fever, weight loss (>10%), and night sweats. Extra-nodal disease (any site) usual, with GI tract, CNS, bone marrow, and liver more frequently affected. GI presentation most common, and NHL should be considered if suspicious symptoms (e.g. dysphagia, GI bleeding/pain).

Diagnosis and staging
- Biopsy of lymph node/lesion, consider bone marrow if cytopaenia.
- Staging by CT/MRI scanning, presence of B symptoms (fever, weight loss, and sweats), CSF indicated if CNS disease and bone marrow aspiration and trephine. ^{18}F-FDG PET scan should be used, but need to be aware of false +ve in HIV patients, particularly with low CD4 count.
- Prognosis depends on a number of factors and is poor if >60 years old, CD4 <100 cells/µL, ↑ LDH, lymph node involvement above and below diaphragm, extra-nodal involvement and/or poor function. Failure to attain complete remission is associated with a poor prognosis.

Management
- MDT, including HIV physician/haematology/oncology.
- *DLBCL*: chemotherapy (improved tolerance if CD4 count >200 cells/µL), usually cyclical. PCP prophylaxis should be taken. Regimen examples include the following.
  - ART+ CHOP (cyclophosphamide, hydroxydaunomycin [doxorubicin], Oncovin® [vincristine], prednisolone) should be given full dose where possible (reduced dose CHOP ↓ remission rate). Addition of G-CSF reduces neutropenia.
  - ART+ infusional chemotherapy—etoposide, prednisolone, vincristine, cyclophosphamide, and doxorubicin or cyclophosphamide, doxorubicin, and etoposide.
  - *Rituximab (monoclonal antibody causing B-cell lysis)*—may improve efficacy in combination with above regimes, but caution if CD4 <50/µL because of significant increase infection, if given consider pre-emptive G-CSF.
  - Previously responding patients should be considered for high-dose chemotherapy and stem-cell transplant if they relapse.

- Reported average complete remission 48%; >80% if good prognostic features, <30% if poor prognostic features.
- *Burkitt's lymphoma*: poorer response seen with above chemotherapy. May require more aggressive regime such as the following.
  - Cyclophosphomide, vincristine, doxorubicin, methotrexate/ifosfomide, etoposide, and cytarabine.
  - Cyclophosphomide, vincristine, doxorubicin, dexamethasone, methotrexate, and cytarabine.

Primary CNS lymphoma

- These are DLBCL or immunoblastic lymphomas confined to the CNS with no systemic involvement. It is EBV-induced, and is ×1000 more frequent in those with HIV infection. Significantly lower incidence in the ART era.
- Survival has ↑ since the introduction of ART, although its optimal use during chemotherapy has not been established.
- Associated with very low CD4 count (<50 cells/μL in 75%) and history of OIs. Usually presents with confusion, amnesia, lethargy. In addition, focal symptoms may appear (e.g. seizures, hemiparesis, cranial nerve palsies, and aphasia).

Diagnosis

Difficult to distinguish from cerebral toxoplasmosis.

- *CT/ MRI*: single (α50%) vs multiple lesions (former suggests PCL as only α20% of those with toxoplasmosis have a single lesion).
- Fundal and slit-lamp examination (20% have ocular involvement).
- *Lumbar puncture for*:
  - lymphoma cells
  - EBV DNA using PCR +ve in α90% of CNS lymphoma, but not specific.
- Toxoplasma serology (toxoplasma unlikely if negative serology).
- Combined EBV detection in CSF and hyperactive lesion on single-photon emission CT has a very high sensitivity and specificity. If available, may make brain biopsy unnecessary.
- Brain biopsy confirms the diagnosis.
- Failure to respond to 2 weeks anti-toxoplasma treatment equates to a presumptive diagnosis of PCL.

Management

- Initially, consider anti-toxoplasma therapy in any space-occupying lesion.
- ART ↑ survival, but inferior to that of other lymphomas.
- Whole-brain radiotherapy (usually with short-term dexamethasone to reduce oedema) for symptomatic palliation.
- Combined radiotherapy and chemotherapy, e.g. high-dose methotrexate and other agents that cross the blood–brain barrier.

Prognosis still poor and partly dependent on control of OIs.

Primary effusion lymphoma (body cavity lymphoma)

Accounts for 5% of HIV-associated lymphoma. Usually seen in MSM, and associated with HHV 8 and co-infection with EBV in >50%. Characteristic features include involvement of the pleural, pericardial, and abdominal cavities as lymphomatous effusions in the absence of a solid tumour mass. Cytological examination of fluid, looking for typical immunophenotype and HHV8 is required. HHV-8 viral load is helpful when high suggestive and should fall with successful treatment. Associated with multicentric Castleman's disease

Ideal treatment strategy unclear. Treat with chemotherapy (e.g. CHOP or single-agent chemotherapy), interferon alfa α. Anti-CD20 monoclonal antibody (rituximab) may also be used as first-line therapy, for relapse, or following chemotherapy. Addition of ART improves survival.

Multicentric Castleman's disease

Induced by HHV-8 in HIV infection. Characterized by recurrent lymph-adenopathy, multiple organ involvement, hepatosplenomegaly, systemic symptoms (fever, malaise, anorexia, and weight loss), effusions, and some-times KS. May occur on ART and with CD4>200 cells/μl. Neuropathy and pancytopaenia seen in some. Histological examination confirms the diag-nosis and HHV-8 viral load is helpful (>1000 copies/mL suggestive) and may predict relapse. Progression to NHL may occur.

Ideal treatment strategy unclear. Rituximab may be used as first-line therapy, for relapse, or following chemotherapy. Treat aggressive dis-ease with chemotherapy (e.g. CHOP or single-agent chemotherapy) with rituximab, interferon alfa α. ART should be given.

Hodgkin's disease

Although not an AIDS-defining illness, incidence is increased ×10–20 fold compared with HIV –ve population. Tends to be more aggressive, with the mixed cellularity subtype predominating. Associated with EBV infection, usually developing with CD4 counts of 200–300 cells/μL.

Presents with lymphadenopathy (glands often very large), Pel–Ebstein fever, anaemia, and systemic symptoms. Diagnosed by lymph node or bone marrow histology (Reed–Sternberg cells). Must have full staging assessment and bone marrow biopsy.

Treatment
- ART.
- First-line chemotherapy is doxorubicin, bleomycin, vinblastine, and dacarbazine + involved field radiotherapy.

Prognosis
ART combined with chemotherapy improves prognosis; disease-free sur-vival and complete remission rates approach those of HIV –ve patients.

Invasive cervical carcinoma

Added to the AIDS case definition in 1993, following reports showing ↑ prevalence of cervical dysplasia with HPV infection and immuno-suppression (usually severe). Cervical intra-epithelial neoplasia (CIN) is more common and recurs more in HIV +ve ♀, especially if CD4 <200/μL. Incidence of ICC in ♀ with HIV not declining.

HIV +ve ♀ should have annual cervical smear. The age range for cervical smear should be the same as for HIV –ve individuals (25yrs-64yrs).

ICC should be managed as for ♀ without HIV infection. Abnormal cy-tology should be investigated by colposcopy with biopsy of suspicious areas. Mild dyskaryosis (CIN I) should be followed every 3–6 months as spontaneous regression is common. Standard treatment for moderate/se-vere dyskaryosis (CIN II and III) consists of lesional ablation or excision. Treatment is less effective in patients with high HIV VL, not on ART and CD4 <200 cells/μl.

Anal carcinoma

Anal cancer is ×40 more frequent and occurs at younger age in HIV +ve individuals and in MSM HIV +ve. However, the excess risk amongst HIV +ve MSM is difficult to quantify as anal receptive sexual intercourse is a strong independent risk factor for the two conditions. Similar to cervical cancer, high-grade HPV is an important aetiological factor. HIV +ve individuals with anal HPV infection are significantly more likely to develop high-grade dyskaryosis or anal carcinoma if they acquire other local infections (e.g. gonorrhoea, syphilis, HSV).

Diagnosis and treatment

Similar to the female cervix, the anal canal has a TZ at the junction of the anal squamous and rectal columnar epithelia. HPV infection of metaplastic cells ↑ tendency to oncogenic transformation in the anal TZ and, thus, the development of cancer.

Anal cancer is preceded by pre-cancerous changes, AIN. The role of anal cytology and anoscopy to detect pre-cancerous changes is not yet defined. Patients should be encouraged to report any anal symptoms (bleeding, pain, discharge), and be clinically examined and referred to local specialists units, preferably with the ability to perform high-resolution anoscopy, for examination under anaesthetic (EUA) and biopsy. ART does not appear to alter AIN progression or the incidence of invasive cancer.

Anal carcinoma is treated as for those without HIV with chemoradiotherapy. CT chest, abdomen, and pelvis with MRI pelvis should be performed. Limited data are available on management of anal dyskaryosis, but current practice suggests that treatment (by excision or laser ablation) should only be considered if severe dyskaryosis (AIN3).

Leiomyosarcoma

↑ Rate in children with HIV when, unlike HIV in uninfected children, tumours are induced by EBV.

Lung cancer

The incidence of non-small-cell lung cancer, and to some extent adenocarcinoma, in HIV +ve individuals is higher than in age-matched HIV −ve controls. This difference is not explained by smoking alone. Compared with HIV −ve individuals, lung cancer usually occurs at a younger age and with advanced disease. Similar to HIV −ve individuals, it presents with cough, chest pain, haemoptysis, and dyspnoea. ART does not improve survival; median time is 4 months. Patients with operable or locally advanced disease should be treated similar to HIV −ve individuals and ART should be commenced if they are not already on it. Patients with metastatic disease may have palliative chemotherapy (poorly tolerated).

Hepatocellular carcinoma

Generally seen in context of HCV and/or HBV co-infection. Overall, poor prognosis (28% 1-year survival) in HIV +ve patients. Presents at later stage and with more aggressive tumours than HIV −ve patients.

Screening with 6-monthly liver ultrasound and AFP should be offered to HBV or HCV co-infected patients with cirrhosis and HBV patients with severe fibrosis. Patients risk is ↑ by alcohol, male sex, Asian/African origin, family history of HCC and high HBV VL.

Local resection, liver transplantation should be offered if appropriate. Radiofrequency ablation, or chemoembolization and sorafenib may be offered to bridge to transplant or as palliative treatment.

HIV: management

Introduction 622
When to start 623
How to start 625
Adherence 626
What to start 627
Monitoring and follow up 633
Vaccinations 638
Switching antiretroviral therapy 639
Stopping antiretroviral therapy 639
Antiretroviral side effects 640
Immune response 642
Antiretroviral drug–drug interactions 643
HIV drug resistance 645
Prophylaxis against infections 650

Introduction

ART has dramatically improved prognosis and life expectancy of PLWH. Many of the newer antiretrovirals (ARVs) are better tolerated with several combination tablets available, improving quality of life and reducing pill burdens.

The main principles of management of PLWH include:

- engaging and maintaining patients in regular follow-up with HIV specialist care
- prognosis improved by early initiation of ART, regardless of CD4 count, VL or symptoms
- patient views, social history and lifestyle, medical history, mental health, co-medications, and recreational drug use should be considered when choosing ARV regimen.
- patient readiness and adherence support should be discussed.
- baseline resistance testing, HLAB*57:01 status, co-infection, e.g. with HBV, HCV, or TB will also influence drug choice.

With effective ART, PLWH are living longer and many of the issues seen in routine follow-up are co-morbidities seen in the general population, social issues, and mental health issues, as well as problems with polypharmacy and drug–drug interactions. Side effects of ART can still be problematic; for some, direct symptoms of HIV or opportunistic infections are less common.

When to start

Early initiation of treatment is associated with improved outcomes, and is recommended to all, irrespective of CD4 count, with the possible exception of elite controllers with stable high CD4 counts. However, patients need to be ready to take on the commitment of lifelong treatment, as poor adherence and breaks from treatment are associated with worse outcomes.

Primary HIV infection

PHI is defined as the first 6 months following acquisition of the virus. PHI may be diagnosed according to symptoms of seroconversion, previous −ve HIV test within the last 6 months, history of HIV contact, etc. During PHI, the HIV VL is at its highest and there is, therefore, a high risk of transmission. Initiating treatment during this phase reduces the reservoir of HIV, which can improve long-term outcomes.

Treatment as prevention

Strong evidence (including PARTNER study) has shown that PLWH who have sustained viral suppression with good adherence to effective ART will not transmit HIV infection. Condoms are still recommended to protect against other STIs and unplanned pregnancy.

Opportunistic infections

People presenting with CD4 count <200 cells/µL, AIDS defining infection, or other serious infection, should be started on ART within 2 weeks. This has been shown to improve survival; however, those with intracranial OIs, particularly cryptococcal meningitis, may be more at risk of developing immune reconstitution disorders, so consider delaying ART initiation.

Chronic infection

Where a patient is not ready to commit to treatment, or for other reasons where it is thought best to delay initiation, treatment may be delayed until before the CD4 count is <350 cells/µL

In asymptomatic patients, the likelihood of developing AIDS over a 3-year period can be predicted according to VL and CD4 count (Fig. 55.1) CD4 count is the best indicator of OI risk, but high VLs are associated with more rapid rates of CD4 fall. Patients who have not done so already should be strongly encouraged and supported to start ART when they have:
- symptomatic HIV
- neurological symptoms
- AIDS-defining illness regardless of CD4 count
- Before CD4 count reaches 350 cells/µL or <14%.

Hepatitis B or C co-infection

ART should be offered to all patients with HBV or HCV co-infection. ART should not be delayed, particularly if HBV requires treatment and should be initiated before treatment for HCV where this is required, unless CD4 count >500 cells/µL.

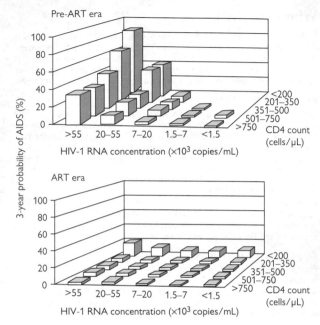

Fig. 55.1 Prognosis according to CD4 cell count and viral load in the pre-ART and ART eras.

Reprinted from *The Lancet*, **360**, Egger M. et. al. Prognosis of HIV-1-infected patients starting highly active antiretroviral therapy: a collaborative analysis of prospective studies, 119–129. Copyright (2002) with permission from Elsevier.

TB co-infection

In patients diagnosed with TB and HIV infection, simultaneously, anti-tuberculosis treatment (ATT) should be initiated as soon as possible. Treatment of HIV should be started as soon as possible; however, it can be complicated by drug interactions with ATT, so if the CD4 count is >100 cells/μL, ART may be delayed until 8–12 weeks into ATT. If CD4 <50 cells/μL, ART should be started within 2 weeks, where possible.

Malignancy

All PLWH diagnosed with a malignancy, whether or not it is HIV associated, should commence ART alongside any cancer specific therapy. Drug–drug interactions must be taken into account

How to start

Many factors should be considered prior to treatment initiation. Discussion with the patient regarding the advantages of treatment, uninterrupted life-long treatment, the importance of adherence, and ways to support this, potential for drug interaction, including recreational drugs and important side effects. Involvement of patient in decision-making is essential.

Baseline blood tests as a minimum should include:
- CD4 count and VL
- HIV viral resistance testing
- Human leucocyte antigen (HLA) B*57:01 if abacavir considered
- FBC, renal, including eGFR, and LFTs.

Patient history
- co-morbidities (renal, liver, cardiovascular, osteoporosis, psychiatric, substance misuse)
- co-infection (HBV, HCV, TB)
- pregnancy, pregnancy planning, and contraceptive needs
- drug history, including over the counter and recreational drugs.

Regimen specific factors
- potential side effects
- genetic barrier to resistance
- DDIs
- convenience
- cost.

Top tip
Always check for drug interactions using a reliable database, such as the University of Liverpool HIV Drug Interactions website. Advise patients and GPs to check for drug interactions before introducing new medications ℘www.hiv-druginteractions.org

Adherence

Treatment adherence is essential for successful viral suppression as sub-therapeutic drug levels select for HIV-resistant mutations arising from error-prone viral replication. Improving adherence is more cost effective than managing the consequences of poor compliance. Most patients are non-adherent sometimes and this is influenced by various factors, intentional, or unintentional:

• cultural/social beliefs
• mental health
• drugs and alcohol abuse
• stigma of taking medication
• relationship with healthcare team
• symptoms and side effects
• socioeconomic status and poor diet.

Supporting adherence

• Involve patients in treatment decisions and help them understand the reasons for taking medication, as well as possible adverse effects.
• Enquire about adherence in a non-judgmental way, whenever ART is discussed, prescribed, or dispensed.
• Address barriers, such as culture/beliefs, psychosocial factors, drugs, and alcohol use.

Interventions to improve adherence

Address any misconceptions or concerns regarding treatment. If side effects are an issue, alternative dosing, timing, regimen, or simplification should be considered. Some side effects may be treated through, e.g. nausea or diarrhoea, and may need further medication to control. Practical solutions, such as pill apps, alarms, text message reminders, and medication boxes can help. Adherence support from specialist nurses, pharmacists, or peer support groups should be considered.

Top tip

When enquiring about adherence ask, 'When was the last time you missed your medication?' or 'How many times have you missed your medicines in the last month?' rather than 'Do you take all your medicines'.

What to start

There are currently 6 different classes of antiretroviral drugs that inhibit the virus at different stages of viral replication (Fig. 55.2):

- interaction with CD4 receptors–fusion/CCR5 inhibitors
- inhibition of reverse transcriptase, which converts viral RNA to pro-viral DNA –NRTI and NNRTI;
- inhibition of post-transcribed viral DNA into the host DNA-integrase inhibitors;
- inhibition of protease involved in assembly of infective virions–protease inhibitors (PIs).

Combination therapy

Triple therapy is the standard of care. There are now over 30 licensed ARVs with many combination tablets available (Table 55.1). Treatment choice is guided by the differing tolerability, side effects, drug interactions, impact on co-pathologies, as well as individual resistance profile, VL, CD4 count, and convenience. Recommended treatment combinations includes 2 NRTIs (the backbone) + a third agent from another class of ARV (Table 55.2). Dual therapy regimes are being studied and effective regimes include DTG/RPV as a switch and DTG/3TC in naive patients with VL <100,000.

Common characteristics of ARVs are outlined in Table 55.3, including prescribing restrictions.

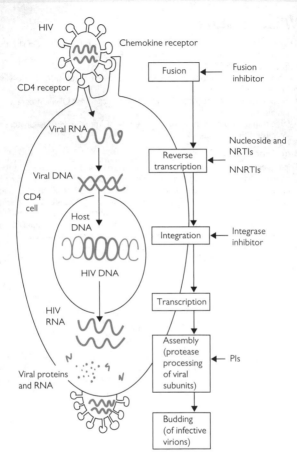

Fig. 55.2 HIV life cycle and points of drug action.

Table 55.1 Antiretroviral combination tablets

Combination tablet		Drug components
Triple combinations	Atripla®	tenofovir DF/emtricitabine/efavirenz
	Biktarvy®	bictegravir/tenofovir AF/emtricitabine
	Eviplera®	tenofovir DF/emtricitabine/rilpivirine
	Genvoya®	tenofovir AF/emtricitabine/elvitegravir/cobicistat (COBI)
	Odefsey®	tenofovir AF/emtricitabine/rilpivirine
	Stribild®	tenofovir DF/emtricitabine/elvitegravir/COBI
	Symtuza™	darunavir/COBI/tenofovir AF/emtricitabine
	Triumeq®	abacavir/lamivudine/dolutegravir
	(Trizivir)®	(abacavir/lamivudine/zidovudine)
Dual combinations	Combivir®	zidovudine/lamivudine
	Descovy®	tenofovir AF/emtricitabine
	Evotaz™	atazanavir/COBI
	Juluca®	dolutegravir/rilpivirine
	Kaletra®	lopinavir/ritonavir
	Kivexa®	abacavir/lamivudine
	Rezolsta®	darunavir/COBI
	Truvada®	tenofovir DF/emtricitibine

Table 55.2 Recommended first-line ARV regimens

	Preferred choice	Alternative
Backbone	Tenofovir[1] + emtricitibine	Abacavir[2] + lamivudine
Plus third agent	Atazanavir/ritonavir	Efavirenz
	Elvitegravir/COBI	
	Darunavir/ritonavir	
	Darunavir/COBI	
	Dolutegravir	
	Raltegravir (RAL)	
	Rilpivirine[2]	

[1] Tenofovir disoproxil fumarate or Tenofovir alafenamide.

[2] ➔ Table 55.3 for prescribing restrictions.

Table 55.3 Characteristics of commonly used antiretrovirals

ARV	Dosing*	Prescribing considerations
NRTIs		
Abacavir (ABC)	600 mg od	❶ Avoid if +ve for HLA*B57:01. Hypersensitivity reaction associated with HLA*B57:01 can be fatal. Do not re-challenge
		Avoid if VL >100K, unless combined with boosted DTV. Caution if CVS risk or hepatic impairment
Emtricitabine (FTC)	200 mg cap od	Dose reduce if eGFR <50. Avoid FTC/TDF if eGFR<30
		SEs rare
		Rarely lactic acidosis, hepatic steatosis
Lamivudine (3TC)	300 mg od	Dose reduce if eGFR <50
		SEs rare: lactic acidosis, hepatic steatosis
Tenofovir disoproxil fumarate (TFD)	300 mg od	Dose reduce if eGFR <50. Avoid if eGFR<30. Caution if osteoporosis
		Can cause renal impairment and altered bone metabolism
Tenofovir alafenamide (TAF)	25 mg od	Approved as part of fixed drug combinations, ❷ Table 55.1
		↓↓ dose compared with TDF so ↓ adverse effects on bone and kidneys
Zidovudine (AZT)	300 mg bd	↓ Dose if eGFR <15
		IV or oral administration
		Bone marrow suppression, myopathy, lactic acidosis, hepatic steatosis
NNRTIs		
Efavirenz (EFV)	600 mg od	Avoid if history of mental illness or neurological symptoms
		↓ Cost as generics available
		CNS (vivid dreams) and psychiatric SEs (depression, suicidality), ↑ lipids, rash
Rilpivirine (RPV)	25 mg od	Avoid if VL>100K as ↑ failure rate
		Should be taken with ≥350 kcal meal
		↓ SE than EFV. No significant drug–drug interactions (DDI) with hormonal contraceptive
		CNS, lipid, and rash side effects

Table 55.3 (Contd.)

ARV	Dosing*	Prescribing considerations
Nevirapine (NVP)	**200** mg bd	Avoid if CD4 >250♀ or CD4>400♂
		SE rash, Steven–Johnson's, hepatitis
Etravirine (ETV)	**200** mg bd	No dose adjustment for renal or hepatic impairment
		↑ Barrier to resistance
		Rash, diarrhoea
Integrase inhibitors (INI)		
Elvitegravir (EVG)	**150** mg od in Stribild® varies with regimen	Administered with COBI. Avoid Stribild® if eGFR <70 and in severe hepatic impairment
		Comes as part of STR Stribild®
		DDI due to COBI
Dolutegravir (DTV)	**50** mg od	Avoid co-administration with bi-ionic cations (Ca^{2+}, Mg^{2+}, etc.)
		↑ Genetic barrier to resistance
		↓ SEs, ↓ DDI
		Insomnia, headache
Raltegravir (RAL)	**400** mg bd or **1200** mg od	BD or OD dosing. Avoid co-administration with bi-ionic cations (Ca^{2+}, Mg^{2+}, etc.)
		Well tolerated, ↓ DDI
		Compliance issues
Bictegravir	**50** mg od	INI in Biktarvy part of fixed dose regimen
		Biktarvy has high genetic barrier to resistance
		↓ DDI
PIs#		
Atazanavir (AZV)	**300/400** mg od	Administer with ritonavir (RTV) or COBI (300 mg when boosted,)
		>10-year safety data in pregnancy
		↑ Bilirubin, ↑ PR interval, DDI
Darunavir (DRV)	**800** mg od	Administer with RTV or COBI. Not recommended in severe liver failure.
		↑ barrier to resistance, ↑ half life
		GI side effects, lypodystrophy, DDI
Entry inhibitors		
Enfuvirtide (ENF)	**90** mg SC bd	Licensed for treatment failure, rarely used. Useful when other options exhausted as part of salvage regime
		Injection site reactions common, hypersensitivity, ↑ pneumonia

(Continued)

Table 55.3 (*Contd.*)

ARV	Dosing*	Prescribing considerations
Maraviroc (MVC)	Dose depends on ARV regimen	Only effective if CCR5 Tropic. Requires tropism testing (VL must be >1000)
		Useful when other options exhausted as part of salvage regime
Pharmacokinetic boosters		
Cobicistat (COBI)	**150** mg od	Must be co-administered with ARV. Booster only. No ARV activity alone
		Reduces dose of boosted ARV
		Alters creatinine clearance without affecting renal function. DDIs
RTV	**100** mg od	Used as a booster in combination with other PI
		GI side effects. DDIs

*Oral unless otherwise stated.

#Other PIs are available—they are rarely used first-line, but are still used by some patients.

Monitoring and follow-up

Side effects of ARVs are common; however, many resolve within a few weeks, while others can persist. Psychosocial issues are often present and can impact on well-being and compliance. Also, with effective modern therapy, people living with HIV are ageing, with consequent co-morbidities common. Routine review aims to detect any issues arising and dealing with them in order to promote psychological and physical well-being, and quality of life (See Table 55.4 for suggested schedules).

Routine tests

- Renal (+ eGFR), liver and bone profiles, and FBC are measured routinely in order to detect adverse effects of ARVs. If eGFR ↓ urine protein/creatinine ratio should be measured.
- Lipids and HbA1c are measured annually in patients >40 in order to detect signs of metabolic syndrome as HIV and ART adversely affect cardiovascular risk
- CD4 cell count usually ↑ with ↓ VL, initially as a result of re-circulated reserves. Long-term CD4 count depends on the ability of the thymus to produce new T cells. Immune reconstitution is variable and often depends on the extent of immunosuppression at the time of ART initiation.
- VL suppression to <1000 copies/mL is usually achievable by 4 weeks regardless of initial VL or ARV regimen, and VL <50 copies/mL is a sign of successful treatment, which should be achieved by 3–6 months. Ongoing VL monitoring is required to ensure ongoing treatment success.

Therapy specific tests

- TDF can cause renal tubular toxicity with phosphate wasting and rarely Fanconi's syndrome; therefore, careful renal monitoring is required and switching therapy may be required if renal function declines or there is evidence of renal tubular dysfunction. TAF does not have this same effect as renal tubular cell uptake and dosing is significantly less.
- HLAB*57:01 typing should be performed prior to considering abacavir treatment. HLAB*57:01 is present in 5% Caucasians, but rare in sub-Saharan Africans and is associated with hypersensitivity reaction. If HLAB*57:01 positive abacavir should not be started.
- Tropism testing should be carried out only if treatment with maraviroc (CCR5 antagonist) is being considered. Routine testing is not indicated, and tropism can change over time so historic tests would need repeating. Only patients with CCR5 tropic virus should be started on maraviroc.

Monitoring CD4 cell count

Perform CD4 cell count at baseline. If ART not initiated, monitor yearly if CD4 >500 cells/mL and 6 monthly if <500 cells/mL.

For patients established on ART
- If CD4 <200 cells/mL monitor 3–6-monthly
- If CD4 200–350 measure 6–12-monthly
- If CD4 cell count >350 for >1 year routine monitoring not required.

Table 55.4 Schedule of routine monitoring and investigations

Assessment of patients starting and established on ART	Baseline	2–4 weeks	12 weeks	6 monthly	Annual	3-yearly	As indicated
History							
• Medical history	✓						
• Mental health					✓		
• Neurocognitive				✓			
• Sexual history, partners					✓		
• Children				✓			✓
• Contraception, conception							✓
Social history	✓						
Smoking, alcohol, deprivation					✓		
Travel history	✓						
• IGRA[2,1]							✓
• Tropical screen[1]							✓
Medication	✓						
• Prescribed					✓		
• Recreational							
• Non-prescribed							✓
• Herbal							

• Adherence	✓	✓	✓			
• Side effects	✓	✓	✓			✓
Vaccination history	✓			✓		
Family history	✓					
Patient ideas/concerns	✓					
Examination						
• General physical	✓					✓
• Blood pressure				✓		
• BMI[3]				✓		
Investigations						
• Viral load[4]	✓	✓	✓	✓		✓
• CD4 count[5]	✓	✓				✓
• HIV resistance	✓	✓				✓
• HLAB*57:01	✓					
• Tropism	✓					
Viral serology						
• Hep A						✓
• Hep B						✓
• Hep C						

(Continued)

Table 55.4 (*Contd.*)

Assessment of patients starting and established on ART	Baseline	2–4 weeks	12 weeks	6 monthly	Annual	3-yearly	As indicated
• Measles[1]							
• Varicella[1]							
• Rubella[1]							
STI screen + syphilis	✓		✓[6]				✓
• Blood monitoring	✓				✓		
• FBC							
• U&E, eGFR		✓	✓				
• LFT, Bone		✓	✓				
• Lipids, HbA1c >40							
Urinalysis	✓			✓			
Cervical cytology ♀25–64	✓				✓		
Risk assessments							
• Cardiovascular >40 years	✓				✓		
• Fracture risk >50 years						✓	

[1]Depending on travel/vaccination history; [2]interferon gamma release assay (IGRA); [3]body mass index (BMI); [4]if ART being used for 'treatment as prevention'; [5]Monitoring CD4 cell count box → 'Monitoring CD4 cell count', p. 633;[6] depending on sexual risks.

Therapeutic drug monitoring (TDM)

Routine TDM is not recommended, although in certain situations it may be useful:

- *Drug interactions*: to monitor plasma concentrations, which may be altered by drug interactions.
- Children, pregnant ♀, and in older patients where pharmacokinetics may be altered.
- Extremes of weight.
- *Unexplained VL* ↑: TDM in therapeutic range does not exclude non-adherence, but absent or low levels can help confirm it.
- Blood sampling (plasma) should ideally be at the end of the dosing interval (Cmin) in patients established on treatment ≥14 days.

Vaccinations

People with HIV with CD4<200 have ↓ response to non-replicating vaccines and risk of vaccination-related disease with replicating vaccines. PLWH are at increased risk of other vaccine preventable infections such as HBV, HAV, pneumococcal illness, influenza so these should be routinely offered and/or immunity checked (see Table 55.5).

- If CD4 <200 replicating vaccinations contraindicated.
- If CD4 200-350 immune response is suboptimal so balance urgent need for immunization with better response when ↑CD4.
- Co-administration of replicating vaccines not advised – give 4 weeks apart.
- Replicating vaccines should not be given ≤2 weeks before or ≤12 weeks after blood products containing antibodies.

Table 55.5 Vaccinations for people living with HIV

	Infection	Vaccine type	Recommendation
Recommended	Hepatitis B	Subunit	All non-immune
	Hepatitis A	Inactivated	All at risk
	Influenza	Inactivated	All annually
	Pneumococcal	PCV13 Conjugated	All once
Caution	Measles, mumps, rubella	Live attenuated	Avoid if CD4 <200
	Varicella		If CD4 >200 give as per Green Book recommendations ◆ Further information, below
	Herpes zoster		
	Yellow fever		
Avoid	Influenza	Live attenuated	Intranasal; not preferred
	Typhoid	Live attenuated	Contraindicated
	TB	BCG	Contraindicated

Further information

- The Green Book (immunization against infectious disease): ℘ www.gov.uk/government/collections/immunisation-against-infectious-disease-the-green-book
- British HIV Association guideline on use of vaccines in HIV positive adults: ℘ https://www.bhiva.org/vaccination-guidelines

Switching antiretroviral therapy

Switching ARVs may be necessary for a number of reasons, such as side effects/toxicity, adherence issues, or failing therapy. Considerations depend on whether or not VL is suppressed and whether there are any drug interactions between the original regimen and the new regimen ARVs. In particular, NNRTIs efavirenz and nevirapine are enzyme inducers, with effects likely to last for a while after drug cessation.

- If VL is fully suppressed direct switch can be made.
- If switching to PI or integrase inhibitor (INI), direct switch can be made.
- If viral replication ongoing and switching away from NNRTI, switch to boosted PI (COBI or RTV)-containing regimen, and not to other NNRTI.
- For other switches in the presence of ongoing viral replication, seek specialist advice.[1]

Stopping antiretroviral therapy

Stopping ART is not recommended, but in rare circumstances, such as drug toxicity, intercurrent illness, patient choice, or post-partum, it may be necessary. Due to differing half-life of different ARVs, stopping all drugs simultaneously may lead to effectively mono- or dual- therapy of the drugs with longer half-life, which can lead to drug resistance. The different approaches include:[1]

- stopping simultaneously if PI-based regimen or regimen containing ARVs with similar half-lives
- staggered stopping for regimen containing ARVs with long and short half-lives
- replacing all ARVs with boosted PI (e.g. darunavir with RTV or COBI) for 4 weeks if regimen contains ARVs with long and short half-lives, e.g. NNRTI and NRTI regime.

1 See also ♒ http://www.bhiva.org/HIV-1-treatment-guidelines.aspx

Antiretroviral side effects

Many side effects historically associated with ARVs were caused by drugs that have been discontinued or rarely used. Newer agents tend to be better tolerated, but side effects are still common, and side effects of discontinued ARVs may persist.

ABC hypersensitivity

Occurs in 4% (almost always associate with HLAB*57:01), usually within first 6 weeks. Usually presents with >2 of GI symptoms, headache, fever, rash, abnormal LFTs, myalgia, respiratory symptoms, and eosinophilia. If suspected, discontinue ABC immediately, give supportive care. Symptoms resolve within 24–48 hours, rash may take longer. *Do not* re-challenge with ABC as risk of mortality.

Gastrointestinal disturbance

Nausea and diarrhoea are common, especially in the first days/weeks of most ARVs, but especially PIs, which may cause persistent diarrhoea. Anti-emetics and/or loperamide may alleviate symptoms.

Hepatotoxicity

Can be caused by most ARVs. ↑ ♂ and those with other risk factors, e.g. alcohol excess, HBV/HCV co-infection. Graded 1 (ALT 2–3× normal upper limit) to 4 (>10× normal upper limit). Most common with DDI, stavudine (D4T), AZT, ABC, NVP, EFV, and RTV. If minor abnormality only monitoring required. If severe, stop offending ARV. If caused by ABC or NVP, do not re-challenge.

Lipodystrophy

Found in ~4% untreated PLWH.
- *Lipohypertrophy*: central adiposity, 'buffalo hump', lipomas, ↑ neck circumference—associated with PIs.
- *Lipoatrophy*: peripheral and facial subcutaneous fat loss—associated with older NRTIs particularly D4T, can be stigmatizing.
- *Dyslipidaemia*: ↑ total cholesterol and/or ↑ triglycerides—reported in <80% taking ARVs, associated with PIs, especially RTV, and older PIs.

Mitochondrial toxicity

May present with nausea/vomiting, abdominal pain, hepatic steatosis, myopathy, neuropathy, lactic acidosis. Mainly associated with AZT, D4T, and DDI. Switch to alternative ARVs and supportive care recommended.

Neuropathy

Distal symmetric polyneuropathy (DSP) can be difficult to distinguish from HIV-related DSP, but tends to be painful, more sudden, and progressive. Discontinue offending ARV and, if needed, offer pain relief with tricyclic antidepressants or gabapentin.

Neuro-psychiatric

Can manifest as depression and other mood disorders, insomnia, vivid dreams, dizziness. Common with EFV and DTV. May settle or patients become accustomed, but can persist long term. Switch to alternative ARV if severe or affecting quality of life.

Rash

Rash is common especially with NNRTIs and ABC ⟴ Table 55.3. NVP rash, typically maculopapular, affecting trunk, occurs in first 2 weeks of therapy and risk is minimized by half-dose induction for first 2 weeks. Mild rash does not require intervention and will usually settle. Antihistamine for symptom relief. If severe or SJS (mucous membranes involved) switch to alternative ARV.

Renal impairment and Fanconi's syndrome

Renal tubular dysfunction, tubule-interstitial nephritis, and Fanconi syndrome are most commonly associated with TDF, but also ATV. ↓ eGFR, proteinuria or persistent significant hypophosphataemia may be initial signs. Switch to alternative ARV if possible.

↑ Creatinine seen with DTV, RAL, COBI, RPV, RTV occurs 2–4 weeks after starting, is non-progressive, and due to altered creatinine transport. It is not associated with altered kidney function.

Immune reconstitution

ART leads to ↓ viral replication and ↓ VL, with subsequent ↑ CD4, initially due to ↑ memory cells followed by ↑ naïve CD4 cells. CD8 cells initially ↑, but then ↓. ART causes ↓ HIV specific immune response, but ↑ immune response to other pathogens, with ↓ OIs with ↑ CD4. Lower CD4 nadir usually results in slower and less complete immune recovery.

Immune reconstitution inflammatory response

Aetiology is thought to be the result of immune reconstitution with abnormal response to an underlying pathogen. It is characterized by worsening or appearance of new clinical signs/symptoms after initiation of ART, and is not the result of treatment failure, drug hypersensitivity, malignancy, or other disease processes. It may appear as a paradoxical worsening after treatment of a known OI, such as TB (paradoxical IRIS), or as symptoms of a previously unknown OI (unmasking IRIS). It appears ≤12 weeks after ART and occurs in 11–36% TB/HIV co-infected patients. IRIS is also seen with CMV, MAC, HCV, HSV, cryptococcal meningitis, and progressive multifocal leucoencephalopathy.

Clinical features of TB IRIS include fever, lymphadenopathy +/−overlying redness, worsening pulmonary lesions, pleural effusion/ascites, abscesses cutaneous lesions, CNS tuberculoma. May be transient or last for months. It is more likely if low nadir CD4 with rapid ↑ CD and rapid ↓ VL following ART, disseminated infection and early ART initiation.

Management

Exclude other cause, start/continue treatment of OI. If severe, high dose corticosteroids (e.g. 1–1.5 mg/kg prednisolone) may be required for variable duration. May recur when steroids discontinued, so gradual reduction recommended.

Antiretroviral drug–drug interactions

Interactions with ARVs are common, so always check for DDIs before co-administering ॐ www.hiv-druginteractions.org.

Common interactions are described in Table 55.6.

Table 55.6 Important and common ARV drug interactions

Co-med	ARV	Effect	Action
Antimicrobials			
• Rifamycins	Most	↓ ARV ↑ Rifampicin	Avoid rifampicin, use rifabutin cautiously. Dose adjust ARV and Rif as necessary[1]
• HCV DAAs[2]	many	Complex	Prescribe with caution
Steroids, including inhaled steroids	PIs COBI EFV	↑ steroid ❶ Iatrogenic Cushing's ↓ steroid	Caution, may require dose adjustment. Monitor closely for systemic SE. Beclometasone has no DDIs with ARVs
Proton pump inhibitors	ATV RPV	↓ ARV	Do not co-administer
Antacids	PIs RAL RPV	↓ ARV	Avoid with RAL. Separate DTV, ATV, RPV from antacid ≤6 hours[3]
Recreational			
• Amphetamine • Cocaine • GHB[4]	PIs COBI RPV ATV	↑ toxicity of recreational drug ↓ ATV	Ensure patient is aware of potential for interactions that could either ↑ toxicity of recreational drug or ↓ efficacy of ARV
• Cannabis	EFV	↑ cannabis	
Contraceptives	PIs EFV	↓ Contraceptive efficacy	ATV/r + COCP containing ≥30 mcg estradiol can be co-administered. IUD/IUS + DMPA are safe to co-administer.
Opiates	PIs EFV	↓ Opiate	May need ↑ opiate dose
Statins	PIs Cobi EFV	↑ statin ↓ Statin	*Do not* co-administer PI + simvastatin. Otherwise, monitor lipids/toxicity
Benzodiazepines	PIs COBI EFV	↑ Sedation	*Do not* co-administer with oral midazolam. Caution with others
Anti-depressants	PIs EFV RPV	↑ or ↓ antidepressant	❶ St John's wort contraindicated. Use others with caution, monitor for side effects

[1]See Ⓢ www.bhiva.org/TB-HIV-coinfection-guidelines.aspx; [2]hepatitis C direct-acting antivirals; [3]see Ⓢ www.hiv-druginteractions.org; [4]gamma-hydroxybutyrate.

HIV drug resistance

There are different mechanisms for ARV drug resistance:
- Intrinsic drug resistance, such as HIV-2 resistance to NNRTIs.
- Transmitted drug resistance (TDR) occurs when the transmitted HIV has resistance mutations. In the UK, TDR rate is 10%, greatest in London. TDR for integrase inhibitor (INI) is very low.
- Resistance may also be acquired following poor adherence, drug interaction or poor absorption leading to treatment failure.
- ~70% of virological failure is not due to ARV resistance, but 2° to poor adherence, DDI, or malabsorption.

Development of HIV drug resistance

HIV has a high rate of replication (unhindered 10^{8-10} virions produced daily) and replication is error-prone with one mutation on average per replication cycle. Therapeutic drug levels will reduce resistance mutations occurring by inhibiting viral replication and suppressing existing mutations if they are not resistant to all drugs in the ARV regimen. However, if drug levels are sub-therapeutic, the on-going viral replication will select for mutations that can overcome the ARVs present. Resistance to some ARVs occurs with only a small number of mutations (low barrier to resistance, e.g. NNRTIs), while others require several cumulative mutations to develop before resistance is seen (high barrier to resistance, e.g. boosted PIs). Even with undetectable VL, low-level replication may allow resistance to develop. Compensatory mutation reverses ↓ viral fitness resulting from other mutations. Some mutations induce resistance to certain agents, while simultaneously producing hypersusceptibility to others (e.g. M184V causes resistance to 3TC, but ↑ sensitivity to AZT). Drug resistance has been demonstrated in up to 25% of patients on ART.

Resistance mutations

Resistance mutations are described using a number referring to the affected codon in the HIV genome, preceded by a letter referring to the wild type amino acid, and followed by a letter referring to the mutant amino acid, e.g. L74V is a mutation at codon 74 where leucine has been replaced by valine. (For examples, see Table 55.7.)

Resistance mutations are variable in their effect upon viral fitness and their effectiveness in pervading ARV therapy. Resistance can occur rapidly within weeks if only a single mutation confers resistance, e.g. K103N (NVP/EFV-resistant mutation). A mutation may also confer resistance to other ARVs within the same class e.g. M184V (ABC/3TC/FTC resistance). Other mutations may only confer resistance when multiple mutations have accumulated, so resistance develops slowly or not at all, e.g. PI resistance mutations.

Many mutations ↓ viral fitness, e.g. DTV-resistance mutations. However, resistance mutations confer a selective advantage by ↓ susceptibility to antiviral agents, thereby enabling the mutant quasi-species to proliferate under treatment with those agents. Compensatory mutations, e.g. 30N (nelfinavir resistance) may be required to ↑ viral fitness.

Table 55.7 Examples of resistance mutations

Major NRTI mutations

	Non-TAMs					TAMs[1]						MDR[2]	
Codon	65	70	74	115	184	41	67	70	210	215	219	69	151
Wild type	K	K	L	Y	M	M	D	K	T	T	K	T	Q
3TC/FTC	R				VI								
ABC	R	E	VI	F	VI	L			W	FY		Ins*	M
TDF	R	E		F		L		R	W	FY		Ins	M
AZT/D4T						L	N	R	W	FY	QE	Ins	M

Major PI mutations

Codon	30	32	33	46	47	48	50	54	76	82	84	88	90
Wild type	D	V	L	M	I	G	I	I	L	V	I	N	L
ATV		I		IL			L	V		A	V	S	M
DRV		I	F		VA		V	LM	V	F	V		

Major NNRTI mutations

Codon	100	101	103	106	138	181	188	190	230
Wild type	L	K	K	V	E	Y	Y	G	M
EFV/NVP	I	EP	NS	AM		CIV	LCH	ASE	L

RPV	I	EP			AGKQ	CIV		L		ASE	L

Major INI mutations

Codon	66	92	138	140	143	148	155	263
Wild type	T	E	E	G	Y	Q	N	R
RAL	AK	Q	KAT	SAC	RCH	HRK	H	K
DTV	K	Q	KAT	SAC		HRK	H	K

*Insertion at codon 69.

[1]Thymidine analogue mutations (TAM) develop under selective pressure from AZT/D4T.

[2]Multidrug resistant mutations. 151 Complex usually occurs with other accessory mutations.

Letters represent the different amino acids. Those in bold represent mutations that cause reduction in ARV susceptibility, those in plain text reduce susceptibility in combination with other mutations.

Drug resistance patterns

K65R mutation (selected by TDF, ABC and DDI) confers resistance to TDF, ABC, and 3TC and ↑ susceptibility to AZT and D4T. This mutation develops rapidly when regimens combining TDF with two of ABC, DDI, or 3TC are given to the treatment naïve. Co-existence of K65R and M184V ↑ resistance to ABC and DDI, but retains suscepti-bility to TDF, AZT, and D4T. Multiple mutations may interact. Resulting resistance patterns can be predicted by matching with resistance profile databases. This is provided by commercial resistance tests.

Databases of resistance profiles are available at:
• *Stanford Database*: ℘ http://hivdb.stanford.edu
• *ANRS*: ℘ http://www.hivfrenchresistance.org
• *REGA*: ℘ http://rega.kuleuven.be/cev/regadb/download

Persistence of mutation/resistance

When treatment that selected for resistant quasi-species is discontinued, wild-type virus usually becomes predominant within 2 months. Drug-resistant mutants occasionally remain dominant, e.g. 41L (zidovudine), but usually cease to be detectable by standard assay. How-ever, they may still persist as minority quasi-species, e.g. 90M (PI), or latent integrated proviral DNA (archived resistance). Therefore, standard assays may not exclude drug resistance, if carried out >1 month after stopping a failing regimen, and may not detect TDR, if performed long after HIV acquisition. Interpretation of resistance mutations must take into account previous treatment history and previous resistance reports.

Resistance testing

Standard resistance assays require VL >500 copies/mL and cannot detect minority species. Expert advice is needed to interpret the results.

Genotyping

Viral genes are sequenced to identify key mutations known to confer (alone or with others) resistance. Current methodology only detects viral mutants comprising at least 20–30% of the total population. Analysis is based on known correlation between genotype and phenotype from previous studies. Results are normally available in 2–4 weeks.

Phenotyping

Viral cell cultures are set up with increasing concentrations of ARTs to determine IC_{50}, the concentration of drug required to inhibit viral replication by 50%. Cut-off value indicates by what factor the IC_{50} of an HIV isolate can be ↑, while still being classified as susceptible, compared with a wild-type control. IC_{50} above this value indicates resistance. Phenotyping is not available in the UK.

Clinical application of resistance testing

Resistance testing is recommended in the following circumstances:
• At diagnosis to identify transmitted resistance.
• Before treatment initiation, including during pregnancy.
• Suboptimal virological response to treatment (<0.5 log_{10} ↓ in 1 month).
• At each treatment failure, to guide choice of next regimen.
• If treatment is discontinued to detect mutations that may later be archived.

Management of virological failure

Definitions

- Virological failure is viral rebound >200 copies/mL or failure to achieve initial viral suppression.
- Viral rebound is failure to maintain VL below level of detection.
- Low level viraemia (LLV) is persistent VL 50-200
- Viral blip is VL 50-200, preceded and followed by undetectable VL.
- Incomplete viral response is never achieving suppressed VL after ≥24 weeks treatment.

Investigating suspected virological failure

Investigate virological failure, rebound, incomplete response or LLV:

- Check drug adherence, side effects/toxicity
- Address factors affecting drug exposure e.g. drug/food interactions, pharmacokinetics (pregnancy, co-morbidities), liver/renal disease).
- Resistance test on failing treatment or <4weeks of stopping.
- Review previous resistance tests and treatment history.
- Tropism/HLAB*57:01 test if MVC/ABC being considered.
- Change regimen as soon as viral resistance confirmed to avoid accumulation of mutations.

Treatment options following confirmed viral resistance

Treatment switch should be considered when there have been ≥2 consecutive VL >400 copies/mL, having excluded other explanations. The new regimen should be tailored according to available resistance reports and previous treatment history.

- For complex resistance seek expert advice, consult HIV MDT.
- New regimen should include ≥2 active drugs, preferably 3, to include boosted PI (ideally DRV) and ≥1 of INI, MVC, or ENF.
- *First-line failure with no resistance*: switch to PI/r or PI/c +2NRTI.
- *First-line failure with limited resistance (NRTI+/-NNRTI)*: switch to new boosted PI regimen + ≥1 active drug, e.g. INI/MVC.
- *Failure of first-line boosted PI+2NRTI regimen with limited PI mutations*: switch to alternative boosted PI (+2NRTI), + 2 other active agents.

DO NOT

- Interrupt treatment.
- Intensify current regimen with only1 new active drug.
- Switch from boosted PI + 2NRTI to INI or NNRTI as third agent if NRTI mutations present or suspected.

Prophylaxis against infections

Here, we consider conditions in which 1° prophylaxis and post-exposure prophylaxis should be considered. If the patient has been treated for a condition and 2° prophylaxis is being considered, refer to information for the infection in question.

Primary prophylaxis

This is where the patient is at risk of an infection and prophylactic treatment is required to prevent it.

Pneumocystis jiroveci
- Prophylaxis recommended if CD4 <200 or CD4% <14.
- *First line*: co-trimoxazole 480–960 mg daily (desensitization schedules are shown in Table 55.8).
- *Alternative*: Dapsone 50–200 mg daily *plus* pyrimethamine 50 mg weekly (to protect against toxoplasmosis) *plus* folinic acid 15 mg weekly *or* atovaquone 750 mg bd.
- Should be continued until CD4 >200 for 3 consecutive months.

Toxoplasmosis
- Recommended if CD4 <200 and positive serology.
- *First line and second line*: as for PCP.
- Continue until CD4 >200 consistently.

Table 55.8 Suggested desensitization schedule for co-trimethoprim/sulfamethoxazole (T/S)

Day	Dose	T/S
1	1 mL of 1:20 paediatric suspension	0.4 mg/2 mg
2	2 mL of 1:20 paediatric suspension	0.8 mg/4 mg
3	4 mL of 1:20 paediatric suspension	1.6 mg/8 mg
4	8 mL of 1:20 paediatric suspension	3.2 mg/16 mg
5	1 mL of paediatric suspension	8 mg/40 mg
6	2 mL of paediatric suspension	16 mg/80 mg
7	4 mL of paediatric suspension	32 mg/160 mg
8	8 mL of paediatric suspension	64 mg/320 mg
9	1 tablet	80 mg/400 mg
10	1 double strength tablet	160 mg/800 mg

Thereafter 1 double strength tablet 3 days a week until CD4 >200 cell/µL for at least 3 months.

Reprinted from Absar N, Daneshvar H, Beall G. (1994) Desensitization to trimethoprim/sulfamethoxazole in HIV-infected patients *J Allergy Clin Immunol*, 93, 1001–5 . © 1994 with permission from Elsevier.

Mycobacterium avium complex
- Recommended if CD4 <50.
- *First line*: azithromycin 1250 mg weekly.
- Can be discontinued when CD4 >50 for 3 months.

Malaria
Should be offered if travelling to endemic area.

Penicilliosis (P. marneffei)
- If CD4 <100 consider prophylaxis with itraconazole if travelling to southeast Asia or south China where it is endemic.

Post-exposure prophylaxis
- Diptheria, *Haemophilus influenza*, meningococcus, pertussis.
- Contacts should be offered antibiotic prophylaxis and vaccination.
- HAV.
- Contacts should be offered HAV vaccination if HAV IgG negative if within 1 week of jaundice in index case.
- If CD4 <200 HAV-specific immunoglobulin is recommended if within 14 days of exposure.
- HBV.
- Following exposure, urgently determine HBV immunity.
- No prophylaxis required if good immunity/past infection.
- If suboptimal immunity, offer booster.
- If non-immune offer rapid vaccination course, plus HBV-specific immunoglobulin regardless of CD4 count.

Influenza
Oseltamivir or inhaled zanamivir for post-exposure within 48 and 36 hours of exposure, respectively.

Measles
Urgently request measles IgG. If measles IgG –ve and CD4 >200, measles vaccine within 3 days or HNIG within 6 days is recommended. If CD4 <200 offer NHIG regardless of measles immunity.

Polio
If immunocompromised and inadvertently given oral polio vaccine (OPV), contact with OPV recipient, or wild-type polio, give HNIG unless known to be seropositive to all 3 polio types

Varicellas zoster
Prophylaxis with chickenpox vaccine or Varivax should be given within 3-5 days of exposure. If CD4<400 varicella immunoglobulin should be given within 7–10 days of significant exposure.

Further information

British HIV Association guidelines ℘ www.bhiva.org/guidelines
   The Green Book: Immunization against infectious disease: ℘ https://www.gov.uk/government/collections/immunisation-against-infectious-disease-the-green-book

HIV: pregnancy

Introduction 654
Pre-conception 654
ART in pregnancy and labour 655
Obstetric considerations 656
Neonatal interventions 657
Infant feeding 658

Introduction

In the UK in 2011 the prevalence of HIV was 2.2 per 1000 ♀ giving birth. Routine antenatal HIV screening began in 2000, with national uptake >97% since 2011. Most cases of perinatal HIV transmission occur from undiagnosed ♀. Without intervention, the risk of vertical transmission of HIV from mother to child is between 25% and 45% and can occur *in utero* (20%), during delivery (45–50%) and during breastfeeding (30–35%). With the effective use of ART, ♀ with VL<50 are now recommended vaginal delivery, if no obstetric contraindications. With current medical, obstetric, and neonatal management, transmission rates are now 0.1% in the UK.

Pre-conception

Treatment as prevention (⊃ Chapter 55, 'Treatment as prevention', p. 623) has dramatically reduced the risk of transmission following UPSI, so couples wishing to conceive naturally can be advised that risk of transmission from UPSI is zero providing all the following conditions are met:

- HIV +ve partner is adherent to effective ART.
- HIV +ve partner has had VL <200 copies/ml for >6 months.
- Both partners are monogamous.

Folic acid and vitamin D should be advised as for women without HIV. Choice of cART for ♀ should have good pregnancy safety profile.

Assisted conception to reduce risks of transmission

Availability is increasingly limited and generally advice is as above, but some couples may need further counselling and advice if VL >200 copies/ml.

HIV-positive ♀ with HIV-negative ♂ partner
Self-administered insemination into the vagina around the fertile window using sperm ejaculated into a spermicide-free condom.

HIV-positive ♂ with HIV negative ♀ partner
- Sperm washing with artificial insemination.
- Using donor sperm for artificial insemination.

Fertility treatment and adoption

♀ with HIV have a higher rate of infertility compared with HIV –ve ♀. PLWH, either in same-sex or heterosexual relationships, have the same rights as HIV-negative people to access fertility services and adoption.

ART in pregnancy and labour

Screening
- HIV screening should be part of routine antenatal care.
- Re-offer HIV screening at 28 weeks to ♀ previously untested.
- All pregnant ♀ with HIV should have sexual health screening.

ART in pregnancy

Conceiving with cART
♀ conceiving on effective cART should continue with it, except PI mono-therapy should be intensified, and D4T + DDI is contraindicated, DTG may be associated with neural tube defects.

Starting cART in pregnancy
When to start
Immediately if 28 weeks pregnant. All should start by 24 weeks gestation, early 2nd trimester if VL >30K, or earlier if VL >100K.

If CD4 >350 *and* VL<10K AZT monotherapy may be considered, but is not recommended.

What to start
NRTI backbone (TDF+FTC or ABC+3TC or AZT+3TC) *plus* ATV/r or EFV or as alternatives Rilpivirine, RAL (400 mg bd) or DRV/r (bd). Avoid cobicistat regimes.

Unsuppressed on cART or late presenting ♀ not taking cART
- If presenting after 28 weeks not on cART start treatment immediately.
- If VL >100K start cART that includes RAL.
- If in labour, not on cART, give stat NVP *and* start AZT+3TC +RAL.
- IV infusion of AZT during labour if VL unknown or >1000.
- If pre-term labour <34 weeks, give double-dose TDF to load infant.
- If presenting in labour with no HIV test, perform rapid testing.

Elite controllers
Untreated women with CD4 >350 and VL <50 can be treated with AZT monotherapy and have vaginal delivery.

Discontinuing ART post-partum
This is not recommended, but if considered refer to ➔ Chapter 55, 'anti-retroviral therapy', p. 639. Initiating PI-based regimen preferred if discontinuation is considered. Perform viral resistance test after short-course ART.

Hepatitis B and hepatitis C co-infection
See sections ➔ Chapter 25, 'Hepatitis B virus infection', pp. 313–17; 'Hepatitis C virus infection', pp. 318–21; Chapter 43, 'HIV: hepatitis virus co-infection', pp. 507–12. Avoid entecavir and HCV treatment in pregnancy/breast feeding.

Monitoring of pregnant women with HIV
- Newly diagnosed pregnant ♀ require no additional investigations.
- Check VL after 2–4 weeks for those starting cART, and for all ♀ at least once every trimester, and at 36 weeks, and delivery.
- Check CD4 at baseline and delivery as a minimum.
- Monitor liver function at each antenatal visit.
- If viral suppression not achieved by 36 weeks investigate:
  - adherence check and drug history/interactions
  - consider resistance testing and/or therapeutic drug monitoring
  - optimize/intensify treatment regimen

Obstetric considerations

Antenatal management

National guidelines for antenatal management should be followed, regardless of HIV status, with the following additional considerations:

- *Foetal ultrasound*: standard national guidelines should be followed. No additional scanning required.
- *Trisomy 21 screening*: combined trisomy 21 screening at 11^{+0}–13^{+6} weeks gestation is recommended. For late presenters, triple or quadruple trisomy 21 screening should be offered, but there is ↑ false positive rate in HIV+ ♀ due to ↑ βHCG, ↑ αFP, and ↓ UE3 levels.
- *Invasive foetal testing*: invasive prenatal foetal procedures (e.g. amniocentesis or chorionic villous sampling) should be delayed until VL<50. If delay not possible, ♀ should be started on cART, including RAL and stat dose NVP given 2–4 hours prior to procedure.
- *External cephalic version*: if required, can be offered if VL<50 and no obstetric contraindications.

Labour and delivery

Mode of delivery

Women taking cART with VL<50 at ≥36 weeks are recommended vaginal delivery, including vaginal delivery after previous caesarian section, unless obstetric contraindications. If VL 50–399 pre-labour caesarian section (PLCS) should be considered. If VL≥400, PLCS recommended. Women on AZT monotherapy should proceed with PLCS, irrespective of VL, except elite controllers ➔ Chapter 56, 'Elite controllers', p. 655. Planned PLCS for PMCT should be performed at 38–39 weeks gestation.

Instrumental delivery

Where vaginal delivery is recommended, this should proceed as for HIV-uninfected, including amniotomy, scalp electrodes, foetal blood sampling, instrumental delivery, and episiotomy if required. No ↑ transmission has been seen with these practices where VL<50.

Pre-labour rupture of membranes at term (at ≥37 weeks)

If VL<50, expedite delivery (<4 hours), with induction of labour and low threshold for treating intra-partum pyrexia. If VL ≥1000, proceed to immediate caesarian section. If latest VL 50–999 consider immediate caesarian section depending on actual VL and trajectory.

Premature rupture of membranes and preterm labour

Premature delivery is ↑ in ♀ with HIV. In PROM at 34–37 weeks manage as for 37+ and follow national guidelines for premature PROM. If <34 weeks give steroids according to national guidelines, optimize virological control, and involve MDT in decisions on timing of delivery.

Neonatal interventions

Baby PEP

- If cART >10 weeks, VL <50 copies/mil >2 measurements 4 weeks apart and at 36 weeks AZT monotherapy for 2 weeks. If VL <50 copies/ml at 36 weeks but cART <10 weeks or VL >50 in previous measurements give AZT for 4 weeks.
- Triple therapy for 4 weeks in infant is advised if mother had detectable VL at time of delivery. AZT, 3TC, and NVP are the most commonly used in neonates.
- Baby PEP should be started as soon as possible/<4hrs.

Prophylaxis

Babies at high risk of transmission and those with detectable HIV DNA/RNA at birth should be given prophylactic co-trimoxazole from age 4 weeks.

Vaccinations

Should be in line with routine national immunization schedule.

Infant HIV testing

- Infants should be tested <48 hours post-delivery, 2 weeks (if on cART) at 6 and 12 weeks with HIV DNA/RNA PCR.
- HIV antibody at 18–24 months to check for late post-natal infection.
- For breastfed infants ➔ Chapter 56, 'Infant feeding', p. 658.

Infant feeding

In the UK, all ♀ with HIV should be advised not to breastfeed, due to the risk of HIV transmission to the infant.

Women with low income may be eligible for free formula milk via their HIV service provider or local authority.

Breastfeeding against medical advice

- Mother with fully suppressed VL should be advised to exclusively breastfeed (except during weaning), and to discontinue as early as possible, but before 6 months at the latest.
- Monitor infant HIV VL at 2 weeks and then monthly monitoring of mother and infant HIV VL is required and 4 and 8 weeks post breastfeeding.
- Infant PEP should not be continued beyond the standard 4 weeks, even if breastfeeding continues.
- Mother should continue ARVs until ≥1 week after completing breast-feeding.
- If mother develops mastitis, intercurrent illness affecting ARV absorption, has poor ARV compliance, or detectable VL she should be advised to discontinue breastfeeding.
- If mother has HIV viraemia and is/plans to breastfeed, this is a child protection concern and may require social services referral if the mother cannot be persuaded to follow advice.

Further information

Refer to national guidelines, e.g. British HIV Association pregnancy guidelines: M www.bhiva.org/pregnancy-guidelines

HIV: travel

Planning 660
Vaccination 661
Food and water 662
Travellers' diarrhoea 662
Other precautions 662

Planning

Travel, particularly to developing countries, may carry substantial risks of infection, e.g. malaria, salmonella, hepatitis viruses, and cryptosporidiosis. Infections, especially relevant for those with immunodeficiency, include Leishmaniasis, *Penicillium marneffei*, coccidioidomycosis, histoplasmosis and blastomycosis. Many developing countries have high rates of TB.

Few countries ban tourist travel for PLWH, but a larger number have entry restrictions for longer stays, or prevent them from settling there. Useful advice and information by country available at: ℘ www.travelhealthpro.org. uk/factsheet/29/hiv-and-aids. Specific information should be sought from relevant consulates.

Travel risk in relation to degree of immune deficiency, range of potential pathogens, and availability of medical care need to be discussed and evaluated with the patient. Cost of healthcare and treatment must be considered, and adequate insurance cover arranged. Adequate medications should be given, supplemented with a confidential letter, containing essential information about treatment may prevent problems with customs. Rehydration sachets and standby therapy for GI infections and malaria may be indicated. If travel crosses time zones, either remain on UK time for taking medication for the entire trip or adjust in 1-hour steps before/during travel; an alternative is to take medications earlier as unlikely to cause harm. Interruptions to ART are harmful and should be avoided

A newly started ART regimen should be known to be effective and well tolerated before travelling.

Vaccination

Preparation for travel should include a review and updating of routine vaccinations (see Table 57.1). Special precautions are required for certain areas, such as Africa, the Middle East, Asia and south America. Details are available at ℘ www.dh.gov.uk/travellers).

There is no ↑ incidence of adverse reactions to inactivated vaccines, although their protective efficacy may be ↓.

Live vaccines and live attenuated vaccines should not be given if CD4 <200 mm³, and risk vs benefit should be discussed if CD 250–350/mm³. Yellow fever vaccine is a live attenuated vaccine with uncertain safety and efficacy in HIV infection. WHO recommends immunization for asymptomatic HIV-infected people travelling to endemic areas, but there is insufficient evidence to advise those with symptomatic infection. A certificate of exemption is needed for those who cannot be immunized if travel is necessary. Pregnant women should be discouraged from travelling to yellow fever destinations that pose a true risk of infection.

For vaccinated individuals, the importance of infection avoidance (e.g. insect bites) and infection control (e.g. handwashing and food hygiene) should continue to be emphasized. PLWH should be advised that the level and duration of vaccine-induced protection might be reduced relative to HIV-negative individuals.

Cholera vaccine has little protective value.

Table 57.1 Travel vaccination and HIV infection

Vaccine	Asymptomatic HIV	Symptomatic HIV
Polio (inactive)	Yes	Yes
Meningococcus (ACWY)	Yes	Yes
Hepatitis A	Yes	Yes
Hepatitis B	Yes	Yes
Rabies	Yes	Yes
Tetanus	Yes	Yes
Yellow fever	Yes (CD4 >350 cells/μL) Discuss (CD4 200–350 cells/μL)	No (CD4 <200 cells/ μL)
Japanese encephalitis	Yes	Yes
Typhoid	Yes	Yes
Tuberculosis (BCG)	No (CD4 >200 cells/mm³)	No

Food and water

Those with CD4 <250 cells/μL are at ↑ risk from GI pathogens (crypto-sporidiosis, salmonella, etc.). Particular care should be taken with raw fruit/vegetables, undercooked or raw seafood/meat, tap water/ice, unpasteurized milk/dairy products, and food/ beverages purchased from street vendors. Safe products include thoroughly cooked food, fruit peeled by the traveller, bottled/canned drinks (especially carbonated), hot coffee/tea, or water brought to the boil and simmered for 1 minute. If local tap water must be used and cannot be boiled, the use of a water filtration unit, with added chlorine or iodine ↑ its safety. Water-borne infections (e.g. cryptosporidiosis, giardiasis) may also result from ingesting water during recreational water activities, therefore, swimming in contaminated water (sewage, animal waste) should be avoided.

Travellers' diarrhoea

Prophylactic antimicrobials against travellers' diarrhoea are not routinely recommended (side effects, promotion of drug-resistant organisms), but if risk/benefit analysis favours their use, options include fluoroquinolones, e.g. ciprofloxacin 500 mg daily and co-trimoxazole (trimethoprim, sulfamethoxazole) 960 mg daily (resistance common in tropical areas). Antibiotics may be carried for empirical therapy if significant diarrhoea develops (e.g. ciprofloxacin 500 mg bd for 3–7 days). Anti-peristaltic agents, e.g. loperamide, are useful (except if diarrhoea is bloody or associated with pyrexia), but should be discontinued if symptoms persist >48 hours. Seek medical advice if failure to respond, blood in the stool, pyrexia/ rigors, or dehydration.

Other precautions

Advice should be given about other preventive measures for anticipated exposure, e.g. malaria prophylaxis and protection against arthropod vectors. Avoid direct soil and sand contact with skin by wearing shoes, protective clothing, and using towels on beaches to avoid hook worm, strongyloidosis, and cutaneous larva migrans. Avoid swimming in freshwater in areas of risk for schistosomiasis.

Recreational travel is commonly associated with sexual encounters. Newly acquired STIs, including HIV superinfection, can compromise the underlying HIV infection. A supply of condoms should be carried, as availability at the destination may be limited and of dubious quality.

Index

Tables, figures, and boxes are indicated by an italic *t*, *f*, and *b* following the page number.

A

abacavir (ABC) hypersensitivity reaction 640
acalculous cholecystitis 506
access to clinics 6
accessory proteins 459*t*
aciclovir resistance and anogenital herpes 285
Actinomyces israelii 79, 171
actinomyces-like organisms (ALOs) 179
adenovirus 93–94
adoption 654
adrenal function 574–75
advance decisions/statements 36
Age of Legal Capacity (Scotland) Act 1991: 21
agglutination and syphilis 127
aggressive patients 48
aims of GUM services 4
amiodarone and epididymo-orchitis 195
amoebiasis: *Entamoeba histolytica* 253, 265–66
Amsel's criteria 220, 221*t*
anaemia 604–5
anal canal and anogenital warts 301–2
anal carcinoma 618
anal diseases 501–2
anal problems and sexual problems 435
anaphylactic shock 133
angiokeratomas 346
angular cheilitis 489–90
animals, sex with 51
anogenital blisters or ulcers in children 112*t*
anogenital dermatoses 345–56
common benign lesions/anomalies 346
degenerative condition 347
genital allergic contact hypersensitivity 348*b*
infective conditions 347
inflammatory conditions 348–51
malignant conditions 356
premalignant conditions 354–55

topical treatments 356, 356*t*
ulcerative conditions 352–53
anogenital herpes 277–89
aetiology 278
clinical features 280–81
diagnosis 282
epidemiology and transmission 279
and HIV 289*b*
and male condoms 406*b*
management 283–85
pregnancy and neonatal infection 286–88
terminology 278
ulceration, causes of 281*b*
anogenital infections and gonorrhoea 139, 147
anogenital squamous cell carcinoma 292*t*
anogenital ulceration 87*f*, 87*b*
anogenital warts 291–304
aetiology 292
in children 112*t*, 115
clinical features 294
diagnosis 295, 295*t*
epidemiology and natural history 293
HIV 304*b*
human papilloma virus types in lesions 292*t*, 302–3*b*, 304*b*
management 297–303
frequently asked questions 297–99*b*, 302–3*b*
general principles 297–99
sexual partners 301
special situations 301–2
specific treatments 299–301
treatment algorithm 298*f*, 299*f*
vaccine 302–3
pregnancy and infection in neonates and children 101, 296
relative frequency of location of 294*t*
transmission 293
anorectal stimulation 50
anorectal syndrome 249

anterior uveitis 517
antibiotics
and genital candidiasis 236
and oral contraceptives 414*b*
sexual assault management 108*b*
sexually acquired reactive arthritis 210
antibodies and anogenital herpes 282
antifungals 490
antiretroviral drugs
for HIV during pregnancy and labour 655
and hormonal contraception 414*b*
antiviral management and anogenital herpes 284, 285
aortitis 121–22
aphthous ulcers 352, 491
arousal with body fluids 50
arthralgia 597
arthritis 118, 205, 210 11
gonococcal 143
HIV-associated 597
psoriatic 598
reactive 598
septic 599
see also sexually acquired reactive arthritis
assisted conception 654
Atopobium vaginae 215
attendance confirmation 7
atypia 358
availability of services 6
azoles and genital candidiasis 242*b*

B

B19 parvovirus 604–5
bacillary angiomatosis 554–55
bacillary dysentery 264
bacteria 264
aerobic 215
anaerobic 215
bacterial infection and HIV 489, 524*b*, 554–55, 565, 567*b*
bacterial pneumonia 527
bacterial vaginosis (BV) 65, 94, 213–24
aetiology 215–16

bacterial vaginosis (BV)
(*Contd.*)
altered vaginal
discharge 85*f*
anaerobic and *G. vaginalis*
-associated balanitis/
balanoposthitis 224
-associated organisms in
pelvic inflammatory
disease 171
associations 217
children 115
clinical features 217
complications 218
diagnosis 220, 221*t*
HIV 224*b*
management 222–23
microscopy accuracy 75*t*
pregnancy 98
bacteriuria,
asymptomatic 270
balanitis and
balanoposthitis 83*f*,
224, 241
Bancroftian filariasis 253
Bartholinitis and Bartholin's
cyst and abscess 142,
153, 380
Behçet's disease 195, 352
biliary tract disease 505
biological false-positive reactions and syphilis 125*b*
bone marrow
infiltration 604–5
bone mineral
dysfunction 579
boric acid 243
breastfeeding 147, 158,
222, 338
HIV 658
Brucella spp. 194
Brugia malayi 194
bullous impetigo 554

C

Caesarean section and anogenital herpes 288
calcium 578–79
Campylobacter infection 264
Candida spp. 66
candidal
endophthalmitis 520
candidal oesophagitis 493
candidiasis 94
accuracy of
microscopy 75*t*
altered vaginal
discharge 85*f*
cutaneous 555–56
epidemiological treatment
for contacts 91*t*

erythematous 489–90
hyperplastic 489–90
oral 489–90
pharyngeal 489–90
pregnancy 98
pseudomembranous
489–90
see also genital candidiasis
candour, professional
duty of 31
capacity 19
cardiovascular disease 593
cardiovascular disorders
see HIV: cardiovascular
disorders
catheterized patients
and urinary tract
infection 270
CD4 count 462, 633, 633*b*
cellular response and HIV
primary infection 481
cerebral disorders 542–43
cerebral toxoplasmosis
(*Toxoplasma gondii*) 543
cerebrospinal fluid
examination and
syphilis 127–28, 128*t*
cerebrovascular disease 549
cervical cytology technique
and guidance 360*b*
cervical neoplasia 357–64
chlamydia 153
classification 361*t*
clinical features 359
diagnosis 362
glandular intra-epithelial
(CGIN) 358, 362, 363
HIV and cervical
carcinoma 364
intra-epithelial (CIN) 358,
361*t*, 362, 363
invasive cervical
carcinoma 358, 362
management 363
pregnancy 364
primary prevention 363
risk factors 359
screening 46, 360
cervical polyp 380
cervical warts 301–2
cervicitis 203, 217
cervix, histology of the
normal 358
chancroid 87*f*, 91*t*,
94, 246–47
chaperones and intimate
examinations 32, 32*b*
'chemsex' 504–5
children 48
anogenital warts 112*t*, 115
assessment for risk 23*b*
bacterial vaginosis 115

chlamydia 114
competence 20–21
consent 20–22, 111
gonorrhoea 114
herpes 114
HIV 114
protection issues 21
sexual assault 110–15,
110–15*b*
sexual exploitation 24–25,
25*b*, 26*b*
sexually transmitted
infections 111
syphilis 114–15
trichomoniasis 115
see also infant; neonates/
neonatal; prepubertal
infection
Chlamydia trachomatis 64,
86*f*, 94, 149–59
aetiology 150
bacterial
vaginosis 216, 217
children 114
clinical features 152–53
complications 153
diagnosis 156–57
epidemiological treatment
for contacts 91*t*
epidemiology and
transmission 151
epididymo-
orchitis 194, 197
lymphogranuloma
venereum 248
and male condoms 406*b*
management 158–59
nucleic acid amplification
test 64, 107–8*t*, 156
pelvic inflammatory
disease 171
point of care tests 76
pregnancy and the
neonate 98, 154–55
sexually acquired reactive
arthritis 203
cholangiopathy,
HIV-associated 505
circumcision and anogenital
herpes 285
cirrhosis 504–5
cisgender 42
clinic-based tests 71–72
Clinical Commissioning
Groups 60
clinical psychology and vulval
pain syndromes 371
clitoridectomy 29*b*
coagulation disorders 606
coliform enteric bacteria and
epididymitis 194
colposcopy 362

coming out 44
commensals 79–80
competence (of
children) 20–21
computed tomography
angiography and syph-
ilis 128
condoms and anogenital
herpes 285
confidentiality 17, 38
confounders 79–80
congenital infection and
syphilis 119, 123–24,
124b, 129, 132
conjunctival infection/
conjunctivitis
chlamydia 153, 154, 158
gonococcal 147
gonorrhoea 139, 141
sexually acquired reactive
arthritis 205
conjunctival
microvasculopathy 515
conjunctival squamous cell
carcinoma 516
connective tissue/auto-
immune diseases 567b
consent 18–19, 31
children 20–22, 111
forensic assessment for
sexual assault 109
contact dermatitis 348
contact slips 9–11
contraception 381–416
cautions and contraindications 417–27t, 416
coitus interruptus
('withdrawal') 408
combined hormonal
contraceptives including
combined pill, vaginal
ring, and patch 417–
27t, 384–86, 385b,
386t, 415
copper intra-uterine de-
vice 417–27t, 400–1,
401t, 410
depot
medroxyprogesterone
acetate 417–27t, 415
diaphragms and caps 402
efficacy 383t
emergency 409–10
female condom 403
female sterilization 411,
412b, 414
fertility awareness
methods 407
and genital candidiasis 236
HIV-positive
women 414–15
IMP 417–27t

implants 394–95,
395t, 415
injectable 391–93, 393t
intra-uterine devices 415
lactational amenorrhoea
method 408
levonorgestrel intra-uterine
system 417–27t,
397–98, 399t, 409
male condom 405,
406b, 414
male sterilization: vasectomy 413, 413b, 414
progestogen-only pill
417–27t, 388–89, 389t,
390b, 409, 415
spermicides 404
transgender/non-binary
people 46
UK Medical eligibility criteria for contraceptive
use guidelines 417–27t
ulipristal acetate
emergency
contraception 409–10
contract referral 9–11
core (HIV structure) 458
co-receptors 462
court appearances 37
cowperitis and abscess 141
Coxsackie virus B 194
cranberry juice 275–76
Criminal Law
(Consolidation)
(Scotland) Act
1995: 27–28
criminalization of HIV
transmission 35
cryotherapy 298f, 299f,
300–1, 613
cryococcosis 556
cryptosporidiosis:
Cryptosporidium
spp. 265, 495–96
cystitis 271
Cystoisospora belli (formerly
Isospora belli) 497
cystoisosporiasis 497
cytomegalovirus (CMV) 94,
194, 264, 326
and HIV 488, 518–19
oesophagitis 494
pneumonitis 537
retinitis 518–19

D

Data Protection Act
1998: 34
death 36
death certificates 36
deinfibulation 29b

demographic risk
factors 48–49
dermatological disorders
see HIV: dermatological
disorders
dermatological infection and
sexually acquired reactive
arthritis 206, 211
dermatophytosis 556
desensitization and genital
candidiasis 243
diabetes mellitus and genital
candidiasis 236
diarrhoea and travellers with
HIV 662
diathermy 300–1
diffuse idiopathic lymphocytic syndrome
(DILS) 597
dilated cardiomyopathy 591
disability 6
disseminated gonococcal infection (DGI) 142, 147
distal symmetric
polyneuropathy 548
distressed patient 48
doctors 4
donovanosis see granuloma
inguinale
drug/drugs
-associated cardiovascular
disorders 593
-facilitated sexual
assault 102
reactions and dermato-
logical disorders in
HIV 562
and renal
disease 586, 587t
resistance and genital
candidiasis 241
resistance and
HIV 645–49
resistance testing 648
side effects in HIV
management 640–41
toxicity and
anaemia 604–5
toxicity and
neuropathy 547
use of during sex 51
dyskaryosis 358
dyslipidaemia 576–77, 640
dyspareunia 434, 440
dysphagia investigations 493
dysuria 272

E

Ebola 327
ecthyma 554
ectopic pregnancy 174

ectopic sebaceous glands (Fordyce spots) 346
eczema 558
ejaculation
  1–2 hours before coitus 438–39
  retarded 439–40
ejaculatory pain 440
elderly patients and urinary tract infection 271
electrocautery 300–1
electrolytes 578–79
electronic technology 34
electrosurgery 300–1
emotional implications of Kaposi's sarcoma 612
Encephalitazoon intestinalis 496
endemic treponematoses 255–58
  endemic syphilis (bejel, dichuchwa) 258
  management 258
  pinta 257
  yaws (framboesia, pian, buba) 257
endocarditis 148, 591
endocrine disturbances in HIV 572, 573–75
endometritis 153
enteric diseases 94, 495–500
  causes of diarrhoea 500b
  chronic diarrhoea evaluation in HIV 499f
  cryptosporidiosis 495–96
  cystoisosporiasis 497
  HIV enteropathy 498–500
  microsporidiosis 496
  salmonellosis 497–98
  shigellosis 498
  enteritis 261, 262
Enterocytozoon bieneusi 496
enthesitis 205, 210–11
entry inhibitors 630t
envelope (HIV structure) 458
enzyme immunoassay (EIA)
  chlamydia 64, 156
  syphilis 126t, 127
  eosinophilic pustular folliculitis 559
epidemiological studies 31
epidermal naevi 346
epidermoid cysts 346
epididymal cysts 379
epididymo-orchitis 193–200
  aetiology 194–95
  clinical features 196
  complications 196
  diagnosis 198, 198b, 199t

epidemiological treatment for contacts 91t
  investigations 197
  management 200
  episcleritis 205
Epstein–Barr virus (EBV) 94, 324, 324b, 610
Equality Act 2010: 610–42
erectile dysfunction 436–38, 437t
erythema 348
  multiforme 353, 562
  nodosum 206
erythrasma 347
erythroderma 562
Escherichia coli 194
ethical, medico-legal, and sociocultural issues 15–39
  confidentiality 17
  consent 18–19, 31
  death 36
  electronic technology 34
  female genital mutilation 29–30
  HIV-infected healthcare workers 35
  intimate examinations and chaperones 32
  legislation 38–39
  partner notification issues 35
  sexual offences 27–28
  statements and court appearances 37
  evidence and sexual assault 109
excoriation 348
expressed prostatic secretions (EPS) 186b
extra-genital infection 57–58
extra-mammary Paget's disease 354
eye disorders *see* HIV: eye disorders
eyelashes and pediculosis 344

F

factitious illness 431
Fanconi's syndrome 641
female genital mutilation 29–30, 29b
female to male (FtM) 43
females *see* women
fertility treatment 654
fibrates 577–78
filarial organisms 194
Fitz–Hugh–Curtis syndrome *see* perihepatitis

fixed drug eruption 349
5-fluorouracil 5% cream 300–1
focal neurological signs and symptoms 541b
folliculitis 554
food and water for travellers with HIV 662
foreign bodies 274b
forensic assessment/ testing and sexual assault 104, 109
Fraser Ruling (Gillick competence) 20, 21
free treatment 59
fungal infection 194, 489–90, 524b, 535–36, 555–56, 565, 567b

G

gabapentin 370t
Gardnerella vaginalis 215
gastrointestinal disorders *see* HIV: gastrointestinal disorders
gastrointestinal disturbance 640
gender diversity 41–46
  sexual health 46
  terminology 43–45
gender dysphoria 43
gender expression 43
gender non-conforming 43
Gender Recognition Act 2004: 45
gender role 43
genderqueer 43–44
general examination 55
genetic susceptibility and HIV disease progression 463
genital allergic contact hypersensitivity 348b
genital anomalies 377–80
genital candidiasis 233–44
  aetiology 234
  chronic mucocutaneous 238b
  clinical features 237–38
  diagnosis 239
  epidemiology and transmission 235
  and HIV 244b
  management 241–43
  predisposing factors 236
  standard antimycotics 242b
  see also vulvo-vaginal candidiasis, recurrent
genital infections
  chlamydia 158

epididymo-orchitis 194
and gonorrhoea 147
see also mucopurulent
cervicitis; non-
gonococcal urethritis;
tropical genital and
sexually acquired
infections
genital lesions and sexu-
ally acquired reactive
arthritis 206
genital lumps and bumps
89*f*
genital reassignment/recon-
structive surgery 44–45
genital stimulation using
mouth 50
genotyping 648
giant condyloma of Buschke
and Lowenstein 294
giardiasis: *Giardia
duodenalis* 265
glans penis material 74
gonadal function 573–74
gonococcal dermatitis 142
gonorrhoea 86*f*, 95, 137–48
accuracy of
microscopy 75*t*
aetiology 138
children 114
clinical
features 140–42, 140*t*
complications 141–42
diagnosis 145–46
epidemiological treatment
for contacts 91*t*
epidemiology and
transmission 139
and HIV infection 148
infectivity and clearance
rates 139*b*
and male condoms 406*b*
management 147–48
point of care tests 76
pregnancy and the
neonate 98, 143–44
*see also Neisseria
gonorrhoeae*
Gram-negative diplococci
(GNDC) 73, 74
Gram-stained smear 71
cervical 73
urethral 74
from urine 74
vaginal 73*f*
granuloma
inguinale 95, 251–52
anogenital ulceration 87*f*
and epidemiological treatment for contacts 91*t*
granulomatous
diseases 567*b*
granulomatous orchitis 195

group B β-haemolytic
streptococci 79
Guinea worm
infestation 253

H

haemangioma 346
haematological
disorders 604–6
haematospermia 183*b*
haematuria 270–71
haemoglobin 273
Haemophilus ducreyi 246
Haemophilus influenzae 97
*Haemophilus
parainfluenzae* 194
hair follicles, prominent
346
head and neck
carcinoma 292*t*
headaches and HIV 541*b*
health advisers (HAs) 5,
5*b*, 9–11
healthcare workers,
HIV-infected 36
Helicobacter pylori
infection 264
hepatic disease 504–5,
504*b*
hepatic steatosis 504–5
hepatitis A virus (HAV) 95
epidemiological treatment
for contacts 91*t*
vaccination 478
hepatitis B virus (HBV) 95
co-infection with
HIV 509–10, 510*b*,
610, 623, 655
epidemiological treatment
for contacts 91*t*
immunization and
sexual assault
management 107*t*
and male condoms 406*b*
pregnancy 98–99
vaccination 478
hepatitis C virus (HCV) 95
co-infection with
HIV 511–12, 511*b*,
512*b*, 610, 623, 655
immunization and
sexual assault
management 107*t*
pregnancy 99
hepatocellular carcinoma
(HCC) 619
hepatotoxicity 640
herbal treatment and ano-
genital herpes 285
herpes simplex virus
(HSV) 65–66, 95
anal 501

anogenital
ulceration 87*f*, 87*b*
children 114
and HIV 487, 553
pregnancy 99
see also anogenital herpes
herpes zoster (shingles) 547
herpes zoster
ophthalmicus 515
hidradenitis-like plaques 554
hidradenitis suppurativa 351
high-grade squamous
intraepithelial lesions of
the genital tract 354–55
histoplasmosis 556
HIV 96
anogenital herpes 289*b*
anogenital warts 304*b*
assessment 477–78
-associated wasting
syndrome 580
bacterial vaginosis 224*b*
cervical carcinoma 364
children 114
chlamydia 159
clinical indicator
conditions 471*b*
clinical staging 466–67,
466*t*, 467*t*
desensitization schedule
for trimethoprim–
sulfamethoxazole 650*t*
diagnosis and
assessment 469–78
endocrine
disturbances 572
epidemiological treatment
for contacts 91*t*
epididymo-orchitis 200*b*
genital candidiasis 244*b*
gonorrhoea 148
hepatitis virus
co-infection 507–12
-infected healthcare
workers 36
and male condoms 406*b*
metabolic
disorders 572, 576–79
*Molluscum
contagiosum* 308
natural history of untreated
infection 468, 468*f*
pelvic inflammatory
disease 179
point of care tests 77
-positive women and
contraception 414–15
post-test
counselling 476, 476*b*
pregnancy 99
prophylaxis and sexual
assault manage-
ment 107*t*, 108*b*

HIV (*Contd.*)
prostatitis/chronic pelvic pain syndrome 191*b*
psychological aspects 430, 441*b*
-related anaemia 604–5
scabies 335
sexually acquired reactive arthritis 212*b*
and syphilis co-infection 135
testing
infants 657
and risk assessment 471–75, 471*b*, 472–74*b*, 473*t*, 474*t*
transgender/non-binary people 46
transmission, criminalization of 35
and trichomoniasis 232*b*
HIV: cardiovascular disorders 589–93
cardiac neoplasia 592
cardiovascular disease 593
dilated cardiomyopathy 591
drug-associated disorders 593
endocarditis 591
myocarditis 590
pericardial effusion 590
pulmonary hypertension 592
venous thrombosis 592
HIV: dermatological disorders 471*b*, 551–62
bacterial infections 554–55
drug reactions 562
fungal infections 555–56
inflammatory conditions 558
neoplasia 560–61
pruritic follicular and papular eruptions 559
scabies 557
viral infections 553–54
HIV: epidemiology 449–54
biological implications of types and subtypes 452
history 450
origin 451
prevalence 453, 453*t*
risk factors and transmission routes 454, 454*t*
HIV: eye disorders 513–21
anterior segment of eye 517
neuro-ophthalmic manifestations 521
ocular surface and adnexa 515–16

posterior segment of eye 518–20
HIV: gastrointestinal disorders 485–506
anal diseases 501–2
biliary tract disease 505
hepatic disease 504–5, 504*b*
pancreatic diseases 503
see also enteric diseases; oral diseases
HIV: malignancies 609–19, 624
anal carcinoma 618
hepatocellular carcinoma 619
Hodgkin's disease 617
invasive cervical carcinoma 617
Kaposi's sarcoma 611–13
leiomyosarcoma 618
lung cancer 618
multicentric Castleman's disease 617
non-Hodgkin's lymphoma 614–16
HIV: management 621–51
adherence 626
antiretroviral drug–drug interactions 643, 644*t*
antiretroviral side effects 640–41
characteristics of commonly used antiretrovirals 630*t*
chronic infection 623
combination therapy 627, 629*t*
drug resistance 645–49
entry inhibitors 630*t*
HIV life cycle and points of drug action 628*f*
immune reconstitution 642
initial treatment 625
integrase inhibitors 630*t*
monitoring and follow-up 633–37, 634*t*
non-nucleoside reverse transcriptase inhibitor 630*t*
nucleoside/nucleotide reverse transcriptase inhibitor 630*t*
opportunistic infections 623
pharmacokinetic boosters 630*t*
primary infection 623
prognosis according to CD4 cell count and viral load 624*f*
prophylaxis against infections 650–51, 650*t*

protease inhibitor 630*t*
recommended first-line antiretroviral regimens 629*t*
stopping antiretroviral therapy 639
switching antiretroviral therapy 639
vaccinations 638, 638*t*
virological failure 649
HIV: musculoskeletal disorders 595–601
immunity pathogenesis 596
infections 599
inflammatory arthropathies 597–98
muscle disease 601
neoplasia 600
osteopenia and osteoporosis 600
rheumatic disease 601
HIV: neurological disorders 539–49
autonomic neuropathy 545
cerebral disorders 542–43
cerebrovascular disease 549
meningitis 544
neoplastic disease 549
neurosyphilis 549
peripheral nerve disease 547–48
spinal cord disease 546
symptom complexes 541*b*
HIV: pathogenesis 457–63
factors influencing disease progression 463
genetic organization 459, 459*t*
receptors 462
replicative cycle 460–61
binding/attachment 460
fusion 460
integration 460
maturation 461
proviral transcription and translation 461
reverse transcription 460
budding 461
structure 458, 458*f*
HIV: pregnancy 653–58
antenatal management 656
antiretroviral treatment 655
infant feeding 658
labour and delivery 656
monitoring 655
neonates 657

pre-conception 654
screening 655
see also contraception
HIV: prevention 443–47
post-exposure prophy-
laxis 445–46,
445*b*, 446*b*
pre-exposure prophy-
laxis 446, 447, 447*b*
treatment as 623
HIV: primary
infection 479–84
clinical features of acute
seroconversion
illness 482, 483*t*
diagnosis 484, 484*b*
immune responses 481
management 484
prevalence of acute sero-
conversion illness 482
HIV: pyrexia of unknown
origin 563–70
aetiology 565
diagnosis 566–67
management 568
Mycobacterium avium
complex 569
visceral leishmaniasis
570
HIV: renal
disorders 581–88
acute renal failure and HIV
seroconversion 585
assessment 582
drugs and renal
disease 586, 587*t*
end-stage renal
disease 588
HIV-associated
nephropathy 583
immune-mediated renal
disease 584
interstitial nephritis 585
thrombotic
microangiopathy 585
HIV: respiratory
disorders 524–25
bacterial pneumonia 527
chest X-ray
appearances 526*t*
cytomegalovirus
pneumonitis 537
mediastinal and hilar
lymphadenopathy 537
pneumocystis
pneumonia 528–30
pulmonary
aspergillosis 535–36
pulmonary
cryptococcosis 535
pulmonary vascular
disease 537–38
spectrum of illnesses
524*b*

tuberculosis 531–33
HIV: reticulo-endothelial
disorders 471*b*, 603–7
haematological
disorders 604–6
persistent generalized
lymphadenop-
athy 607, 607*b*
HIV: travel 659–62
diarrhoea 662
food and water 662
planning 660
vaccination 661, 661*t*
Hodgkin's disease 617
hormonal factors and genital
candidiasis 236
human herpes virus-8
(HHV8) 95, 329, 610
human papilloma virus
(HPV) 96
and anal disease 501–2
anogenital and male
condoms 406*b*
and anogenital
warts 292*t*, 304*b*
DNA triage 360
and HIV 488–89, 554,
610
human T-cell lymphotropic
virus 1 (HTLV-1) 328
-associated
myelopathy 546
humoral response and HIV
primary infection 481
hyfrecation 300–1
hyperglycaemia 577–78
hypernatraemia 578
hypersensitivity and
condoms 405
hypersensitivity and
dermatoses 348
hypersensitivity and drug reactions 527, 560, 628–9,
631, 638, 640
hypersensitivity and genital
candidiasis 237–8, 241
hypersensitivity and sca-
bies 335, 343
hypertrophic
osteoarthropathy
597–98
hyphae 239
hypochondriasis 431
hyponatraemia 578
hypophosphataemia 578–79
hyporeninaemic
hypoaldosteronism 578
hypospadias 378

I

idiopathic calcinosis of the
scrotum with multiple
nodules 346

imiquimod 5% cream 298*f*,
299*f*, 299–300
immature patients 21
immune-mediated renal
disease 584
immune reconstitution
syndrome 534, 642
immune recovery in-
flammatory response
(IRIS) 601, 642
immune-recovery
uveitis 517
immunity, impaired and
genital candidiasis 236
immunity pathogenesis in
HIV 596
incest 27–28
indecent exposure 27
indecent/sexual assault 27
infant
feeding and HIV in
pregnancy 658
pneumonia 159
serology 129
infectious mononucleosis-
like illness 482
infertility and pelvic inflammatory disease 174
infibulation 29*b*
inflammatory
arthropathies 597–98
inflammatory conditions and
HIV-related dermato-
logical disorders 558
inflammatory demyelinating
neuropathy (Guillain–
Barré syndrome) 548
influenza
prophylaxis 651
vaccination 478
inguinal syndrome
248–49
inherited diseases 567*b*
integrase inhibitors
(INIs) 630*t*, 646*t*
integrated sexual health
services 2–3
interferon 300–1, 613
interpreters 6
interstitial nephritis 585
intestinal problems and
sexual problems 435
intimate examinations and
chaperones 32, 32*b*
intra-epithelial neo-
plasia 292*t*, 354–55,
502
invasive cervical carcinoma
(ICC) 358, 617
investigations and
microscopy 63–80
accuracy of
microscopy 75*t*
chancroid 247

investigations and microscopy (*Contd.*)
chlamydia 156–57
clinic-based tests 71–72
commensals and confounders 79–80
genital candidiasis 239
gonorrhoea 145–46
HIV 477–78
laboratory testing 64–67, 67*b*
microscope 69
rapid point of care tests 76–78, 76*b*
routine female microscopy 73
routine male microscopy 74
sexual assault investigation 107*t*
slide preparation 70*b*
syphilis 125–29
trichomoniasis 229
iridocyclitis 517
iritis (acute anterior uveitis) 205
irritant dermatitis 348
ivermectin 338

J

Jarisch–Herxheimer reaction 131–32, 133

K

Kaposi's sarcoma (KS) 490–91, 600, 611–13
and cardiac neoplasia 592
and HIV-related dermatological disorders 560
and HIV-related eye disorders 515–16
see also human herpes virus-8 (HHV8)
keratitis, infectious 517
keratoderma blennorrhagica (KB) 206
Klebsiella (*Calymmatobacterium*) *granulomatosis* 251
Klebsiella spp. 194

L

larva migrans, cutaneous 253
laryngeal papilloma 292*t*
laser therapy 300–1
Lassa virus 327
lasting power of attorney 36
leg weakness 541*b*
legislation 38–39
leiomyosarcoma 618
Leishmania spp. 570
leishmaniasis 253
leptothrix 79
leucocyte esterase 273
leukaemia/lymphoma, adult T-cell 328
lichen planus 349–50
lichen sclerosus (LS) 350
linear gingival erythema 489
lipid profiles 633
lipoatrophy 576, 640
lipodystrophy 576–78, 640
lipohypertrophy 576, 640
liposomal chemotherapy 613
Lipschutz ulcers 352
liquid-based cytology 360, 360*b*
living wills 36
Local Authorities commission 60
low-grade squamous intraepithelial lesions of the genital tract 354–55
lung cancer 618
lymphadenopathy, mediastinal and hilar 537
lymphocele 378
lymphogranuloma venereum (LGV) 87*f*, 91*t*, 96, 248–50
lymphomas 491, 560–61, 614–16

M

macular rash 121*b*
malaria prophylaxis 651
malassezia furfur folliculitis 559
malathion 0.5% aqueous lotion 338
male to female (MtF) 43
males *see* men
malignancies *see* HIV: malignancies
malignant conditions and anogenital dermatoses 356
management 59
Marburg haemorrhagic fever virus 327
matrix (HIV structure) 458
measles prophylaxis 651
mechanical aids (sexual problems) 437–38
medical transition 44
melanocytic naevi (moles) 346

men
anogenital warts treatment 299*f*
complications and gonorrhoea 141
general examination 56–57, 57*f*
genital anomalies 378–79
genital candidiasis 238
genital infection and chlamydia 152
genital infection and gonorrhoea 140
microscopy, routine 74
non-gonococcal urethritis 162, 163, 164, 165–67
sexual problems 436–40
trichomoniasis, clinical features of 228
urinary tract infection 272
urogenital infection and sexually acquired reactive infection 205
meningitis 148, 544
aseptic 544
cryptococcal 544
gonococcal 148
Mental Capacity Act 2005: 18–19
metabolic disorders in HIV 572, 576–79
metoidioplasty 44–45
microscopy *see* investigations and microscopy
microsporidiosis 496
mitochondrial toxicity 640
Molluscum contagiosum 96, 305–8, 516
aetiology and epidemiology 306
clinical features 306
diagnosis 307
HIV 308, 554
management 307
mononeuritis multiplex 547
Moraxella catarrhalis 97
morbilliform (erythematous maculopapular) drug eruption 562
mucopurulent cervicitis 91*t*, 161–67
clinical features 163
diagnosis 164
management 167
mucosal melanosis (genital lentiginosis) 346
mucous membrane lesions and secondary syphilis 120

Mullerian duct
anomalies 380
multicentric Castleman's
disease 617
mumps 194
Munchausen's
syndrome 431
muscle disease 601
musculoskeletal disorders
see HIV: musculoskeletal
disorders
musculoskeletal infection
and sexually acquired
reactive arthritis 205
mutations 645–48, 646t
mycobacterial
infection 555, 565
Mycobacterium avium com-
plex (MAC) 534
and HIV 567, 478
prophylaxis 651
Mycobacterium leprae 194
Mycobacterium tubercu-
losis 171, 191, 194
Mycoplasma
genitalium 66, 165b
epidemiological treatment
for contacts 91t
epididymo-
orchitis 194, 197
pelvic inflammatory
disease 171
sexually acquired reactive
arthritis 203
mycoses 191
myelopathy (tropical spastic
paraparesis) 328, 546
myiasis 253
myocarditis 590

N

Nabothian follicles 346
nail pigmentation 562
nails 206
National Health Service Act
1977: 38
necrotizing periodontal
diseases 489
necrotizing stomatitis 489
necrotizing ulcerative
periodontitis 489
Neisseria
gonorrhoeae 65, 138
bacterial
vaginosis 216, 217
epididymo-
orchitis 194, 197
laboratory detection 146
pelvic inflammatory
disease 171
sexual assault
investigation 107t, 108

sexually acquired reactive
arthritis 203
Neisseria meningitidis 79,
97, 194
nematodes 266
neonates/neonatal
anogenital herpes
286–88
anogenital warts 296
chlamydia 154–55, 158–59
gonorrhoea 139,
143–44, 148
group B β-haemolytic
streptococci 374–75
HIV 148, 657
sepsis 148
syphilis 132
vulvovaginitis 227
neoplasia 490–91, 524b,
549, 560–61, 565,
567b, 592, 600
see also intra-epithelial
neoplasia
nephropathy, HIV-associated
(HIVAN) 583
neuritis 547
neuro-cognitive disorder,
HIV-associated 542
neurological disorders
see HIV: neurological
disorders
neurological
manifestations 482
neuropathy 545,
547–48, 640
neuro-psychiatric side
effects 641
neuroses associated with
sexual health 431
neurosyphilis 122, 127–28,
128t, 131, 549
neutropenia 605
NHS England 60
NHS Trusts and Primary
Care Trusts (Sexually
Transmitted Diseases)
Directions 2000: 38
nitrate reductase 273
no referral 9–11
Nocardia spp. 194
nodular regenerative
hyperplasia 504–5
non-binary
people 42, 43–44
sexual health 46
non-gonococcal urethritis
(NGU) 96, 161–67
aetiology 162, 162t
clinical features 163, 163t
diagnosis 164
epidemiological treatment
for contacts 91t
management 165–67

and sexually acquired re-
active arthritis 203
non-Hodgkin's lymphoma
(NHL) 592,
600, 614–16
non-nucleoside reverse
transcriptase inhibitors
(NNRTIs) 630t, 646t
nucleic acid amplification
tests (NAATs) 156
nucleoside/nucleotide re-
verse transcriptase inhibitors (NRTIs) 630t, 646t
nurse specialists/
practitioners 5

O

occupational exposure to
infection 31
oesophageal
diseases 493–94, 493b
oesophagitis, candidal 493
Offences against the Person
Act 35
onchocerciasis 253
onychomycosis 556
ophthalmia
neonatorum 143, 148,
154, 159
ophthalmic infection and
sexually acquired reactive
arthritis 205, 210
opportunist mycobacterial
infections 534
oral diseases 487–92, 487b
bacterial diseases 489
differential diagnosis
of oral–pharyngeal
ulcers 492b
differential diagnosis of
white lesions in oral
cavity 487b
fungal diseases 489–90
neoplasia 490–91
parotid gland
enlargement 492
salivary gland
disease 491–92
viral infections 487–89
oral hairy leukoplakia (OHL)
and HIV 488
oral lesions
and Kaposi's sarcoma
611
and sexually acquired re-
active arthritis 206
oral–pharyngeal
ulcers 492b
oral pigmentation 562
oral sex 93–97, 93–97b
oral ulcers and
cytomegalovirus 488

oral warts and human papilloma virus (HPV) types in lesions 292t
orchitis see epididymo-orchitis
orgasmic dysfunction 434
osteomyelitis 599
osteonecrosis (avascular necrosis) 598
osteopenia 600
osteoporosis 600
ovarian function 574

P

paclitaxel and Kaposi's sarcoma 613
pancreatic diseases 503
pancreatic function 575
pancreatitis 503
papular lesions 121b
paralysis 122
paraphilia 51
paraphimosis 378
parasitic infection 191, 524b, 565, 567b
parotid gland enlargement 492
particle agglutination 77–78
partner notification 9–11, 10t, 35
bacterial vaginosis 222
chancroid 247
chlamydia 159
epididymo-orchitis 200
gonorrhoea 148
granuloma inguinale (Donovanosis) 252
lymphogranuloma venereum 250
mucopurulent cervicitis 167
non-gonococcal urethritis 167
pediculosis 344
pelvic inflammatory disease 179
scabies 338
syphilis 134
patient 48–49
referral 9–11
pearly penile papules 346
pediculosis 97, 339–44
aetiology 341
clinical features 343
diagnosis 344
epidemiological treatment for contacts 91t
epidemiology 343
management 344
transmission 343

pelvic floor exercises 437–38
pelvic inflammatory disease 169–79
aetiology 171
chlamydia 153
clinical features 173
complications and sequelae 174
diagnosis 176–77, 176t, 177b
epidemiological treatment for contacts 91t
epidemiology 172, 172b
gonorrhoea 142
investigations 175
management 178–79
pelvic pain syndrome, chronic see prostatitis/chronic pelvic pain syndrome
pelvic problems and sexual problems 435
pemphigus vulgaris 353
penicillin allergy 133
penicilliosis 556
prophylaxis 651
penile ulceration 562
peri-appendicitis 174
pericardial effusion 590
perihepatitis (Fitz-Hugh–Curtis syndrome) 142, 153, 174
periodontal disease 489
peripheral nerve disease 547–48
peripheral sensation, altered 541b
peri-urethral cellulitis and abscess 141
permethrin 5% cream 338
persistent generalized lymphadenopathy 607, 607b
Peyronie's disease 378
phalloplasty 44–45
pharmacokinetic boosters 630t
pharmacy arrangements 59
pharyngeal infection 139, 141, 147, 153, 158, 489–90
pharynx 58
phenotyping 648
phimosis 378
phobias 431
phosphate 578–79
phosphodiesterase-5 inhibitors 436–37
physiotherapy and vulval pain syndromes 371
piercings 51

pigmentary changes 346
pinta 257
pituitary function 573
plasma cell balanitis (of Zoon) 350
pneumococcal vaccination 478
pneumocystis pneumonia 478, 528–30, 565
prophylaxis 650, 657
podophyllin 15–25% 300–1
podophyllotoxin 298f, 299f, 299–300
point of care tests (POCTs), rapid 76–78, 76b
polio prophylaxis 651
polymerase chain reaction (PCR)
chancroid 247
trichomoniasis 229
polymorphonuclear leucocytes (PMNLs) 73, 74
post-exposure prophylaxis 651
neonates 657
post-mortem testing for sexually transmitted blood-borne infections 31
potassium 578
pregabalin 371t
pregnancy 98–101
anogenital herpes 286–88
anogenital warts 296, 301–2
bacterial vaginosis 222
cervical neoplasia 364
chlamydia 154–55, 158
gonorrhoea 143–44, 147
granuloma inguinale (Donovanosis) 252
hepatitis A virus 311
pelvic inflammatory disease 179
scabies 338
sexually acquired reactive arthritis 211
streptococcal infections 374–75
syphilis 124b, 131–32, 139
test 72b
trichomoniasis 228
urinary tract infection 270
see also HIV: pregnancy
premalignant conditions and anogenital dermatoses 354–55
premature ejaculation 438–39
prepubertal infection 141, 148, 153, 158–59

priapism 379
procaine
  benzylpenicillin 131b, 133
process of
  appointment 7–11
proctitis 90f, 261, 262
proctocolitis and enteric
  sexually acquired
  infections 259–66
  infections not usu-
    ally sexually
    transmitted 264–66
  infections usually sexually
    transmitted 263
  no infection
    demonstrable 263
  sexually transmitted
    causes and clinical
    features 261–62
progressive lumbosacral
  polyradiculopathy 548
progressive multifocal
  leukoencephalopathy
  (PML) 543
progressive outer retinal necrosis (PORN) 519–20
prostatitis/chronic pelvic
  pain syndrome 141, 153,
  174, 181–91
  acute bacterial
    prostatitis 183
  asymptomatic inflamma-
    tory prostatitis 191
  chronic bacterial
    prostatitis 185
  Chronic Prostatitis
    Symptom Index 188b
  expressed prostatic
    secretions 186b
  and HIV 191b
  prostatic massage 186b
  sexually transmitted
    infections 191
  symptoms 182t
protease inhibitors
  (PIs) 630t, 646t
protein 273
Proteus spp. 194
protozoa 265–66
provider referral 9–11
provision of services 4–5
  transgender/non-binary
    people 46
pruritic follicular and
  papular eruptions 559
pruritus 348, 559
pseudohyphae and/or
  spores 239
Pseudomonas aeruginosa 194
psoriasis 349, 558
psychological factors 430
  HIV 441b

psychosexual therapy
  chronic prostatitis/
    chronic pelvic pain
    syndrome 190
  erectile
    dysfunction 436–37
  vulval pain syndromes 371
Public Health (Control of
  Diseases) Act 1984: 39
Public Health (Infectious
  Diseases) Regulations
  1988: 39
public interest 17
Public Interest Disclosure
  Act 1998: 36
pulmonary
  aspergillosis 535–36
pulmonary
  cryptococcosis 535
pulmonary
  hypertension 592
pulmonary vascular
  disease 537–38
pyelonephritis 270
pyoderma
  gangrenosum 353
pyrexia of unknown origin
  see HIV: pyrexia of
  unknown origin
pyuria with no or low bacterial counts 274b

R

rape 27, 48
rash 641
recall 9
recording consultations 34
rectal infection 141,
  152–53, 158
rectum 57–58
referrals 6
registration 7, 7t
regulatory proteins 459t
renal disorders see HIV:
  renal disorders
renal impairment 641
respiratory disorders
  see HIV: respiratory
  disorders
respiratory secretions/lung
  tissue and pneumocystis
  pneumonia 528
respiratory tract infection
  and chlamydia 154
respiratory tract
  organisms 97
reticulo-endothelial dis-
  orders see HIV: reticulo-
  endothelial disorders
retinal
  microvasculopathy 518

retinal necrosis, acute 519
review 59
rheumatic disease 601
risk factors 48–49
routine examination 54

S

sadomasochism 51
'safer sex' 50
saline suspension 71, 74
salivary gland
  disease 491–92
Salmonella spp. 171, 194
salmonellosis 497–98
sarcoidosis 195
scabies 331–38, 557
  aetiology 332
  clinical features 335
  diagnosis 337
  distribution 336f
  epidemiological treatment
    for contacts 91t
  epidemiology 334
  HIV 335
  incognito 335
  management 338
  Norwegian
    (crusted) 335, 338
  transmission 334
  scalded skin
    syndrome 554
scalp abscess 148
Schistosoma
  haematobium 194
schistosomiasis 253
scrotal mass/pain 198b
seborrhoeic
  dermatitis 348–49, 558
seborrhoeic keratosis 346
seizures 541b
seminal vesiculitis 141, 153
sensate focus 434
sensation reduction (premature ejaculation)
  438–39
seroconversion,
  acute (retroviral
  syndrome) 553
service development 2–3
service provision 4–5
  levels of 60–61, 61b
  transgender/non-binary
    people 46
  sex and genital
    candidiasis 237
sex toys 51
sexual activity and abuse
  (children) 22
sexual activity, causing
  person to engage in
  without consent 27

sexual assault 48
  forensic assessment 109
  general principles 102–4
  management 105–8, 105b, 106b, 107t, 108b
  by penetration 27
  sexual contacts, management of 91t, 92t
  see also partner notification
sexual desire/arousal, low 434
sexual health commissioning 60–61
sexual health in primary care 60–61
sexual health promotion 12–13
sexual history 52, 53f
sexual offences 27–28
Sexual Offences Act 1967: 38–28
Sexual Offences Act 2003: 22, 27–28, 38–39
Sexual Offences (Northern Ireland) Order 2008: 27–28
sexual practice, types of 50–51
sexual problems 432
  classification 433
  women 434–35
sexuality and relationship 50
sexually acquired reactive arthritis 201–12
  aetiology 203
  associations 204
  causes of acute painful swollen joints 209b
  chlamydia 153
  clinical features 205–6
  diagnosis 208
  management 210
  natural history 207
  pregnancy 99
sexually acquired viral hepatitis 309–22
  hepatitis A virus 311–12, 316b, 322t
  hepatitis B virus 313–17, 315t, 316t, 316b, 322t
  hepatitis C virus 318–21, 319t, 320t, 322t
  shigellosis 498
sicca syndrome 515
sinecatechins 10–15% extract of green tea leaf 299–300
skin
  lesions and Kaposi's sarcoma 611
  lesions and syphilis 120, 123

rash, drug-related 641
samples 71
tags (achrocordon) 346
warts 292t
social implications of Kaposi's sarcoma 612
social risk factors 48–49
social transition 44
sodium and water 578
Soundex codes 7, 8t
special situations 48
specialized roles of GUM 4
specific antitreponemal immunoglobulin M (IgM) detection 126t, 127
specific genitourinary situations 81–115
  anogenital ulceration 87f, 87b
  balanitis and balanoposthitis 83f
  child sexual assault 110–15, 110–15b
  genital lumps and bumps 89f
  oral sex 93–97, 93–97b
  pregnancy 98–101
  proctitis 90f
  sexual contacts, management of 91t, 92t
  urethritis, symptoms suggesting 82
  vaginal discharge, altered 85–86, 85f, 86f
  vulval irritation/discomfort/pain 84f
  see also sexual assault
spectinomycin 148b
spermatic granuloma 195
spermatoceles 379
spinal cord disease 546
squeeze technique (premature ejaculation) 438–39
standard clinic process 47–61
  examination of men 56–57, 57f
  examination of women 55f, 55–56
  extra-genital infection 57–58
  general examination 55
  management and review 59
  patient 48–49
  routine examination 54
  sexual health commissioning and sexual health in primary care 60–61
  sexual history 52, 53f

sexual practice, types of 50–51
staphylococcal skin infection 554
Staphylococcus aureus 376, 554
statements and court appearances 37
statins 577–78
Stevens–Johnson syndrome (SJS) 353, 562
stop/start (premature ejaculation) 438–39
streptococcal infections 97, 374–75
Streptococcus agalactiae 79, 374–75
Streptococcus pneumonia 194
Streptococcus pyogenes 374
Strongyloides stercoralis 266
structural proteins, major 459t
sub-preputial material 74
symmetrical polyarthritis, acute 597
synthetic prostaglandin E1 agent 437–38
syphilis 97, 117–35
  accuracy of microscopy 75t
  acquired 118, 120–22
  aetiology 118
  anogenital ulceration 87f
  biopsy 128
  cardiovascular 121–22, 130
  children 114–15
  co-infection with HIV 135
  congenital infection 119, 123–24, 124b, 129, 132
  diagnosis and investigations 125–29
  early 118, 123, 134
    clinical features 120–21
    management 130
  endemic (bejel, dichuchwa) 258
  epidemiological treatment for contacts 91t
  epidemiology and transmission 118
  follow-up 134
  gummatous 121, 130
  late 118, 123–24, 134
    clinical features 121–22
    management 130
  latent 118, 121, 130
  and male condoms 406b
  natural history 118
  pregnancy 100, 123–24, 124b, 131–32
  primary 120

secondary 120, 121*b*
sexual assault
    investigation 107*t*
see also neurosyphilis

T

T-cell leukaemia/lymphoma,
    adult 328
tabes dorsalis 122
tenosynovitis 142, 205
termination of preg-
    nancy and bacterial
    vaginosis 223
test results 8
testicular cancer 199*t*
testicular function 573–74
testicular torsion 199*t*
testing in error 31
testosterone (IM or trans-
    dermal) 434, 437–38
threadworms 266, 271
thrombocytopenia 605
thrombotic
    microangiopathy 585
thrombotic
    thrombocytopenic
    purpura 605
thyroid disease 573
tinea infections 347, 556
toxic epidermal
    necrolysis 562
toxoplasma
    retinochoroiditis 520
toxoplasmosis 478
    prophylaxis 650
    transgender people 42, 43
    sexual health 46
    transman 43, 46
transsexual 43
transwoman 43, 46
travel
    expenses,
        reimbursement of 8
    see also HIV: travel
treatment 59
Treponema pallidum 70*b*,
    118, 127, 194
triage 6
trichloroacetic acid
    (TCA) 298*f*, 299*f*, 300–1
Trichomonas vaginalis 66, 76
trichomoniasis 225–32
    accuracy of
        microscopy 75*t*
    aetiology 226
    altered vaginal
        discharge 85*f*
    bacterial vaginosis 217
    children 115
    clinical features 228
    diagnosis 229

epidemiological treatment
    for contacts 91*t*
epidemiology and
    transmission 227
    and HIV 232*b*
    and male condoms 406*b*
    management 230–31
    pregnancy 100
    trimethoprim–
        sulfamethoxazole
        desensitization
        schedule 650*t*
tropical genital and
    sexually acquired
    infections 245–53
    anogenital ulceration 87*f*
    chancroid 246–47
    granuloma inguinale
        (Donovanosis)
        251–52
    lymphogranuloma
        venereum 248–50
    tuberculosis 478, 489,
        531–33, 624
tubo-ovarian and pelvic
    abscess 174
tubular necrosis, acute 582
tumours and possible HIV
    infection 471*b*
typhoid 171, 264

U

ulcerative conditions
    and anogenital
    dermatoses 352–53
Ureaplasma
    urealyticum 194, 203
urethral caruncle 380
urethral channels
    (accessory) 379
urethral material 74
urethral meatus 301–2
urethral strictures and
    fistulae 141
urethral syndrome 271
urethritis, symptoms
    suggesting 82
urinalysis 72
urinary problems and sexual
    problems 435
urinary tract infection
    (UTI) 82, 267–76
    aetiology 268
    diagnosis 273
    epididymo-orchitis 194
    management 275–76
    men 272
    pregnancy 100
    pyuria with no or low bac-
        terial counts 274*b*
    women 269–71

urine
    inspection 71
    pregnancy test 72*b*
urogenital infection and
    sexually acquired re-
    active arthritis 205
urology referral 276
uterine problems and sexual
    problems 435
uveitis
    anterior 517
    immune-recovery 517

V

vaccination and HIV 478,
    638, 638*t*, 661, 661*t*
    neonates 657
vacuolar myelopathy 546
vaginal bleeding
    cervical neoplasia 359
    chlamydia 152, 153
    contraception
        417–27*t*, 392
    transgender/non-binary
        people 46
vaginal discharge 71,
    85*f*, 86*f*
vaginal stenosis, trans-
    gender/non-binary
    people 46
vaginismus 435
vaginitis 79–80
    atrophic 434, 435
    bacillary dysentery 264
    candidiasis 234, 244
    contraception
        417–27*t*, 384–85
    leptothrix 79
    neonate 143
    non-specific *see* bacterial
        vaginosis
    Staphylococcus aureus 376
    streptococcal
        infections 374
    transgender/non-binary
        people 46
    trichomoniasis 228, 229
    urinary tract infections,
        recurrent 269
vaginoplasty 44–45
varicella zoster virus
    (VZV) 478, 488,
    553–54
    prophylaxis 651
varicocele 379
vasculitis 567*b*
Venereal Diseases Act
    1917: 38
Venereal Diseases
    Regulations 1916: 38
venous thrombosis 592

viral encephalitis 542–43
viral infections
  and HIV 553–54,
    565, 567b
  and oral disease 487–89
viruses
  and proctocolitis and en-
    teric sexually acquired
    infections 264
  and prostatitis 191
  and respiratory illnesses in
    HIV 524b
visceral leishmaniasis
  570
vitiligo 346
vulval irritation/discomfort/
  pain 84f
vulval pain
  syndromes 365–72
  aetiology 367
  clinical features 367
  management 368–71,
    370t, 371t

prognosis 372
vulval papillae 346
vulvoplasty 44–45
vulvo-vaginal candidiasis, recurrent 237, 239, 242
vulvo-vaginal problems and
  sexual problems 434
vulvo-vaginitis,
  acute 237, 241

W

warts see anogenital warts
wasting syndrome,
  HIV-associated 580
women
  anogenital warts
    treatment 298f
  general
    examination 55f, 55–56
  genital anomalies 380
  genital candidiasis 237
  genital infection and
    chlamydia 152

genital infection and
  gonorrhoea 140
gonorrhoea 142
microscopy, routine 73
mucopurulent cervi-
  citis 162, 163, 164, 167
sexual problems 434–35
trichomoniasis 228
urinary tract
  infection 269–71
urogenital infection and
  sexually acquired re-
  active arthritis 205
Wuchereria bancrofti 194
Wuchereria pacifica 194

Y

yaws 257
yeast infections 194

Z

Zika 327